Methods of Assessing the
Reinforcing Properties of Abused Drugs

Michael A. Bozarth
Editor

Methods of Assessing the Reinforcing Properties of Abused Drugs

With 207 Illustrations

Springer-Verlag
New York Berlin Heidelberg
London Paris Tokyo

Michael A. Bozarth
Department of Psychology
State University of New York
    at Buffalo
Buffalo, New York 14260
USA

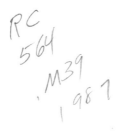

Library of Congress Cataloging in Publication Data
Methods of assessing the reinforcing properties of
    abused drugs.
    Includes bibliographies.
    1. Drug abuse—Psychological aspects.
2. Psychotropic drugs-Psychological aspects.
3. Reinforcement (Psychology)   4. Psychopharmacology—
Research—Methodology.   I. Bozarth, Michael A.
[DNLM: 1. Reinforcement (Psychology).   2. Substance
Dependence—psychology.   WM 270 M5925]
RC564.M39   1987   616.86′3   87-26310

Text prepared by the editor in camera-ready form.
Printed and bound by Edwards Brothers Inc., Ann Arbor, Michigan.
Printed in the United States of America.

9 8 7 6 5 4 3 2 1

ISBN 0-387-96625-0 Springer-Verlag New York Berlin Heidelberg
ISBN 3-540-96625-0 Springer-Verlag Berlin Heidelberg New York

FOREWORD

Drug abuse is a major health problem affecting increasingly larger segments of society. Statistics regarding heroin addiction show that the number of addicts has remained stable for the past decade, but data regarding the use of cocaine reveal a current epidemic with over 5 million Americans using cocaine on a regular basis. With the increased availability of new, less expensive forms of cocaine accompanied by a change in the route of administration (i.e., increased number of people smoking cocaine) and by a change in the social acceptability of its recreational use, a continued rise in cocaine addiction is expected throughout this decade. In addition, there are pronounced cyclic variations in the incidence of abusing other drugs such as phencyclidine, methaqualone, and diazepam.

Traditional views of drug abuse have focused on a variety of factors ranging from genetic to psychodynamic theories. Attempts have been made both to explain drug addiction case-by-case (i.e., develop special theories for each class of abused drug) and to formulate a unifying theory that would include a wide variety of drug classes. The opioids have long been studied as a prototypical class of addictive drugs, and early work focused on the physiological dependence produced by the repeated administration of these drugs. This research provided the basis for one of the first theories that attempted to explain addiction to several classes of drugs based on a single variable--addiction to opioids, ethanol, and barbiturates are all accompanied by strong signs of physiological dependence, and drug-taking behavior was suggested to evolve from the ability of these drugs to abate the withdrawal discomfort associated with abstinence. This theory, emphasizing the physiological dependence produced by these drugs, was very important because it focused on empirical (and not psychodynamic) factors involved in drug addiction.

In the 1960s three major developments helped shape the current view of drug addiction. First, definitions of drug addiction shifted from emphasis on physiological dependence to emphasis on the drug-taking behavior itself. That is, it was recognized that the defining characteristic of an addiction is not the development of physiological dependence but rather the development of compulsive drug-taking behavior. Second, specific psychometric scales were developed to quantify the subjective effects of abused drugs (e.g., the Addiction Research Center Inventory), and considerable attention focused on the mood-altering properties of these drugs. This revealed that a number of addictive drugs share an ability to elevate mood and produce "pleasant" affective changes. Third, experimental techniques were developed that permit studying drug self-administration in laboratory animals. These animals are presumed not to suffer from any predisposing psychological tendencies (e.g., addictive personalities, psychoneuroses), and operant conditioning paradigms have shown that an animal's behavior can be controlled by addictive drugs in much the same manner that food or water can control the behavior of a hungry or thirsty animal. These three factors led to a reassessment of traditional views of drug addiction and helped develop a more empirically oriented, scientific perspective for studying drug addiction.

Considerable research during the past two decades has focused on studying the reinforcing properties of abused drugs. This has led to the development of a number of techniques for assessing drug reward. Many of the procedures involve directly measuring the reinforcing property of a drug (e.g., drug self-administration in both laboratory animals and humans), while other methods study a variety of factors that appear to correspond to drug reinforcement (e.g., subjective effects in humans and drug discrimination in animals). The study of drug reinforcement contributes not only to the screening of new compounds for addiction liability but also to a basic understanding of drug addiction. In addition, studying the ability of pharmacological agents to control behavior may reveal important insights into the nature of brain mechanisms underlying basic motivational processes.

The main objective of this book is to create a compendium of the methods currently used to assess drug reinforcement by providing synopses of these diverse procedures in a single reference. Each of the major methods of studying drug reinforcement has been summarized, and applications of these techniques are illustrated. Although the specific applications of these methods may vary, the methodological considerations outlined in this book should provide a lasting framework for interpreting the results of current experimental findings.

A number of people have contributed to the development of this book. First, the participants in the 1983 Satellite Symposium held in conjunction with the Society for Neuroscience Meeting in Boston provided the initial encouragement that such a book would make an important contribution to research in this field--the success of the interdisciplinary symposium reinforced the notion that individual researchers could greatly benefit from learning about the work done using different methods to address a common problem. Second, Margaret Hamilton and Jim Dalton are thanked for proof reading sections of the book; the elusive typographical errors and omissions that invariably appear in such a volume have been greatly reduced by their efforts. Finally, the encouragement and editorial skills of Valarie Harlan Bozarth are gratefully acknowledged. The fruit of her commitment to facilitating the presentation of scientific material to a diverse audience can be found throughout the pages of this book.

Support for some phases of manuscript preparation came from grants from the National Institute on Drug Abuse (U.S.A.) and the Natural Sciences and Engineering Research Council (Canada).

Michael A. Bozarth

CONTENTS

SELF-ADMINISTRATION STUDIES

CONDITIONING STUDIES

DRUG DISCRIMINATION STUDIES

BRAIN STIMULATION REWARD STUDIES

ASSESSMENT IN HUMANS

OTHER CONSIDERATIONS

LIST OF CONTRIBUTORS

Zalman Amit

Center for Studies in Behavioral Neurobiology,
Department of Psychology, Concordia University,
1455 de Maisonneuve Boulevard West, Montreal, Quebec
H3G 1M8 CANADA

Nancy A. Ator

Department of Psychiatry and Behavioral Sciences,
The Johns Hopkins University School of Medicine,
720 Rutland Avenue, Baltimore, Maryland 21205 U.S.A.

Michael A. Bozarth

Department of Psychology, State University of New York
at Buffalo, Buffalo, New York 14260 U.S.A.

Joseph V. Brady

Department of Psychiatry and Behavioral Sciences,
The Johns Hopkins University, School of Medicine,
720 Rutland Avenue, Baltimore, Maryland 21205 U.S.A.

Chris L. E. Broekkamp

Organon International BV, P.O.B. 20, 5240 OH OSS
HOLLAND

Geoffrey D. Carr

Department of Psychology, University of British
Columbia, 2136 West Mall, Vancouver, British Columbia
V6T 1Y7 CANADA

Marilyn E. Carroll

Department of Psychiatry, University of Minnesota, Box
392 Mayo Memorial Building, 420 Delaware Street S.E.,
Minneapolis, Minnesota 55455 U.S.A.

R. James Collins

The Upjohn Company, Kalamazoo, Michigan 49001 U.S.A.

Francis C. Colpaert

Department of Pharmacology, Janssen Pharmaceutica
Research Laboratories, B-2340 Beerse BELGIUM

Hugh E. Criswell

Department of Psychology, East Tennessee State
University, Box 21970A, Johnson City, Tennessee
37614 U.S.A.

W. Marvin Davis

Department of Pharmacology, University of Mississippi,
School of Pharmacy, University, Mississippi 38677
U.S.A.

Harriet de Wit

Department of Psychiatry, Drug Abuse Research Center,
The University of Chicago, 5841 S. Maryland Avenue,
Chicago, Illinois 60637 U.S.A.

Ralph U. Esposito

Laboratory of Cerebral Metabolism, National Institute
of Mental Health, Building 36, Room 1A-27,
9600 Rockville Pike, Bethesda, Maryland 20205 U.S.A.

Hans C. Fibiger

Department of Psychiatry, University of British
Columbia, Vancouver, British Columbia V6T 1W5 CANADA

George J. Fouriezos

University of Ottawa, School of Psychology, Ottawa,
Ontario K1N 6N5 CANADA

Richard A. Glennon   Department of Medicinal Chemistry, School of Pharmacy, Medical College of Virginia, Virginia Commonwealth University, P.O. Box 581, Richmond, Virginia 23298 U.S.A.

Steven R. Goldberg   Preclinical Pharmacology Branch, NIDA Addiction Research Center, P.O. Box 5180, Baltimore, Maryland 21224 U.S.A.

Roland R. Griffiths   Department of Psychiatry and Behavioral Sciences, The Johns Hopkins University, School of Medicine, 720 Rutland Avenue, Baltimore, Maryland 21205 U.S.A.

Charles A. Haertzen   NIDA Addiction Research Center, P.O. Box 5180, Baltimore, Maryland 21224 U.S.A.

Jack E. Henningfield   NIDA Addiction Research Center, Francis Scott Key Medical Center, 4940 Eastern Avenue, Baltimore, Maryland 21224 U.S.A.

John E. Hickey   NIDA Addiction Research Center, P.O. Box 5180, Baltimore, Maryland 21224 U.S.A.

R. D. Hienz   Department of Psychiatry and Behavioral Sciences, The Johns Hopkins University, School of Medicine, 720 Rutland Avenue, Baltimore, Maryland 21205 U.S.A.

Donald R. Jasinski   Center for Chemical Dependence, Francis Scott Key Medical Center, Baltimore, Maryland 21224 U.S.A.

Chris E. Johanson   Department of Psychiatry, Drug Abuse Research Center, The University of Chicago, 5841 S. Maryland Avenue, Chicago, Illinois 60637 U.S.A.

Rolley E. Johnson   NIDA Addiction Research Center, P.O. Box 5180, Baltimore, Maryland 21224 U.S.A.

Jonathan L. Katz   Preclinical Pharmacology Branch, NIDA Addiction Research Center, P.O. Box 5180, Baltimore, Maryland 21224 U.S.A.

Richard J. Lamb   Department of Psychiatry and Behavioral Sciences, The Johns Hopkins University, School of Medicine, 720 Rutland Avenue, Baltimore, Maryland 21205 U.S.A.

Michael J. Lewis   Department of Psychology, Howard University, Washington, D.C. 20059 U.S.A.

Scott E. Lukas   Alcohol and Drug Abuse Research Center, Harvard Medical School - McLean Hospital, 115 Mill Street, Belmont, Massachusetts 02178 U.S.A.

Richard A. Meisch   Department of Psychiatry, University of Minnesota, Box 392 Mayo Memorial Building, 420 Delaware Street S.E., Minneapolis, Minnesota 55455 U.S.A.

Nancy K. Mello — Alcohol and Drug Abuse Research Center, Harvard Medical School - McLean Hospital, 115 Mill Street, Belmont, Massachusetts 02178 U.S.A.

Jack H. Mendelson — Alcohol and Drug Abuse Research Center, Harvard Medical School - McLean Hospital, 115 Mill Street, Belmont, Massachusetts 02178 U.S.A.

Claude Messier — Laboratoire de Psychophysiologie, Universite de Bordeaux I, 33405 Talence Cedex FRANCE

Edward Nawiesniak — University of Ottawa, School of Psychology, Ottawa, Ontario K1N 6N5 CANADA

Donald A. Overton — Department of Psychology, Weiss Hall, Temple University, 13th Street and Columbia Avenue, Philadelphia, Pennsylvania 19140 U.S.A.

Richard W. Phelps — Cortex Corporation, Wellesley, Massachusetts, U.S.A.

Anthony G. Phillips — Department of Psychology, Univeristy of British Columbia, Vancouver, British Columbia V6T 1W5 CANADA

Linda J. Porrino — NIDA Addiction Research Center, P.O. Box 5180, Baltimore, Maryland 21224 U.S.A.

Larry D. Reid — Department of Psychology, Rensselaer Polytechnic Institute, Troy, New York 12181 U.S.A.

David C. S. Roberts — Department of Psychology, Carleton University, Ottawa, Ontario K1S 5B6 CANADA

Thomas F. Seeger — Division of Neuroscience, Pfizer Central Research, Eastern Point Road, Groton, Connecticut 06340 U.S.A.

Brian R. Smith — Center for Studies in Behavioral Neurobiology, Department of Psychology, Concordia University, 1455 de Maisonneuve Boulevard West, Montreal, Quebec H3G 1M8 CANADA

Stanley G. Smith — Choctaw Community Mental Health Center, Philadelphia, Mississippi U.S.A.

Jane Stewart — Center for Studies in Behavioral Neurobiology, Department of Psychology, Concordia University, 1455 de Maisonneuve Boulevard West, Montreal, Quebec H3G 1M8 CANADA

E. A. Sutherland — Center for Studies in Behavioral Neurobiology, Department of Psychology, Concordia University, 1455 de Maisonneuve Boulevard West, Montreal, Quebec H3G 1M8 CANADA

Derek J. van der Kooy — Department of Anatomy, University of Toronto, Medical Science Building, Toronto, Ontario M5S 1A8 CANADA

James R. Weeks   Experimental Biology, The Upjohn Company, Kalamazoo,
                        Michigan 49001 U.S.A.

Norman M. White   Department of Psychology, McGill University,
                        1205 Dr. Penfield Avenue, Montreal, Quebec H3A 1B1
                        CANADA

Roy A. Wise   Center for Studies in Behavioral Neurobiology,
                        Department of Psychology, Concordia University
                        1455 de Maisonneuve Boulevard West, Montreal, Quebec
                        H3G 1M8 CANADA

Tomoji Yanagita   Preclinical Research Laboratories, Central Institute
                        for Experimental Animals, 1433 Nogawa, Kawasaki,
                        JAPAN 213

Robert A. Yokel   Pharmacy Building, Rose Street, University of Kentucky
                        Medical Center, Lexington, Kentucky 40536-0082
                        U.S.A.

Richard Young   Department of Medicinal Chemistry, School of Medicine,
                        Medical College of Virginia, Virginia Commonwealth
                        University, P.O. Box 581, Richmond, Virginia 23298
                        U.S.A.

K. A. Zito   Department of Anatomy, Faculty of Medicine, University
                        of Toronto, Medical Sciences Building, Toronto,
                        Ontario M5S 1A8 CANADA

CHAPTER 1

INTRAVENOUS SELF-ADMINISTRATION: RESPONSE RATES, THE EFFECTS OF PHARMACOLOGICAL CHALLENGES, AND DRUG PREFERENCE

Robert A. Yokel

Division of Pharmacology and Toxicology
College of Pharmacy
University of Kentucky
Lexington, Kentucky 40536-0053

Abstract

Intravenous self-administration preparations, utilizing a chronic indwelling catheter, have been developed for the rat, rhesus monkey, dog, squirrel monkey, pig, baboon, cat, and mouse. A wide variety of psychoactive drugs has been tested in these animal preparations which are considered to be reliable predictors of the abuse potential of drugs. Maintained self-administration is taken as evidence of reinforcing effect, and therefore abuse potential, and has been reported for most of the drugs that humans abuse. Use of the self-administration technique also predicts that some drugs not widely available for human use would be abused if available. Long-term drug access results in drug-intake patterns and drug-induced effects in animals that are similar to those seen in humans. The self-administration technique has been widely used to determine the neurotransmitter basis of the reinforcing effects of drugs. Drug preference and reinforcement magnitude have been estimated by comparing the self-administration of two or more drugs available under various experimental conditions, including choice procedures, progressive-ratio reinforcement schedules, and chain reinforcement schedules.

Introduction

Intravenous self-administration in experimental animals can be viewed as an operant behavior. The response, usually a lever press, is followed by a drug injection. In the initial work rats were used as experimental subjects. This required development of techniques which did not necessitate restraint. This was first successfully accomplished by Jim Weeks (1962), who developed a swivel and leash arrangement allowing the intravenous injection of drugs in rats, restrained only by the leash attached to the animal's back. The method of Weeks has been modified somewhat over the past 20 years (Pickens & Thompson, 1975; Smith & Davis, 1975; Weeks, 1972) and has been applied to the rhesus monkey (Deneau, Yanagita, & Seevers, 1969; Thompson & Schuster, 1964), the squirrel monkey (Goldberg, 1973; Stretch & Gerber, 1970), the pig (Bedford, 1973), the dog (Jones & Prada, 1973), the baboon (Griffiths, Findley, Brady, Dolan-Gutcher, & Robinson, 1975; Lukas, Griffiths, Bradford, Brady, Daley, & Delorenzo, 1982), the cat (Balster, Kilbey, & Ellinwood, 1976), and the mouse (Criswell & Ridings, 1983).

Basically, a silicone rubber catheter, or less commonly a polyvinyl chloride catheter, is implanted into the internal or external jugular vein or into the femoral vein, and sufficient tubing is inserted so that the catheter ends in or near the atrium of the heart. The tubing is usually passed subcutaneously around the shoulder to exit from either the center of the back or from the top of the head (Balster et al., 1976; van Ree, Slangen, & De Wied, 1978). This intravenous catheter is ultimately connected to a pump, which delivers the intravenous fluid injections from its fluid reservoir. [For details on catheter construction and surgical implantation, see Deneau et al., 1969; Jones and Prada, 1973; Pickens and Dougherty, 1972; Smith and Davis, 1975; or Weeks, 1972, who suggests sources of equipment and supplies useful in setting up this technique.] For animals not restrained in a chair during experimental sessions, a chain, parallel with the tubing, is connected to the jugular catheter connecting the animal to a swivel which is mounted either on the top or on the side of the cage. The chain protects the tubing and provides rigidity; as the animal turns in the experimental chamber, it rotates the fluid swivel. The chain is connected to the animal by a harness around its torso, (Weeks, 1972), a subcutaneously implanted anchor on the animal's back (Pickens & Dougherty, 1972), or an assembly attached to the animal's skull (Balster et al., 1976). Application of this technique to most species has included the use of a padded leather harness or jacket to facilitate connection of the intravenous cannula to the leash. In dogs and primates a hinged or flexible metal tubing is used as the leash to enclose and to protect the fluid tubing and to provide sufficient rigidity to rotate the fluid swivel. If good catheter materials are used, if the catheter is properly implanted, and if preventive measures are taken against the development of a fibrin clot in the catheter tip, the catheter should remain open for weeks to months in rats and perhaps for a year or more in monkeys and dogs. During prolonged periods between self-administration sessions, hourly or daily programmed injections of vehicle or of heparinized saline help to keep the catheter open (Findley, Robinson, & Peregrino, 1972). The experimental preparation is therefore a chronically intravenous catheterized subject that may be semi-restrained in a chair during a self-administration session (e.g., monkeys) or may be allowed to move freely within the experimental chamber (e.g., rats, cats, and dogs). The technique for intravenous self-administration has been applied to other routes of administration, including the oral, intragastric, and intracranial routes (see Amit, Smith, & Sutherland, this volume; Bozarth, this volume; Meisch & Carroll, this volume.)

Self-administration of a drug is claimed to occur when the operant responding which produces the intravenous drug injection by programming equipment or microprocessor-controlled activation of the fluid pump is initiated and maintained. Generally it is concluded that a drug is self-administered if the rate of drug responding is greater than the response rate on a control lever (which does not result in drug injections), if the rate of drug responding is greater than the saline (or vehicle) response rate, or if the response rate is greater in the subject whose response produces drug injections than its yoked control (Davis & Miller, 1963; Pickens, Meisch, & McGuire, 1967). It can be easily determined if responding is being maintained by drug injection (e.g., if the drug is serving as a reinforcer) by turning off the injection pump or by replacing the drug solution in the pump reservoir with a saline (or vehicle) solution. Extinction (an increase in response rate followed by a cessation of responding) should become evident (Pickens & Harris, 1968; Pickens & Thompson, 1968; Weeks, 1962; Winger & Woods, 1973). If the experimental chamber has two or more response levers with only one producing drug injections, then switching the contingencies between the levers (making the drug lever a control lever and vice versa) should result in appropriate switching of responding. If the response requirement is increased from one response (FR-1 or CRF) to 10 responses per injection (FR-10) then one would expect to see an appropriate increase in the response rate providing the drug dose is an adequate reinforcer (Pickens & Harris, 1968). It has been demonstrated that drug responding under partial reinforcement schedules (e.g., fixed-ratio, fixed-interval, etc.) maintains response patterns consistent with the reinforcement schedule--similar to those obtained with traditional reinforcers like food and water (Pickens, Meisch, & Thompson, 1978; Pickens & Thompson, 1972; Spealman & Goldberg, 1978). In fact, by selecting the proper amounts of reinforcers and the appropriate reinforcement schedule, such as a second order schedule, the rate and pattern of responding by squirrel monkeys for food and cocaine are the same (Goldberg, 1973; Goldberg & Kelleher, 1976). However, when barbiturates or phencyclidine are the reinforcers, increasing the response requirement for drug injection results in reduction of the drug consumed--appropriate increases in responding do not result.

If an experimentally naive animal is prepared with a chronic intravenous catheter and drug injections are made available by allowing access to the lever programmed to deliver drug injections, the subject may eventually initiate self-administration of the drug. If the rate exceeds control lever or saline responding, the drug is probably reinforcing. Less stringent demonstrations that a drug can serve as a reinforcer are obtained: (a) when the experimental subject is first made physically dependent on the drug by programmed drug delivery and then allowed to respond for drug injections after the programmed delivery is terminated (Weeks, 1962); (b) when the subject is trained to respond for a traditional reinforcer (e.g., food) before making the drug injection a consequence of the response (Talley & Rosenblum, 1972); (c) when responding is first established with another reinforcing drug before making the drug of study a consequence of the response (i.e., the substitution technique where the drug under investigation is substituted for the training drug either during the same session [Yokel & Wise, 1978] or during a subsequent session [Winger & Woods, 1973; Yokel & Pickens, 1973]); (d) when shock avoidance is used to encourage drug responding (Findley et al., 1972); (e) when the subject is enticed to respond for the study drug by placing food on the response lever to increase the probability of the first few responses (Johanson & Schuster, 1975); (f) when drugs are injected noncontingently as the study drug is first made available for self-administration (Lyness, Friedle, & Moore, 1980); or (g) when the use of partial food deprivation and prior experience with lever pressing for food presentation encourage drug intake (Lang, Latiff, McQueen, & Singer, 1977).

Using the above approaches, a wide variety of compounds has been demonstrated to maintain intravenous self-administration, as listed in Table 1. These compounds are all centrally acting. It is their central action that is responsible for their reinforcement effects (Yokel & Pickens, 1973; Koob, Pettit, Ettenberg, & Bloom, 1984; Woolverton, Goldberg, & Ginos, 1984).

Drugs that humans abuse are not the only compounds that are self-administered by animals, as listed in Table 1. Although the self-administration procedure does have good predictive value and has been used to predict abuse liability (Brady, Griffiths, Hienz, Ator, Lukas, & Lamb, this volume; Clineschmidt, Hanson, Pflueger, & McGuffin, 1977; Schuster, Aigner, Johanson, & Gieske, 1982; Weeks & Collins, this volume; Yanagita, this volume; Yanagita & Takahashi, 1973; Yokel & Pickens, 1973), it seems likely that some of the drugs reported to be self-administered by animals (ACTH, clonidine, and haloperidol) will not be abused by humans, although many of these drugs have positive and negative reinforcing effects depending on the circumstances (Wise,

Yokel, & de Wit, 1976).

Table 1

Examples of Compounds that Maintain
Intravenous Self-Administration in Animals

Compound	Species	Reference
Acetaldehyde	rat	Myers et al., 1982
l-α-Acetylmethadol	rat rhesus monkey	Moreton et al., 1976 Harrigan & Downs, 1978
nor-l-α-Acetylmethadol	rat	Young et al., 1979
dinor-l-α-Acetylmethadol	rat	Young et al., 1979
ACTH	rat	Jouhaneau-Bowers & Le Magnen, 1979
Amobarbital	baboon rat rhesus monkey	Griffiths et al., 1981 Davis & Miller, 1963 Winger et al., 1975
d-Amphetamine	baboon dog rat rhesus monkey squirrel monkey	Griffiths et al., 1975 Risner & Jones, 1975 Pickens, 1968 Deneau et al., 1969 Stretch & Gerber, 1970
l-Amphetamine	dog rat rhesus monkey	Risner, 1975 Yokel & Pickens, 1973 Balster & Schuster, 1973
Apomorphine	rat rhesus monkey squirrel monkey	Baxter et al., 1974 Woolverton et al., 1984 Gill et al., 1973
Barbital	rhesus monkey	Winger et al., 1975
Bromocriptine	rhesus monkey	Woolverton et al., 1984
Buprenorphine	rhesus monkey	Lukas et al., 1984
Bupropion	rhesus monkey	Woods, 1983
Butorphanol	rat	Steinfels et al., 1982
d-N-Butylamphetamine	rhesus monkey	Woolverton et al., 1980
Caffeine*	rat rhesus monkey	Atkinson & Enslen, 1976 Deneau et al., 1969
Cathinone	rhesus monkey	Johanson & Schuster, 1979

Chlordiazepoxide*	rhesus monkey	Yanagita & Takahashi, 1973
Chloroprocaine	rhesus monkey	Woolverton & Balster, 1982
Chlorphentermine*	baboon	Griffiths et al., 1975
	rat	Baxter et al., 1973
Clonidine	rat	Shearman et al., 1977
Clortermine	baboon	Griffiths et al., 1975
Cocaine	baboon	Griffiths et al., 1975
	cat	Balster et al., 1976
	pig	Bedford, 1973
	rat	Pickens, 1968
	rhesus monkey	Deneau et al., 1969
	squirrel monkey	Goldberg, 1973
Codeine	rat	Collins & Weeks, 1965
	rhesus monkey	Deneau et al., 1969
Diazepam*	rhesus monkey	Yanagita & Takahashi, 1973
Diethylpropion	baboon	Griffiths et al., 1975
	rat	Baxter et al., 1973
	rhesus monkey	Johanson et al., 1976a
	squirrel monkey	Gill et al., 1973
Dimethocaine	rhesus monkey	Woolverton & Balster, 1982
Dimethylprocaine	rhesus monkey	Woolverton & Balster, 1982
Dynorphin-[1-13]	rat	Khazan et al., 1983
D-ala^2-Dynorphin-[1-11]	rat	Khazan et al., 1983
D-Enkephalin	rat	Tortella & Moreton, 1980
Enkephalin analog, FK-33-824	rhesus monkey	Mello & Mendelson, 1978
Ethanol*	rat	Smith & Davis, 1974
	rhesus monkey	Deneau et al., 1969
d-N-Ethylamphetamine*	rhesus monkey	Woolverton et al., 1980
Ethyl ketocyclazocine	rat	Young & Khazan, 1983
Etonitazene	rat	Carroll et al., 1979
Fencamfamin	dog	Cone & Risner, 1983
	rhesus monkey	Estrada et al., 1967
Fenetylline	rhesus monkey	Hoffmeister, 1980
Fentanyl	rat	Shearman et al., 1977

Flurazepam*	rat	Collins et al., 1984
Haloperidol*	rat	Glick & Cox, 1975a
Heroin	rat	Blakesley et al., 1972
	rhesus monkey	Harrigan & Downs, 1978
Hexobarbital	rat	Davis et al., 1968
Hydromorphone (dihydromorphine)	rat	Collins & Weeks, 1965
Ketamine	baboon	Lukas et al., 1984b
	dog	Risner, 1982
	rhesus monkey	Moreton et al., 1977
Ketocyclazocine	rat	Young & Khazan, 1983
Mazindol	dog	Risner & Silcox, 1979
	rhesus monkey	Wilson & Schuster, 1976
Meperidine	rat	Collins & Weeks, 1965
Methadone	rat	Collins & Weeks, 1965
	rhesus monkey	Harrigan & Downs, 1978
d-Methamphetamine	cat	Balster et al., 1976
	rat	Pickens et al., 1967
	rhesus monkey	Deneau et al., 1969
	squirrel monkey	Gill et al., 1973
l-Methamphetamine*	rat	Yokel & Pickens, 1973
Methohexital	rat	Pickens et al., 1981
	rhesus monkey	Winger et al., 1975
Methylenedioxyamphetamine (MDA)	baboon	Griffiths et al., 1975
Methylphenidate	baboon	Griffiths et al., 1975
	dog	Risner & Jones, 1975
	rhesus monkey	Wilson et al., 1971
Morphine	dog	Jones & Prada, 1973
	mouse	Criswell & Ridings, 1983
	rat	Weeks, 1962
	rhesus monkey	Thompson & Schuster, 1964
	squirrel monkey	Goldberg et al., 1979
Nalbuphine	rat	Steinfels et al., 1982
Nalorphine*	rat	Collins et al., 1984

Nicotine	baboon	Ator & Griffiths, 1983
	dog	Risner & Goldberg, 1981
	rat	Lang et al., 1977
	rhesus monkey	Deneau & Inoki, 1967
	squirrel monkey	Goldberg et al., 1981
Norcocaine	dog	Risner & Jones, 1980
Oxymorphone	rhesus monkey	Aigner & Balster, 1979
Pentazocine	rat	Steinfels et al., 1982
	rhesus monkey	Hoffmeister & Schlichting, 1972
Pentobarbital	baboon	Griffiths et al., 1981
	rat	Collins et al., 1984
	rhesus monkey	Deneau et al., 1969
Phencyclidine (PCP)	baboon	Lukas et al., 1984
	dog	Risner, 1982
	rat	Carroll et al., 1979
	rhesus monkey	Balster et al., 1973
Phencyclidine analogues	baboon	Lukas et al., 1984b
	dog	Risner, 1982
β-Phenethylamine	dog	Risner & Jones, 1977
Phenmetrazine	baboon	Griffiths et al., 1975
	dog	Risner & Jones, 1975
	rat	Baxter et al., 1973
	rhesus monkey	Wilson et al., 1971
Phentermine	baboon	Griffiths et al., 1976
Pipradrol	rhesus monkey	Wilson et al., 1971
Piribedil (ET 495)	rat	Davis & Smith, 1977
	rhesus monkey	Woolverton et al., 1984
Procaine	rat	Collins et al., 1984
	rhesus monkey	Ford & Balster, 1977
Propiram	rhesus monkey	Hoffmeister & Schlichting, 1972
d-Propoxyphene	rat	Collins et al., 1984
	rhesus monkey	Hoffmeister & Schlichting, 1972
d-N-Propylamphetamine	rhesus monkey	Woolverton et al., 1980
Propylbutyldopamine	rhesus monkey	Woolverton et al., 1984
Secobarbital	baboon	Griffiths et al., 1975
	rhesus monkey	Findley et al., 1972

SPA (1-1-2-diphenyl-1-dimethyl-aminoethane)	rhesus monkey	Estrada et al., 1967
Tetracaine	rhesus monkey	Woolverton & Balster, 1979
Δ^9 THC*	rat rhesus monkey	Takahashi & Singer, 1979 Pickens et al., 1973
Thiamylal*	rhesus monkey	Winger et al., 1975
Wy 13,828	rat	Baxter et al., 1973

*Compounds with equivocal reinforcing properties listed in both
Tables 1 and 2.

Although it is not possible to demonstrate that a drug will not be self-administered (i.e., not serve as a reinforcer) under any condition in any species, some studies have failed to obtain drug self-administration after employing several techniques which should elicit drug self-administration (see Table 2). For example, Harris, Waters, and McLendon (1974) failed to obtain THC self-administration (a) in experimentally naive rhesus monkeys, (b) in drug self-administration experienced monkeys, (c) in monkeys that had received repeated THC injections, and (d) in monkeys that had THC paired with a reinforcing drug (cocaine). The latter two procedures assured that the subjects had experience with THC. However, Deneau and Kaymakcalan (1971) obtained THC self-administration in some of the rhesus monkeys tested after repeated programmed injections and after induction of dependence. THC self-administration was also obtained after replacing the phencyclidine that monkeys were self-administering with THC, although substitution of cocaine by THC did not result in THC self-administration (Pickens, Thompson, & Muchow, 1973). Van Ree et al. (1978) reported self-administration after four days of THC injections. Rats maintained at 80% free-feeding weight and trained to work for food on a fixed interval 1-min schedule have also been reported to self-administer THC (Takahashi & Singer, 1979). Caffeine self-administration has been observed in monkeys by Schuster, Seevers, and Woods (1969) and by Deneau et al. (1969), although not by Hoffmeister and Wuttke (1973) nor by Atkinson and Enslen (1976) in rats.

Patterns of Drug Intake

Once self-administration is initiated a pattern of drug intake often develops. After initiation of stimulant self-administration, drug intake usually continues for a few days before a period of drug abstinence lasting hours or days is self-imposed by the experimental animal. Over weeks or months of unlimited drug access a pattern of alternating drug-intake and drug-abstinence periods is seen. During drug intake periods there is a great increase in the level of behavior (usually stereotypic movements with little locomotion) accompanied by reduced food and water intake and by no sleeping. Food and water intake and sleeping occur during drug abstinence periods. Alternating periods of stimulant drug intake and abstinence have been reported for amphetamine and methamphetamine (Deneau et al., 1969; Pickens & Harris, 1968; Yokel & Pickens, 1973), cocaine (Deneau et al., 1969; Johanson et al., 1976a), caffeine (Deneau et al., 1969), fencamfamin and SPA (Estrada et al.,

Table 2

Examples of Compounds Reported not to Maintain
Intravenous Self-Administration in Animals

Compound	Species	Reference
Aminophenazone	rhesus monkey	Hoffmeister & Wuttke, 1975
Amitriptyline	rhesus monkey	Hoffmeister, 1977
Aspirin	rhesus monkey	Hoffmeister & Wuttke, 1973
Buspirone	rhesus monkey	Balster & Woolverton, 1982
Caffeine*	rhesus monkey	Hoffmeister & Wuttke, 1973
Chlordiazepoxide*	rhesus monkey	Balster & Woolverton, 1982
Chlorphentermine*	rhesus monkey	Yanagita et al., 1969
Chlorpromazine	rat rhesus monkey squirrel monkey	van Ree et al., 1978 Deneau et al., 1969 Gill et al., 1973
Clonazepam	baboon	Griffith et al., 1981
Clorazepate	baboon rhesus monkey	Griffith et al., 1981 Balster & Woolverton, 1982
Cyclazocine	rat rhesus monkey	Collins et al., 1984 Aigner & Balster, 1979
Diazepam*	baboon	Griffiths et al., 1981
Diethylaminoethanol	rhesus monkey	Woolverton & Balster, 1979
Dimethylaminoethanol (Deanol)	rhesus monkey	Woolverton & Balster, 1982
Ethanol*	rat	Collins et al., 1984
N-Ethylamphetamine*	rhesus monkey	Tessel & Woods, 1975
Fenfluramine	baboon dog rat rhesus monkey squirrel monkey	Griffiths et al., 1976 Risner & Silcox, 1981 Baxter et al., 1973 Woods & Tessel, 1974 Gill et al., 1973
Flurazepam*	baboon	Griffiths et al., 1981
d, l-Glaucine.1.5-phosphate	rhesus monkey	Schuster et al., 1982
Haloperidol*	rhesus monkey	Hoffmeister, 1977
αHHC	rhesus monkey	Aigner & Balster, 1979

Imipramine	rhesus monkey	Yanagita et al., 1972
Imipramine-N-oxide	rhesus monkey	Yanagita et al., 1972
Iprindole	rhesus monkey	Yanagita et al., 1972
Levallorphan	rhesus monkey	Aigner & Balster, 1979
Lidocaine	rhesus monkey	Woolverton & Balster, 1979
Maprotiline	rhesus monkey	Yanagita et al., 1972
Mescaline	rhesus monkey	Deneau et al., 1969
l-Methamphetamine*	squirrel monkey	Gill et al., 1973
Methoxyamine	dog	Risner & Jones, 1976b
Medazepam	baboon	Griffiths et al., 1981
Midazolam	baboon	Griffiths et al., 1981
MK-212 (fenfluramine-like drug)	rat	Clineschmidt et al., 1977
Morphine	pig	Bedford, 1973
Nalorphine*	rhesus monkey	Deneau et al., 1969
Naloxone	rat rhesus monkey	van Ree et al., 1978 Goldberg et al., 1971a
Nefopam	rat	Collins et al., 1984
Perphenazine	rhesus monkey	Johanson et al., 1976b
Phenylbutazone	rhesus monkey	Hoffmeister & Wuttke, 1975
Phenobarbital	rat	Collins et al., 1984
Phenylpropanolamine	baboon	Griffiths et al., 1978
Phenytoin	rat	Collins et al., 1984
Pilocarpine	rat	Glick & Cox, 1975b
Piperocaine	rhesus monkey	Woolverton & Balster, 1982
Procainamide	rhesus monkey	Woolverton & Balster, 1979
Propoxycaine	rhesus monkey	Woolverton & Balster, 1982
Protriptyline	rhesus monkey	Yanagita et al., 1972
Scopolamine	rat rhesus monkey	Glick & Cox, 1975b Aigner & Balster, 1979

Δ^9 THC*   rhesus monkey   Harris et al., 1974

Thiamylal*   pig   Bedford, 1973

*Compounds with equivocal reinforcing properties listed in both
Tables 1 and 2.

1967), methylphenidate and phenmetrazine (Risner & Jones, 1975, 1976a),
diethylpropion (Johanson et al., 1976b), and mazindol (Risner & Jones, 1980).
Humans demonstrate similar periods of drug intake (binges) and abstinence
(Kramer, Fischman, & Littlefield, 1967). Stimuli (perhaps internal) normally
initiating a period of drug intake are largely unstudied. However, the ability
of external stimuli, particularly drugs, to initiate a period of self-
administration is a fruitful approach to the evaluation of the stimulus and
reinforcing properties of drugs (see Stewart & de Wit, this volume).

    Self-administration of freely available ethanol is also characterized by
alternating intake and abstinence periods. Withdrawal symptoms, including
convulsions, often appear during the self-imposed drug abstinence periods
(Winger & Woods, 1973). Pentobarbital self-administration is characterized by
a lack of abstinence periods--monkeys consume the maximum amount of drug they
seem to be able to physically obtain (Deneau et al., 1969; Yanagita &
Takahashi, 1970). Intravenous opioid self-administration of unlimited drug
results in a more uniform pattern with fairly constant daily intake mainly
during the light phase (daytime) with less drug intake during the evening.
Animals, like humans, do not exhibit voluntary opioid abstinence periods
(Deneau et al., 1969; Harrigan & Downs, 1978). Self-administration of
phencyclidine, when freely available, results in periods of severe intoxication
sufficient to interfere with further drug responding, alternating with periods
of mild intoxication during which eating and drinking occur. Withdrawal signs
are seen upon drug discontinuation (Balster et al., 1973; Balster & Woolverton,
1980).

    Nearly all intravenously self-administered drugs present the risk of being
consumed by the experimental animal to the point of acute toxicity or death
during periods of unlimited access. Convulsions and self-mutilation have been
seen from stimulants (Deneau et al., 1969; Yokel & Pickens, 1973); severe
intoxication and respiratory depression have been seen from ethanol,
barbiturates, and opioids (Deneau et al., 1969; Harrigan & Downs, 1978; Winger
& Woods, 1973); and convulsions have been seen from codeine (Deneau et al.,
1969). Unlimited access results in a high incidence of fatality when
stimulants are self-administered--most rats and monkeys die within a few weeks
after initiation of drug intake--and a lower but significant incidence of
fatality from depressants.

    Due to the fluctuations in drug intake over time and the risk of acute and
chronic toxicity when the self-administered drug is freely available,
experimenters place restrictions on drug availability. Typically, drug is made
available for self-administration for only a few (1 to 6) hours during daily
sessions or during less frequent sessions when long acting drugs are being
evaluated. In addition, response requirements for drug injections are often
increased beyond a single response.

Regulation of Response Rate

When drug availability is limited to a daily session of several hours, drug intake is usually quite stable from session to session. After a few sessions experimental subjects learn to initiate drug responding as soon as drug becomes available. The stability of the rate of self-administration can be seen from a plot of the number of injections, of the amount of drug consumed, or of the number of responses per session across sessions. The reported data are often the total drug intake or the number of responses during an experimental session. Some investigators report their data in successive 1 hour time periods, which is beneficial when response rate is not uniform throughout the session. For example, with the stimulants amphetamine and cocaine, there is a period at the beginning of the self-administration session where several injections are earned in rapid succession before response rate stabilizes in the second or third hour (e.g., see Figure 1). Resolution of results into 1 hour time blocks is useful to see changes in drug response rate caused by manipulations such as pharmacological probes, particularly when the pharmacological probe may have an onset or duration of action that would not produce uniform pharmacological effects throughout the self-administration session (e.g., see Figures 5 and 6). For drugs that produce very uniform response rates, like cocaine and apomorphine, the use of inter-response times can be a sensitive measure of changes in self-administration rate (Dougherty & Pickens, 1973; Griffiths, Bradford, & Brady, 1979).

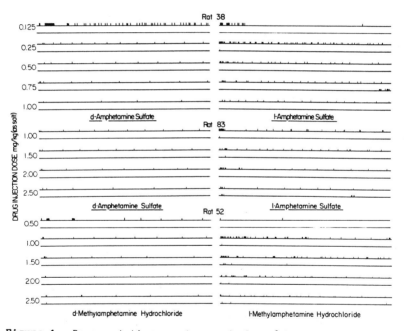

Figure 1: Representative event records from 6 hour sessions of drug lever responding (upper record) and control lever responding (lower record) for several doses of the two optical isomers of amphetamine or methamphetamine. Reprinted with permission from Yokel and Pickens, 1973. Copyright 1973 by the American Society for Pharmacology and Experimental Therapeutics.

Producing a stable response rate by limiting drug access allows manipulation of variables relevant to the reinforcing effects of the drug. For example, if different doses of the drug are available for injection during different sessions, it becomes apparent that below a certain dose the drug will not be self-administered, perhaps being too weak of a reinforcing stimulus. Above a certain dose the drug will not maintain self-administration, perhaps due to aversive properties. The resulting function between the number of responses per session and the dose of the drug injected becomes an inverted U. To the right of the peak of this inverted U-shaped dose response curve (on the descending limb), response rate decreases as the injection dose increases, as shown in Figure 2. If the amount of drug consumed is plotted against the drug dose, then one usually sees a slight increase in drug intake as the drug dose greatly increases. For example, a 50 fold increase in the injection dose of cocaine resulted in only a 5 fold increase in intake (Wilson et al., 1971); an 8 fold increase in d-amphetamine, phenmetrazine and methylphenidate produced no more than a 2.5 fold increase in intake (Risner & Jones, 1975); procaine intake increased 10 fold over a 30 fold increase in dose (Ford & Balster, 1977); sodium amobarbital, methohexital, pentobarbital, and thiopental intake increased less than 2 fold over an 8 fold increase in dose (Goldberg, Hoffmeister, Schlichting, & Wuttke, 1971b; Winger et al., 1975); and a 30 fold

Figure 2: Mean injections per hour and drug intake per hour for intravenous injection of amphetamine and methamphetamine isomers as a function of injection dose. All values are means ±SEM (vertical lines) in micromoles per kilogram of base. SEM in some cases is less than point height. Reprinted with permission from Yokel and Pickens, 1973. Copyright 1973 by the American Society for Pharmacology and Experimental Therapeutics.

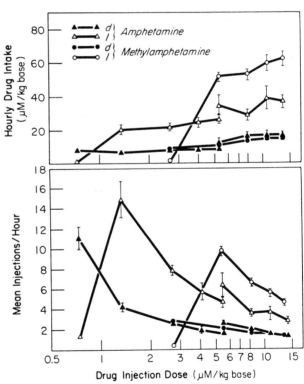

- 13 -

increase in morphine dose produced only a 3 fold increase in intake (Smith, Werner, & Davis, 1976; Weeks & Collins, 1964). Therefore, the increase in drug intake is only 10 to 25% of the increase in injection dose. These results have been taken as evidence that drug intake is being regulated by the animal to produce, over a fairly broad range of doses, a fairly uniform intake.

Several mechanisms have been hypothesized to account for this regulation of drug intake, including an adjustment of response rate to maintain a fairly constant drug level in the animal, a suppression of ongoing behavior by each drug injection in a dose-dependent manner, and a production of aversive effects by the drug injection in a dose dependent manner limiting further intake (Wilson et al., 1971). Support for the maintenance of a minimal drug level as the mechanism regulating drug intake was provided from calculations of whole body amphetamine levels during self-administration in rats. The calculations indicated that the trough levels were always about the same (see Figure 3). That is, rats responded for subsequent drug injections when metabolism had reduced their drug level to a fairly constant, critical level. Obviously, peak drug levels were much greater after larger than smaller drug injections; thus, peak levels were not uniform. When d-amphetamine was compared to l-amphetamine, the former being about 3 times as potent in maintaining self-administration in the rat (Yokel & Pickens, 1973), it was found that the

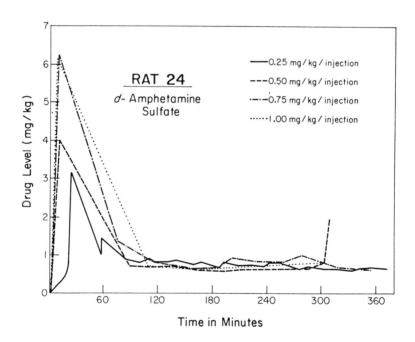

Figure 3: Calculated d-amphetamine whole body drug level during self-administration in a rat. Each point represents the drug level at the time of responding for drug injection. Reprinted with permission from Yokel and Pickens, 1974. Copyright 1974 by Springer-Verlag.

calculated drug level at the time of responding for a subsequent injection was three times higher with l-amphetamine than d-amphetamine. This supports the notion of maintenance of a minimal effect (Yokel & Pickens, 1974). Furthermore, consideration of the first order kinetics of amphetamine metabolism explained the slight increase in intake as drug dose was increased. That is, the larger injection doses merely resulted in more drug being metabolized between drug injections, while the minimal drug level, which perhaps served as a stimulus for drug responding, was maintained. Analysis of amphetamine levels in blood of rats self-administering d- or l- amphetamine demonstrated that across a 4 fold range of injection doses blood amphetamine levels were constant at the time of responding for drug injection and that the levels were about three times higher with the l-isomer, which was 1/3 as potent as the d-isomer (see Figure 4). Cone, Risner, and Neidert (1978) found in the dog that plasma β-phenethylamine levels were relatively constant when a drug response was made.

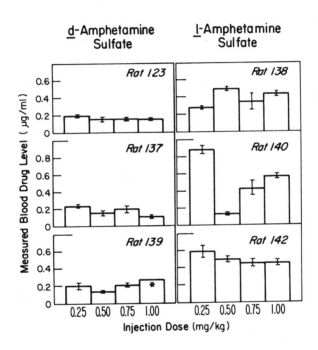

Figure 4: Mean ± SEM of measured blood levels of amphetamine isomers in rats at approximately 2, 4, and 6 hours into a 6 hour session of self-administration of those isomers. * = no replication. Reprinted with permission from Yokel and Pickens, 1974. Copyright 1974 by Springer-Verlag.

- 15 -

The Effects of Pharmacological Challenges

As previously noted, a stable response rate allows manipulation of variables that influence the reinforcing effects of drugs. One approach is the use of pharmacological agents. For example, if the reinforcing drug which the animal is self-administering is given noncontingently before or during a drug self-administration session, there is a suppression of responding (Weeks & Collins, 1964). Unfortunately, a suppression of responding can also be obtained with drugs producing nonspecific behavioral disruption. For example, Wilson and Schuster (1973) found that administration of imipramine, morphine, pentobarbital, d-amphetamine, and phenmetrazine all produced similar decreases in the self-administration of cocaine. However, upon observation, monkeys receiving d-amphetamine, phenmetrazine, and imipramine looked the same as they did during control cocaine self-administration sessions, whereas monkeys receiving morphine or pentobarbital showed gross evidence of depression (e.g., decreased grooming, locomotion, and absence of cocaine-induced stereotypic behaviors). Additionally, d-amphetamine and phenmetrazine produced dose-dependent durations of suppression of cocaine intake. One can conclude from these observations that manipulations increasing or substituting for the reinforcing properties of the drug being self-administered maintain other behaviors but suppress drug responding for a period of time commensurate with the duration of action of the manipulation. By comparison, manipulations which reduce the reinforcing properties of the drug may result in an increased drug intake to compensate for the reduced drug effectiveness, while other behaviors (nondrug responding) remain unchanged. This is well illustrated by demonstrations that increasing doses of nalorphine, naloxone, and naltrexone will initially increase then decrease the rate of morphine and heroin intake in rats and rhesus monkeys (Downs & Woods, 1975; Ettenberg, Pettit, Bloom, & Koob, 1982; Glick, Cox, & Crane, 1975; Goldberg, Hoffmeister, Schlichting, & Wuttke, 1971a; Thompson & Schuster, 1964; Weeks & Collins, 1964). Likewise, antibodies to morphine produce an increase in heroin intake (Killian, Bonese, Rothberg, Wainer, & Schuster, 1978). Although an increased drug intake following a pharmacological challenge may reflect a reduced reinforcement magnitude of the drug, alternative interpretations may need to be ruled out. The pharmacological challenge may increase drug intake by antagonizing an aversive, behaviorally disruptive or toxic action of the self-administered drug or by alteration of the absorption, distribution, biotransformation, or excretion of the self-administered drug (Wilson & Schuster, 1973).

Pharmacological probes that reduce the function of neurotransmitter systems mediating the reinforcing effects of a self-administered drug produce the expected increase in drug intake in the absence of observable changes in nondrug responding behaviors. Amphetamine's pharmacological actions, although many, are all believed to be dependent on catecholaminergic function. Treatment of rats or rhesus monkeys self-administering an amphetamine or cocaine with an inhibitor of catecholamine synthesis (alpha-methyl-para-tyrosine: α mpt) resulted in a temporary increase in drug intake (Baxter, Gluckman, & Scerni, 1976; Pickens, Meisch, & Dougherty, 1968; Wilson & Schuster, 1974). With increases in the dose of α mpt there was a further increase in response rate until a dose of α mpt was reached which produced termination of responding. These results can be interpreted as partial blockade of drug reinforcement effects from doses of α mpt which produced increased drug intake progressing to complete blockade of reinforcement effects from α mpt doses that result in cessation of responding. The results suggest that the animal is able to overcome the blockade of reinforcement effect only to a certain dose of blocking drug; after this dose the blockade cannot be overcome with increases in drug intake, and extinction results. The advantage of using this technique to evaluate the mechanisms of drug reinforcement is that a decrease in reinforcement results in an increase in drug responding and argues against nonspecific disruption of drug responding. With most techniques the response rate reflects reinforcement. When a decreased response rate is seen the experimenter faces the nagging question whether the effect is due to reinforcement reduction or to an effect other than reinforcement reduction. One way to clarify the interpretation of changes in response rate following treatment with a potential reinforcement blocking drug is reviewed by Davis and Smith (this volume).

Further work with more specific pharmacological agents supported the above interpretation that blockade of catecholaminergic function attenuated amphetamine's reinforcing effects. Administration of a fairly specific dopaminergic blocking agent, pimozide, in doses of 0.0625 to 0.25 mg/kg produced a dose-dependent increase in amphetamine intake similar to that produced by αmpt while the characteristic stereotypic behavior of amphetamine self-administration continued. Further increases in the pimozide dose above 0.25 mg/kg produced cessation of responding with loss of amphetamine stereotypic behavior (see Figures 5 and 6).

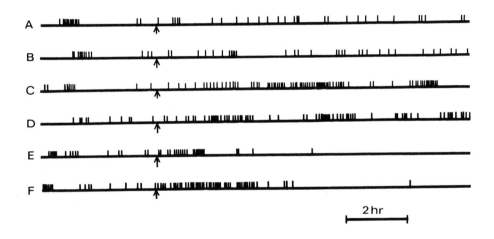

Figure 5: Responding from a representative rat after various manipulations. Each vertical line represents a lever press; arrows mark the experimental manipulations. Manipulations were injections of (A) saline (intraperitoneal), (B) 0.0625 mg/kg of pimozide, (C) 0.125 mg/kg of pimozide, (D) 0.25 mg/kg of pimozide, (E) 0.5 mg/kg of pimozide, and (F) substitution of intravenous saline injections for amphetamine. Reprinted with permission from Yokel and Wise, 1975. Copyright 1975 by the American Association for the Advancement of Science.

Utilization of a dopamine blocker with stereoisomers, one having dopamine blocking activity (+ butaclamol), and the other not (- butaclamol), produced partial and then complete extinction of amphetamine responding with the + isomer only (Yokel & Wise, 1976). An increase in drug responding after lower doses of pimozide and other dopamine blockers (e.g., perphenazine, chlorpromazine, α-flupenthixol, and trifluoperazine) and a decrease in responding after higher doses have been observed in animals self-administering amphetamine, cocaine, phenmetrazine, methylphenidate, pipradrol, SPA, phenethylamine, and mazindol (de Wit & Wise, 1977; Ettenberg et al., 1982; Herling & Woods, 1980; Johanson et al., 1976b; Risner & Jones, 1976b; Risner & Jones, 1977; Risner & Jones, 1980; Risner & Silcox, 1979; Stretch, 1977; Wilson & Schuster, 1968, 1972, 1973) and in animals self-administering morphine (Davis & Smith, 1974a; Hanson & Cimini-Venema, 1972), but not heroin (Ettenberg et al., 1982). The dose-dependent increase, then decrease, in cocaine self-administration following injection of dopamine-receptor blocking drugs has been proposed as a screening method for potential antipsychotic drugs, which presumably block dopamine receptors (Roberts & Vickers, 1984).

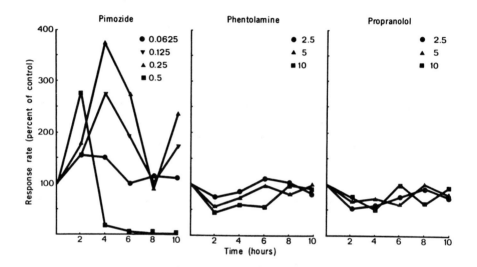

Figure 6: Median response rate for d-amphetamine after intraperitoneal injections of various doses of pimozide, phentolamine, and l-propranolol, expressed in mg/kg body weight. Reproduced with permission from Yokel and Wise, 1975. Copyright 1975 by the American Association for the Advancement of Science.

In comparison, the alpha- and beta-adrenergic blocking drugs phentolamine, phenoxybenzamine, and l-propranolol failed to significantly influence amphetamine, cocaine, or SPA self-administration in the rat (de Wit & Wise, 1977; Yokel & Wise, 1976), dog (Risner & Jones, 1976b; 1980), or rhesus monkey (Wilson & Schuster, 1968; 1974) suggesting that the noradrenergic system was not mediating the reinforcement effects of these stimulants. Neither phenoxybenzamine nor pimozide increased the rate of β-phenethylamine intake (although chlorpromazine did), suggesting a nonadrenergic, nondopaminergic reinforcement mechanism (Risner & Jones, 1977).

A role for cholinergic systems in cocaine and amphetamine self-administration was suggested by Wilson and Schuster (1973) and by Davis and Smith (1974b), who found an increase in cocaine and d-amphetamine self-administration after atropine but not methylatropine administration. De La Garza and Johanson (1982) found an increase in cocaine intake after physostigmine, further supporting this notion. Whether the effects of cholinergic blockade and blockade of acetylcholine metabolism correspond to decreases and increases, respectively, in the reinforcing effects of these stimulants or to other factors regulating drug responding is unclear. A role for a serotonergic mechanism was suggested by Lyness et al. (1980) and by Lyness and Moore (1983) who found that destruction of serotonergic neurons by 5,7-DHT or by injection of metergoline, a serotonergic antagonist, increased the rate of d-amphetamine intake.

The results of studies using drugs as probes could be interpreted several ways. A decrease in response rate produced by the probe could be due to an increase in reinforcement effects of the drug self-administered or to an inhibition of motor behavior interfering with the animal's ability to respond. An increase in response rate produced by the probe may be due to a decrease in reinforcement effects of the drug self-administered, to a reduction in aversive effects of the drug self-administered, or to an increase in motor behavior. One way to rule out the interference effect of changes in motor behavior is to record responding on a control lever or to use a reinforcement schedule requiring concurrent responding for another reinforcer. Another approach is to verify your interpretation of the results by using another behavioral procedure; such methods are discussed in this volume by Davis and Smith and by van der Kooy. Another approach is the study of concurrent self-administration and self-stimulation, which provides simultaneous data from two methods commonly used to evaluate drug reinforcing effects (Bozarth, Gerber, & Wise, 1980; Wise, Yokel, Hansson, & Gerber, 1977). Ultimately, humans could be used as subjects to verify the results obtained from experimental animals. In fact, many of the methods used in animal self-administration have been applied to human self-administration studies, as discussed by Henningfield, Jasinski, and Johnson (this volume) and Mello and Mendelson (this volume). The role of dopaminergic systems and the lack of a role of adrenergic systems in amphetamine reinforcement as demonstrated in animal studies reviewed above were supported by results obtained in human amphetamine abusers. The volunteers rated their subjective euphoria produced by intravenous amphetamine injections. Alpha-methyl-para-tyrosine, chlorpromazine, and pimozide reduced the euphoria, whereas phentolamine and phenoxybenzamine had little effect (Jonsson, 1972; Jonsson, Anggard, & Gunne, 1971; Jonsson, Gunne, & Anggard, 1969).

The influence of neurotransmitter system blockers on the rate of responding for reinforcing drugs suggested another pharmacological approach-- the administration of neurotransmitter agonists. As noncontingent injections of amphetamine temporarily decrease amphetamine intake, would another drug having similar neurotransmitter actions produce the same effect without markedly influencing behaviors other than amphetamine responding? Administration of the dopamine agonists apomorphine and piribedil to rats self-administering d-amphetamine resulted in a temporary cessation in amphetamine responding, with larger doses of dopaminergic agonists producing a longer temporary response cessation (Yokel & Wise, 1978). Administration of the noradrenergic agonists methoxamine and clonidine failed to influence amphetamine intake in the dog and rat (Risner & Jones, 1976b; Yokel & Wise, 1978). Apomorphine, bromocriptine, piribedil, and propylbutyldopamine, all DA_2 receptor agonists, are self-administered, whereas SKF 38393, a DA agonist, is not (Baxter et al., 1974; Davis & Smith, 1977; Gill et al., 1973; Woolverton et al., 1984; Yokel & Wise, 1978). These results suggest that DA_2 receptor activation, rather than DA_1 or noradrenergic activation mediates the reinforcing effects of psychomotor stimulants.

A further approach to the manipulation of neurotransmitter function in elucidating the reinforcement mechanisms of abused drugs is to manipulate the neurotransmitter systems directly. This can be accomplished by stimulation of specific pathways or nuclei of a particular neurotransmitter system or by ablation, either surgically or chemically, as discussed by Roberts and Zito (this volume).

Drug Preference

Clearly then, response rate alone cannot be used to predict reinforcement magnitude or drug preference. To compare two or more doses of the same drug or two or more drugs for their relative reinforcement magnitude (e.g., to ask the simple question whether one is preferred over the other) requires methods more complex than merely looking at response rate. When Deneau et al. (1969) made cocaine and morphine simultaneously available to rhesus monkeys via a double lumen catheter, they found a predominance of cocaine intake during the day and morphine intake at night. Findley et al. (1972) produced a forced choice between two simultaneously available injections by shocking monkeys that failed to self-administer one of the two choices. When secobarbital and saline were choices, secobarbital was preferred. Chlordiazepoxide was preferred over saline, but secobarbital was preferred over chlordiazepoxide when these were the two choices.

One method to compare reinforcers for their relative reinforcement magnitude is to use the discrete trial choice procedure. In the simplest case the animal can select between two levers, either of which, when pressed, results in an injection of the drug paired with the lever. To assure experience with each drug contingency prior to the choice session, training sessions can be conducted prior to the choice session with only one of the choices available in each session. Using this procedure, rats were allowed to self-administer either 0.5 or 1.5 mg/kg cocaine for 6 hours by pressing one of two levers in an operant chamber (the other lever being covered). The following day 6 hours of self-administration of the other dose of cocaine was allowed by pressing the other lever. On the third day both levers were uncovered allowing the choice between the two levers (two cocaine doses) for 6 hours of self-administration. Using a counterbalanced design, this procedure was repeated three times so that the four choice sessions represented the four dose presentation orders and the dose/lever combinations. Figure 7 shows that there was no consistent preference for the larger or smaller dose of cocaine over the other. Further stimulus cues were added during the experiment to facilitate the distinction between the two doses. A similar comparison of 0.5 mg/kg d- vs. 0.5 mg/kg l-amphetamine produced comparable results (i.e., no preference; Yokel & Pickens, unpublished observations). Johanson and Schuster (1975) used a similar discrete trial choice procedure to compare cocaine, methylphenidate, and saline in the rhesus monkey. Both cocaine and methylphenidate were preferred over saline. Higher doses of cocaine were preferred over lower doses. Higher doses of methylphenidate were also preferred over lower doses, although the preference was not as strong as seen between the higher and lower cocaine doses. When cocaine was compared to methylphenidate, the higher dose was always preferred over the lower dose, regardless of the drug.

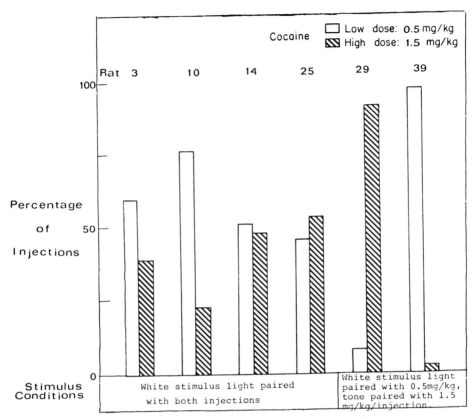

Figure 7: Mean percentage of injections for each of two cocaine doses presented during four 6-hour choice trials in each rat. Additional stimuli were paired with drug injections for rats 29 and 39, as noted on the bottom of the figure. Yokel and Pickens, unpublished observations.

Similar results were obtained using a concurrent schedule involving two response levers and two doses of cocaine where rhesus monkeys could choose between the two doses. Under independent (Iglauer & Woods, 1974) or dependent variable-interval schedules (where the first response on one lever inactivated the second lever until the first lever's schedule was completed; Llewellyn, Iglauer, & Woods, 1976), the higher of two cocaine doses was consistently preferred. Utilizing several different reinforcement schedules, Shannon and Risner (1984) found that cocaine maintained higher response rates than d-amphetamine in the dog, suggesting that cocaine is more reinforcing.

Use of the progressive ratio as a means of evaluating the magnitude of the reinforcement effect of intravenously self-administered drugs was suggested by Yanagita in 1972. The breaking point, or first ratio where responding is not maintained, is considered to reflect reinforcement magnitude. The reinforcing drug injection producing the higher breaking point of the two compared is considered to be the more reinforcing of the pair. Yokel and Pickens (unpublished observations) used an arithmetic progressive-ratio (PR) schedule to compare the breaking points of d- and l-amphetamine. On an arithmetic PR-1 schedule, each response for successive injections increases by 1 (FR-1, FR-2, FR-3, etc.), whereas on a PR-5 schedule each increment is 5 (FR-5, FR-10, FR-15, etc.). By presenting d- and l-amphetamine in a counterbalanced sequence and by incrementing the PR schedule by 1 after each pair of d- and l-amphetamine self-administration sessions until the breaking point was reached within 12 hours for one or both drugs, we were able to compare the two amphetamine isomers for their relative reinforcement magnitudes. Comparison of breaking points suggested that l-amphetamine was as reinforcing as d-amphetamine in the rat whether equal doses (Figure 8, left side) or equipotent doses (Figure 8, right side and Figure 9) were used.

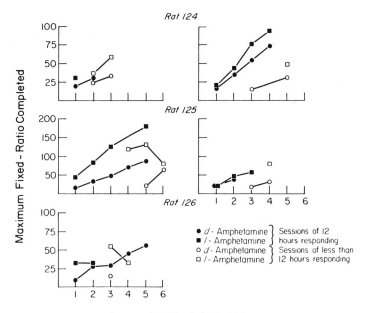

Figure 8: Maximum fixed-ratio completed as a function of progressive ratio value. Left side: equal injection doses. Right side: injection doses chosen to produce equal inter-injection times. (Note: These results were obtained after equal injection dose data had been obtained). Injection doses of d-amphetamine sulfate were 0.5 mg/kg. All injection doses of l-amphetamine sulfate were 0.5 mg/kg (left side) and 1.1 mg/kg for Rat 124 and 1.4 mg/kg for Rat 125 (right side). Yokel and Pickens, unpublished observations.

Griffiths et al. (1975, 1978) have utilized the breaking point generated by increasing the fixed-ratio requirement weekly to compare the reinforcement magnitudes of several stimulants in the baboon. Cocaine and methylphenidate produced comparable breaking points. Lower breaking points (reinforcement magnitude) were produced by diethylpropion and chlorphentermine. Fenfluramine was not self-administered. Comparison of cocaine, d-amphetamine, mazindol, and fenfluramine for their relative reinforcement magnitude in the dog as evidenced by breaking point demonstrated that higher doses were more reinforcing than lower doses and that cocaine was the most reinforcing followed by amphetamine and then mazindol. Fenfluramine did not maintain self-administration (Risner & Silcox, 1981). The breaking point for cocaine seems to increase as the injection dose increases to a point beyond which further increases in dose fail to produce any further increase in the breaking point (Bedford, Bailey, & Wilson, 1978; Griffiths et al., 1979). Breaking points obtained with the progressive-ratio schedule were similar to those obtained with a fixed-ratio schedule (Griffiths et al., 1979).

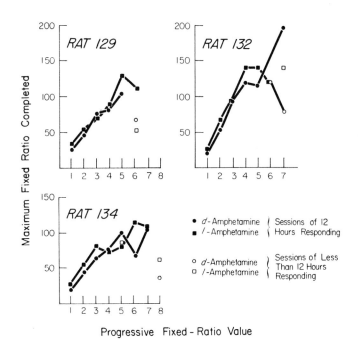

Figure 9: Maximum fixed-ratio completed as a function of progressive-ratio value for injections of d- and l-amphetamine. All injection doses of d-amphetamine were 0.5 mg/kg. Injection doses of l-amphetamine were 2.0 mg/kg for Rat 124 and 1.5 mg/kg for Rats 129 and 132. Yokel and Pickens, unpublished observations.

Comparison of the reinforcement magnitude of opioids using a progressive-ratio schedule demonstrated that higher injection doses produced higher breaking points with codeine and heroin (Hoffmeister, 1979; Lukas et al., 1984). However, with d-propoxyphene, pentazocine and buprenorphine, the increase in breaking point with increased injection dose was less robust. Beyond a point increases in injection dose resulted in decreased breaking points presumably because toxicity results from these higher doses. For codeine the breaking point increased as the dose increased 16,000 times above the minimally effective reinforcing dose. For heroin the breaking point increased up to 500 times the minimally effective dose, but for pentazocine and d-propoxyphene the breaking point increased as the dose increased only to 50 or 70 times the minimally effective injection dose, suggesting a lower reinforcement potential (Hoffmeister, 1979). Applications of the progressive-ratio method of measuring the relative reinforcement magnitude of two drugs may require equipotent drug doses to obtain meaningful results.

A novel method to compare the reinforcement magnitude of two drugs was developed by Hoffmeister (1980) where drug responding occurs at the end of a chain of reinforcement schedules in which food is earned in the first two of the three components of the chain. This procedure allows the analysis of any influence of previous drug injection on schedule of nondrug (e.g., food) responding. With this procedure cocaine, d-amphetamine, and phenmetrazine were found to be better reinforcers than fenetylline, which had only weak reinforcing properties.

Conclusions

Since the initial observation that rats would lever press for intravenous injections of morphine, the technique of intravenous drug self-administration has been widely applied and tested. Modifications of Weeks' original technique have been applied to at least seven other species, four of which (rhesus and squirrel monkey, dog and baboon) have been extensively used to evaluate the reinforcing potential, and therefore abuse potential, of over 100 psychoactive compounds. Self-administration techniques are considered useful in predicting drug abuse potential due to the strong concordance between human and animal drug self-administration.

When allowed unlimited drug access, animals develop patterns of drug intake that produce toxicity similar to that seen in humans. Limited drug access (short daily sessions) is required to obtain the stable drug intake rate desired to study the mechanisms of drug reinforcement. The use of pharmacological challenges has received considerable attention, in attempts to elucidate the mechanisms responsible for the reinforcing effects of abused drugs. The use of behavioral approaches to estimate the magnitude of the reinforcing effect, and therefore the preference of one drug over another, has received less attention.

The self-administration technique seems to be the procedure most clearly modeling the human drug abuser. As with any experimental approach, the results obtained from self-administration studies need to be interpreted cautiously to avoid arriving at the wrong conclusion.

Acknowledgment

I thank Elisabeth Bascom for her skillful typing of this review.

References

Aigner, T. G., & Balster, R. L. (1979). Rapid substitution procedure for intravenous drug self-administration studies in rhesus monkeys. Pharmacology Biochemistry & Behavior, 10, 105-112.

Atkinson, J., & Enslen, M. (1976). Self-administration of caffeine by the rat. Arzneimittel-Forschung/Drug Research, 26, 2059-2061.

Ator, N. A., & Griffiths, R. R. (1983). Nicotine self-administration in baboons. Pharmacology Biochemistry & Behavior, 19, 993-1003.

Balster, R. L., Johanson, C. E, Harris, R. T., & Schuster, C. R. (1973). Phencyclidine self-administration in the rhesus monkey. Pharmacology Biochemistry & Behavior, 1, 167-172.

Balster, R. L., Kilbey, M. M., & Ellinwood, E. H., Jr. (1976). Methamphetamine self-administration in the cat. Psychopharmacologia, 46, 229-233.

Balster, R. L., & Schuster, C. R. (1973). A comparison of d-amphetamine, l-amphetamine, and methamphetamine self-administration in rhesus monkeys. Pharmacology Biochemistry & Behavior, 1, 67-71.

Balster, R. L., & Woolverton, W. L. (1980). Continuous-access phencyclidine self-administration by rhesus monkeys leading to physical dependence. Psychopharmacology, 70, 5-10.

Balster, R. L., & Woolverton, W. L. (1982). Intravenous buspirone self-administration in rhesus monkeys. Journal of Clinical Psychiatry, 43, Dec., 34-39.

Baxter, B. L., Gluckman, M. I., & Scerni, R. (1973). Differential self-injection behavior produced by fenfluramine versus other appetite inhibiting drugs. Federation Proceedings, 32, 754.

Baxter, B. L., Gluckman, M. I., & Scerni, R. A. (1976). Apomorphine self-injection is not affected by alpha-methylparatyrosine treatment: Support for dopaminergic reward. Pharmacology Biochemistry & Behavior, 4, 611-612.

Baxter, B. L., Gluckman, M. I., Stein, L., & Scerni, R. A. (1974). Self-injection of apomorphine in the rat: Positive reinforcement by a dopamine receptor stimulant. Pharmacology Biochemistry & Behavior, 2, 387-391.

Bedford, J. A. (1973). Drug self-administration in the pig. Dissertation Abstracts International, 34, 1767-B.

Bedford, J. A., Bailey, L. P., & Wilson, M. C. (1978). Cocaine reinforced progressive-ratio performance in the rhesus monkey. Pharmacology Biochemistry & Behavior, 9, 631-638.

Blakesley, B. C., Dinneen, L. C., Elliott, R. D., & Francis, D. L. (1972). Intravenous self-administration of heroin in the rat: Experimental technique and computer analysis. British Journal of Pharmacology, 45, 181P.

Bozarth, M. A., Gerber, G. J., & Wise, R. A. (1980). Intracranial self-administration as a technique to study the reward properties of drugs of abuse. Pharmacology Biochemistry & Behavior, 13(Suppl. 1), 245-247.

Carroll, M. E., France, C. P., & Meisch, R. A. (1979). Food deprivation increases oral and intravenous drug intake in rats. Science, 205, 319-321.

Clineschmidt, B. V., Hanson, H. M., Pflueger, A. B., & McGuffin, J. C. (1977). Anorexigenic and ancillary actions of MK-212 (6-chloro-2-[1-piperazinyl]-pyrizine; CPP). Psychopharmacology, 55, 27-33.

Collins, R. J., & Weeks, J. R. (1965). Relative potency of codeine, methadone and dihydromorphinone to morphine in self-maintained addict rats. Naunyn-Schmiedebergs Archiv fur Experimentelle Pathologie und Pharmakologie, 249, 509-514.

Collins, R. J., Weeks, J. R., Cooper, M. M., Good, P. I., & Russell, R. R. (1984). Prediction of abuse liability of drugs using IV self-administration by rats. Psychopharmacology, 82, 6-13.

Cone, E. J., & Risner, M. E. (1983). The reinforcing properties of fencamfamine HC1 (F, "fake cocaine") in the dog. Pharmacologist, 25, 199.

Cone, E. J., Risner, M. E., & Neidert, G. L. (1978). Concentrations of phenethylamine in dog following single doses and during intravenous self-administration. Research Communications in Chemical Pathology and Pharmacology, 22, 211-232.

Criswell, H. E., & Ridings, A. (1983). Intravenous self-administration of morphine by naive mice. Pharmacology Biochemistry & Behavior, 18, 467-470.

Davis, J. D., Lulenski, G. C., & Miller, N. E. (1968). Comparative studies of barbiturate self-administration. The International Journal of the Addictions, 3, 207-214.

Davis, J. D., & Miller, N. E. (1963). Fear and pain: Their effect on self-injection of amobarbital sodium by rats. Science, 141, 1286-1287.

Davis, W. M., & Smith, S. G. (1974a). Noradrenergic basis for reinforcement associated with morphine action in nondependent rats. In J. M. Singh & H. Lal (Eds.), Drug addiction Vol 3: Neurobiology and influences on behavior (pp. 155-168). Miami: Symposia Specialists.

Davis, W. M., & Smith, S. G. (1974b). Central cholinergic influence on self-administration of morphine and amphetamine. Life Sciences, 16, 237-246.

Davis, W. M., & Smith, S. G. (1977). Catecholaminergic mechanisms of reinforcement: Direct assessment by drug self-administration. Life Sciences, 20, 483-492.

De La Garza, R., & Johanson, C. E. (1982). Effects of haloperidol and physostigmine on self-administration of local anesthetics. Pharmacology Biochemistry & Behavior, 17, 1295-1299.

Deneau, G. A., & Inoki, R. (1967). Nicotine self-administration in monkeys. Annals New York Academy of Sciences, 142, 277-279.

Deneau, G. A., & Kaymakcalan, S. (1971). Physiological and psychological dependence to synthetic Δ^9 tetrahydrocannabinol (THC) in rhesus monkeys. Pharmacologist, 13, 246.

Deneau, G., Yanagita, T., & Seevers, M. H. (1969). Self-administration of psychoactive substances by the monkey. Psychopharmacologia, 16, 30-48.

de Wit, H., & Wise, R. A. (1977). Blockade of cocaine reinforcement in rats with the dopamine receptor blocker pimozide, but not with the noradrenergic blockers phentolamine or phenoxybenzamine. Canadian Journal of Psychology, 31, 195-203.

Dougherty, J., & Pickens, R. (1973). Fixed-interval schedules of intravenous cocaine presentation in rats. Journal of the Experimental Analysis of Behavior, 20, 111-118.

Downs, D. A., & Woods, J. H. (1975). Fixed-ratio escape and avoidance-escape from naloxone in morphine-dependent monkeys: Effects of naloxone dose and morphine pretreatment. Journal of the Experimental Analysis of Behavior, 23, 415-427.

Estrada, U., Villarreal, J. E., & Schuster, C. R. (1976). Self-administration of stimulant drugs as a function of the dose per injection. Committee on Problems of Drug Dependence, Appendix 27, 5056-5059.

Ettenberg, A., Pettit, H. O., Bloom, F. E., & Koob, G. F. (1982). Heroin and cocaine intravenous self-administration in rats: Mediation by separate neural systems. Psychopharmacology, 78, 204-209.

Findley, J. D., Robinson, W. W., & Peregrino, L. (1972). Addiction to secobarbital and chlordiazepoxide in the rhesus monkey by means of a self-infusion preference procedure. Psychopharmacologia, 26, 93-114.

Ford, R. D., & Balster, R. L. (1977). Reinforcing properties of intravenous procaine in rhesus monkeys. Pharmacology Biochemistry & Behavior, 6, 289-296.

Gill, C. A., Hill, H. H., Holz, W. C., & Zirkle, C. L. (1973). Squirrel monkey self-injection. Presented to a satellite symposium of the Committee on Problems of Drug Dependence, personal communication.

Glick, S. D., & Cox, R. S. (1975a). Self-administration of haloperidol in rats. Life Sciences, 16, 1041-1046.

Glick, S. D., & Cox, R. D. (1975b). Dopaminergic and cholinergic influences on morphine self-administration in rats. Research Communications in Chemical Pathology and Pharmacology, 12, 17-24.

Glick, S. D., Cox, R. S., & Crane, A. M. (1975). Changes in morphine self-administration and morphine dependence after lesions of the caudate nucleus in rats. Psychopharmacologia, 41, 219-224.

Goldberg, S. R. (1973). Comparable behavior maintained under fixed-ratio and second-order schedules of food presentation, cocaine injection or d-amphetamine injection in the squirrel monkey. Journal of Pharmacology and Experimental Therapeutics, 186, 18-30.

Goldberg, S. R., Hoffmeister, F., Schlichting, U., & Wuttke, W. (1971a). Aversive properties of nalorphine and naloxone in morphine-dependent rhesus monkeys. Journal of Pharmacology and Experimental Therapeutics, 179, 268-276.

Goldberg, S. R., Hoffmeister, F., Schlichting, U. U., & Wuttke, W. (1971b). A comparison of pentobarbital and cocaine self-administration in rhesus monkeys: Effects of dose and fixed-ratio parameter. Journal of Pharmacology and Experimental Therapeutics, 179, 277-283.

Goldberg, S. R., & Kelleher, R. T. (1976). Behavior controlled by scheduled injections of cocaine in squirrel and rhesus monkeys. Journal of the Experimental Analysis of Behavior, 25, 93-104.

Goldberg, S. R., Spealman, R. D., & Goldberg, D. M. (1981). Persistent behavior at high rates maintained by intravenous self-administration of nicotine. Science, 214, 573-576.

Goldberg, S. R., Spealman, R. D., & Kelleher, R. T. (1979). Enhancement of drug-seeking behavior by environmental stimuli associated with cocaine or morphine injections. Neuropharmacology, 18, 1015-1017.

Griffiths, R. R., Bradford, L. D., & Brady, J. V. (1979). Progressive ratio and fixed ratio schedules of cocaine-maintained responding in baboons. Psychopharmacology, 65, 125-136.

Griffiths, R. R., Brady, J. V., & Snell, J. D. (1978). Relationship between anorectic and reinforcing properties of appetite suppressant drugs: Implications for assessment of abuse liability. Biological Psychiatry, 13, 283-290.

Griffiths, R. R., Findley, J. D., Brady, J. V., Dolan-Gutcher, K., & Robinson, W. W. (1975). Comparison of progressive-ratio performance maintained by cocaine, methylphenidate and secobarbital. Psychopharmacologia, 43, 81-83.

Griffiths, R. R., Lukas, S. E., Bradford, L. D., Brady, J. V., & Snell, J. D. (1981). Self-injection of barbiturates and benzodiazepines in baboons. Psychopharmacology, 75, 101-109.

Griffiths, R. R., Winger, G., Brady, J. V., & Snell, J. D. (1976). Comparison of behavior maintained by infusions of eight phenylethylamines in baboons. Psychopharmacology, 50, 251-258.

Hanson, H. M., & Cimini-Venema, C. A. (1972). Effects of haloperidol on self-administration of morphine in rats. Federation Proceedings, 31, 503.

Harrigan, S. E., & Downs, D. A. (1978). Self-administration of heroin, acetylmethadol, morphine, and methadone in rhesus monkeys. Life Sciences, 22, 619-624.

Harris, R. T., Waters, W., & McLendon, D. (1974). Evaluation of reinforcing capability of delta-9-tetrahydrocannabinol in rhesus monkeys. Psychopharmacologia, 37, 23-29.

Herling, S., & Woods, J. H. (1980). Chlorpromazine effects on cocaine-reinforced responding in rhesus monkeys; reciprocal modification of rate-altering effects of the drugs. Journal of Pharmacology and Experimental Therapeutics, 214, 354-361.

Hoffmeister, F. (1977). Reinforcing properties of perphenazine, haloperidol and amitriptyline in rhesus monkeys. Journal of Pharmacology and Experimental Therapeutics, 200, 516-522.

Hoffmeister, F. (1979). Progressive-ratio performance in the rhesus monkey maintained by opiate injections. Psychopharmacology, 62, 181-186.

Hoffmeister, F. (1980). Influence of intravenous self-administered psychomotor stimulants on performance of rhesus monkeys in a multiple schedule paradigm. Psychopharmacology, 72, 41-59.

Hoffmeister, F., & Goldberg, S. R. (1973). A comparison of chlorpromazine, imipramine, morphine and d-amphetamine self-administration in cocaine-dependent rhesus monkeys. Journal of Pharmacology and Experimental Therapeutics, 187, 8-14.

Hoffmeister, F., & Schlichting, U. U. (1972). Reinforcing properties of some opiates and opioids in rhesus monkeys with histories of cocaine and codeine self-administration. Psychopharmacologia, 23, 55-74.

Hoffmeister, F., & Wuttke, W. (1973). Self-administration of acetylsalicylic acid and combinations with codeine and caffeine in rhesus monkeys. Journal of Pharmacology and Experimental Therapeutics, 186, 266-275.

Hoffmeister, F., & Wuttke, W. (1975). Further studies on self-administration of antipyretic analgesics and combinations of antipyretic analgesics with codeine in rhesus monkeys. Journal of Pharmacology and Experimental Therapeutics, 193, 870-875.

Iglauer, C., & Woods, J. H. (1974). Concurrent performances: Reinforcement by different doses of intravenous cocaine in rhesus monkeys. Journal of the Experimental Analysis of Behavior, 22, 179-196.

Johanson, C. E., & Balster, R. L. (1978). A summary of the results of self-administration studies using substitution procedures in primates. Bulletin on Narcotics, 30, 43-54.

Johanson, C. E., Balster, R. L., & Bonese, K. (1976a). Self-administration of psychomotor stimulant drugs: The effects of unlimited access. Pharmacology Biochemistry & Behavior, 4, 45-51.

Johanson, C. E., Kandel, D. A., & Bonese, K. (1976b). The effects of perphenazine on self-administration behavior. Pharmacology Biochemistry & Behavior, 4, 427-433.

Johanson, C. E., & Schuster, C. R. (1975). A choice procedure for drug reinforcers: Cocaine and methylphenidate in the rhesus monkey. Journal of Pharmacology and Experimental Therapeutics, 193, 675-688.

Johanson, C. E., & Schuster, C. R. (1979). Self-administration of cathinone and its effects on schedule-controlled responding in the rhesus monkey. Federation Proceedings, 38, 436.

Jones, B. E., & Prada, J. A. (1973). Relapse to morphine use in dog. Psychopharmacologia, 30, 1-12.

Jonsson, L. E. (1972). Pharmacological blockade of amphetamine effects in amphetamine dependent subjects. European Journal of Clinical Pharmacology, 4, 206-211.

Jonsson, L. E., Anggard, E., & Gunne, L. M. (1971). Blockade of intravenous amphetamine euphoria in man. Clinical Pharmacology and Therapeutics, 12, 889-896.

Jonsson, L. E., Gunne, L. M., & Anggard, E. (1969). Effects of alpha-methyltyrosine in amphetamine-dependent subjects. Pharmacologia Clinica, 2, 27-29.

Jouhaneau-Bowers, M., & Le Magnen, J. (1979). ACTH self-administration in rats. Pharmacology Biochemistry & Behavior, 10, 325-328.

Khazan, N., Young, G. A., & Calligaro, D. (1983). Self-administration of dynorphin-[1-13] and D-Ala^2-dynorphin-[1-11] (kappa opioid agonists) in morphine (mu opioid agonist)-dependent rats. Life Sciences, 33(Suppl. 1) 559-562.

Killian, A., Bonese, K., Rothberg, R. M., Wainer, B. H., & Schuster, C. R. (1978). Effects of passive immunization against morphine on heroin self-administration. Pharmacology Biochemistry & Behavior, 9, 347-352.

Koob, G. F., Pettit, H. O., Ettenberg, A., & Bloom, F. E. (1984). Effects of opiate antagonists and their quaternary derivatives on heroin self-administration in the rat. Journal of Pharmacology and Experimental Therapeutics, 229, 481-486.

Kramer, J. C., Fischman, V. S., & Littlefield, D. C. (1967). Amphetamine abuse. Pattern and effects of high doses taken intravenously. Journal of the American Medical Association, 201, 305-309.

Lang, W. J., Latiff, A. A., McQueen, A., & Singer, G. (1977). Self-administration of nicotine with and without a food delivery schedule. Pharmacology Biochemistry & Behavior, 7, 65-70.

Llewellyn, M. E., Iglauer, C., & Woods, J. H. (1976). Relative reinforcer magnitude under a nonindependent concurrent schedule of cocaine reinforcement in rhesus monkeys. Journal of the Experimental Analysis of Behavior, 25, 81-91.

Lukas, S. E., Bree, M. P., Mello, N. K., & Mendelson, J. H. (1984). Relative reinforcing properties of buprenorphine, heroin, and methadone in macaque monkeys. Pharmacologist, 26, 239.

Lukas, S. E., Griffiths , R. R., Bradford, L. D., Brady, J. V., Daley, L., & Delorenzo, R. (1982). A tethering system for intravenous and intragastric drug administration in the baboon. Pharmacology Biochemistry & Behavior, 17, 823-829.

Lukas, S. E., Griffiths, R. R., Brady, J. V., & Wurster, R. M. (1984). Phencyclidine-analogue self-injection by the baboon. Psychopharmacology, 83, 316-320.

Lyness, W. H., Friedle, N. M., & Moore, K. E. (1980). Increased self-administration of d-amphetamine after destruction of 5-hydroxytryptaminergic neurons. Pharmacology Biochemistry & Behavior, 12, 937-941.

Lyness, W. H., & Moore, K. E. (1983). Increased self-administration of d-amphetamine by rats pretreated with metergoline. Pharmacology Biochemistry & Behavior, 18, 721-724.

Mello, N. K., & Mendelson, J. H. (1978). Self-administration of an enkephalin analog by rhesus monkey. Pharmacology Biochemistry & Behavior, 9, 579-586.

Moreton, J. E., Meisch, R. A., Stark, L., & Thompson, T. (1977). Ketamine self-administration by the rhesus monkey. Journal of Pharmacology and Experimental Therapeutics, 203, 303-309.

Moreton, J. E., Roehrs, T., & Khazan, N. (1976). Drug self-administration and sleep-awake activity in rats dependent on morphine, methadone, or l-alpha-acetylmethadol. Psychopharmacology, 47, 237-241.

Myers, W. D., Ng, K. T., & Singer, G. (1982). Intravenous self-administration of acetaldehyde in the rat as a function of schedule, food deprivation and photoperiod. Pharmacology Biochemistry & Behavior, 17, 807-811.

Pickens, R. (1968). Self-administration of stimulants by rats. The International Journal of the Addictions, 3, 215-221.

Pickens, R., & Dougherty, J. (1972). A method for chronic intravenous infusion of fluids in unrestrained rats. Reports from the Research Laboratories of the Department of Psychiatry, University of Minnesota, 1-29.

Pickens, R., & Harris, W. C. (1968). Self-administration of d-amphetamine by rats. Psychopharmacologia, 12, 158-163.

Pickens, R., Meisch, R. A., & Dougherty, J. A., Jr. (1968). Chemical interactions in methamphetamine reinforcement. Psychological Reports, 23, 1267-1270.

Pickens, R., Meisch, R., & McGuire, L. E. (1967). Methamphetamine reinforcement in rats. Psychonomic Science, 8, 371-372.

Pickens, R., Meisch, R. A., & Thompson, T. (1978). Drug self-administration: An analysis of the reinforcing effects of drugs. In L. L. Iversen, S. D. Iversen, & S. H. Snyder (Eds.), Handbook of psychopharmacology, (Vol. 12, pp. 1-37). New York: Plenum Press.

Pickens, R., Muchow, D., & De Noble, V. (1981). Methohexital-reinforced responding in rats: Effects of fixed ratio size and injection dose. Journal of Pharmacology and Experimental Therapeutics, 216, 205-209.

Pickens, R., & Thompson, T. (1968). Cocaine-reinforced behavior in rats: Effects of reinforcement magnitude and fixed-ratio size. Journal of Pharmacology and Experimental Therapeutics, 161, 122-129.

Pickens, R., & Thompson, T. (1972). Simple schedules of drug self-administration in animals. Drug addiction: Experimental pharmacology (Vol. 1). Mount Kisco, New York: Futura.

Pickens, R., & Thompson, T. (1975). Intravenous preparations for self-administration of drugs by animals. American Psychologist, 30, 274-276.

Pickens, R., Thompson, T., & Muchow, D. C. (1973). Cannabis and phencyclidine self-administration by animals. In L. Goldberg & F. Hoffmeister (Eds.), Psychic dependence (78-86). New York: Springer-Verlag.

van Ree, J. M., Slangen, J. F., & De Wied, D. (1978). Intravenous self-administration of drugs in rats. Journal of Pharmacology and Experimental Therapeutics, 204, 547-557.

Risner, M. E. (1975). Intravenous self-administration of d- and l-amphetamine by dog. European Journal of Pharmacology, 32, 344-348.

Risner, M. E. (1982). Intravenous self-administration of phencyclidine and related compounds in the dog. Journal of Pharmacology and Experimental Therapeutics, 221, 637-644.

Risner, M. E., & Goldberg, S. R. (1981). Behavior maintained by intravenous injection of nicotine in beagle dogs. Presented at the American Psychological Association Annual Meeting, Los Angeles.

Risner, M. E., & Jones, B. E. (1975). Self-administration of CNS stimulants by dog. Psychopharmacologia, 43, 207-213.

Risner, M. E., & Jones, B. E. (1976a). Characteristics of unlimited access to self-administered stimulant infusions in dogs. Biological Psychiatry, 11, 625-634.

Risner, M. E., & Jones, B. E. (1976b). Role of noradrenergic and dopaminergic processes in amphetamine self-administration. Pharmacology Biochemistry & Behavior, 5, 477-482.

Risner, M. E., & Jones, B. E. (1977). Characteristics of β-phenethylamine self-administration by dog. Pharmacology Biochemistry & Behavior, 6, 689-696.

Risner, M. E., & Jones, B. E. (1980). Intravenous self-administration of cocaine and norcocaine by dogs. Psychopharmacology, 71, 83-89.

Risner, M. E., & Silcox, D. L. (1979). Mazindol self-administration by dog. Presented at the American Psychological Association Annual Meeting, New York.

Risner, M. E., & Silcox, D. L. (1981). Psychostimulant self-administration by beagle dogs in a progressive-ratio paradigm. Psychopharmacology, 75, 25-30.

Roberts, D. C. S., & Vickers, G. (1984). Atypical neuroleptics increase self-administration of cocaine: An evaluation of a behavioral screen for antipsychotic activity. Psychopharmacology, 82, 135-139.

Schuster, C. R., Aigner, T., Johanson, C. E., & Gieske, T. H. (1982). Experimental studies of the abuse potential of d, l-glaucine.1.5-phosphate in rhesus monkeys. Pharmacology Biochemistry & Behavior, 16, 851-854.

Schuster, C. R., Woods, J. H., & Seevers, M. H. (1969). Self-administration of central stimulants by the monkey. In F. Sjoqvist & M. Tottie (Eds.), Abuse of central stimulants (pp. 339-347). New York: Raven Press.

Shannon, H. E., & Risner, M. E. (1984). Comparison of behavior maintained by intravenous cocaine and d-amphetamine in dogs. Journal of Pharmacology and Experimental Therapeutics, 229, 422-432.

Shearman, G., Hynes, M., Fielding, S., & Lal, H. (1977). Clonidine self-administration in the rat: A comparison with fentanyl self-administration. Pharmacologist, 19, 171.

Smith, S. G., & Davis, W. M. (1974). Intravenous alcohol self-administration in the rat. Pharmacological Research Communications, 6, 397-402.

Smith, S. G., & Davis, W. M. (1975). A method for chronic intravenous drug administration in the rat. In S. Ehrenpreis & A. Neidle (Eds.), Methods in narcotic research (pp. 3-32). New York: Marcel Dekker.

Smith, S. G., Werner, T. E., & Davis, W. M. (1976). Effect of unit dose and route of administration on self-administration of morphine. Psychopharmacology, 50, 103-105.

Spealman, R. D., & Goldberg, S. R. (1978). Drug self-administration by laboratory animals: Control by schedules of reinforcement. Annual Review of Pharmacology, 18, 313-339.

Steinfels, G. F., Young, G. A., & Khazan, N. (1982). Self-administration of nalbuphine, butorphanol and pentazocine by morphine post-addict rats. Pharmacology Biochemistry & Behavior, 16, 167-171.

Stretch, R. (1977). Discrete-trial control of cocaine self-injection behaviour in squirrel monkeys: Effects of morphine, naloxone, and chlorpromazine. Canadian Journal of Physiology and Pharmacology, 55, 778-790.

Stretch, R., & Gerber, G. J. (1970). A method for chronic intravenous drug administration in squirrel monkeys. Canadian Journal of Physiology and Pharmacology, 48, 575-581.

Takahashi, R. N., & Singer, G. (1979). Self-administration of Δ^9 - tetrahydrocannabinol by rats. Pharmacology Biochemistry & Behavior, 11, 737-740.

Talley, W. H., & Rosenblum, I. (1972). Self administration of dextropropoxyphene by rhesus monkeys to the point of toxicity. Psychopharmacologia, 27, 179-182.

Tessel, R. E., & Woods, J. H. (1975). Fenfluramine and N-ethylamphetamine: Comparison of the reinforcing and rate-decreasing actions in the rhesus monkey. Psychopharmacologia, 43, 239-244.

Thompson, T., & Schuster, C. R. (1964). Morphine self-administration, food reinforced, and avoidance behaviors in rhesus monkey. Psychopharmacologia, 5, 87-94.

Tortella, F. C., & Moreton, J. E. (1980). D-ala^2-methionine-enkephalinamide self-administration in the morphine dependent rat. Psychopharmacology, 69, 143-147.

Weeks, J. R. (1962). Experimental morphine addiction: Method for automatic intravenous injections in unrestrained rats. Science, 138, 143-144.

Weeks, J. R. (1972). Long-term intravenous infusion. In R. D. Myers (Ed.), Methods in psychobiology (Vol. 2, pp. 155-168). New York: Academic Press.

Weeks, J. R., & Collins, R. J. (1964). Factors affecting voluntary morphine intake in self-maintained addicted rats. Psychopharmacologia, 6, 267-279.

Wilson, M. C., Hitomi, M., & Schuster, C. R. (1971). Psychomotor stimulant self-administration as a function of dosage per injection in the rhesus monkey. Psychopharmacologia, 22, 271-281.

Wilson, M. C., & Schuster, C. R. (1968). Pharmacological modification of the self-administration of cocaine and SPA in the rhesus monkey. Committee on Problems of Drug Dependence, 5610-5617.

Wilson, M. C., & Schuster, C. R. (1972). The effects of chlorpromazine on psychomotor stimulant self-administration in the rhesus monkey. Psychopharmacologia, 26, 115-126.

Wilson, M. C., & Schuster, C. R. (1973). The effects of stimulants and depressants on cocaine self-administration behavior in the rhesus monkey. Psychopharmacologia, 31, 291-304.

Wilson, M. C., & Schuster, C. R. (1974). Aminergic influences on intravenous cocaine self-administration by rhesus monkeys. Pharmacology Biochemistry & Behavior, 2, 563-571.

Wilson, M. C., & Schuster, C. R. (1976). Mazindol self-administration in the rhesus monkey. Pharmacology Biochemistry & Behavior, 4, 207-210.

Winger, G., Stitzer, M. L., & Woods, J. H. (1975). Barbiturate-reinforced responding in rhesus monkeys: Comparisons of drugs with different durations of action. Journal of Pharmacology and Experimental Therapeutics, 195, 505-514.

Winger, G. D., & Woods, J. H. (1973). The reinforcing property of ethanol in the rhesus monkey: I. Initiation, maintenance and termination of intravenous ethanol-reinforced responding. Annals New York Academy of Sciences, 215, 162-175.

Wise, R. A., Yokel, R. A., Hansson, P. A., & Gerber, G. J. (1977). Concurrent intracranial self-stimulation and amphetamine self-administration in rats. Pharmacology Biochemistry & Behavior, 7, 459-461.

Wise, R. A., Yokel, R. A., & de Wit, H. (1976). Both positive reinforcement and conditioned aversion from amphetamine and from apomorphine in rats. Science, 191, 1273-1275.

Woods, J. H. Personal communication to J. D. Griffith. Bupropion: Clinical assay for amphetamine-like abuse potential. The Journal of Clinical Psychiatry, 44, 206-208.

Woods, J. H., & Tessel, R. E. (1974). Fenfluramine: Amphetamine congener that fails to maintain drug-taking behavior in the rhesus monkey. Science, 185, 1067-1069.

Woolverton, W. L., & Balster, R. L. (1979). Reinforcing properties of some local anesthetics in rhesus monkeys. Pharmacology Biochemistry & Behavior, 11, 669-672.

Woolverton, W. L., & Balster, R. L. (1982). Behavioral pharmacology of local anesthetics: Reinforcing and discriminative stimulus effects. Pharmacology Biochemistry & Behavior, 16, 491-500.

Woolverton, W. L., Goldberg, L. I., & Ginos, J. Z. (1984). Intravenous self-administration of dopamine receptor agonists by rhesus monkeys. Journal of Pharmacology and Experimental Therapeutics, 230, 678-683.

Woolverton, W. L., Shybut, G., & Johanson, C. E. (1980). Structure-activity relationships among some d-N-alkylated amphetamines. Pharmacology Biochemistry & Behavior, 13, 869-876.

Yanagita, T. (1972). An experimental framework for evaluation of dependence liability of various types of drugs in monkeys. Fifth International Congress on Pharmacology. Symposium: Drugs and Society, 133-134.

Yanagita, T., Ando, K., Takahashi, S., & Ishida, K. (1969). Self-administration of barbiturate, alcohol (intragastric) and CNS stimulants (intravenous) in monkeys. Committee on Problems of Drug Dependence, 31st Meeting, 6039-6050.

Yanagita, T., & Takahashi, S. (1970). Development of tolerance to and physical dependence on barbiturates in rhesus monkeys. Journal of Pharmacology and Experimental Therapeutics, 172, 163-169.

Yanagita, T., & Takahashi, S. (1973). Dependence liability of several sedative-hypnotic agents evaluated in monkeys. Journal of Pharmacology and Experimental Therapeutics, 185, 307-316.

Yanagita, T., Takahashi, S., & Oinuma, N. (1972). Drug dependence liability of tricyclic antidepressants evaluated in monkeys. Japanese Journal of Clinical Pharmacology, 3, 289-294.

Yokel, R. A., & Pickens, R. (1973). Self-administration of optical isomers of amphetamine and methylamphetamine by rats. Journal of Pharmacology and Experimental Therapeutics, 187, 27-33.

Yokel, R. A., & Pickens, R. (1974). Drug level of d- and l-amphetamine during intravenous self-administration. Psychopharmacologia, 34, 255-264.

Yokel, R. A., & Wise, R. A. (1975). Increased lever pressing for amphetamine after pimozide in rats: Implications for a dopamine theory of reward. Science, 187, 547-549.

Yokel, R. A., & Wise, R. A. (1976). Attenuation of intravenous amphetamine reinforcement by central dopamine blockade in rats. Psychopharmacology, 48, 311-318.

Yokel, R. A., & Wise, R. A. (1978). Amphetamine-type reinforcement by dopaminergic agonists in the rat. Psychopharmacology, 58, 289-296.

Young, G. A., & Khazan, N. (1983). Self-administration of ketocyclazocine and ethylketocyclazocine by the rat. Pharmacology Biochemistry & Behavior, 19, 711-713.

Young, G. A., Steinfels, G. F., & Khazan, N. (1979). Pharmacodynamic profiles of l-alpha-acetylmethadol (LAAM) and its N-demethylated metabolites, nor-LAAM and dinor-LAAM, during self-administration in the dependent rat. Journal of Pharmacology and Experimental Therapeutics, 210, 453-457.

CHAPTER 2

SCREENING FOR DRUG REINFORCEMENT USING INTRAVENOUS SELF-ADMINISTRATION IN THE RAT

James R. Weeks and R. James Collins

The Upjohn Company
Kalamazoo, Michigan 49001

ABSTRACT

The reinforcing activity of 31 psychoactive drugs was evaluated. Drugs were offered by intravenous self-administration to groups of naive rats. Reinforcement is indicated by an injection rate greater than that for rats offered only saline. Two similar protocols were used. In the first protocol, rats were offered drug at a selected dose for 5 days, then the dose was reduced by one log unit (to 0.1 times the initial dose) for an additional 4 days. In the second protocol, saline only was offered the first 3 days to eliminate rats with high or low operant rates, and the dose was reduced 0.5 log unit (to 0.32 times the initial dose) instead of one log unit. An empirical score, based on the injection rates during the last 3 days of each period, describes the reinforcing activity. Replicate tests using both protocols gave similar scores. Literature data for reinforcing activity in monkeys was available for 27 of the drugs tested. Results for rats and monkeys agreed for 24 of the 27 drugs. Nalorphine and ethylketazocine were reinforcers only in rats, and ethanol was a reinforcer only in monkeys.

INTRODUCTION

Assessment of abuse liability is an important consideration in the development of new psychoactive drugs. It is now well accepted that drugs which are reinforcing in animals by intravenous self-administration may have abuse liability in humans (Griffiths & Balster, 1979; Griffiths, Bigelow, & Henningfield, 1980; Griffiths, Brady, & Bradford, 1979; van Ree, 1979; Schuster & Thompson, 1969; Thompson & Unna, 1977). Monkeys have been the preferred species, and regulatory agencies in some countries specify testing in monkeys. Cost and limited availability of monkeys or other sub-human primates preclude testing of compounds early in the drug development process. A reliable method using rodents would be very desirable.

Any protocol for screening compounds for a pharmacological activity may be viewed as a special form of a biological assay. Both screens and bioassays require a dose-related assessment of the activity with adequate statistical controls. In a screen less precise measures are tolerable, and significance levels can be less stringent than the conventional 5% level. False positives are more likely to occur, but results from screens are followed with more testing to eliminate them. Implied in a screening test is the ability to test relatively large numbers of compounds without excessive cost or labor.

Several pharmacological classes of drugs are reinforcing by self-administration. When substances are tested early in the development process, knowledge of their pharmacology may be very limited. Accordingly, the screening method should be applicable without change across pharmacological classes. Drug-naive animals should be used.

We have recently devised a method for assessing reinforcing activity in rats (Collins, Weeks, Cooper, Good, & Russell, 1984). The method is suitable for several pharmacological classes of abused drugs, has a firm statistical basis, and gives a dose-related measure of reinforcing activity. Naive rats were offered test drugs by intravenous self-administration, without shaping or accessory cues, for several days and then the dose was reduced. Reinforcing activity was indicated by injection rates greater than those of control rats offered only saline. Activity was assessed in four ways: (1) an empirical score based on the injection rates for the two doses, (2) the number of rats reinforced (at either dose), (3) a comparison of the group mean injection rates to the rate for control rats self-injecting only saline, and (4) the presence of physical dependence. The data were gathered over a period of several years. At first we used a motor-driven syringe (Weeks & Collins, 1976). Syringes were often emptied when injection rates exceeded a few hundred a day. Later, a pneumatic-operated syringe with a fluid reservoir was developed which allowed unlimited numbers of injections (Weeks & Collins, 1981). After initial studies were completed, the protocol was modified to decrease the variability of the assay. These protocols will be referred to as "old" and "new," respectively. Thirteen drugs were re-tested using the new protocol. Since the protocols were very similar and the data were evaluated in the same manner, comparison of such results served to test the reproducibility of the method.

If the rat is a satisfactory alternate species for predicting abuse liability, results obtained must parallel those obtained in the monkey. Thirty-one different psychoactive drugs were studied. The reinforcing activity in the monkey had been reported in the literature for 27 of these drugs. Results in the rat were compared to these reports. The reader is referred to the publication by Collins et al. (1984) for details on interpretation of results and statistical validation of some aspects of the tests.

MATERIALS AND METHODS

Subjects

Rats were Sprague-Dawley origin females, ranging from 250 to 400 g. At least 6 days before use, rats were prepared with chronic venous cannulas (Weeks, 1972). After completion of the protocol, cannulas were considered functional if either blood could be withdrawn or the rat lost consciousness immediately following rapid injection of 3 to 5 mg/kg of sodium methohexital.

Apparatus

Experimental cages were standard individual hanging cages in a stainless steel rack similar to that used for prolonged intravenous infusions (Weeks, 1979). A lever switch (No. 121-03, BRS/LVE, 5301 Holland Drive, Beltsville, MD 20705), with the return spring removed to reduce operating pressure, was amounted on the rear wall of the cage 4 cm above the floor. It was essential to shield the paddle on the lever. Rats wore a saddle connected to a cannula feed-through swivel (see Weeks, 1977, for details of the lever switch and saddle). Each lever press resulted in a drug injection delivered by either a motor-driven or pneumatic syringe (Weeks, 1977, 1981; Weeks & Collins, 1976). The motor-driven syringe delivered injection volumes of 320 (initial dose) or 100 (reduced dose) µl/kg at 10.8 µl/second. The pneumatic syringe delivered only 100 µl/kg in about 0.5 second. Since 1979 we have used the pneumatic syringe exclusively (Ledger Technical Services, 2626 Lomond Drive, Kalamazoo, MI 49008). The total daily number of injections was noted at 8:00 a.m. ± 20 minutes, and any changes in experimental conditions were completed by no later than 9:30 a.m.

Most drugs were prepared in physiological saline. Drug forms and special solvents are noted in Collins et al. (1984). Doses of drugs were those of their respective salts, except for cyclazocine, ketamine, and pentazocine which were expressed as the free base.

Protocols

The duration of the test was 13 days for both protocols. Rats were weighed initially, on return to the home cage after completion of the protocol, and again 24 hours later (initial, final, and withdrawal weights, respectively).

In the old protocol naive rats had been offered drug at an initial dose for 5 days, then the dose was reduced one log unit (to 0.1 the initial dose) for 4 days. A fixed-ratio (FR) schedule of FR-2 and FR-4 for two additional days each completed the protocol. Results for FR testing did not contribute to evaluation as a reinforcing agent and will not be discussed.

In the new protocol naive rats were offered 100 µl/kg of saline for 3 days, then the drug at an initial dose for 5 days, and finally the dose was reduced by 0.5 log unit (to 0.32 the initial dose) for 5 additional days. Rats averaging less than 4 or more than 50 injections per day of saline were rejected.

The dose selected for the first test was arbitrary, based upon known pharmacological effects of the drugs in rats. In subsequent tests, doses were increased or decreased in 0.5 log increments.

Controls were groups of 30 rats offered saline for 13 days. Separate controls were used for the motor-driven syringe old protocol, pneumatic syringe old protocol, and pneumatic syringe new protocol.

Evaluation of Reinforcing Activity

We showed earlier (Weeks & Collins, 1979) that daily injection rates of saline and morphine are log-normally distributed between rats. Analysis of 125 rats receiving only saline for 13 days supported the hypothesis that injection rates within rats are also log-normally distributed (Collins et al., 1984). Accordingly, each daily injection rate x was analyzed after the transformation log $(x + 1)$ and the means expressed as the antilog - 1.

An empirical score was used to express the reinforcing activity of compounds in each individual rat. It was based on the injection rate for the last 3 days for the two drug doses compared to the same time periods for the appropriate saline controls. The 90% confidence limits for the number of injections of saline were calculated for both doses by the one-sample t-test.

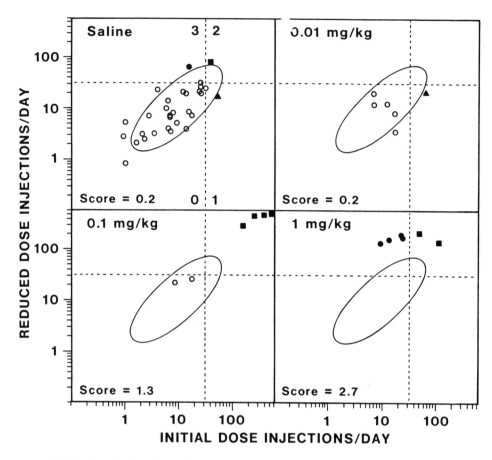

Figure 1: Injection rates and scores for rats self-administering saline and morphine using the pneumatic syringe and new protocol. The ellipse is the 90% confidence limits for saline control rats based upon the bivariate distribution of injection rates corresponding to the initial and reduced dose periods. The dashed lines represent the 90% confidence limits for saline self-administration for the initial and reduced doses individually. The scores for points falling in each quadrant formed by these lines are shown with the saline data. Open circles, score 0; solid triangles, score 1; solid squares, score 2; and solid circles, score 3. Note that injection rates are plotted to a logarithmic scale.

In addition, the 90% confidence ellipse, based upon the bivariate normal distribution, was calculated (Morrison, 1967). Rats whose mean injection rates were within either of these limits scored 0. A score of 1 signified that reinforcing activity was present only at the initial dose. A score of 2 signified that the reinforcing activity was present at both doses, therefore the initial dose was higher on the dose-response curve. A score of 3 signified that the initial dose was so high on the dose-response curve that responding was maintained at a rate not significantly greater than saline but became significantly greater when the dose was reduced. We have shown that self-injection rates of large doses of morphine fall within the saline range for many rats (Weeks & Collins, 1979).

Figure 1 illustrates the scoring system for saline and morphine doses of 0.01, 0.1 and 1 mg/kg on the new protocol. The dashed lines are the 90% confidence limits for saline injections for the initial and reduced doses, and the ellipse is the 90% confidence limit based upon the bivariate distribution. Three of the 30 saline rats fell outside these limits and so received a score, which would be expected at the 90% significance level. At 0.01 mg/kg of morphine, only one of six rats received a score. At 0.1 mg/kg, four of six rats were reinforced, each with a score of 2. The average daily injection rates for three of these four rats was over 250 per day for both doses, but the two non-reinforced rats took less than 30 injections per day. At 1 mg/kg all six rats were reinforced, four of them scoring 3. At the reduced dose all six rats took over 100 injections per day, but those rats scoring 3 took less than 25 injections per day on the initial dose.

Evaluation of Group Mean Injection Rates

If injection rates of most rats tested are only somewhat greater than saline, few if any would receive a score, yet the group mean could still be significantly greater than saline. The significance of this difference was calculated using Hotelling's T^2 statistic, which takes into consideration the bivariate analysis using data from both doses (Morrison, 1967).

Evaluation of Physical Dependence

A withdrawal weight loss significantly greater than that of saline controls was considered evidence of physical dependence. Significance was calculated using a one-tailed t-test.

RESULTS

Thirty-one psychoactive drugs were tested, 21 of them at more than one initial dose. Drugs were selected from several pharmacological classes. To illustrate dose-response relationships and correlation of results from the two protocols, drugs are divided into pharmacological classes (Johanson & Balster, 1978) and their mean scores plotted graphically (see Figure 2). Sixteen active drugs were tested at more than one dose. For some drugs further increases in the dose did not give a greater score, since the maximal effect was being approached. The relation to dose was not clear for methohexital, perhaps because lower doses had not been tested. Higher doses of methohexital might not yield valid results, since even at the doses tested some rats were nearly anesthetized. With those drugs which caused convulsions at toxic doses (e.g., meperidine, cocaine, methamphetamine, and nicotine), deaths from overdosage occurred at the higher doses tested.

The score versus log dose was analyzed as a linear regression for nine studies in which three or more doses of each drug were used. The slopes all had a common value (p = 0.98), and an estimate of the common slope ($\pm$ SD) was 0.98 $\pm$ 0.1 (Collins et al., 1984). In other words, for each ten-fold (log 1) increase in dose the score increased about 1 unit.

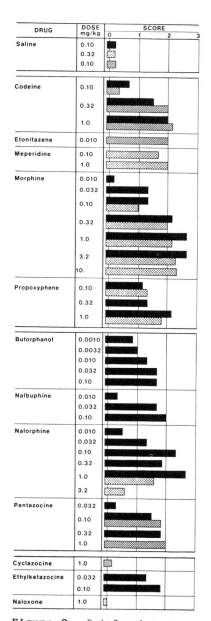
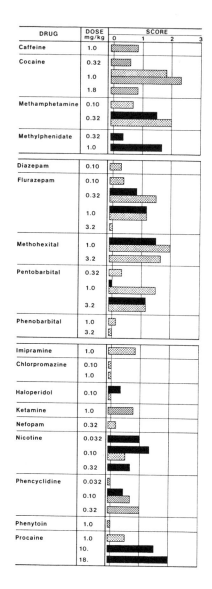

Figure 2: Reinforcing scores. **Column 1:** controls, narcotic agonists, mixed agonist-antagonists, and antagonists. **Column 2:** psychomotor stimulants, CNS depressants, and miscellaneous drugs. Saline doses are ml/kg. Protocol and syringe codes: solid = new, pneumatic; cross hatch = old, motor; diagonal = old, pneumatic. Reproduced with permission from Collins et al., 1984. Copyright 1984 by Springer-Verlag.

For mean scores greater than 1.3, mean injection rates for all rats taken as a group differed from saline (p = 0.01). However, scores are based on performance of individual rats, wherewith the injection rate must be three or more times greater than saline to achieve statistical significance. If several rats had injection rates greater than saline but not significantly different as individuals, the compound still could have reinforcing activity. Grouped data may resolve this uncertainty. In Figure 1 the probability for the mean injection rates differing from saline was 0.5 for morphine at 0.01 mg/kg. The score of 0.2 was probably due only to chance. However, for nalorphine (3.2 mg/kg, old protocol, motor syringe) the mean score was only 0.6, but the group data had differed significantly from saline (p = 0.003). Likewise, for ketamine (1 mg/kg, old protocol, pneumatic syringe) the mean score was 0.6, but the group data had been significantly different from saline (p = 0.001).

Results of a screening test must give consistent results when repeated. Generally two to three years elapsed between tests on old and new protocols. The two protocols differed only in minor details and the scores were calculated in the same manner. Analysis of the old and new protocol scores for the same drugs and doses as a linear regression yielded a correlation coefficient of 0.7, and neither the slope nor intercept differed significantly from unity (p > 0.05). The test method clearly yielded consistent, reproducible results.

Experimental data have been summarized in tabular form by Collins et al. (1984). For each drug, dose, and protocol, values are given for the mean injection rates, the mean weight changes, the number of rats reinforced out of the total tested, the significance level of the grouped data, and the mean scores. On specific request to R. J. Collins, we can supply the raw data.

DISCUSSION

Johanson and Balster (1978) have summarized world-wide tests for reinforcing activity of psychoactive drugs in monkeys using substitution procedures. Monkeys were trained to self-administer a reinforcing drug, such as cocaine or codeine, usually in 2- to 4-hour sessions. The test drug or vehicle was substituted, and the drug was considered active as a reinforcer when the injection rate for the test drug had been maintained at a rate significantly greater than when vehicle was substituted. When laboratories disagreed, we considered the drug active. In addition to the drugs in this report, ethylketazocine (ethyl cycloketazocine) was reported inactive (Woods, Smith, Medzihradsky, & Swain, 1979) and nicotine, although inactive in the substitution test described above, was active when offered by continuous self-administration (Yanagita, 1977). We considered nicotine as active in the monkey. In our rat studies, a drug was considered active if it met all of the following criteria at any dose: (1) at least half of the rats scored 1 or more, (2) the mean score was 1 or more, and (3) the significance level of the grouped data was 0.05 or less.

Results for monkeys were available for all drugs we tested except diazepam, phenobarbital, nefopam, and phenytoin. Results in the two species agreed for 24 of the 27 drugs compared. The exceptions were nalorphine and ethylketazocine (inactive in monkeys but active in rats) and ethanol (active in monkeys but inactive in rats). Cyclazocine, naloxone, caffeine, imipramine, chlorpromazine, and haloperidol were inactive in both species, and the remaining 16 drugs were active in both species.

Screening for reinforcing activity of psychoactive drugs in rats gives, with few exceptions, results which parallel those obtained with monkeys. The use of rats makes practical the evaluation of new psychoactive drugs for potential abuse early in their development.

REFERENCES

Collins, R. J., Weeks, J. R., Cooper, M. M., Good, P. I., & Russell, R. R. (1984). Prediction of abuse liability of drugs using intravenous self-administration by rats. Psychopharmacology, 82, 6-13.

Griffiths, R. R., & Balster, R. L. (1979). Opioids: Similarity between evaluation of subjective effects and animal self-administration results. Clinical Pharmacology and Therapeutics, 25, 611-617.

Griffiths, R. R., Bigelow, G. E., & Henningfield, J. E. (1980). Similarities in animal and human drug-taking behavior. In N. K. Mello (Ed.), Advances in substance abuse (Vol. 1, pp. 1-90). Greenwich, CT: JAI Press.

Griffiths, R. R., Brady, J. V., & Bradford, L. D. (1979). Predicting the abuse liability of drugs with animal drug self-administration procedures: Psychomotor stimulants and hallucinogens. In T. Thompson & P. B. Dews (Eds.), Advances in behavioral pharmacology (Vol. 2, pp. 163-208). New York: Academic Press.

Johanson, C. W., & Balster, R. L. (1978). A summary of the results of a drug self-administration study using substitution procedures in rhesus monkeys. Bulletin of Narcotics, 20, 43-54.

Morrison, D. F. (1967). Multivariate statistical methods. San Francisco: McGraw-Hill.

van Ree, J. M. (1979). Reinforcing stimulus properties of drugs. Neuropharmacology, 18, 963-969.

Schuster, C. W., & Thompson, T. (1969). Self-administration of and behavioral dependence on drugs. Annual Review of Pharmacology, 9, 483-502.

Thompson, T., & Unna, D. R. (Eds.). (1977). Predicting dependence liability of stimulant and depressant drugs. Baltimore: University Park Press.

Weeks, J. R. (1972). Long-term intravenous infusion. In R. D. Myers (Ed.), Methods in psychobiology (Vol. 2, pp. 155-168). London: Academic Press.

Weeks, J. R. (1977). The pneumatic syringe: A simple apparatus for self-administration of drugs by rats. Pharmacology Biochemistry & Behavior, 7, 559-562.

Weeks, J. R. (1979). A method for administration of prolonged intravenous infusion of prostacyclin (PGI_2) to unanesthetized rats. Prostaglandins, 17, 495-499.

Weeks, J. R. (1981). An improved pneumatic syringe for self-administration of drugs by rats. Pharmacology Biochemistry & Behavior, 14, 573-574.

Weeks, J. R., & Collins, R. J. (1976). Changes in morphine self-administration induced by prostaglandin E$_1$ and naloxone. Prostaglandins, 12, 11-19.

Weeks, J. R., & Collins, R. J. (1979). Dose and physical dependence as factors in the self-administration of morphine by rats. Psychopharmacology, 65, 171-177.

Woods, J. H., Smith, C. B., Medzihradsky, F., & Swain, H. H. (1979). Preclinical testing of new analgesic drugs. In R. E. Beers & E. G. Bassett (Eds.), Mechanisms of pain and analgesic compounds, (pp. 429-445). New York: Raven Press.

Yanagita, T. (1977). Brief review on the use of self-administration techniques for predicting drug dependence potential. In T. Thompson & K. R. Unna (Eds.), Predicting dependence liability of stimulant and depressant drugs, (pp. 231-242). Baltimore: University Park Press.

ADDENDUM

The screening test described above is based upon the activity of the drug, i.e., the dose required to reinforce self-administration. The strength of such a reinforcement is another factor in abuse liability. The latter has been evaluated in monkeys using progressive-ratio programs. Since this chapter was submitted, we have completed preliminary studies evaluating the rat in a progressive-ratio program. Groups of naive rats were offered morphine under a continuous reinforcement schedule for 5 days, then on a fixed-ratio schedule increased daily to the break point (less than 4 injections in one day). Results were expressed as the mean of the daily steps to the breaking point. A progressively decreasing geometric progression was used, the initial increment being log 0.20 (1.58 fold), decreasing 4.5 percent each step. This decreasing increment prevented excessively large (arithmetic) increases in the work requirement, which might compromise discrimination between different strength reinforcements at higher ratios. Thus, in this series, steps 13 and 20 are FR-100 and FR-473, respectively, but without the decreasing increment they would have been FR-398 and FR-10,000.

Results for morphine are summarized in the table. The mean breaking points are linearly related to the log dose (b = 4.4, r = 0.69). However, the protocol used may not be the most suitable. It is time-consuming, and at the lower fixed ratios some rats may consume toxic quantities of drug. J. E. Moreton (personal communication) has suggested that instead of a daily increase in fixed ratios, the ratio be increased after a set number of reinforcements. Likewise, the 5-day continuous reinforcement training period could be amended to allow starting the progressive-ratio program when the daily injection rate exceeded a specified number of injections. These preliminary studies suggest that the rat is a suitable species for progressive-ratio studies on reinforcing drugs.

Table 1

The Relative Strength of Reinforcement of Different Doses of
Morphine Sulfate Using the Progressive-Ratio Method

Dose mg/kg	Number of Rats	Steps to Breaking Point Mean ± S.E.	Approximate FR (by interpolation)
0.032	10	8.0 ± 1.32	23
0.10	10	11.1 ± 1.53	60
0.32	10	12.7 ± 1.07	92
1.0	10	15.0 ± 0.39	165
3.2	10	17.1 ± 0.82	265

CHAPTER 3

ASSESSING DRUGS FOR ABUSE LIABILITY
AND DEPENDENCE POTENTIAL IN LABORATORY PRIMATES

J. V. Brady, R. R. Griffiths, R. D. Hienz, N. A. Ator,
S. E. Lukas, and R. J. Lamb

Department of Psychiatry and Behavioral Sciences
The Johns Hopkins University School of Medicine
720 Rutland Avenue
Baltimore, Maryland 21205

ABSTRACT

Distinctions between abuse liability and dependence potential are developed within the context of an assessment approach focusing upon the reinforcing, discriminative, and eliciting properties of drugs as the basis for an effective technology to evaluate a broad range of pharmacological agents. Procedures and outcomes from extensive studies with primates assessing drug self-administration, drug discrimination, physiological dependence, and behavioral toxicity are described and discussed.

INTRODUCTION

The practices associated with preclinical assessment of abused drugs have generally relied upon a characterization of their physicochemical structure and physiological activity in relationship to known standards of pharmacological equivalence (Martin, 1977). The increasingly prominent role of behavioral methodologies has extended the range of such evaluations and provided a more comprehensive basis for analysis of a drug's functional properties. The resulting advances in knowledge about drug actions, and particularly in research technology, have made possible an operational approach to pharmacological assessment of abused drugs and have called attention to the need for reappraisal of traditional concepts and definitions in the field. The distinction between physical and psychic or psychological dependence, for example, has long since outlived its usefulness, and even the dichotomy between physical and behavioral factors has not provided a completely satisfactory framework for analyzing the essential dimensions of drug-related problems. And while the terms dependence and abuse are generally considered preferable to addiction as a basis for operational analysis, terminological ambiguities persist.

The word dependence, for example, continues to be widely used in at least two quite different ways. In the scientific and technical literature, the term dependence or, more precisely, physical dependence is used with specific reference to the chemical and biological effects which follow repeated exposure to a drug resulting in tolerance and an abstinence syndrome when the drug is withdrawn (e.g., Clouet & Iwatsubo, 1975; Cochin, 1970; Eddy, 1973; Kalant, LeBlanc, & Gibbins, 1971). Less technically, however, dependence or, more commonly, drug dependence is often used synonymously with the term abuse to refer to a range of complex phenomena frequently characterized as "loss of voluntary control over drug-taking," "compulsive drug use," and "reduced range of behavioral options." In contemporary research literature, however, the term abuse is used more operationally to refer to the behavioral changes (e.g., drug-seeking and drug discriminating) which precede or accompany self-administration of a pharmacologic agent (e.g., Brady, 1981; Brady & Griffiths, 1977; Griffiths, Bigelow, & Henningfield, 1980; Woods, Young, & Herling, 1982). In a broader context, drug abuse references generally incorporate the adverse physiological, behavioral, and/or social effects of such drug self-administration as well (Schuster & Fischman, 1975).

The relevance and importance of maintaining an operational distinction between the terms dependence (i.e., physical dependence or, perhaps more appropriately, physiological dependence) and abuse reside in the fact that, from the perspective of drug evaluation, their defining properties are not coextensive, they do not invariably occur together, and the methods for their assessment differ. Determinations of dependence potential, based primarily upon measures of tolerance and withdrawal, do not necessarily predict a drug's abuse liability as measured by the generation and maintenance of drug-seeking and drug-taking behaviors. There are compounds (e.g., propranolol) which produce tolerance and an abstinence syndrome after drug withdrawal but which do not give rise to drug-seeking or drug self-administration (Ambrus, Ambrus, & Harrison, 1951; Crandall, Leake, Loevenhart, & Muehlberger, 1931; Jaffe, 1980; Myers & Austin, 1929; Rector, Seldin, & Copenhaver, 1955). On the other hand, drug-seeking and drug self-injection performances can be maintained in strength by use patterns and doses of drugs (e.g., cocaine) which produce no significant degree of tolerance or withdrawal (Johanson, Balster, & Bonese, 1976; Jones & Prada, 1977; Schuster & Woods, 1967).

Interactions between physiological dependence and drug abuse are, of course, commonplace. Changes in drug-seeking and drug-taking often occur as sequelae to both the acute effects of a pharmacological agent and to the tolerance and withdrawal effects which follow more chronic drug exposure (Musto, 1973). Conversely, the chemical and biological changes which define physical dependence can as well be sequelae to the self-administration of abused drugs (Jaffe, 1980). But the relative contributions of these distinguishable processes to drug-related problems can vary widely with different pharmacologic agents as a function of dose, environmental circumstances, and previous drug history (Mendelson & Mello, 1982). Moreover, the methods used to assess a pharmacologic agent's dependence potential and abuse liability, both in laboratory animals and humans, are quite distinct.

The temporal ordering of physiological and behavioral changes in relationship to the drug intake event provides an operational basis for characterizing the range of a pharmacologic agent's functional properties and for differentiating its dependence potential and abuse liability as well. A convenient and useful framework for such drug evaluation focuses upon the changes or events antecedent to repeated drug-taking, on the one hand, and those consequent to it, on the other. Operationally, measures of the reactive biochemical, physiological, and behavioral changes which follow as consequences of repeated drug intake provide an effective means of assessing dependence potential, while measures of the proactive drug-seeking and drug-discriminating behaviors which occur as antecedents to habitual drug use can reliably index a pharmacologic agent's abuse liability. Significantly, the conceptual and methodological bases for developing laboratory procedures for pharmacological assessment within the framework of this operational approach derive from the data base provided by systematic analysis of the stimulus properties of drugs.

- 46 -

Over the past two decades, an extensive research literature focusing on the reinforcing, discriminative, and eliciting stimulus properties of drugs has provided an effective technology for evaluating the abuse liability and dependence potential of a broad range of pharmacological agents. Most notably, experimental procedures for the generation and maintenance of drug self-administration performances based upon the reinforcing properties of chemical substances have now become the mainstays of abuse liability assessment in both animals and human research volunteers. More recently, techniques for differentiating between drugs based upon their discriminative properties have added an important dimension to abuse liability evaluation by expanding the scope of drug discrimination methodologies for the operational measurement of self-report (i.e., "subjective") effects in laboratory animals as well as in humans. And, finally, procedures based upon the eliciting properties of drugs continue to provide for the assessment of a pharmacological agent's dependence potential as measured by the biochemical, physiological, and behavioral sequelae, both acute and chronic, to drug exposure. Indeed, the relevance and importance of a drug's eliciting properties have also been emphasized by the increasingly prominent role of behavioral toxicity assessment procedures in the comprehensive pharmacological evaluation of both dependence potential and abuse liability.

ASSESSING THE REINFORCING PROPERTIES OF DRUGS

Research over the past decade has demonstrated that there is a good correspondence between the range of chemical compounds self-injected by laboratory animals and those abused by humans (Brady & Griffiths, 1976a, 1976b, 1977; Brady, Griffiths, & Winger, 1975; Griffiths, Brady, & Snell, 1978a, 1978b; Griffiths, Lukas, Bradford, Brady, & Snell, 1981; Griffiths, Winger, Brady, & Snell, 1976; Griffiths et al., 1980). Moreover, the variables of which such drug administration are a function (e.g., dose, response requirement, schedule of availability, environmental conditions, past history) have been found to exert their influence in a similar fashion independently of the type of substance maintaining the performance or the species of organism involved (Griffiths et al., 1980). This cross-species and cross-substance generality has provided the basis for assessing the reinforcing properties of a range of drugs and the procedures developed with laboratory primates for this purpose have been previously described in detail (Brady & Griffiths, 1976a, 1976b, 1977, Brady, Griffiths, & Hienz, 1983; Brady et al., 1975; Griffiths, Ator, Lukas, & Brady, 1983; Griffiths, Bradford, & Brady, 1979; Griffiths, Brady, & Bradford, 1979; Griffiths et al., 1978a).

Briefly, mature male baboons (Papio anubis) are adapted to a standard harness/tether system (Lukas, Griffiths, Bradford, Brady, Daley, & DeLorenzo, 1982) and are individually housed in sound-attenuated chambers with water and the opportunity to respond for food continuously available. After initial behavioral training on a progressive-ratio paradigm with food reinforcement, each subject is surgically prepared with a chronic silastic catheter in the internal jugular, femoral, or axillary vein. The catheter is passed subcutaneously, exited at the middle of the back, and attached to a valve system which allows for the slow continuous administration of heparinized saline via a peristaltic pump to maintain catheter patency. Drugs are injected into the valve system near the animal by means of a second peristaltic pump and then flushed into the animal with saline from a third pump. This system necessitates a delay of approximately 20 seconds between the onset of drug delivery and actual injection into the vein. All drugs are delivered within a 2-minute period, however, and the volume of drug solution per injection as well as the injection duration remain constant throughout an experiment.

The availability of a drug for self-injection by the animal is indicated by the illumination of a jewel light directly over a standard Lindsley lever mounted on the baboon's work panel which compromises the back wall of the cage housing. The light remains illuminated until completion of a fixed-ratio requirement (e.g., FR-160), on the Lindsley manipulandum, at which time the drug injection begins. A time-out period of 3 hours follows each injection. Thus, a maximum of eight injections is possible each day.

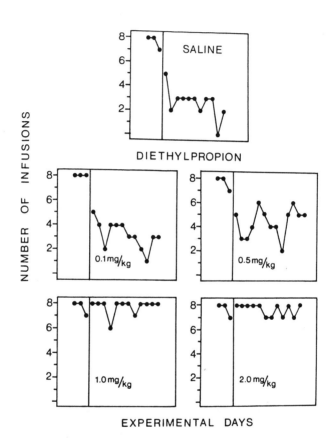

Figure 1: Daily pattern of self-injection maintained by various doses of diethylpropion HCl and saline in the same subject. The initial 3-day period of each determination shows the self-injection performance maintained by cocaine HCl (0.4 mg/kg) prior to substitution of saline or the indicated dose of diethylpropion. Reproduced with permission from Brady and Griffiths, 1983.

A substitution procedure is utilized to determine whether an unknown compound will maintain self-injection behavior. Self-injection performance is first established with cocaine at a dose of 0.32 mg/kg/injection. After 3 consecutive days of cocaine availability, during which six or more injections are taken each day, a specified dose of the test drug or saline is substituted for the cocaine. At least 12 days of access to each dose of drug or saline is permitted. Cocaine is then reinstated, and when the criterion of 3 consecutive days of six or more injections per day has been met, another dose or another drug is substituted. The order of exposure to drugs, saline, and different doses is mixed; all animals are given at least 12 days of access to saline during the examination of different drugs at different doses. This basic approach thus provides a standardized procedure for evaluating the reinforcing properties of drugs.

A progressive-ratio procedure is used to measure a drug's relative reinforcing efficacy by determining the maximum amount of responding (i.e., work) that can be maintained by the compound. Progressive-ratio experiments involve first introducing a drug on a low response requirement (e.g., FR-160) to obtain a high and stable drug self-injection performance. The response requirement is then systematically increased until the rate of drug self-injection falls below a criterion level which defines the breaking point. The sequence of fixed-ratio values typically includes: 160, 320, 640, 1280, 2400, 3600, 4800, 6000, and 7200. After the breaking point is determined, the response requirement on the Lindsley lever is lowered, and the original performance recovers prior to replication of the experiment or substitution of another dose of drug.

Figure 1 presents illustrative data obtained with the substitution procedure in examining a range of doses of the substituted phenylethylamine, diethylpropion, in one baboon. The figure shows that when saline or a low dose (0.1 mg/kg) of diethylpropion was substituted for cocaine, the self-injection performance decreased during the 12-day substitution period until the subject self-administered only two or three injections per day. At a dose of 0.5 mg/kg diethylpropion, self-administration performance was maintained at an average rate of about five injections per day, which was higher than saline but lower than the preceding cocaine control periods. Finally, the figure shows that at the highest doses tested (1.0 and 2.0 mg/kg), the number of injections per day was stable and was comparable to that during the cocaine control period (seven or eight injections per day).

Figure 2 also presents illustrative data from the substitution procedure showing daily patterns of self-injection performance maintained by saline and several doses of phentermine in three baboons. The figure shows that when saline was substituted for cocaine, the number of injections per day progressively decreased. At a dose of 0.5 mg/kg, phentermine self-injection performance was maintained at levels similar to cocaine control levels. At a dose of 1.0 mg/kg, self-injection performance was also maintained in all three animals; however, drug intake was characterized by a cyclic pattern in which a number of consecutive days of self-injection at a high rate (six or more injections per day) was followed by several consecutive days at a lower rate and then by a return to the higher rate. Previous experiments (Griffiths et al., 1976; Pickens & Thompson, 1971) have documented a virtually identical cyclic pattern of self-injection performance with d-amphetamine.

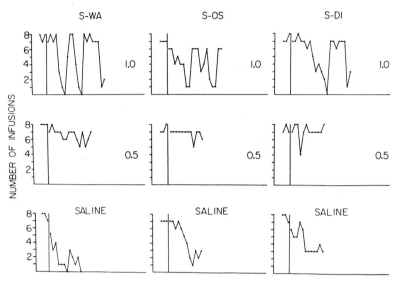

Figure 2: Daily pattern of self-injection maintained by saline or phentermine in three baboons. Ordinates: number of injections. Abscissae: experimental days. Intravenous injections were delivered upon completion of 160 lever presses; a 3-hour time-out followed each injection, permitting a maximum of eight injections per day. The initial 3-day period of each determination shows the number of injections maintained by cocaine prior to substitution of saline or the indicated dose (mg/kg/injection) of phentermine. Reproduced with permission from Griffiths, Brady, and Bradford, 1979. Copyright 1979 by Academic Press.

Figure 3 presents the chemical structures, and Figure 4 the mean levels of self-injection for the 14 phenylethylamines evaluated. As shown in Figure 4, of all the drugs examined d-amphetamine was the most potent, maintaining levels of self-administration above saline at doses of 0.05 and 1.0 mg/kg. Phentermine, diethylpropion, phenmetrazine, phendimetrazine, benzphetamine, and MDA all maintained levels of self-administration above saline at doses of 0.5 and 1.0 mg/kg. l-Ephedrine, clortermine, and chlorphentermine were the least potent of the drugs which maintained performance, supporting self-injection rates above saline control levels at doses of 3.0 and 10.0 mg/kg (l-ephedrine), 3.0 and 5.0 mg/kg (clortermine), and 2.5 and 5.0 mg/kg (chlorphentermine). In contrast to most of the other phenylethylamines that maintained self-administration behavior, the pattern of self-administration with l-ephedrine was particularly unstable and was characterized by either an erratic or cyclic pattern over days. Finally, fenfluramine, PMA, DOM, and DOET were not self-administered at a rate higher than saline at any of the doses studied (means of the determinations at each dose did not exceed the range of saline values).

Figure 3: Chemical structures of the 14 phenylethylamines tested to determine whether they maintained drug self-administration. Reproduced with permission from Griffiths, Brady, and Bradford, 1979. Copyright 1979 by Academic Press.

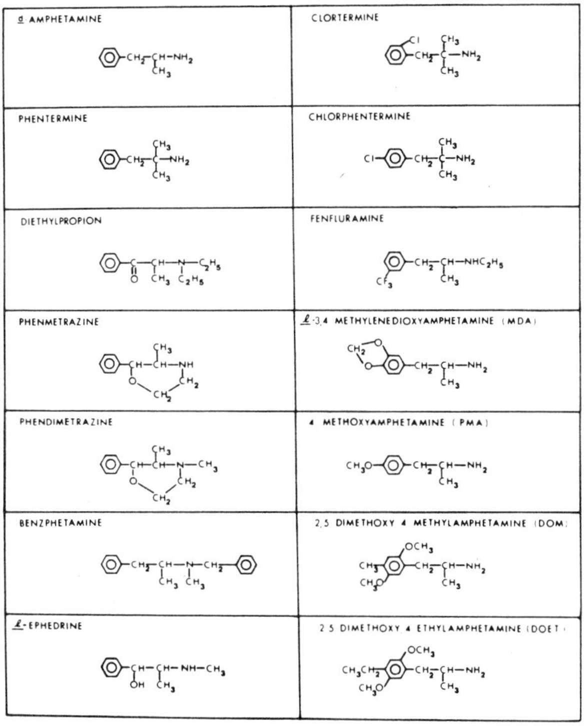

A comparison of Figures 3 and 4 provides some information about structure-activity relationships of phenylethylamines. Other laboratory studies (Tessel, Woods, Counsell, & Basmadjian, 1975a; Tessel, Woods, Counsell, & Lu, 1975b) have demonstrated that the ability of a series of N-ethylamphetamines substituted at the meta position of the phenyl ring either to increase locomotor activity in mice or to increase isolated guinea-pig atrial rate is inversely related to the size of the meta-substituted groups. In a subsequent study (Tessel & Woods, 1975), it was demonstrated that N-ethylamphetamine maintained self-injection performance in rhesus monkeys, whereas fenfluramine (meta-trifluoromethyl-N-ethylamphetamine) failed to maintain self-injection performance. These results indicate that the failure of fenfluramine to maintain self-injection behavior is attributable to its meta-trifluoromethyl group. The results obtained with the present series of phenylethylamines extend these findings and suggest that ring substitutions in general may decrease the potency of the phenylethylamines in maintaining self-injection behavior. The seven compounds shown in the right columns of Figures 3 and 4 had substitutions on the phenyl ring; generally, these compounds were less potent (on a mg/kg basis) in maintaining self-injection than the compounds in the left columns of Figures 3 and 4, which did not have ring substitutions.

Figures 5, 6, 7, 8, and 9 present additional results from assessing the reinforcing properties of a range of other centrally active drugs using the substitution procedure described above.

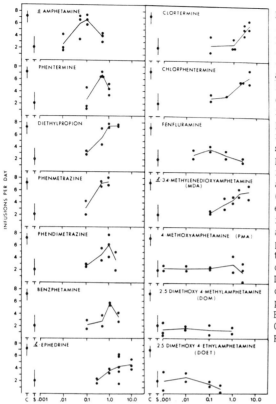

Figure 4: Average number of injections per day with 14 phenylethylamines. Intravenous injections were delivered upon completion of 160 lever presses: a 3-hour time-out followed each injection permitting a maximum of eight injections per day. C indicates mean of all the 3-day periods with cocaine which immediately preceded every substitution of a phenylethylamine or saline. S indicates mean of Days 8 to 12 after substitution of saline (two saline substitutions in each of 15 animals). Brackets indicate ranges of individual animal's means. Drug data points indicate mean of Days 8 to 12 after substitution of a drug for individual animals. Lines connect means at indicated doses of drug. Reproduced with permission from Griffiths, Brady, and Bradford, 1979. Copyright 1979 by Academic Press.

The reinforcing efficacy of a selected series of CNS stimulants was systematically exhausted using the progressive-ratio procedure described above. Figure 10 shows the results of the progressive-ratio breaking point determinations over a range of doses of fenfluramine, chlorphentermine, diethylpropion, and cocaine. Doses of fenfluramine (0.02, 0.1, 0.5 and 2.5 mg/kg) did not maintain criterion-level self-injection performance in the two baboons tested and therefore were assigned breaking point scores of zero. As shown in Figure 10, chlorphentermine maintained self-injection performance at some of the intermediate doses tested (1.0, 3.0, 5.6 mg/kg) in three baboons. In all three animals, lower and higher doses failed to maintain criterion-level self-injection performance. In the fourth baboon tested (SA), chlorphentermine did not maintain self-injection performance at the doses tested (1.0, 3.0, 5.6 mg/kg). As shown in Figure 10, 0.1 mg/kg diethylpropion did not maintain self-injection performance, while at doses ranging from 1.0 to 10.0 mg/kg, the drug maintained self-administration in all five baboons tested. Therefore, the dose-breaking point function obtained for diethylpropion was an inverted U-shaped curve with a peak at 1.0 or 3.0 mg/kg. Finally, Figure 10 shows that the 0.01 mg/kg cocaine dose did not maintain performance; the 0.03 mg/kg dose maintained performance in three of the four baboons tested; and doses of 0.1, 0.4, and 1.0 mg/kg maintained self-injection behavior in all five baboons. Examination of the figure reveals that, for the four baboons that were exposed to a number of intermediate doses of cocaine, the breaking point values generally increased as doses increased up to 0.1 or 0.4 mg/kg.

Figure 5: Average number of injections per day as a function of dose of cocaine, caffeine, and nicotine. Details of the experiments are presented in the legend for Figure 4. Reproduced with permission from Griffiths, Brady, and Bradford, 1979. Copyright 1979 by Academic Press.

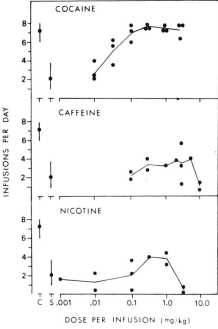

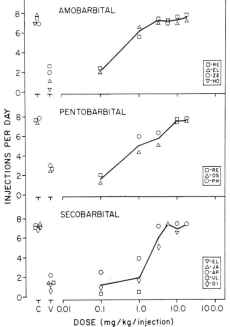

Figure 6: Average number of injections per day as a function of dose of three barbiturates. Details of the experiments are presented in the legend of Figure 4. Reproduced with permission from Griffiths, Lukas, Bradford, Brady, and Snell, 1981. Copyright 1981 by Springer-Verlag.

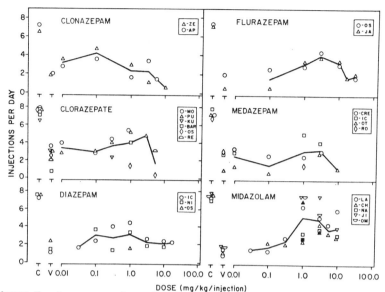

Figure 7: Average number of injections per day as a function of dose of six benzodiazepines. Details of the experiment are presented in the legend of Figure 4. Reproduced with permission from Griffiths, Lukas, Bradford, Brady, and Snell, 1981. Copyright 1981 by Springer-Verlag.

Comparisons of the maximum breaking points maintained by the different drugs indicate that for a given baboon cocaine generally maintained the highest breaking points, followed in order by diethylpropion, chlorphentermine, and fenfluramine. More specifically, data presented in Figure 10 show that some doses of cocaine maintained higher average breaking points in a given baboon than all the doses of diethylpropion, chlorphentermine and fenfluramine tested. Similar within animal comparisons reveal that some doses of diethylpropion maintained higher breaking points than all doses of chlorphentermine and fenfluramine and, finally, that some doses of chlorphentermine maintained higher breaking points than all doses of fenfluramine.

Although the progressive-ratio procedure provides a useful measure of the relative reinforcing efficacy of drugs, the procedure is quite time consuming. An alternative procedure was therefore examined to determine whether it might provide a more efficient alternative to the progressive-ratio procedure. Specifically, the alternative procedure involved measuring stable response rates on a drug-maintained fixed-ratio schedule. A study was undertaken to determine whether fixed-ratio schedules and progressive-ratio schedules would provide similar information about the relative reinforcing efficacy of different cocaine doses. The progressive-ratio procedure was identical to that previously described. On the fixed-ratio schedule, 160 responses were required for each injection. Each injection was followed by a time-out of either 3 or 12 hours. Each dose of cocaine was available for at least 15 days and until response rates showed no trends. Figure 11 shows that with the 3-hour time-out, the dose-breaking point function on the progressive ratio schedule (left-hand column) was similar to the dose-response rate function on the fixed-ratio

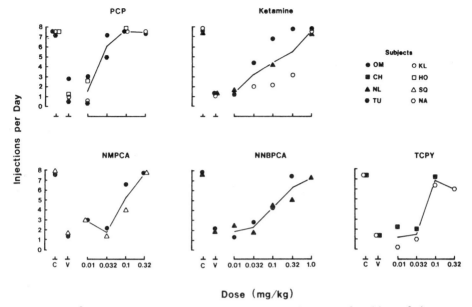

Figure 8: Average number of injections per day as a function of dose of five phencyclidine-analogue compounds. Details of the experiment are described in the legend of Figure 4. Reproduced with permission from Lukas, Griffiths, Brady, and Wurster, 1984. Copyright 1984 by Springer-Verlag.

schedule (center column). As shown, these dose-effect functions were inverted U-shaped curves characterized by a graded ascending limb (0.01 to 0.32 mg/kg) and by a downturn at the highest dose (3.0 to 4.0 mg/kg). On the fixed-ratio schedule, the downturn in the dose response rate function was probably attributable to a cumulative drug effect, as revealed by manipulation of the time-out duration (i.e., 3 or 12 hours), by analysis of sequential interresponse time distribution, and by cumulative response records. Overall, the study showed that these fixed-ratio and progressive-ratio schedules provide similar information about the relative reinforcing efficacy of different cocaine doses and that both schedules may be useful in the assessment of drug reinforcing efficacy.

Utilizing information collected during the initial screening of drugs, it has been possible to develop another potentially valuable dimension for ranking the abuse liability of anorectic drugs. The rationale for this analysis is similar to that for the Therapeutic Index, which provides a measure of the toxicity of a drug in terms of a ratio expressing the relationship between the therapeutic or effective dose and a dose which produces a given toxic effect. In the present case, the anorectic-reinforcement ratio (Griffiths et al., 1978b) provides a means of rank ordering drugs in terms of a ratio between two doses--a dose which produces a specified anorectic effect ("therapeutic" effect) and a dose which produces a specified reinforcing effect ("toxic" effect). Clearly, the most desirable anorectic drug would have potent anorectic properties but minimal reinforcing properties. An undesirable

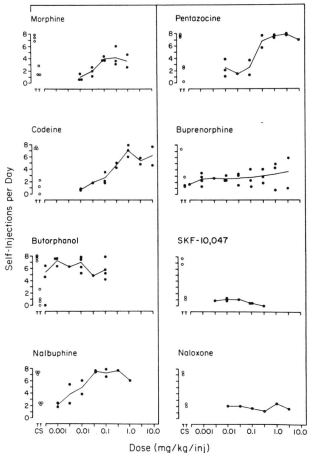

Figure 9: Average number of injections per day as a function of dose of eight opioid agonist and antagonist compounds. Details of the experiment are presented in the legend of Figure 4.

anorectic drug would be a weak anorectic but a powerful reinforcer. Undoubtedly, existing anorectic drugs fall on a continuum between these extremes; a quantitative measure of this continuum is provided by the anorectic-reinforcement ratio. A number of substituted phenylethylamines and cocaine have been evaluated using this measure.

The analysis of the reinforcing properties of a drug requires examination of a substantial range of doses. The lowest reinforcing dose maintaining self-injection performance at FR-160 provided the denominator of the anorectic-reinforcement ratio (Table 1, Column B). Concurrent assessments were made of the anorectic effects of these compounds, and the dose which suppressed food intake to 50% of saline control levels was calculated individually for all compounds. These calculated values are shown in Table 1, Column C and provided the numerator for the anorectic-reinforcement ratio.

Table 1, Column D and the filled bars of Figure 12 show the resulting anorectic-reinforcement ratios (based upon adjustment to an arbitrarily assigned d-amphetamine value of 1.0) derived from the relationship between food suppression dose (i.e., Column C, numerator) and criterion·reinforcing dose

Figure 10: Breaking point values for doses of fenfluramine, chlorphentermine, diethylpropion, and cocaine in five baboons. Ordinates: breaking points. Abscissae: dose (mg/kg/injection). Each point represents a single breaking point observation. Lines connect the means of the breaking point observations at different doses of drug. Filled circles indicate data obtained during the first exposure to a drug dose. Unfilled circles indicate data obtained during a second exposure to a drug dose. Reproduced with permission from Griffiths, Brady, and Snell, 1978a. Copyright 1978 by Springer-Verlag.

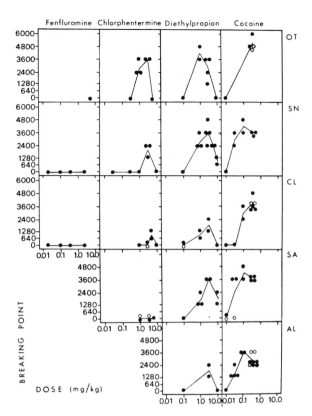

(i.e., Column B, denominator) for each of the drugs studies. The ratio values range from a low of zero for fenfluramine and phenylpropanolamine to a high of 14.81 for cocaine and reflect the fact that compounds with high ratio values are more potent reinforcers (relative to their anorectic potency) than compounds with lower ratio values. To provide more information about anorectic potency of the drugs, an alternative set of values was derived by utilizing the lowest recommended daily human anorectic doses. These doses appear in Column E of Table 1 and provide the numerator for computing a comparative set of ratio values (Column F). Since cocaine is not used clinically as an anorectic, no entry appears in Column E. Comparisons of the values in Columns D and F (also the striped bars vs. the filled bars of Figure 10) show the correspondence between the ratios based upon these two independent measures of anorectic potency.

ASSESSING THE DISCRIMINATIVE STIMULUS PROPERTIES OF DRUGS

There is now abundant evidence that both laboratory animals and humans can be trained to respond differentially in the presence of different stimulus conditions, whether the stimuli are presented exteroceptively (e.g., vision, audition) or interoceptively as in the case of drugs (Colpaert & Rosecrans, 1978). In the typical drug discrimination experiment, for example, differential reinforcement procedures are used to strengthen one response

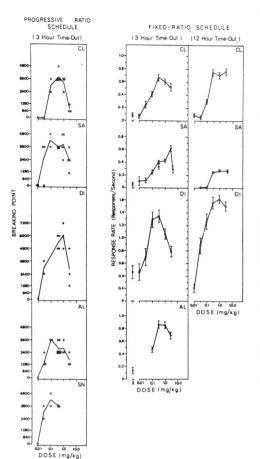

PROGRESSIVE RATIO
SCHEDULE
(3 Hour Time-Out)

FIXED-RATIO SCHEDULE
(3 Hour Time-Out) (12 Hour Time-Out)

BREAKING POINT

RESPONSE RATE (Responses/Second)

DOSE (mg/kg)

DOSE (mg/kg)

DOSE (mg/kg)

Figure 11: LEFT-HAND COLUMN: Breaking point values for doses of cocaine in five baboons; Y-Axis = cocaine dose (mg/kg/injection), log scale. Each point represents a single breaking point observation. Lines connect at means at different doses of drug. **RIGHT-HAND COLUMN:** Response rates maintained by saline and various cocaine doses in four baboons on an FR-160 schedule with either a 3-hour or 12-hour time-out following each injection; Y-Axis = responses per second; X-Axis = cocaine dose (mg/kg/injection), log scale; S = saline. Data points and brackets indicate mean response rate ± SEM for the last 25 injections, except for the data points for SA at 0.32 and 0.1 mg/kg with the 12-hour time-out, which are based on the last 12 injections. Unfilled circles = data obtained during first exposure to a drug dose; filled circles = data obtained during second exposure to a drug dose. Reproduced with permission from Griffiths, Bradford, and Brady, 1979. Copyright 1979 by Springer-Verlag.

(e.g., pressing the left lever) after a certain drug dose is administered and a different response (e.g., pressing the right lever) after saline or the drug vehicle alone is administered. The presence or absence of the training drug comes to set the occasion for making one of two (or more) responses, only one of which will be reinforced (e.g., produce food) in any given training session (see reviews by Colpaert, this volume; Overton, this volume; Schuster & Balster, 1977; Winter, 1978). This procedure permits study not only of the discriminability of individual drugs (Overton, 1982a) but also of the range of drugs that will occasion the same response as the training drug in tests of drug stimulus generalization. Drugs that are pharmacologically similar to the training drug generally occasion responding similar to that under the training drug condition at some doses, while drugs from different classes do not (Colpaert & Rosecrans, 1978; Schuster & Balster, 1977). Such cross-drug test procedures may be operationally analogous to the assessment of self-reported comparisons of drug effects in experienced human drug users (Haertzen & Hickey, this volume; Hill, Haertzen, Wolbach, & Miner, 1963).

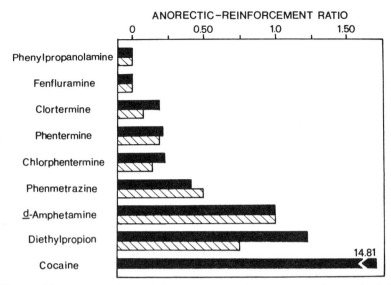

Figure 12: Anorectic-reinforcement ratios for cocaine and eight anorectic drugs. Filled bars show data derived entirely from baboon experiments. Striped bars show data derived from both human clinical information and baboon experiments. Compounds with high ratio values are more potent reinforcers (relative to their anorectic potency) than compounds with lower ratio values. Reproduced with permission from Griffiths, Brady, and Snell, 1978b. Copyright 1978 by the Society of Biological Psychiatry.

Procedures for assessing sedative-hypnotics as discriminative stimuli have been developed for baboons and used as part of an overall assessment of novel psychoactive compounds (Ator & Griffiths, 1983). Some baboons were trained to discriminate the benzodiazepine lorazepam, and others were trained to discriminate the barbiturate pentobarbital in a two-lever drug discrimination procedure. Sessions were 20 minutes long with a 60-minute presession time-out that served as the pretreatment time. Under training conditions food delivery depended on 20 consecutive responses on one lever when the session was preceded by the training drug or on the other lever under no-drug or vehicle conditions. Test sessions were interspersed among training sessions after criterion performance had been maintained for the last 4 of at least 10 sessions of alternation of drug and no-drug conditions. Criterion performance was defined as 96 to 100% of the total session responses on the reinforced lever in the absence of 20 or more consecutive responses on the nonreinforced lever before the first pellet delivery of the session. Test sessions were also 20 minutes long and 20 consecutive responses on either lever produced food. Under test conditions, then, the baboon was always "right." Alternative procedures have been reported in which responding under test conditions was never reinforced (e.g., Barry & Krimmer, 1978) or in which the first completed response sequence determined the lever that would remain the reinforced lever for the entire session (Colpaert, Niemegeers, & Janssen, 1976b).

Table 1

Anorectic-Reinforcement Ratio for Eight Phenylethylamine
Anorectic Drugs and Cocaine

A Drug	B Lowest Reinforcing Dose in Baboon (mg/kg/infusion)	C Dose Suppressing Baboon Food Intake 50% (mg/kg/day)	D Ratio C/B	E Lowest Recommended Human Anorectic Dose (mg/day)	F Ratio E/B
Cocaine	0.03	17.0	15.74	--	--
Diethylpropion	0.5	23.0	1.28	75	0.75
d-Amphetamine	0.05	1.8	1.0	10	1.0
Phenmetrazine	0.5	7.4	0.41	50	0.50
Chlorphentermine	2.5	20.3	0.23	77.9	0.16
Phentermine	0.5	3.7	0.21	18.7	0.19
Clortermine	3.0	21.0	0.19	50	0.08
Fenfluramine	∞	7.0	0	60	0
Phenylpropanolamine	∞	49.1	0	75	0

Calculation of doses is described in text. All doses are expressed
on the basis of the hydrochloride salts except for d-amphetamine
which is expressed as the sulfate. To facilitate comparison, ratios
were adjusted to an arbitrarily assigned d-amphetamine value of 1.0.
Reproduced with permission from Griffiths, Brady, and Snell, 1978b.
Copyright 1978 by the Society of Biological Psychiatry.

When tested with other doses of the training drug, the baboons responded
predominantly on the drug lever following all but the lowest doses tested.
Equivalent cross-drug generalization between the lorazepam- and pentobarbital-
trained baboons did not occur, however. Pentobarbital-trained baboons responded
predominantly on the drug lever after both pentobarbital and lorazepam, but the
lorazepam-trained baboons responded predominantly on the drug lever only after
lorazepam and not after pentobarbital (Ator & Griffiths, 1983). Similar
asymmetries have been found with other training drugs (fentanyl/apomorphine,
Colpaert, Niemegeers, & Janssen, 1976a; nalorphine/cyclazocine, Hirschhorn,
1977; ethanol/diazepam, Jarbe & McMillan, 1983; ethanol/pentobarbital, York,
1978). Further work is needed to establish the determinants and limits of such
asymmetries, but it has been shown that other benzodiazepines (e.g.,
alprazolam, diazepam, triazolam) occasioned drug lever responding in the
lorazepam-trained baboons but, like pentobarbital, phenobarbital did not.
Indeed, there is considerable interest in the possibility of manipulating
training conditions in order to produce greater or lesser specificity in drug
stimulus generalization (Barry & Krimmer, 1978; Overton, 1978; 1982b). To the
extent that greater specificity can be attained as the result of training with
certain drugs, it may be possible to gain a better understanding of those
structural variables that determine the discriminative stimulus properties of
individual compounds.

Figure 13 shows the results of an experiment in which two compounds, CPDD
0001 and CPDD 0002, were studied under "blind" conditions in lorazepam-trained
baboons. The drugs had been received for assessment from the Committee on

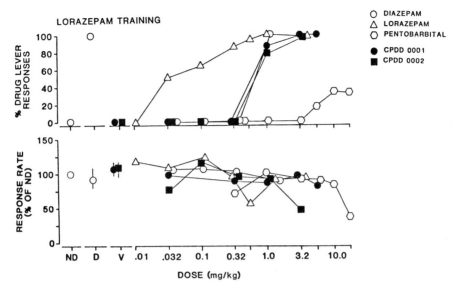

Figure 13: Mean percentage of drug-lever responding (upper panel) and response rate expressed as percentage of mean response rate in no drug training sessions (lower panel) for three baboons trained to discriminate lorazepam (1.0 mg/kg). Connected points represent mean data for test sessions with lorazepam, diazepam, pentobarbital, and two compounds studied under blind conditions (CPDD 0001 and 0002). CPDD 0001 and 0002 were revealed to be the benzodiazepines, diazepam and bromazepam, respectively. Points over ND and D represent responding in the no drug and drug training sessions, respectively, that preceded test sessions; V indicates test sessions conducted with drug vehicle. Vertical bars around D and ND points indicate ranges.

Problems of Drug Dependence without any accompanying information about their chemical structure or pharmacological activity. The results summarized in Figure 13 include drug discrimination data previously obtained with lorazepam, diazepam, and pentobarbital for comparison and show that both CPDD compounds occasioned 100% drug lever responding in all baboons. When the "blind" was broken, the drugs were revealed to be the benzodiazepines diazepam (CPDD 0001) and bromazepam (CPDD 0002). It was of interest that the results with diazepam when studied "blind" were completely consistent with diazepam results obtained earlier under "nonblind" conditions.

That the discriminative stimulus function of drugs may be mediated by specific populations of receptors has been suggested by studies in which discriminative stimulus effects were antagonized by compounds known to be competitive antagonists in a variety of other preparations (e.g., morphine, Shannon & Holtzman, 1976; nicotine, Meltzer, Rosecrans, Aceto, & Harris, 1980). It also has been shown that the discriminative stimulus effects of diazepam and lorazepam, but not pentobarbital, were antagonized by the imidazodiazepine derivative Ro 15-1788 (Ator & Griffiths, 1983; Herling & Shannon, 1982); and diazepam and lorazepam also were antagonized by the pyrazoloquinolone CGS 8216 (Ator & Griffiths, 1985; Shannon & Herling, 1983). The results with CGS 8216

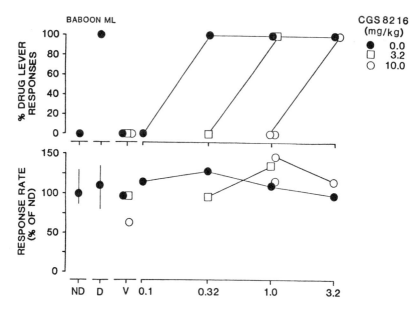

Figure 14: Interactions of CGS 8216 with lorazepam in a baboon trained to discriminate lorazepam 1.0 mg/kg (i.m.) from the no-drug (ND) condition. Drug lever responding (upper panel) is shown as a percentage of total session responding in test sessions after administration of lorazepam alone (filled symbols) and in combination with doses of CGS 8216 (p.o.). Pretreatment time was 60 minutes for both drugs. Overall response rates (lower panel) in those test sessions are presented as percentages of the mean rate in the ND training sessions immediately preceding test sessions. Points at ND and D represent mean responding in the no-drug and drug training sessions, respectively, that immediately preceded test sessions; V indicates administration of the lorazepam vehicle. Vertical bars around ND and D points indicate ranges unless the mean was encompassed by the data point.

and lorazepam in the baboon, illustrated in Figure 14, show that CGS 8216 produced a complete shift to the no-drug lever in a dose-related manner, and this antagonism was surmountable with higher doses of lorazepam.

Systematic study of the time course of the drug discrimination stimulus effects has been approached either by varying the pretreatment time before the test session (e.g., Winger & Herling, 1982) or by reinstating the test procedure at intervals after the initial test session. This latter procedure is illustrated in Figure 15 which presents further data from the study with the benzodiazepine antagonist CGS 8216 in combination with lorazepam (Ator & Griffiths, 1985). Following a test session with the usual pretreatment time of 1 hour, the experimental procedure was reinstated under test conditions at 3, 5, 7, 9, 11, 13, and 15 hours after drug or vehicle administration. Figure 15 shows consistent responding on the no-drug lever across these test sessions

Figure 15: Cumulative records of responding in 10-minute test sessions conducted at 1, 3, 5, 7, 9, 11, 13, and 15 hours after drug or vehicle administration in a baboon trained to discriminate lorazepam (1.0 mg/kg). Lorazepam was administered intramuscularly and CGS 8216 was administered orally. In these test sessions, pellet delivery depended on 20 consecutive responses on either lever. The upper pen in each record stepped upward with each drug-lever response and the lower pen deflected with each response on the no-drug lever; the upper pen deflected with all pellet deliveries, regardless of the lever on which responding occurred. The recorder did not run during the 2-hour intervals between test sessions; the upper pen reset to baseline after either 175 responses or at the end of the test session.

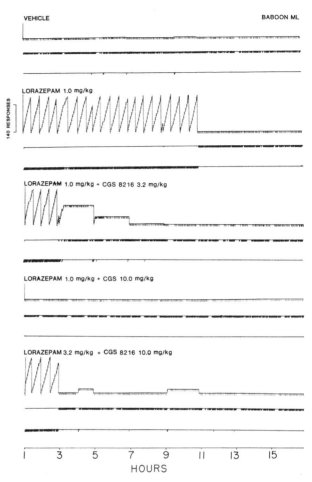

after drug vehicle. After lorazepam (1.0 mg/kg), however, responding shifted from the drug to the no-drug lever by 11 hours post administration. When CGS 8216 (10.0 mg/kg) was administered in combination with this dose of lorazepam, there was complete antagonism of lorazepam (i.e., all responding was on the no-drug lever after the usual pretreatment time of 1 hour and across the entire 15-hour period). With a higher dose of lorazepam (3.2 mg/kg), however, the CGS 8216 antagonism was surmountable (i.e., all responding occurred on the drug lever at the 1-hour test time); but the time course procedure revealed a late onset of CGS 8216 antagonism at this dose combination (i.e., responding shifted from the lorazepam lever to the no-drug lever during subsequent test sessions). Because such a shift never occurred by 3 hours after administration of this dose of lorazepam alone, the results of the time course procedure suggest an increasing effect of CGS 8216 across time.

The results of the time course procedure shown in Figure 15 also serve to illustrate that, contrary to the oft-stated hypothesis that once pellet delivery occurs it precludes switching levers (i.e., the "win-stay, lose shift" strategy, Barry & Krimmer, 1978; Colpaert et al., 1976b; Goudie, 1977), baboons trained and tested under the conditions described do exhibit responding on both levers under some test conditions. This has been shown at lower and intermediate doses of drugs as well as with time-course procedures for a number of drugs (Ator & Griffiths, 1983; unpublished observations). For example, in the study with Ro 15-1788 (Ator & Griffiths, 1983), it was found that over time the effects of the antagonist apparently decreased and drug lever responding emerged. The time course of this effect of Ro 15-1788 and of lorazepam was consistent with other data for the time course of these compounds in humans (Darragh, Lambe, Kenny, Brick, Taaffe, & O'Boyle, 1982; Greenblatt, Shader, Divoll, & Harmatz, 1981) and emphasizes the impressive degree to which a drug can exert discriminative control of behavior.

ASSESSING THE ELICITING PROPERTIES OF DRUGS

In addition to evaluating a pharmacologic agent's reinforcing and discriminative stimulus properties, the assessment of abuse liability and dependence potential requires analysis of the physiological and behavioral changes, both acute and chronic, which are elicited following drug administration. Substances with only minimal, if any, disruptive physiological/behavioral effects are not generally regarded as having significant dependence potential or abuse liability even though their use may be widespread (e.g., caffeine in tea or coffee). In contrast, compounds self-administered even sparingly which are associated with disruptive physiological/behavioral changes are considered to have high abuse liability (e.g., lysergic acid diethylamide: LSD). Drugs may fall anywhere on the continua defined by these assessment parameters, and a comparative evaluation of drug dependence potential and/or abuse liability is greatly enhanced by an interactive analysis of reinforcing, discriminative, and eliciting functions.

Physiological Dependence

The methods used for assessment of physiological dependence of the opioid-type have been extensively described, and their effectiveness as predictors of physiological dependence potential has been well documented (e.g., Deneau, 1956; Seevers, 1936; Seevers & Deneau, 1963; Villarreal, 1973). Substitution tests are often conducted first to assess the suppression of withdrawal signs in opiate-dependent animals denied their usual dose of morphine. If such procedures indicate only equivocal dependence potential, primary (or direct) dependence and precipitated withdrawal tests are conducted in which animals are treated chronically with drug and observed for withdrawal signs after drug administration is stopped or after administration of an opioid-antagonist (e.g., naloxone).

Physiological dependence on sedative-hypnotics, anxiolytics, and alcohols is potentially more dangerous than dependence on opioids, because sedative withdrawal can be life threatening. Withdrawal signs from sedatives, in particular from the benzodiazepines, can occur in patients taking therapeutic doses for prolonged periods of time when drug treatment is suddenly stopped (Petursson & Lader, 1981; Pevnick, Jasinski, & Haertzen, 1978; Rifkin, Quitkin, & Klein, 1976; Tyrer, Rutherford, & Hugget, 1981; Winokur, Rickels, Greenblatt, Snyder, & Schatz, 1980). In contrast to the opioids, however, sedatives have received relatively less systematic study from the perspective of dependence potential. Phenobarbital, pentobarbital, barbital, alcohol, chloroform, meprobamate, diazepam, chlordiazepoxide, oxazolam, and lorazepam have been shown to suppress barbital withdrawal signs and/or to produce direct physiological dependence in rhesus monkeys (Yanagita & Miyasato, 1976; Yanagita & Takahashi, 1970, 1973; Yanagita, Takahashi, & Oinuma, 1975). In contrast, benzoctamine, perlapine, and methaqualone have been reported by these same investigators neither to suppress barbital withdrawal nor to produce direct physiological dependence, and the results of these laboratory animal studies (with the possible exception of the methaqualone findings) are in general agreement with what is known about the dependence potential of these compounds in man.

The physiological dependence-producing properties of benzodiazepines and benzodiazepine-like compounds have been studied using baboons (Papio anubis) implanted with intragastric catheters, protected by a harness-tether system that allows the animal virtually unrestricted movement (Lukas et al., 1982). The baboons are housed in modified primate cages and have ad libitum access to food and water. Two methods are currently employed to evaluate the dependence potential of benzodiazepines and benzodiazepine-like compounds. The first, precipitated-withdrawal, involves administration of the test compound via a continual intragastric injection using a peristaltic pump. After daily administration (e.g., 7 to 10 days), the benzodiazepine antagonist Ro 15-1788 (5 mg/kg) is administered. The baboons are then evaluated for the presence of precipitated-withdrawal signs for 1 to 2 hours after the administration of the antagonist. The second method, a direct dependence test, involves continued daily administration of the test compound for a period of weeks (e.g., 35 to 40 days) followed by abrupt termination of drug administration and observation for withdrawal signs.

When diazepam (20 mg/kg/day) was administered for 7 days followed by Ro 15-1788, withdrawal signs were observed (Lukas & Griffiths, 1982). These signs included bruxism, retching, vomiting, abnormal posturing, and occasional limb tremor. After 35 days of diazepam administration, the antagonist-precipitated signs were more intense and additional withdrawal signs were observed including lip-licking, nose-rubbing, head and body tremors, preconvulsive posturing, and, on one occasion, convulsions. Table 2 summarizes the results obtained when diazepam administration was stopped after 45 days and the baboons were observed for spontaneously occurring withdrawal signs. The indicated signs first appeared by Day 6 or 7, peaked on Days 9 and 10, and had essentially disappeared by the 15th day after cessation of diazepam administration. Signs of spontaneous withdrawal included nose-rubbing, abnormal postures, limb-tremor, and head and body tremor, but no convulsions were seen. Figure 16 shows that starting 8 days after diazepam administration was discontinued and until the end of the 15-day observation period, food-intake was reduced to 25% of normal.

These observations have been extended in a systematic investigation of intensity of the Ro 15-1788 precipitated-withdrawal syndrome as a function of the diazepam dose and duration of treatment (Lukas & Griffiths, 1983). Baboons were exposed to 20 mg/kg/day diazepam for different lengths of time ranging from 1 hour to 35 days. No precipitated withdrawal signs were seen after 1 hour of diazepam exposure. After 1 day of diazepam exposure, however, a significant number of precipitated withdrawal signs were observed, and these were most intense in baboons which previously had been exposed to benzodiazepines. In general, as the duration of diazepam exposure increased, the number and severity of withdrawal signs increased. In a second series of studies, various doses of diazepam ranging from 0.125 to 20 mg/kg/day were administered for a fixed period of 7 days. At doses of diazepam as low as 0.25 mg/kg/day, Ro 15-1788 administration precipitated withdrawal signs at the end of this 7-day treatment period. As the diazepam dose increased, the number and

Table 2

TIME COURSE OF SPONTANEOUS WITHDRAWAL FROM DIAZEPAM[*]

	1	2	3	4	5	6	7	8	9	10	11	12	13	14	15
NORMAL BODY POSTURE	O ● / ■ □	—	—	—	—	—	—	—	—	—	—	—	—	—	→
LACRIMATION						O									
BRUXISM			O			O	■	■	■				O ●		O
LIP LICKING				O									O		
NOSE RUBBING		O ●		●	O / ■	O	O / ■	O / ■	□ ■ □ ■			O / ■	O ●	O ●	O ●
YAWNS (THREATS)		O					O / □		O / ■ □	O ● / ■ □		O / ■ □	O ● / ■ □	O / ■	O ●
RETCHING															
VOMITING															
HEAD TREMOR					O				O ●						
LIMB TREMOR					O	■	O / ■ □	■ □	O / ■ □	O / ■ □	■ □	O ● / O	O / ■	■	O
BODY TREMOR									O / □	O	□				

CONSECUTIVE DAYS

[*]20 mg/kg/day, i.g. for 45 days

Symbols indicate that the withdrawal sign occurred one or more times in the time block except for yawns for which 4 or more were required. Data shown are for 10 minute observation periods at noon. Body postures are described in Lukas and Griffiths (1982). Individual subjects are indicated by different symbols: PH, O ; AL, ● ; SA, ■ ; and JE, □ .

severity of the precipitated withdrawal signs also increased. These results suggest that even doses of diazepam within the therapeutic range may produce physiological dependence after only brief periods of treatment.

Behavioral Toxicity

Procedures for assessing the behavioral toxicity of a range of abused drugs in terms of their sensory/motor effects have been previously described in detail (Brady, Bradford, & Hienz, 1979; Hienz & Brady, 1981; Hienz, Lukas, & Brady, 1981). The basic methodology focuses on a reaction time (RT) technique that has been used extensively with primates as an index of sensory function (Moody, 1970; Pfingst, Hienz, Kimm, & Miller, 1975a; Pfingst, Hienz, & Miller, 1975b). Briefly, laboratory baboons are required to press and hold down a lever for a variable time, following which a signal is presented (e.g., a white light flash or tone burst). Release of the lever within 1.5 seconds following the onset of the signal is then reinforced with food presentation (190 mg banana pellets). The reaction time is the time elapsed between the onset of the signal and the release of the lever and has been found to be inversely related to stimulus intensity, decreasing as stimulus intensity increases. This relationship between reaction time and stimulus intensity is a naturally occurring one, needs no prior training, and is distinctly advantageous as a measure of sensory function. In addition, the procedure is easily employed with either auditory or visual stimuli, can be used to obtain stimulus detection thresholds, and can be easily modified, when required, to extend research into other areas of possible drug effects (e.g., auditory frequency and intensity discrimination). There is also an already existing large data base on auditory reaction time with a number of primate species, including the baboon.

FOOD INTAKE DURING SPONTANEOUS WITHDRAWAL FROM DIAZEPAM

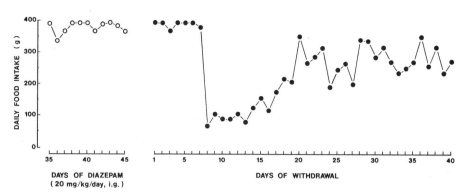

Figure 16: Effects of spontaneous withdrawal from diazepam on food intake. Average daily food intake in grams is shown for the four baboons for which withdrawal effects are summarized in Table 2.

The use of reaction time has allowed for the separation of sensory deficits from extreme motor deficits by requiring that an animal hold a lever down for a considerable period of time prior to stimulus presentation. Thus, for example, an ataxic subject would produce a number of <u>premature lever releases</u> as compared to a normal subject. Further, since variability of reaction times in primates is generally quite small, changes resulting from administration of specific compounds are readily detected. The measurement of the threshold levels for pure tones in primates, however, has been demonstrated not to change greatly when different reaction time criteria are used for estimating detection (Pfingst et al., 1975b). Thus, a compound that produced a motor deficit resulting in longer reaction times would not necessarily cause an increase in sensory threshold estimates unless the deficit was debilitating enough to be detectable by the monitoring of premature releases. Both small and large motor effects of specific compounds can thus be separated from purely sensory effects.

The use of both auditory and visual stimuli in the reaction time procedure has provided for the assessment of drug-related changes in specific sensory systems. If drug-related changes occur in auditory reaction times but not in visual reaction times, for example, the observed effects can be attributed specifically to changes in the auditory system. Further, drug-related changes that produce consistently longer reaction times to near-threshold auditory stimuli, and not to high intensity auditory stimuli, provide a laboratory primate analogue of the clinical phenomenon of loudness recruitment, which typically occurs as a result of a brief exposure to intense sounds (temporary threshold shift; Moody, 1973).

The sequence of events during each reaction time trial was as follows. In the presence of a flashing cue light (5/second), a lever press changed the flashing red light to a steady red light that remained steady as long as the animal held the response lever in the down position. At varying intervals (ranging 1.0 to 7.3 seconds) following initiation of this maintained holding response, a test stimulus (white light on the circular patch or tone burst

- 67 -

through the speaker) was presented for 1.5 seconds. Release of the lever within the 1.5 second test stimulus interval delivered a single banana pellet and initiated a 1 second intertrial interval (ITI) during which no stimuli were presented and lever responses re-initiated the ITI. Incorrect responses (i.e., lever presses prior to test stimulus onset or after the 1.5 second test stimulus interval) were punished with a 2 to 5 second time-out, followed by a return to the ITI without reinforcement. Following the ITI, the flashing red cue light signaled initiation of the next trial in the series of several hundred which comprised each daily 2 to 3 hour experimental session. Asymptotic levels of performance on this procedure typically required 2 to 3 months of such daily training sessions. Auditory and visual testing sessions were conducted separately.

Auditory and visual thresholds were determined by randomly varying the intensity of the test stimuli from trial to trial (method of constant stimuli) and examining detection frequencies (i.e., percent correct lever releases) at each intensity. For the auditory modality (where the baboon detects tones across a range of frequencies extending to 40 kHz), four intensity levels (10 dB apart) of a 16.0 kHz pure tone were used, with the lowest level set just below the animal's estimated threshold. Interspersed among the "test" trials were a series of "catch" trials during which no tone was presented in order to measure the false alarm or "guessing" rate. For the visual modality, four intensity levels (0.5 log density units apart) of the white light were used with the lowest level again set just below the animal's estimated threshold. Again, catch trials with no light were programmed to occur intermittently. In addition, sessions involving visual and auditory threshold determinations were preceded by a 15-minute "warm-up" with the various stimulus intensities to be used in the session.

For both the auditory and visual threshold determinations, each test session was divided into four blocks of 140 trials with each of the four intensity levels plus catch trials presented randomly approximately 28 times during each block. This provided four independent within-session estimates of the sensory thresholds and functions relating reaction time to intensity. Sensory thresholds were determined from percent correct detections at each intensity by interpolating to that intensity producing a detection score halfway between the false alarm rate and 100%. Stable auditory thresholds were based on determinations from three successive test sessions with estimates which varied by no more than 4 dB. Stable visual thresholds were based on determinations from three successive test sessions with estimates which varied by no more than 0.2 log density units. In both cases threshold stability required a false alarm rate below 30% and no systematic changes in the data. Since reaction time distributions are typically skewed due to the physiological limits on lever release time, the measure of central tendency employed for such distributions was the median, with variability reported in terms of the interquartile range. All drugs were administered intramuscularly at the beginning of each experimental session, followed by a 30-minute delay (dark adaptation and warm-up) before formal threshold determinations were begun. Saline control sessions were conducted between drug sessions, and a return to baseline performance was required during these intervening saline control sessions before further drug administrations.

Figure 17 shows the orderly reaction time-lengthening effects of increasing doses of amobarbital sodium (i.e., 3.2, 10.0, 17.0 mg/kg, i.m.) as a function of light intensity in the baboon. The functions relating reaction time to stimulus intensity (latency-intensity functions) were recorded at the peak action time of 1 to 2 hours after drug administration and show the

Figure 17: Median reaction time as a function of visual stimulus intensity after saline and the indicated doses of amobarbital for one animal. Reproduced with permission from Brady, Griffiths, and Hienz, 1983.

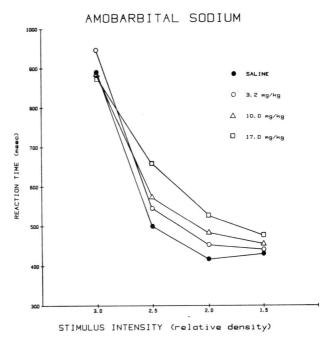

AMOBARBITAL SODIUM

● SALINE

○ 3.2 mg/kg

△ 10.0 mg/kg

□ 17.0 mg/kg

REACTION TIME (msec)

STIMULUS INTENSITY (relative density)

systematic relationship between drug dose and reaction time at all but the lowest (i.e., threshold) intensity. Even at the highest intensities where response variability was minimal, the orderly progression of longer reaction times with increasing doses is apparent.

Figure 18 illustrates the differential dose-dependent effects of pentobarbital upon absolute auditory and visual thresholds, on the one hand, and the similar effects upon auditory and visual reaction times, on the other hand, for three animals. All data points are the average of at least two determinations with each animal at each dose, and represent the difference between those values at peak drug action time and the corresponding saline values during the preceding day's control session. Reaction time values are for auditory stimuli presented at approximately 25 dB above the auditory thresholds and for visual stimuli presented at 1.25 log relative density units above the visual thresholds. The 95% confidence limits of the variability for all saline sessions preceding a drug session are shown to the left in each graph for each animal. Consistent elevations in visual thresholds and in both visual and auditory reaction times were observed following doses of 10.0 and 17.0 mg/kg with no change in auditory thresholds over this same dose range for two of three baboons.

Figure 19 illustrates the nature of these differential threshold changes in more detail and shows individual auditory and visual psychometric functions and their corresponding reaction time functions at peak drug action time for animal IK after pentobarbital administration over the dose range 1.0 to 17.0 mg/kg. Percent correct lever releases and reaction times for correct releases are plotted as a function of stimulus intensity in dB sound pressure level (SPL) for the auditory functions (top) and in log relative density units for

- 69 -

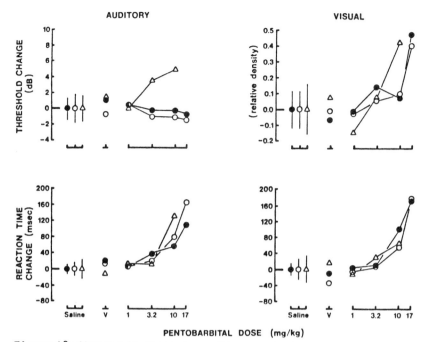

Figure 18: Changes in absolute auditory and visual thresholds and their respective median reaction times for three animals as a function of pentobarbital dose. The 95% confidence limits in variability for all saline sessions preceding a drug session are shown to the left in each graph for each animal. Values obtained following vehicle administration are marked "V." Reproduced with permission from Hienz, Lukas, and Brady, 1981. Copyright 1981 by Ankho International, Inc.

the visual functions (bottom). The saline points were similarly derived from the control sessions conducted on days preceding each drug session. At the highest dose (17.0 mg/kg), pentobarbital produced different effects upon auditory and visual thresholds, though similar increases occurred in both auditory and visual reaction times. The clear shift in the visual threshold function shown in Figure 19 (bottom) at the 17.0 mg/kg dose occurred in the absence of any change in the auditory threshold function (Figure 19, top)-- under identical drug conditions. Also, the drug-induced reaction time increases were approximately parallel shifts for both the auditory and the visual curves.

Similar changes in visual psychometric functions have been observed following doses of d-methylamphetamine, as shown in Figure 20 which presents percent correct lever releases as a function of stimulus intensity for both the previous day's saline session (dashed lines) and the 0.32 mg/kg d-methylamphetamine drug session (solid lines) for one animal. As with pentobarbital, the d-methylamphetamine-induced visual threshold elevations occurred in the absence of any change in auditory sensitivity. Changes in reaction time were, however, quite dissimilar to those produced by

Figure 19: Changes in individual auditory and visual psychometric functions and their corresponding reaction time functions during the time of peak drug effect for animal IK over the dose range of 1.0 to 17.0 mg/kg pentobarbital. Filled circles represent data from drug sessions; open circles represent data similarly derived from the preceding day's saline control session. Reproduced with permission from Hienz, Lukas, and Brady, 1981. Copyright 1981 by Ankho International, Inc.

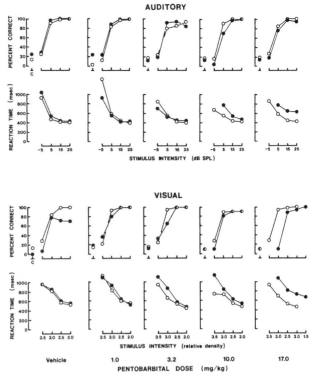

pentobarbital, with d-methylamphetamine frequently having reaction time-shortening effects, as shown in Figure 21. Auditory reaction times for 0.1 (see Figure 21, left) and 0.32 (see Figure 21, right) mg/kg doses of d-methylamphetamine (solid lines) are compared to the total range of saline control session reaction times (shaded areas) for a single animal. Similar reaction time-decreasing effects of the drug were observed for visual reaction times as well.

Figure 22 further compares these progressive decreases in visual reaction time over time (lower panel) with the time course of changes in visual thresholds (upper panel) following this animal's first and second exposures at 0.1 mg/kg d-methylamphetamine. Reaction time became progressively shorter from 60 to 100 minutes after drug injection, while threshold elevations occurred within the first 40 minutes following drug injection--before significant changes in reaction times occurred. And recovery to control threshold values occurred by 100 minutes post-drug, a time when the greatest shortening in reaction times was observed. Clearly, d-methylamphetamine has a differential effect on the sensory and motor components of the psychophysical performance.

The psychophysical profile of the prototypical benzodiazepine, diazepam, is shown in Figure 23. Auditory and visual thresholds, as well as reaction times, were measured in three baboons as a function of dose (0.1, 0.32, 1.0, 3.2, 10.0 mg/kg) at peak drug action time 1 to 2 hours following intramuscular administration. The range of saline control values is shown by the vertical lines on each point. Clear effects upon reaction time and visual thresholds

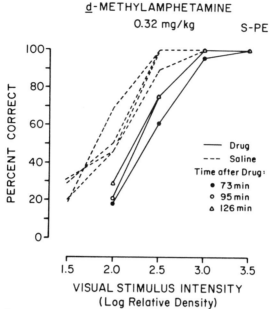

Figure 20: Percent correct lever releases as a function of visual stimulus intensity following a 0.32 mg/kg dose of d-methylamphetamine in animal PE, with time after drug as a parameter (solid lines). Similar data from the immediately preceding saline control day are shown for comparison (dashed lines).

were observed as a function of dose, and auditory thresholds were similarly affected. For the most part, all three effects--lengthened reaction times, visual threshold elevations, and auditory threshold elevations--appeared in a dose-dependent manner with progressively greater decrements through the range from 1.0 to 10.0 mg/kg. In contrast, observations with chlordiazepoxide over approximately the same dose range (1.0 to 32.0 mg/kg) used in the pentobarbital (Figure 18) and diazepam (Figure 23) experiments revealed only modest elevations in auditory thresholds and reaction times at the highest dose (32.0 mg/kg) and no elevations of visual threshold at any of the indicated doses.

To examine the consequences of long-term benzodiazepine administration, repeated diazepam injections were given on a daily schedule followed immediately by daily determinations of visual threshold and visual reaction times. Figure 24 presents changes in visual thresholds (top) and median reaction times for visual stimuli (bottom) over 21 consecutive days of daily intramuscular administration. Successive within-session estimates of visual thresholds and median reaction times are plotted for each session, and these within-session points are connected with solid lines for drug days and with dotted lines for saline days. Thus each series of two to five connected data points represents one day's data for changes in visual threshold (top graph) and changes in visual reaction time (bottom graph). Day 1 shows the acute effects of 0.32 mg/kg diazepam on visual reaction times, a small but consistent increase in reaction time, with no apparent changes in visual thresholds. Tolerance to the drug's effects on reaction times developed gradually, and by

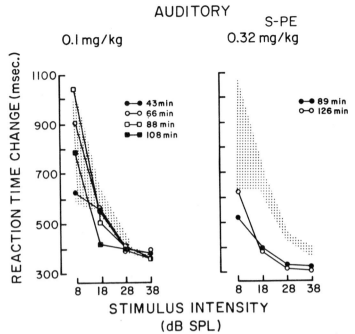

Figure 21: Latency-intensity functions showing median reaction time as a function of auditory stimulus intensity for animal PE following the second exposures to 0.1 mg/kg (left) and 0.32 mg/kg (right) d-methylamphetamine, with time after drug administration as the parameter. Shaded areas encompass total range in median reaction times for each drug day's immediately preceding saline control day.

Day 6 reaction times were back to normal values. Starting at Day 15 an anomalous decrease in visual reaction times occurred, possibly related to the appetite-inducing properties of the drug. (We have previously shown that large changes in deprivation can shift baseline reaction times.) Diazepam was withheld from the animal starting on Day 22, and reaction times then approximated normal values, although the within-session variability increased considerably during the withdrawal period. Visual thresholds continued to show little change.

This general picture of reaction time effects, the development of tolerance to these effects, and highly variable changes in reaction times during withdrawal was magnified somewhat at the daily dose of 1.0 mg/kg diazepam shown in Figure 25. Again, visual thresholds showed little or no change during either drug administration or withdrawal periods, while the initial effect of this dose of diazepam on reaction time was slightly greater, with tolerance to this reaction-time-increasing effect developing over 10 days as compared to 6 days for the 0.32 mg/kg dose. When the drug was stopped, reaction times showed a progressive and pronounced increase that peaked at Day 10 following cessation of the drug, with a gradual recovery following. Again, during this withdrawal period the variability of within-session estimates of reaction times was extreme.

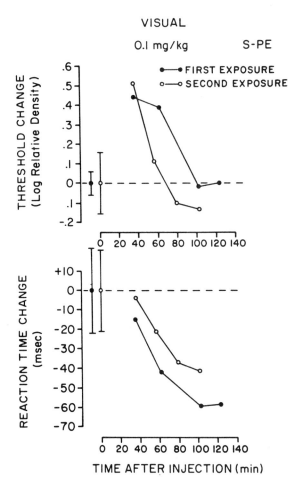

VISUAL

0.1 mg/kg   S-PE

Figure 22: Changes in visual threshold (top) and reaction times to visual stimuli (bottom) as a function of time after injection following first and second exposures to 0.1 mg/kg d-methylamphetamine in animal PE. Vertical bars indicate ± 2 standard deviations of variability for each preceding saline control day.

Increasing the dose again to 3.2 mg/kg diazepam produced even more pronounced effects on visual reaction times. The cumulative effects of the drug on reaction time peaked at Day 2, while the first clear effects on visual thresholds occurred on Days 4 and 5. Initial recovery from the reaction time effects was evident by Day 6 but not completed until Day 21. Stopping drug administration again produced an immediate effect upon reaction time, with complete recovery from this effect not occurring for 19 days after drug administration was stopped.

A procedure has been developed for an interactive analysis of the disruptive eliciting effects of abused drugs upon sensory/motor functions, on the one hand, and for their reinforcing effects in maintaining self-administration, on the other. The reinforcement/toxicity ratio (Brady & Griffiths, 1983) compares the relative potency of a drug as a reinforcer with its relative potency in eliciting disruptive sensory/motor effects. A drug with potent reinforcing properties (i.e., maintains self-injection at relatively low doses) but which produces disruptive effects only at relatively high doses would have a low reinforcement/toxicity ratio, whereas a drug that

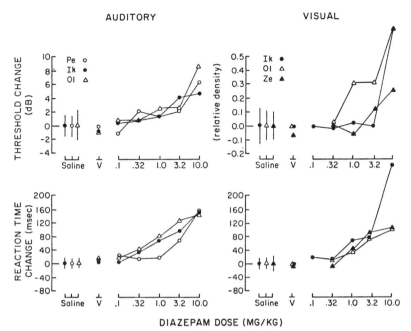

Figure 23: Changes in absolute auditory and visual thresholds and their respective median reaction times for three animals as a function of diazepam dose. The 95% confidence limits for all saline sessions are shown to the left in each graph for each animal. Values obtained following vehicle administration are marked "V."

maintains self-injection only at relatively high doses but produces disruptive sensory/motor effects at relatively low doses would have a high reinforcement/toxicity ratio. The measure thus provides a potentially useful preclinical assessment of the extent that self-administration of a compound may disrupt basic sensory/motor processes as well.

The reinforcing properties of a series of barbiturates, benzodiazepines, stimulants, and dissociative anesthetics were evaluated with laboratory baboons to determine the dose of each compound that maintained criterion self-administration. The procedure for determining reinforcing properties has been previously described in detail (Griffiths et al., 1979; 1981) and involved the initial establishment of drug self-administration with cocaine followed by substitution of saline or another drug for cocaine as described above. A 3-hour time-out period followed each injection, permitting a maximum of eight injections per day. When saline or low doses of drugs were substituted, the number of injections taken decreased over successive days. When higher doses of the drugs were substituted for cocaine, however, the self-injection rate was reliably maintained above saline control levels. Figure 26, for example, shows the effects of dose on the number of pentobarbital injections per day self-administered by two baboons and illustrates the procedure used for determining the criterion reinforcing dose values.

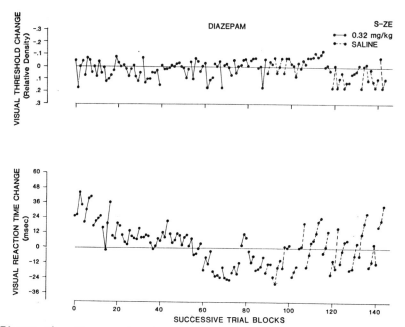

Figure 24: Changes in visual thresholds (top graph) and visual reaction times (bottom graph) over 21 consecutive days of daily intramuscular administration of 0.32 mg/kg diazepam and for subsequent days of saline administration. Threshold and reaction time changes from baseline are plotted for each successive block of trials within each session, and within-session points are connected by solid lines on drug days and by dashed lines on saline days. Reproduced with permission from Brady et al., 1984.

All drugs were also evaluated to determine the criterion dose which produced a 50% change in auditory and/or visual thresholds and/or a 10% change in motor reaction time. The procedures for determining such sensory/motor toxicity have been previously described in detail (Brady et al., 1979; Hienz & Brady, 1981; Hienz et al., 1981) and involved training baboons to perform the reaction time procedure described above. Figure 27 shows an example of the effects of pentobarbital dose on visual thresholds in three baboons and illustrates the determination of toxic doses.

Table 3 and Figure 28 summarize the relationships revealed by the reinforcement/toxicity ratios for amobarbital, pentobarbital, secobarbital, d-methylamphetamine, triazolam, diazepam, phencyclidine (PCP), and ketamine. With a ratio value of 1.0 representing equality between reinforcing and toxic drug doses, Table 3 and Figure 28 show that all three barbiturates, d-methylamphetamine, and the short-acting benzodiazepine triazolam are characterized by both sensory and motor ratio values below 1.0, indicating that the disruptive sensory/motor changes occurred at doses well above the criterion reinforcing dose. A consistent relationship between the sensory and motor effects of these compounds is also apparent because the motor effects appear at lower doses than the sensory effects (i.e., motor ratios higher than sensory

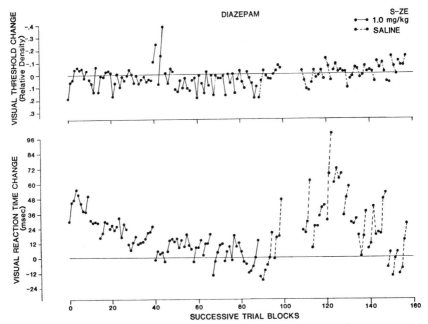

Figure 25: Changes in visual thresholds (top graph) and visual reaction times (bottom graph) over 21 consecutive days of daily intramuscular administration of 1.0 mg/kg diazepam and for subsequent days of saline administration. Further description as in Figure 24. Reproduced with permission from Brady et al., 1984.

ratios). A similar relationship between motor and sensory effects also characterizes the long-acting benzodiazepine diazepam, but disruptive motor effects appear at doses well below those required to maintain self-administration (i.e., motor ratio greater than 1.0). In the case of the dissociative anesthetics, PCP and ketamine are readily differentiated from the other compounds by a reversal of the relationship between sensory and motor effects seen with the other compounds. For PCP and ketamine sensory changes appear at doses below those which produce motor effects (i.e., sensory ratios higher than motor ratios). And PCP appears unique among the compounds thus far studied because both sensory and motor ratio values are greater than 1.0, indicating that the criterion self-administration dose is higher than the doses which produce significant behavioral toxicity.

CONCLUSIONS

The studies with laboratory primates reviewed in this chapter have documented the efficacy of a range of experimental methods and procedures for assessing the reinforcing, discriminative, and eliciting properties of drugs. The good correspondence between the drugs which generate and maintain self-injection in the baboon and those that are abused by man argues convincingly for the validity and utility of abuse liability assessment procedures based upon the reinforcing functions of drugs. In addition, the rapidly developing

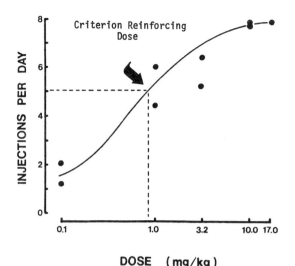

Figure 26: Daily pentobarbital self-injections as a function of dose. The criterion dose for self-administration (dotted line) was halfway between the performance maintained by saline (i.e., 1 to 2 injections/day) and the maximal performance on cocaine (i.e., 7 to 9 injections/day). Reproduced with permission from Brady, Lukas, and Hienz, 1983.

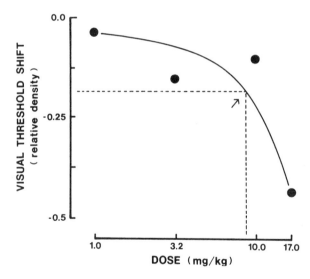

Figure 27: Visual threshold shift as a function of pentobarbital dose. Values are the means of three baboons. The criterion sensory threshold toxicity dose (dotted line) was halfway between central and maximal change. Reproduced with permission from Brady, Lukas, and Hienz, 1983.

Table 3

Reinforcement/Toxicity Ratios for Three Barbiturates, One Stimulant, Two Benzodiazepines, and Two Dissociative Anesthetics

A	B	C	D	E	F
Drug	Criterion Reinforcing Dose (mg/kg)	Criterion Reaction-TIme Toxicity Dose (mg/kg)	Reinforcement Reaction-Time Toxicity Ratio (B/C)	Criterion Sensory-Threshold-Toxicity Dose (mg/kg)	Reinforcement/ Sensory Threshold Toxicity Ratio (B/E)
Amobarbital	0.44	5.9	0.07	11.75	0.04
Pentobarbital	1.44	4.5	0.32	9.0	0.16
Secobarbital	1.80	3.3	0.55	6.2	0.29
d-methylamphetamine	0.052	0.08	0.65	0.14	0.37
Triazolam	0.01	0.017	0.59	0.065	0.15
Diazepam	3.2	0.65	4.92	6.1	0.52
Phencyclidine	0.05	0.041	1.22	0.023	2.17
Ketamine	0.39	2.0	0.20	0.4	0.98

Determination of doses is described in text. The criterion reinforcing doses in column B were derived by multiplying the actual doses by a constant that corrects for differential absorption rates and makes the I.V. self-administration doses more comparable to the I.M. toxicity doses.

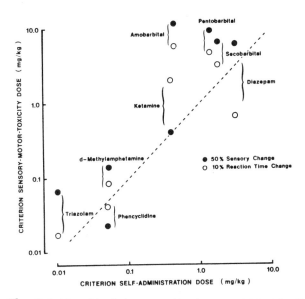

Figure 28: Relationship between criterion sensory and motor toxicity doses and criterion self-administration doses for three barbiturates, two benzodiazepines, two dissociative anesthetics, and a stimulant. The broken diagonal line represents equality between the reinforcing and toxic doses. Reproduced with permission from Brady et al., 1984.

experimental methodologies for differentiating between drugs on the basis of their discriminative functions enhance the laboratory animal testing procedures by operationalizing the subjective self-report domain which has long been the mainstay of abuse liability assessment armamentaria with human test subjects.

Standards in the area of dependence potential evaluation on the other hand have, of course, been set for many decades on the basis of the eliciting functions associated with the biochemical, physiological, and behavioral sequelae of repeated drug administration to laboratory animals. The recent pharmacological development of an extended range of agonist, antagonist, and mixed agonist-antagonist compounds, however, has greatly increased the sensitivity and precision (not to mention the speed) with which animal experimental methods for evaluating the eliciting properties of drugs have provided valid and reliable assessments of a pharmacologic agent's dependence potential in humans.

These studies also show the relevance and importance of evaluating a drug's eliciting functions as they are expressed in the form of behavioral toxicity now recognized as an essential defining feature of comprehensive assessment approaches involving both abuse liability and dependence potential. The increasingly prominent role and scope of these behavioral methodologies in virtually all aspects of drug assessment have extended the range of dependence potential and abuse liability evaluations and provided a more comprehensive and coherent framework for analysis of drug action in relationship to known standards of pharmacological equivalence.

ACKNOWLEDGMENTS

Research reported in this chapter was supported in part by the National Institute on Drug Abuse Contract 271-83-4023, NIDA grants DA01147, DA02490 and DA00018. Many people have contributed to the studies reported here. We would like especially to thank R. Wurster, J. Snell, R. Atkinson, D. Bowers, B. Campbell, E. Cook, L. Daley, D. Spicer, and P. Thiess. We thank D. Sabotka and J. Nierenberg for their help in preparation of this manuscript.

REFERENCES

Ambrus, J. L., Ambrus, C. M., & Harrison, J. W. E. (1951). Effect of histamine desensitization on histamine induced gastric secretion of guinea pigs. Gastroenterology, **18**, 249.

Ator, N. A., & Griffiths, R. R. (1983). Lorazepam and pentobarbital drug discrimination in baboons: Cross-drug generalization tests and interaction with Ro 15-1788. Journal of Pharmacology and Experimental Therapeutics, **226**, 776-782.

Ator, N. A., & Griffiths, R. R. (1985). Lorazepam and pentobarbital discrimination: Interactions with CGS 8216 and caffeine. European Journal of Pharmacology, **107**, 169-181.

Barry, H., III, & Krimmer, E. C. (1978). Similarities and differences in discriminative stimulus effects of chlordiazepoxide, pentobarbital, ethanol and other sedatives. In F. C. Colpaert & J. A. Rosecrans (Eds.), Stimulus properties of drugs: Ten years of progress (pp. 31-51). Amsterdam: Elsevier.

Brady, J. (1981). Common mechanisms in substance abuse. In T. Thompson & C. Johanson (Eds.), Behavioral pharmacology of human drug dependence (National Institute on Drug Abuse Research Monograph 37, pp. 11-20). Washington, DC: U.S. Government Printing Office.

Brady, J. V., Bradford, L. D., & Hienz, R. D. (1979). Behavioral assessment of risk-taking and psychophysical functions in the baboon. Neurobehavioral Toxicology, 1, 73-84.

Brady, J. V., & Griffiths, R. R. (1976a). Behavioral procedures for evaluating the relative abuse potential of CNS drugs in primates. Federation Proceedings, 35, 2245-2253.

Brady, J. V., & Griffiths, R. R. (1976b). Drug maintained performance and the analysis of stimulant reinforcing effects. In E. H. Ellinwood & M. M. Kilbey (Eds.), Cocaine and other stimulants (pp. 599-613). New York: Plenum Press.

Brady, J. V., & Griffiths, R. R. (1977). Drug-maintained performance procedures and the assessment of drug-abuse liability. In T. Thompson & K. Unna (Eds.), Predicting dependence liability of stimulant and depressant drugs (pp. 165-184). Baltimore: University Park Press.

Brady, J. V., & Griffiths, R. R. (1983). Testing drugs for abuse liability and behavioral toxicity: Progress report from the laboratories at the Johns Hopkins University School of Medicine. In L. S. Harris (Ed.), Problems of drug dependence, 1982 (National Institute on Drug Abuse Research Monograph 43, pp. 99-124). Washington, DC: U.S. Government Printing Office.

Brady, J. V., Griffiths, R. R., & Hienz, R. D. (1983). Testing drugs for abuse liability and behavioral toxicity: Progress report from the laboratories at the Johns Hopkins University School of Medicine. In L. S. Harris (Ed.), Problems of drug dependence, 1982 (National Institute on Drug Abuse Research Monograph 43, pp. 99-124). Washington, DC: U.S. Government Printing Office.

Brady, J. V., Griffiths, R. R., Hienz, R. D., Bigelow, G. E., Emurian, H. H., Lukas, S. E., Ator, N. A., Nellis, M. J., Ray, R. L., Pearlson, G. D., Liebson, I., Funderburk, F., Jasinski, D. R., Henningfield, J., & Johnson, R, E. (1984). Abuse liability and behavioral toxicity assessment: Progress report from the Behavioral Biology Laboratories of the Johns Hopkins University School of Medicine. In L. S. Harris (Ed.) Problems of drug dependence, 1983 (National Institute on Drug Abuse Research Monograph 49, pp. 92-108). Washington, DC: U.S. Government Printing Office.

Brady, J. V., Griffiths, R. R., & Winger, G. (1975). Drug-maintained performance procedures and the evaluation of sedative hypnotic dependence potential. In F. Kagan, T. Harwood, K. Rickels, A. Rudzik, & H. Sorer (Eds.), Hypnotics: Methods of development and evaluation (pp. 221-235). New York: Spectrum.

Brady, J. V., Lukas, S. E., & Hienz, R. D. (1983). Relationship between reinforcing properties and sensory/motor toxicity of CNS depressants: Implications for the assessment of abuse liability. In L. S. Harris (Ed.), Problems of drug dependence, 1982 (National Institute on Drug Abuse Research Monograph 43, pp. 196-202). Washington, DC: U.S. Government Printing Office.

Clouet, D. H., & Iwatsubo, K. (1975). Mechanism of tolerance to and dependence on narcotic analgesic drugs. Annual Review of Pharmacology and Toxicology, 15, 49-71.

Cochin, J. (1970). Possible mechanisms in development of tolerance. Federation Proceedings, 29, 19-27.

Colpaert, F. C., Niemegeers, C. J. E., & Janssen, P. A. J. (1976a). Fentanyl and apomorphine: Asymmetrical generalization of discriminative stimulus properties. Neuropharmacology, 15, 541-545.

Colpaert, F. C., Niemegeers, C. J. E., & Janssen, P. A. J. (1976b). Theoretical and methodological considerations on drug discrimination learning. Psychopharmacologia, 46, 169-177.

Colpaert, F. C., & Rosecrans, J. A. (Eds.). (1978). Stimulus properties of drugs: Ten years of progress. Amsterdam: Elsevier.

Crandall, L. A., Leake, C. D., Loevenhart, A. S., & Muehlberger, C. W. (1931). Acquired tolerance to and cross tolerance between the nitrous and nitric acid esters and sodium nitrite in man. Journal of Pharmacology and Experimental Therapeutics, 41, 103.

Darragh, A., Lambe, R., Kenny, M., Brick, I., Taaffe, W., & O'Boyle, C. (1982). Ro 15-1788 antagonizes the central effects of diazepam in man without altering diazepam bioavailability. British Journal of Clinical Pharmacology, 14, 677-682.

Deneau, G. A. (1956). An analysis of factors influencing the development of physical dependence to narcotic analgesics in the rhesus monkey with methods for predicting physical dependence liability in man. Unpublished doctoral dissertation, University of Michigan.

Eddy, N. B. (1973). The national council involvement in the opiate problem: 1928-1971. Washington, DC: National Academy of Sciences.

Goudie, A. J. (1977). Discriminative stimulus properties of fenfluramine in an operant task: An analysis of its cue function. Psychopharmacology, 53, 97-102.

Greenblatt, D. J., Shader, R. I., Divoll, M., & Harmatz, J. S. (1981). Benzodiazepines: A summary of pharmacokinetic properties. British Journal of Clinical Pharmacology, 11, 11S-16S.

Griffiths, R. R., Ator, N. A., Lukas, S. E., & Brady, J. V. (1983). Experimental abuse liability assessment of benzodiazepines. In E. Usdin, P. Skolnick, J. F. Tallman, Jr., D. Greenblatt, & S. M. Paul (Eds.), Pharmacology of benzodiazepines (pp. 609-618). London: MacMillan Press.

Griffiths, R. R., Bigelow, G. E., & Henningfield, J. H. (1980). Similarities in animal and human drug-taking behavior. In N. K. Mello (Ed.), Advances in substance abuse (Vol. 1, pp. 1-90). Greenwich, CT: JAI Press.

Griffiths, R. R., Bradford, L. D., & Brady, J. V. (1979). Progressive ratio and fixed ratio schedules of cocaine-maintained responding in baboons. Psychopharmacology, 65, 125-136.

Griffiths, R. R., Brady, J. V., & Bradford, L. D. (1979). Predicting the abuse liability of drugs with animal drug self-administration procedures: Psychomotor stimulants and hallucinogens. In T. Thompson & P. B. Dews (Eds.), Advances in behavioral pharmacology (Vol. 2, pp. 163-208). New York: Academic Press.

Griffiths, R. R., Brady, J. V., & Snell, J. D. (1978a). Progressive ratio performance maintained by drug infusions: Comparison of cocaine, diethylpropion, chlorphentermine and fenfluramine. Psychopharmacology, 56, 5-13.

Griffiths, R. R., Brady, J. V., & Snell, J. D. (1978b). Relationship between anorectic and reinforcing properties of appetite suppressant drugs: Implications for assessment of abuse liability. Biological Psychiatry, 13, 283-290.

Griffiths, R. R., Lukas, S. E., Bradford, L. D., Brady, J. V., & Snell, J. D. (1981). Self-injection of barbiturates and benzodiazepines in baboons. Psychopharmacology, 75, 101-109.

Herling, S., & Shannon, H. E. (1982). Ro 15-1788 antagonizes the discriminative stimulus effects of diazepam in rats but not similar effects of pentobarbital. Life Sciences, 31, 2105-2112.

Hienz, R. D., & Brady, J. V. (1981). Psychophysical profiles differentiate drugs of abuse. In L. S. Harris (Ed.), Problems of drug dependence, 1980 (National Institute on Drug Abuse Research Monograph 34, pp. 226-231). Washington, DC: U.S. Government Printing Office.

Hienz, R. D., Lukas, S. E., & Brady, J. V. (1981). The effects of pentobarbital upon auditory and visual thresholds in the baboon. Pharmacology Biochemistry & Behavior, 15, 799-805.

Hill, H. E., Haertzen, C. A., Wolbach, A. B., Jr., & Miner, E. J. (1963). The Addiction Research Center Inventory: Standardization of scales which evaluate subjective effects of morphine, amphetamine, pentobarbital, alcohol, LSD-25, pyrahexyl and chlorpromazine. Psychopharmacologia, 4, 167-183.

Hirschhorn, I. D. (1977). Pentazocine, cyclazocine and nalorphine as discriminative stimuli. Psychopharmacology, 54, 289-294.

Jaffe, J. H. (1980). Drug addiction and drug abuse. In A. G. Gilman, L. S. Goodman, & A. Gilman (Eds.), The pharmacological basis of therapeutics (6th Edition, pp. 535-584). New York: MacMillan.

Jarbe, T. U. C., & McMillan, D. E. (1983). Interaction of the discriminative stimulus properties of diazepam and ethanol in pigeons. Pharmacology Biochemistry & Behavior, 18, 73-80.

Johanson, C. E., Balster, R. L., & Bonese, K. (1976). Self-administration of psychomotor stimulant drugs: The effects of unlimited access. Pharmacology Biochemistry & Behavior, 4, 45-51.

Jones, B. E., & Prada, J. A. (1977). Drug seeking behavior in the dog: Lack of effect of prior passive dependence on morphine. Drug and Alcohol Dependence, 2, 287-294.

Kalant, H., Leblanc, A. E., & Gibbins, R. J. (1971). Tolerance to and dependence on some non-opiate psychomotor drugs. Pharmacological Reviews, 23, 135-191.

Lukas, S. E., & Griffiths, R. R. (1982). Precipitated withdrawal by a benzodiazepine receptor antagonist (Ro 15-1788) after 7 days of diazepam. Science, 217, 1161-1163.

Lukas, S. E, & Griffiths, R. R. (1984). Precipitated diazepam withdrawal in baboons: Effects of dose and duration of diazepam exposure. European Journal of Pharmacology, 100, 163-171.

Lukas, S. E., Griffiths, R. R., Bradford, L. D., Brady, J. V., Daley, L., & DeLorenzo, R. (1982). A tethering system for intravenous and gastric drug administration in the baboon. Pharmacology Biochemistry & Behavior, 17, 823-829.

Lukas, S. E., Griffiths, R. R., Brady, J. V., & Wurster, R. M. (1984). Phencyclidine-analogue self-injection by the baboon. Psychopharmacology, 83, 316-320.

Martin, W. R. (Ed.). (1977). Drug addiction I. (Handbook of Experimental Pharmacology, Vol. 45/I). Berlin: Springer-Verlag.

Meltzer, L. T., Rosecrans, J. A., Aceto, M. D., & Harris, L. S. (1980). Discriminative stimulus properties of the optical isomers of nicotine. Psychopharmacology, 68, 283-286.

Mendelson, J. H., & Mello, N. K. (1982). Commonly abused drugs. In Harrison's principle of internal medicine (pp. 1541-1546). New York: McGraw Hill.

Moody, D. B. (1970). Reaction time as an index of sensory function. In W. C. Stebbins (Ed.), Animal psychophysics: The design and conduct of sensory experiments (pp. 277-302). New York: Appleton.

Moody, D. B. (1973). Behavioral studies of noise-induced hearing loss in primates: Loudness recruitment. Advances in Oto-Rhino-Laryngology, 20, 82-101.

Musto, D. F. (1973). The American disease--Origins of narcotic control. New Haven, CT: Yale University Press.

Myers, H. B., & Austin, V. T. (1929). Nitrate toleration. Journal of Pharmacology and Experimental Therapeutics, 36, 227.

Overton, D. A. (1978). Status of research on state-dependent learning--1978. In J. C. Colpaert & J. A. Rosecrans (Eds.), Stimulus properties of drugs: Ten years of progress (pp. 559-562). Amsterdam: Elsevier.

Overton, D. A. (1982a). Comparison of the degree of discriminability of various drugs using the T-maze drug discrimination paradigm. Psychopharmacology, 76, 385-395.

Overton, D. A. (1982b). Multiple drug training as a method for increasing the specificity of the drug discrimination procedure. Journal of Pharmacology and Experimental Therapeutics, 221 , 166-172.

Petursson, H., & Lader, M. H. (1981). Withdrawal from long-term benzodiazepine treatment. British Medical Journal, 283, 643-645.

Pevnick, J. S., Jasinski, D. R., & Haertzen, C. A. (1978). Abrupt withdrawal from therapeutically administered diazepam: Report of a case. Archives of General Psychiatry, 35, 995-998.

Pfingst, B. E., Hienz, R. D., Kimm, J., & Miller, J. (1975a). Reaction-time procedure for measurement of hearing. I. Suprathreshold functions. Journal of the Acoustic Society of America, 57, 421-430.

Pfingst, B. E., Hienz, R. D., & Miller, J. (1975b). Reaction-time procedure for the measurement of hearing. II. Threshold functions. Journal of the Acoustic Society of America, 57, 431-436.

Pickens, R., & Thompson, T. (1971). Characteristics of stimulant drug reinforcement. In T. Thompson & R. Pickens (Eds.), Stimulant properties of drugs (pp. 177-192). New York: Appleton.

Rector, F. C., Seldin, D. W., & Copenhaver, J. H. (1955). The mechanism of ammonia excretion during ammonium chloride acidosis. Journal of Clinical Investigation, 24, 20.

Rifkin, A., Quitkin, F., & Klein, D. F. (1976). Withdrawal reaction to diazepam. Journal of the American Medical Association, 236, 2172-2173.

Schuster, C. R., & Balster, R. L. (1977). The discriminative stimulus properties of drugs. In T. Thompson & P. B. Dews (Eds.), Advances in behavioral pharmacology (Vol. 1, pp. 85-138). New York: Academic Press.

Schuster, C. F., & Fischman, M. W. (1975). Amphetamine toxicity: Behavioral and neuropathological indices. Federation Proceedings, 34, 1845-1851.

Schuster, C. R., & Woods, J. H. (1967). Morphine as a reinforcer for operant behavior: The effects of dosage per injection. Report to the Committee on Problems of Drug Dependence, Washington, DC: National Academy of Science.

Seevers, M. H. (1936). Opiate addiction in the monkey. I. Methods of study. Journal of Pharmacology and Experimental Therapeutics, 56, 147-156.

Seevers, M. H., & Deneau, G. A. (1963). Physiological aspects of tolerance and physical dependence. In W. S. Root & F. G. Hofman (Eds.), Physiological pharmacology (Vol. 1). New York: Academic Press.

Shannon, H. E., & Herling S. (1983). Antagonism of the discriminative effects of diazepam by pyrazoloquinolines in rats. European Journal of Pharmacology, 92, 155.

Shannon, H. E., & Holtzman, S. G. (1976). Evaluation of morphine in the rat. Journal of Pharmacology and Experimental Therapeutics, 198, 54-65.

Tessel, R. E., & Woods, J. H. (1975). Fenfluramine and N-ethylamphetamine: Comparison of the reinforcing and rate-decreasing actions in the rhesus monkey. Psychopharmacologia, 43, 239-244.

Tessel, R. E., Woods, J. H., Counsell, R. E., & Basmadjian, G. P. (1975a). Structure-activity relationships between meta-substituted N-ethyl-amphetamines and isolated guinea-pig atrial rate. Journal of Pharmacology and Experimental Therapeutics, 192, 319-326.

Tessel, R. E., Woods, J. H., Counsell, R. E., & Lu, M. (1975b). Structure-activity relationships between meta-substituted N-ethylamphetamines and locomotor activity in mice. Journal of Pharmacology and Experimental Therapeutics, **192**, 310-318.

Tyrer, P., Rutherford, D., & Hugget, T. (1981). Benzodiazepine withdrawal symptoms and propranolol. Lancet, 520-522.

Villarreal, J. E. (1973). The effects of morphine agonists and antagonists on morphine-dependent rhesus monkeys. In H. W. Kosterlitz, H. O. J. Collier, & J. E. Villarreal (Eds.), Agonist and antagonist actions of narcotic analgesic drugs (pp. 73-93). Baltimore: University Park Press.

Winger, G., & Herling, S. (1982). Discriminative stimulus effects of pentobarbital in rhesus monkeys. Tests of stimulus generalization and duration of action. Psychopharmacology, **76**, 172-176.

Winokur, A., Rickels, K., Greenblatt, D. J., Snyder, P. J., & Schatz, N. J. (1980). Withdrawal reaction from long-term, low-dosage administration of diazepam: A double-blind, placebo-controlled case study. Archives of General Psychiatry, **37**, 101-105.

Winter, J. C. (1978). Drug-induced stimulus control. In D. E. Blackman & D. J. Sanger (Eds.), Contemporary research in behavioral pharmacology (pp. 209-237). New York: Plenum Press.

Woods, J. H., Young, A. M., & Herling, S. (1982). Classification of narcotics on the basis of their reinforcing, discriminative and antagonist effects in rhesus monkeys. Federation Proceedings, **41**, 221-227.

Yanagita, T., & Miyasato, K. (1976). Dependence potential of methaqualone tested in rhesus monkeys. CIEA Preclinical Report, **2**, 63-68.

Yanagita, T., & Takahashi, S. (1970). Development of tolerance to and physical dependence on barbiturates in rhesus monkeys. Journal of Pharmacology and Experimental Therapeutics, **172**, 163-169.

Yanagita, T., & Takahashi, S. (1973). Dependence liability of several sedative-hypnotic agents evaluated in monkeys. Journal of Pharmacology and Experimental Therapeutics, **185**, 307-316.

Yanagita, T., Takahashi, S., & Oinuma, N. (1975). Drug dependence potential of lorazepam (WY 4036) evaluated in the rhesus monkey. CIEA Preclinical Reports, **1**, 1-4.

York, J. L. (1978). A comparison of the discriminative stimulus effects of ethanol, barbital, and phenobarbital in rats. Psychopharmacology, **60**, 19-23.

CHAPTER 4

INTERPRETATION OF LESION EFFECTS ON STIMULANT SELF-ADMINISTRATION

D. C. S. ROBERTS AND K. A. ZITO*

Department of Psychology
Carleton University
Ottawa, Ontario, Canada K1S 5B6

ABSTRACT

A number of studies have employed the lesion approach to understand the neural mechanisms which underlie drug self-administration behavior. In general, two strategies have been used. One method examines the effect of lesions on acquisition of the self-administration response. Changes in drug reward are inferred by comparing differences in the acquisition rates between lesioned and control animals. Alternately, some have used a within subject design and analyzed the effects of lesions on previously established self-administration behavior. To date, only simple schedules of reward (i.e., fixed ratio or continuous reinforcement) have been used in conjunction with the lesion technique. The difficulty in interpreting changes in drug intake or rate of acquisition is discussed with reference to stimulant self-administration data generated in several laboratories. The importance of characterizing the extent and specificity of the lesion and of choosing the most appropriate postlesion test period is also emphasized.

INTRODUCTION

How do drugs of abuse act on the brain to produce their reinforcing effects? This is one of the most interesting and perhaps one of the most difficult questions in the field of neuropsychopharmacology. It is complicated for two reasons. First, most abused drugs have many effects unrelated to reward which are produced at sites throughout the nervous system. The task is to separate these irrelevant responses from those actions in the specific loci responsible for reward. One method which has enjoyed some success has been to lesion different neural systems in an attempt to selectively block the drug reward. This approach requires either the evaluation of drug reward before and after the lesion or the comparison of lesioned with nonlesioned control animals. Such comparisons imply that reward strength can be quantified and that any change in reinforcement may be detected and measured. This is the second complication. There appears to be a lack of consensus on how to measure reward strength. While the concept of reinforcement seems straightforward, methods for quantifying reward remain contentious.

*Present address for K. A. Zito: Department of Anatomy, University of Toronto, Toronto, Ontario, Canada M5S 1A8.

Over the past few decades several different approaches have been used to assess the reinforcing properties of abused drugs. These methods involve brain stimulation, drug discrimination, conditioned reinforcement, conditioned place preference, and intravenous or intracerebral self-administration. Some applications of these approaches are represented in this volume. Although each of these techniques has added to our knowledge of reinforcement, ultimately the characterization of the neural substrates of reward will depend on convergent evidence from all these procedures rather than from one idealized strategy.

This chapter will focus on the self-administration technique as a method to evaluate the effects of lesions on the rewarding effects of psychomotor stimulants. Self-administration studies have proven valuable for evaluating the abuse potential of new drugs. Such studies have shown that drugs that are typically abused by humans are also self-administered by laboratory animals. It should be noted that although such a demonstration may indicate whether a drug is rewarding or not, it does not necessarily measure reinforcement magnitude. Attempts at evaluating the degree of reward strength, therefore, typically require more complex tasks or complicated schedules of reinforcement.

Several potential measures have been offered in the self-administration literature to quantify stimulant reinforcement. For example, the "cost" of the drug in terms of energy or amount of behavior elicited for an infusion has been proposed as one method to measure drug reward. In such studies a progressive-ratio is typically employed and the number of responses required to produce a reinforcement (until the animal eventually fails to respond) is used as a dependent measure. The value where responding falls below a specific criterion is defined as the break point of responding (for an example of this technique the reader is referred to Bedford, Bailey, & Wilson, 1978; Brady, Griffiths, Hienz, Ator, Lukas, & Lamb, this volume; Griffiths, Bradford, & Brady, 1979; Griffiths, Brady, & Snell, 1978; Griffiths, Findley, Gutcher, & Robinson, 1975; Hoffmeister, 1979; Yanagita, 1973, this volume; Yokel, this volume). The break point of responding has been shown to vary systematically with several motivational conditions (e.g., degree of food deprivation, concentration or volume of liquid reinforcer) and has therefore been argued to provide an index of the relative strength of a reinforcer (Hodos, 1961; Hodos & Kalman, 1963).

Drug cost may also be manipulated by employing an electric shock to suppress drug self-administration (Grove & Schuster, 1974; Smith & Davis, 1974). With this method response suppression produced by concurrent shock may be overcome by progressively increasing the dose of the drug (Johanson, 1977). This technique should, therefore, make possible the determination of drug reward strength by measuring the amount of shock animals are willing to tolerate concomitantly with the drug injection. This method, unfortunately, could be confounded by possible analgesic or anxiolytic effects produced by the drug under study.

Concurrent schedules have also been used to evaluate the relative reinforcing properties of various reinforcement relationships. With this technique two equally valued variable interval schedules are made available on two separate operants. The relative response rates produced at each lever are apparently indicative of reinforcement magnitude. This approach has been applied to intravenous self-administration procedures to compare the response rates produced at each lever for two doses of the same drug (Iglauer, Llewellyn & Woods, 1976; Iglauer & Woods, 1974). This method does not lend itself to lesion work, however, because we are most interested in comparing pre- versus post-lesion self-administration behavior. The technique may be useful if a change in relative value between one drug affected by lesion (e.g., cocaine) to another not affected by the lesion (e.g., apomorphine) could be detected, although we are unaware of any studies that have used matching of two different drugs instead of two doses of the same drug.

None of these rather difficult methodologies have so far been used in conjunction with lesion techniques. Future studies may well require these procedures; however, for a number of reasons the studies to date have restricted themselves to simple schedules of drug reward. The continuous reinforcement schedule (CRF), in which each response produces an intravenous injection, is the most basic variation of the self-administration procedure. Intuitively, it makes sense to employ the most elementary approach available (i.e., the most fundamental schedule of drug reward) prior to superimposing other factors which may complicate the analysis unnecessarily (e.g., concurrent shock, more complicated schedules of reinforcement).

Additionally, chronic lesions, whether neurotoxic, radiofrequency, or electrolytic, all require extensive postoperative testing to observe long-term degenerative or compensatory physiological changes. The inclusion of complicated schedules of reinforcement, which may require many days of training before establishment of stable baseline performances, increases the probability of extending the experiment beyond the limits of the intravenous implant. Therefore, due to the technical difficulties inherent in the self-administration technique itself, unnecessary time-consuming procedures should be kept at a minimum. There exists a delicate balance between including those factors which are absolutely essential to the experiment and omitting those which may be unnecessary.

Lastly, aversively motivated behaviors and those maintained by partial reinforcement schedules may make unnecessary response demands on subjects. The more complicated the behavioral response or the more motorically demanding, the more susceptible the behavior is to disruption from secondary effects (e.g., motor impairment). For this reason a simple, stable, on-going behavior is desirable because it eliminates unnecessary masking of effects that may be attributable to the effect of lesions. In general, therefore, most studies have typically employed a CRF schedule, relying on rate and pattern of self-administration. It should be noted that most researchers would agree that rate of self-administration does not measure drug reward, although it does provide a useful starting point for investigating lesion effects.

This chapter discusses both the relative merits and shortcomings of the self-administration technique as a method of assessing the effects of lesions on psychomotor stimulant reward. Particular attention will be drawn to the difficulties in interpreting results obtained with the self-administration technique as well as various control procedures that must be included in the design to rule out nonspecific lesion effects. Experiments which have examined the effects of lesions to monoaminergic systems on stimulant self-administration will be reviewed as a vehicle to explain the conclusions which can be drawn concerning the neuroanatomical and/or neurochemical basis of stimulant reward.

SELF-ADMINISTRATION BEHAVIOR

When provided with the opportunity, laboratory animals will acquire and maintain a lever response to receive a stimulant injection in a pattern very similar to human stimulant abuse (Kramer, Fischman, & Littlefield, 1967). When given unlimited access, all species of laboratory animals show a cyclic pattern of intake (e.g., Deneau, Yanagita, & Seevers, 1969; Johanson, Balster, & Bonese, 1976) with periods of abstinence alternating with periods of high drug intake ("binges"). Daily drug intake, therefore, varies considerably. By contrast, when access to the drug is restricted (e.g., 4 hours/day), a highly reliable and stable rate of responding is observed. Animals will self-administer very close to the same amount of drug each day for many weeks.

Although the mechanisms governing rate of self-administration are not fully understood, response rate typically has been used as the dependent variable. Animals apparently attempt to maintain a constant level of drug effect by increasing drug intake when drug impact is reduced and by decreasing intake when drug impact is increased (see Yokel, this volume). Typically, at the beginning of each session several injections are taken in quick succession after which responding becomes regularly spaced with little variation in the time between infusions (Pickens, 1968; Pickens & Thompson, 1968). Animals may exhibit variability in the rate of drug intake among animals, although the pattern is quite regular from day to day within a single subject. In instances where stimulant reinforcement is totally removed or suppressed, animals will display extinction-like behavior, initially increasing their rate followed by a total cessation of responding (Roberts, Koob, Klonoff, & Fibiger, 1980; Yokel & Wise, 1975, 1976). Thus the self-administration technique is particularly useful because it produces a stable behavior that can be quantified and qualified both preoperatively as a baseline behavior and postoperatively as a dependent measure of the effects of various forms of neuroanatomical disruption.

Although there are many variations of the self-administration technique, considering the procedure more generally, a limited number of ways for investigating the neurobiology of stimulant reward become evident. One approach is to examine the acquisition of the self-administration response (e.g., LeMoal, Stinus, & Simon, 1979; Lyness, Friedle, & Moore, 1980; Singer, Wallace, & Hall, 1982). A second is to examine the effects of particular lesions on the maintenance of self-administration behavior. Possibly the most basic approach requires that subjects acquire a stable self-administration response for the drug prior to surgery, then following surgery animals are again given the opportunity to self-administer. This methodology permits the comparison or pre- and post-operative behavior within a single subject and minimizes the effects of individual differences in rate and pattern of self-administration behavior that are likely to be found among subjects.

EFFECTS OF 6-HYDROXYDOPAMINE LESIONS ON COCAINE SELF-ADMINISTRATION

We have investigated the effects of 6-hydroxydopamine (6-OHDA) induced lesions on cocaine self-administration in a variety of neuroanatomical regions over the past several years, and we have found that this behavior appears to be extremely resistant to such lesions.

For example, injections of 6-OHDA into the dorsal tegmental bundle, the major ascending noradrenergic (NA) fiber system, do not significantly influence the rate or pattern of cocaine self-administration (see Figure 1, injection site 1). This seems remarkable since this treatment reduces NA content of the hippocampus and cortex to 4% of control levels and in the hypothalamus to 28% (Roberts, Corcoran, & Fibiger, 1977). These lesions do not, however, significantly affect dopamine levels. Inasmuch as near total depletion of telencephalic NA has no effect in the rate of cocaine self-administration, it appears that NA does not play an important role in this behavior. This

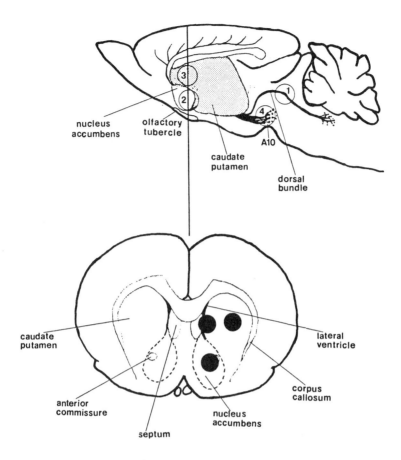

Figure 1: Sagittal projection of the ascending dorsal noradrenergic bundle and the mesolimbic dopaminergic system depicting four lesion sites (upper panel). The lower panel displays a coronal section of the rat brain depicting three 6-hydroxydopamine injection sites into dopaminergic terminal fields that have been tested for their effects on cocaine self-administration. Coronal view corresponds to section A 8920. Reproduced with permission from König and Klippel, 1970.

conclusion is in agreement with pharmacological evidence reviewed by Yokel (this volume).

We have also noted that responding for cocaine infusions is particularly resistant to 6-OHDA lesions in a variety of dopamine-rich areas. Figure 1 (lower panel) displays a coronal section of the rat brain depicting three 6-OHDA injection sites into dopaminergic terminal fields that have been tested for their effects on cocaine self-administration. Only one of these injection

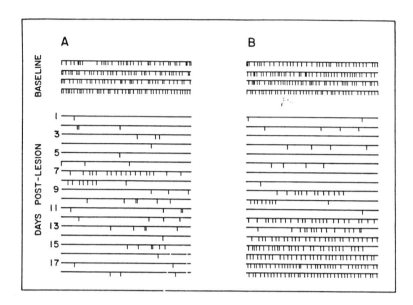

Figure 2: Event records of cocaine self-administration in two rats before and after 6-OHDA infusions into the nucleus accumbens. Each line represents one daily 3-hour session. **A**: An example of one rat (No. 60) which did not resume cocaine self-administration. **B**: An example of a rat (No. 62) which gradually recovered baseline self-administration rate. Reprinted with permission from Roberts, Koob, Klonoff, and Fibiger, 1980. Copyright 1980 by Ankho International, Inc.

sites produces a significant effect on this behavior. The lower circle represents the target for nucleus accumbens injections. The upper, medial circle represents an infusion site which should control for damage caused by leakage of the neurotoxin up the side of the injection needle or into the lateral ventricle. The lateral site was designed to investigate the effect of dopamine depletion of the caudate nucleus.

Neither of the two dorsally placed injections affected either the rate or pattern of cocaine self-administration (Roberts & Koob, unpublished observations). In contrast to the lack of effect produced by these lesions and those to the ascending NA fibers, bilateral 6-OHDA injections into dopaminergic terminal fields in the nucleus accumbens or the DA cell bodies which project to the accumbens (see Figure 1, upper panel, sites 2 and 4) produced a significant alteration in both rate and pattern of responding for cocaine.

Figure 2 displays the effects of such injections on cocaine self-injection for 18 days postlesion. These data illustrate several interesting aspects and problems. First, we see an abrupt cessation of responding, with animals typically taking only 1 or 2 injections on the days immediately following surgery. Second, over a period of several days some animals (e.g., Figure 2, right panel) begin to resume their intake, indicating that the drug continues to have rewarding properties. And third, the rate at which they begin to self-administer is less than prelesion rates. This final observation raises the question about the lesion causing an increase or a decrease in the reward strength of cocaine. The following sections address each of these issues.

Motor Deficits

The simplest explanation for the failure of the animals to respond for cocaine on the day following the lesion is that nonspecific effects of the lesion exist unrelated to reward. Inasmuch as the integrity of central dopaminergic neurons is known to be important in the motor aspect of operant responding (Clavier & Fibiger, 1977; Fibiger, Carter, & Phillips, 1976), it is reasonable to assume that the animals may have been incapable of responding. To examine this possibility, animals were trained to lever press for food on a variable ratio 2.5 schedule of reinforcement and, after their responding had stabilized, stereotaxically injected 6-OHDA into the nucleus accumbens. Although operant responding for food was observably depressed especially on the first day after the lesion, animals were capable of making an average of 55 responses on the food lever in 15 minutes (Roberts et al., 1977). This is far in excess of the responses necessary to self-administer the drug.

These results indicate that animals subjected to 6-OHDA lesions of the nucleus accumbens are probably capable of responding; however, the data do not rule out the possibility that the induced lesion caused a malaise which would inhibit self-administration of any drug. If nucleus accumbens lesions were to disrupt the self-administration of all agents, this would argue that the observed effect was due to a nonspecific mechanism. We have tested this possibility in a separate experiment by examining the effects of the lesion on the pattern of self-administration of two drugs (cocaine and apomorphine; Roberts et al., 1977).

Apomorphine, which has been shown to be reliably self-injected (Baxter, Gluckman & Scerni, 1976; Baxter, Gluckman, Stein, & Scerni, 1974), was chosen as an alternate drug because it is known to be a direct-acting dopamine agonist. Cocaine is thought to act as an indirect agonist: that is, it potentiates the action of dopamine by blocking synaptic reuptake and, therefore, requires intact presynaptic terminals to have an effect. Infusions of 6-OHDA into the nucleus accumbens cause preferential degeneration of the presynaptic catecholamine element but spare the postsynaptic target cell. This treatment should therefore disrupt cocaine self-administration but should leave apomorphine self-administration unaffected. However, if the lesion is shown to disrupt the self-administration of both drugs, then one would have to conclude that the effect was nonspecific.

With this procedure baseline intake for both apomorphine (0.06 mg/kg/injection) and cocaine (0.75 mg/kg/injection) was initially established. Each animal was given access to cocaine for several days (4 hours/day) until daily intake stabilized; then the animals were switched to several days of apomorphine self-administration. The cocaine baseline was again checked prior to surgery.

Following 6-OHDA lesions of the nucleus accumbens, responding for cocaine is disrupted; however, animals displayed a regular response pattern for apomorphine. This double drug baseline procedure helps demonstrate that animals can and will respond and that there are no trivial reasons (e.g., cannula problems) for the effect on cocaine self-administration. Infusions of

6-OHDA into the ventral tegmental area (VTA: the origin of the DA innervation of the nucleus accumbens) also disrupt cocaine self-administration, and the two-drug control procedure has also been used in these experiments to show that animals will continue to respond for apomorphine (Roberts & Koob, 1982).

The apomorphine self-administration results demonstrate that 6-OHDA/accumbens-lesioned animals are capable of responding but will not self-inject cocaine on the first few days following 6-OHDA lesions of the nucleus accumbens. Eventually, however, the animals begin to show signs of a regular self-administration pattern. This recovery begins with a slow self-administration rate which can approach prelesion drug intake. The interpretation of these data is problematic.

Interpretation of Rate Changes

A decrease in the unit dose of cocaine has been shown to produce an increase in response rate (Pickens & Thompson, 1968; Yokel, this volume). Accordingly, an increase in responding may indicate a decrease in reward value. This argument has been used to interpret the increases in stimulant intake observed following neuroleptic pretreatment (de Wit & Wise, 1977; Yokel & Wise, 1975, 1976). Apparently, a partial blockade of dopamine receptors induced by neuroleptics produces a reduction in drug impact, an effect analogous to lowering the drug dose.

If the dopamine terminals in the nucleus accumbens are essential to the rewarding effects of stimulant drugs and if many of these terminals are destroyed by the 6-OHDA treatment, then should we not expect that animals display an increase in self-administration rate rather than a decrease? Why should lesions of the accumbens cause a decrease in rate while neuroleptics cause an increase? Could not the suppressed response rates observed in lesioned animals be interpreted as a potentiation of the drug effect?

The answers to these questions must lie in the assumption that rate of self-administration is in a state of equilibrium, being controlled not only by the rewarding effects of the drug but also by aversive (toxic) properties and other limiting factors (e.g., stereotypy, competing response patterns). We might assume that the animal increases its intake (and therefore its blood or brain levels) to the point where the aversive effects outweigh the rewarding effects. A hypothetical relationship between positive and aversive components at various drug levels is depicted in Figure 3a. Of course the curves could have a variety of shapes, but the figure is simply intended to illustrate that at lower blood levels the predominant effect of the drug may be rewarding, while at higher blood levels the predominant effect could be aversive. Increases or decreases in the injection dose would not alter this relationship; therefore, the animal behaviorally compensates for changes in dose to maintain almost exactly the same optimal drug level.

In the case of response rate increases following neuroleptic treatment, there is an important difference. Animals increase their overall drug intake (not simply their response rate), which presumably causes a substantial increase in the amount of drug in the system. This could imply that blockade of dopaminergic receptors affects not only the positive but also the aversive actions. This relationship is depicted in Figure 3b. The slope of both the rewarding and aversive curves is reduced. If all these effects are mediated by dopamine, then neuroleptic pretreatment should attenuate all aspects of the drug injection, which would indeed by equivalent to reducing the dose.

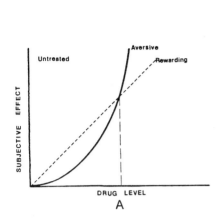

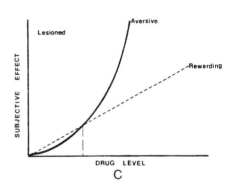

Figure 3: Hypothetical relationships between positive and aversive components at various drug levels illustrating that at low drug levels the rewarding effects outweigh the aversive effects while at higher drug levels the reverse is true. For further discussion see text.

Conversely, lesions to specific nuclei may attenuate individual actions of the drug and potentially affect either the rewarding effects or the aversive effects specifically. By altering the balance between the rewarding and punishing effects, changes in rate in either direction may be expected. Figure 3c illustrates an example of a specific attenuation of the rewarding effects with no change in the aversive effects. Note that the range in which the rewarding effects of the drug predominate is much smaller. The upper bound is greatly reduced which demands a lower rate of intake. In the case of lesions, therefore, a lower rate of intake is not paradoxical and may reflect a specific attenuation of the rewarding effects.

Recovery of Self-Administration

As noted earlier, lesioned animals will frequently recover their self-administration rate, often stabilizing at prelesion levels. We have attempted to relate this recovery to the extent of the 6-OHDA-induced depletions and have found that the greater the dopamine loss in the nucleus accumbens the longer the animal takes to recover. Animals that sustain the greatest degree of dopamine loss (greater than 90%) often fail to recover at all. These data emphasize the importance of achieving complete lesions of the system of interest. Many compensatory changes can reverse the effects of the lesions such as supersensitivity, increased turnover of transmitter in the remaining terminals, regrowth, and compensation by other systems. Thorough depletions

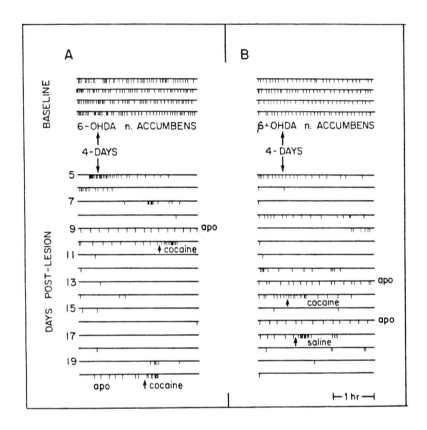

Figure 4: Event records of cocaine self-administration after 6-OHDA infusions into the nucleus accumbens or saline substitution. Each line represents one daily 3-hour session. Downward pen deflections indicate drug injections. **A:** Example of cessation of responding for cocaine 5 days after 6-OHDA treatment. On postlesion Day 9, regular responding is evident for apomorphine. On Days 10 and 20, cocaine was substituted for apomorphine, which produced an initial burst of responding followed by cessation. **B:** Another example of extinction of cocaine self-administration 5 days after 6-OHDA treatment. Apomorphine self-administration is shown on Days 13, 14, 16 and 17. Reprinted with permission from Roberts, Koob, Klonoff, and Fibiger, 1980. Copyright 1980 by Ankho International, Inc.

are essential, particularly since it has been shown in other systems that partial lesions can either fail to block the drug response or even in some cases potentiate it.

Towards this end the neurotoxic action of intracerebral infusions of 6-OHDA may be potentiated by administering the monoamine oxidase inhibitor pargyline. This treatment inhibits the metabolism of 6-OHDA and allows for more thorough depletion of noradrenergic or dopaminergic systems (Kostrzewa & Jacobowitz, 1974). Some degree of specificity may also be achieved by lesioning individual fiber pathways at the point of greatest separation between other catecholamine systems (e.g., dorsal NA bundle, see Figure 1). This is not possible with the DA system due to the considerable intermixing of NA and DA fibers as they ascend. However, NA fibers can be spared from the toxic effects of 6-OHDA by pretreatment with desipramine (DMI), thereby permitting a specific lesion to dopaminergic systems (Roberts, Zis, & Fibiger, 1975).

We have used these pharmacological tools to investigate the effects of more complete and specific depletions of DA from the nucleus accumbens. Because DMI and pargyline could have residual pharmacological effects for several days, animals were not tested until the fifth day post lesion. This strategy produced quite different results from those previously observed. That is, in the first day of testing an extinction-like pattern of responding was observed. Animals displayed bursts of responding followed by occasional "sampling" of the lever (see Figure 4). This is in contrast to the complete failure of animals to respond more than one or two times when tested the day following the lesion (cf. Figure 2).

One explanation for these effects is that until the 6-OHDA-induced degeneration is complete, cocaine may have a pharmacological action on the degenerating terminals. In fact, it has been shown that the blockade of amphetamine and cocaine-induced locomotor activity following 6-OHDA accumbens lesions follows a pattern very similar to that observed in the self-administration studies. Unless a severe depletion of DA is achieved, no blockade of the drug-induced locomotor response is observed (Joyce & Roberts, unpublished observations). Furthermore, the blockade of the locomotor response is not permanent but recovers in many animals just as does the self-administration behavior (Kelly, Saviour, & Iversen, 1975). Interestingly, when tested immediately following 6-OHDA injections, stimulants can elicit vigorous and bizarre behaviors (Creese & Iversen, 1975). This may explain the suppressed self-administration for cocaine immediately after the lesion, if this interaction of drug with degenerating terminals is aversive.

The results observed in both the self-administration and locomotor activity studies are probably interpretable if one considers that at least two mechanisms take place following a lesion--degeneration and recovery. It is difficult to assess the time course for each of these neuroanatomical/neurochemical changes or the degree to which they may interact. It appears that any results observed in the first few days after the lesion are confounded by neuronal degeneration, and that alterations in a drug response may be due to an interaction with a degenerating system rather than on one which has been destroyed.

On the other hand, if the animals are not tested until several weeks after the lesions, compensatory mechanisms may mask the "true" lesion effect. If one assumes that degenerative effects are limited to the first few days and that the influence of compensatory mechanisms is minimal for two weeks, then testing during this middle period best reflects the treatment effect. Of course there may be no appropriate testing period if the lesions are incomplete because recovery processes may already be influencing the results as degeneration proceeds.

ACQUISITION OF SELF-ADMINISTRATION

Another approach that has been used to investigate stimulant reward has been to examine the acquisition curve of animals learning to self-administer the drug. If it is assumed that animals will only acquire the self-administration response when the drug injection is rewarding, then failure to acquire the task following lesions of specific neural pathways supposedly reflects an attenuation or blockade of the reinforcing properties of the drug. A reduction of the rewarding effects should, therefore, retard the acquisition of self-administration behavior. Conversely, the stronger the reward, the faster the acquisition; therefore, faster acquisition may reflect a potentiation of the reinforcing effects. Examples of both accelerated and retarded acquisition of stimulant self-administration employing a variety of lesion techniques may be found in the literature.

5,7-Dihydroxytryptamine (5,7-DHT)

Lyness et al. (1980) have shown that animals injected with 5,7-DHT in the lateral cerebral ventricles self-injected more amphetamine from the first day of training and their intake stabilized at a higher level. Interestingly, the number of sessions required before the lesioned animals stabilized did not differ from controls, indicating that acquisition was not in fact enhanced. The locus of this effect is uncertain. Since 5,7-DHT injections into the nucleus accumbens exaggerate the hyperactive response to amphetamine (Pycock et al., 1978), Lyness et al. (1980) tested the possibility that serotonin depletion from this nucleus may mediate the effect. Injection of 5,7-DHT into the accumbens had no effect on the acquisition of amphetamine self-administration. Therefore, the involvement of serotonin in the acquisition of stimulant self-administration is as yet undefined.

Radiofrequency Lesions

A similar strategy, but a different lesion technique, was used by LeMoal et al. (1979). They reported that radiofrequency lesions to the mesolimbic DA cell bodies of the ventral tegmental area (VTA) result in an improved acquisition of (+)-amphetamine self-administered by rats. Following a one month recovery period from the lesion, animals were catheterized and allowed to self-administer amphetamine every other day for a 12-hour session. Lever pressing for amphetamine evolved dramatically with an extreme sensitivity to the drug and with enhanced acquisition of the operant response (see Figure 5a). The authors have suggested that this acquisition paradigm may be particularly useful for revealing pre-existing vulnerability to amphetamine and "psychopathology which leads to addiction" (p. 158).

These results, however, are inconsistent with literature which suggests that DA is the critical neurotransmitter involved in stimulant reinforcement. If mesolimbic DA is necessary for the rewarding value of amphetamine, then destruction of these perikarya should have resulted in a slower rate of acquisition of amphetamine self-administration or in a total failure to acquire the response.

One possible explanation for these findings may be the inability to have performed a complete lesion of the mesolimbic-cortical DA projection with the radiofrequency method, unlike the total destruction of DA terminals that may be obtained employing 6-OHDA. In studies employing the 6-OHDA lesion technique, destruction of DA terminals results in a failure to acquire self-infusion of amphetamine (Lyness et al., 1979). Experimentally naive rats pretreated with

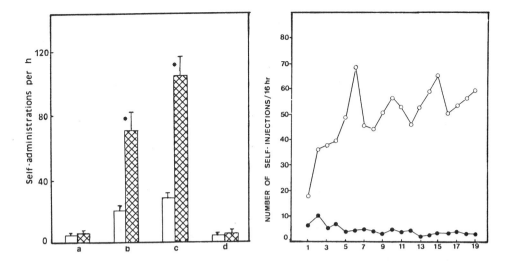

Figure 5A: (+)Amphetamine self-administration (0.75 mg/kg (+)amphetamine per 100 administrations) in rats after radiofrequency lesions of the dopaminergic meso-cortico-limbic (A10) cell group lying in the ventral mesencephalic tegmentum (VMT) surrounding the interpeduncular nucleus (lesioned against controls: *p < 0.001, Student's t-test). **a,** Operant session; **b,** first (+)amphetamine session; **c,** second (+)amphetamine session; **d,** saline; open bars, Controls; n = 20; hatched bars, VMT-A10 lesioned; n = 27. Reprinted with permission from LeMoal, Stinus, and Simon, 1979. Copyright 1979 by MacMillan Journals Ltd.

Figure 5B: Effect of 6-OHDA-induced lesions of DA nerve terminals in nucleus accumbens on the acquisition of d-amphetamine self-administration. Self-administration studies were started 14 days after the bilateral injection of vehicle (o) or 6-OHDA (●) into the nucleus accumbens of rats (four rats in each group). Each symbol represents the mean number of self-injections of d-amphetamine (0.125 mg/kg/injection; FR-1) made during 19 consecutive daily 16-hour sessions. Adapted from Lyness, Friedle, and Moore, 1979. Copyright 1979 by Ankho International, Inc.

6-OHDA in the nucleus accumbens did not acquire self-administration behavior despite only a 95% depletion of accumbens DA; this is true even when they are allowed access for the drug for up to 19 days (see Figure 5B). It is also possible that the one month recovery period allowed by LeMoal et al. (1979) in combination with damage to other nondopaminergic systems could also account for the apparent discrepancy.

The results from these and other studies which employ the acquisition technique inevitably pose the question of what an animal must learn during self-administration acquisition. It must be that animals not only learn that pressing a lever produces an injection but also that responding too often will produce toxic effects. Animals sometimes self-administer lethal doses during the first training session and some lesions appear to increase the likelihood that an animal will take a toxic overdose. Therefore, does the amount of drug taken on the first day necessarily reflect anything useful? Possibly not, although it does appear that a high intake on the first day does predict a higher level of drug intake once the animal has stabilized its pattern of intake. Conversely, a low level may indicate a low stabilization rate or a lesser likelihood that an animal will acquire the behavior. However, neither of these outcomes are predictive of the amount of time an animal will require before intake stabilization. It may be that the rate of acquisition measures something different from the ultimate level of stable intake.

CONCLUSIONS AND RECOMMENDATIONS

In general, then, the self-administration procedure has proven a particularly useful technique to the extent that it produces a stable behavior that can be quantified and qualified both preoperatively as a baseline behavior and postoperatively as a dependent measure of the effects of various lesions. Its use, however, should be approached with some degree of caution. The relative value of any behavioral task is dependent upon the types of questions being posed by the experimenter. For example, the processes involved in acquisition may not be the same as those responsible for the maintenance of the behavior.

Although one of the more attractive features of self-administration behavior is its apparent simplicity, the mechanisms which govern it are exceedingly complex. It would be preferable to view the behavior as a combination or sequence of responses and cognitive events, perhaps mediated by distinct neurochemical systems, which interact to produce the self-administration response. Accordingly, when a disruption in the response is observed, it could be due to the absence of a single neurobiological event or perhaps a breakdown in a complex patterns of events. We should expect that many systems may be critical and should, therefore, be cautious in our interpretations when a disruption is observed. Many systems may also be redundant. Therefore, a failure to disrupt the response or a recovery of the response may indicate compensation of other constituents.

With appropriate lesioning techniques the self-administration procedure is a valuable research tool in the analysis of drug reward. However, there are three important factors which will determine its worth. Firstly, the choice of the lesioning procedure is critical. Electrolytic or radiofrequency lesions seem inappropriate for questions involving specific transmitter systems. With regard to neurotoxins, their value is directly proportional to their specificity in destroying only identifiable classes of cells. Regardless of the nature of the lesion, the importance of allotting sufficient time for recovery cannot be overemphasized. Incomplete lesions can produce bizarre effects due to long-term regeneration or supersensitivity of damaged systems. Complete degeneration of cell bodies, axon terminals, etc. is essential if the behavioral data is to be of any use.

Secondly, the behavioral data cannot be interpreted unless the lesion is adequately characterized. In the case of 6-OHDA and 5,7-DHT, this requires biochemical data to determine the extent of the lesion. It would seem appropriate to investigate also the pattern of cell or terminal field damage through histochemical methods. For other neurotoxins such as ibotenic or kainic acid lesions, complete histology is essential.

Lastly, the behavioral effect must be characterized. It is an important question whether a lesion-induced disruption of self-administration for one drug is specific to that drug or is a more general phenomenon. Dose-response curves may be worthwhile but they may not always be possible to generate if the behavior is changing following the lesion or if the animal fails to self-administer at all. In all cases it is preferable to test subjects as long as is practical for recovery in order that the behavioral effect produced by the lesion can be fully characterized. This is feasible particularly if the experimental design is not unnecessarily complicated.

ACKNOWLEDGMENTS

Supported by the Medical Research Council (Grant MA7374) and the Natural Sciences and Engineering Research Council (Grant A7471) of Canada.

REFERENCES

Baxter, B. L., Gluckman, M. I., Stein, L., & Scerni, R. A. (1974). Self-injection of apomorphine in the rat: Positive reinforcement by a dopamine receptor stimulant. Pharmacology Biochemistry & Behavior, 2, 387-391.

Baxter, B. L., Gluckman, M. I., & Scerni, R. A. (1976). Apomorphine self-injection is not affected by alpha-methylparatyrosine treatment: Support for dopaminergic reward. Pharmacology Biochemistry & Behavior, 4, 611-612.

Bedford, J. A., Bailey, L. P., & Wilson, M. C. (1978). Cocaine reinforced progressive ratio performance in the rhesus monkey. Pharmacology Biochemistry & Behavior, 9, 631-638.

Clavier, R. M., & Fibiger, H. C. (1978). On the role of ascending catecholaminergic projections in intracranial self-stimulation of the substantia nigra. Brain Research, 131, 271-286.

Creese, I., & Iversen, S. D. (1975). The pharmacological and anatomical substrates of the amphetamine response in the rat. Brain Research, 83, 419-436.

Deneau, G., Yanagita, T., & Seevers, M. H. (1969). Self-administration of psychoactive substances by the monkey. Psychopharmacologia, 16, 30-48.

de Wit, H., & Wise, R. A. (1977). Blockade of cocaine reinforcement in rats with the dopamine receptor blocker pimozide, but not with noradrenergic blockers phentolamine and phenoxybenzamine. Canadian Journal of Psychology, 31, 195-203.

Fibiger, H. C., Carter, D. A., & Phillips, A. G. (1976). Decreased intracranial self-stimulation after neuroleptics or 6-hydroxydopamine: Evidence for mediation by motor deficits rather than by reduced reward. Psychopharmacology, 47, 21-27.

Griffiths, R. R., Findley, J. D., Brady, J. V., Gutcher, K., & Robinson, W. W. (1975). Comparison of progressive-ratio performance maintained by cocaine, methylphenidate and secobarbital. Psychopharmacology, 43, 81-83.

Griffiths, R. R., Bradford, L. D., & Brady, J. V. (1979). Progressive ratio and fixed ratio schedules of cocaine-maintained responding in baboons. Psychopharmacology, 65, 125-136.

Griffiths, R. R., Brady, J. V., & Snell, J. C. (1978). Progressive ratio performance maintained by drug infusions: Comparison of cocaine, diethylpropion, chlorphentermine, and fenfluramine. Psychopharmacology, 56, 5-13.

Grove, R. N., & Schuster, C. R. (1974). Suppression of cocaine self-administration by extinction and punishment. Pharmacology Biochemistry & Behavior, 2, 199-208.

Hodos, W. (1961). Progressive ratio as a measure of reward strength. Science, 134, 943-944.

Hodos, W., & Kalman, J. (1963). Effects of increment size and reinforcer volume on progressive ratio performance. Journal of Experimental Analysis of Behavior, 6, 387-392.

Hoffmeister, F. (1979). Progressive-ratio performance in the rhesus monkey maintained by opiate infusions. Psychopharmacology, 62, 181-186.

Iglauer, C., & Woods, J. H. (1974). Concurrent performances: Reinforcement of different doses of intravenous cocaine in the rhesus monkey. Journal of Experimental Analysis of Behavior, 22, 179-196.

Iglauer, C., Llewellyn, M. E., & Woods, J. H. (1976). Concurrent schedules of cocaine injection in rhesus monkeys: Dose variations under independent and non-independent variable interval procedures. Pharmacological Review, 27, 367-383.

Johanson, C. E. (1977). The effect of electric shock on responding maintained by cocaine injections in a choice procedure in the rhesus monkey. Psychopharmacology, 53, 277-282.

Johanson, C. E., Balster, R. L., & Bonese, K. (1976). Self-administration of psychomotor stimulant drugs: The effects of unlimited access. Pharmacology Biochemistry & Behavior, 4, 45-51.

Kelly, P. H., Saviour, P., & Iversen, S. D. (1975). Amphetamine and apomorphine responses in the rat following 6-OHDA lesions of the nucleus accumbens septi and corpus striatum. Brain Research, 94, 507-522.

König, J. F. R., & Klippel, R. A. (1970). The rat brain: A stereotaxic atlas of the forebrain and lower parts of the brainstem. Baltimore: Williams & Wilkins.

Kostrzewa, R. M., & Jacobowitz, D. M. (1974). Pharmacological actions of 6-OHDA. Pharmacological Reviews, 26(3), 199-288.

Kramer, J. C., Fishman, V. S., & Littlefield, D. C. (1967). Amphetamine abuse: Pattern and effects of high doses taken intravenously. Journal of the American Medical Association, 201, 305-309.

LeMoal, M., Stinus, L., & Simon, H. (1979). Increased sensitivity to (+)amphetamine self-administered by rats following meso-cortico-limbic dopamine neurone destruction. Nature, 280, 156-158.

Lyness, W. H., Friedle, N. M., & Moore, K. E. (1979). Destruction of dopaminergic nerve terminal in nucleus accumbens: Effect on d-amphetamine self-administration. Pharmacology Biochemistry & Behavior, 11, 553-556.

Lyness, W. H., Friedle, N. M., & Moore, K. E. (1980). Increased self-administration of d-amphetamine after destruction of 5-hydroxytryptamine neurons. Pharmacology Biochemistry & Behavior, 12, 937-941.

Pickens, R. (1968). Self-administration of stimulants by rats. International Journal of Addiction, 3, 215-222.

Pickens, R., & Thompson, T. (1968). Cocaine-reinforced behavior in rats: Effects of reinforcement magnitude and fixed ratio size. Journal of Pharmacology and Experimental Therapeutics, 161, 122-129.

Pycock, C. J., Horton, R. W., & Carter, C. J. (1980). Interactions of 5-hydroxytryptamine and γ-aminobutyric acid with dopamine. In P. J. Roberts, G. N.Woodruff, & L. L. Iversen (Eds.), Advances in biochemical psychopharmacology (Vol. 19, pp. 323-341). New York: Raven Press.

Roberts, D. C. S., Corcoran, M. E., & Fibiger, H. C. (1977). On the role of ascending catecholamine systems in self-administration of cocaine. Pharmacology Biochemistry & Behavior, 6, 615-620.

Roberts, D. C. S., & Koob, G. F. (1982). Disruption of cocaine self-administration following 6-hydroxydopamine lesions of the ventral tegmental area in rats. Pharmacology Biochemistry & Behavior, 17, 901-904.

Roberts, D. C. S., Koob, G. F., Klonoff, P., & Fibiger, H. C. (1980). Extinction and recovery of cocaine self-administration following 6-hydroxydopamine lesions of the nucleus accumbens. Pharmacology Biochemistry & Behavior, 12, 781-787.

Roberts, D. C. S., Zis, A. P., & Fibiger, H. C. (1975). Ascending catecholamine pathways and amphetamine-induced locomotor activity: Importance of dopamine and apparent non-involvement of norepinephrine. Brain Research, 93, 441-454.

Singer, S. G., Wallace, M., & Hall, R. (1982). Effects of dopaminergic nucleus accumbens lesions on the acquisition of schedule induced self-injection of nicotine in the rat. Pharmacology Biochemistry & Behavior, 17, 579-581.

Smith, S. G., & Davis, W. M. (1974). Punishment of amphetamine and morphine self-administration behavior. Psychological Record, 24, 477-480.

Yanagita, T. (1973). An experimental framework for evaluation of dependence liability in various types of drugs in monkeys. Bulletin on Narcotics, 1, 25-27.

Yokel, R. A., & Wise, R. A. (1975). Increased lever pressing for amphetamine after pimozide in rats: Implication for a dopamine theory of reward. Science, 187, 547-549.

Yokel, R. A., & Wise, R. A. (1976). Attenuation of intravenous amphetamine reinforcement by central dopamine blockade in rats. Psychopharmacology, 48, 311-318.

CHAPTER 5

SECOND-ORDER SCHEDULES OF DRUG INJECTION

Jonathan L. Katz and Steven R. Goldberg

NIDA Addiction Research Center
P.O. Box 5180
Baltimore, MD   21224
and
Department of Pharmacology and Experimental Therapeutics
University of Maryland School of Medicine
Baltimore, MD   21201

Introduction

One of the most noteworthy features of the behavior of human drug abusers is the extent to which their behavioral repertoire consists of responses maintained by procurement, preparation, and the ultimate administration of drug. Since abusers can be totally consumed with drug-seeking and drug-oriented behaviors and since drug abuse is obviously maladaptive, many theories of drug addiction and abuse have emphasized what were thought to be fundamental pathologies in personality or motivations unique to the drug abuser. However, as Sidman (1960) noted many years ago, pathological states in behavior, as in medicine, can be manifestations of normal processes which are determined, lawful extensions of normal functioning in what is often an atypical environment. Excessive behavior maintained by drug, therefore, may be functionally no different from other behavior but maintained in an environment that promotes its predominance. Following the above interpretation, laboratory studies can examine the extent to which drug-seeking or drug-taking behavior is different from behavior maintained by other stimulus events. A related question is whether the reinforcing effects of drugs are fundamentally different from the reinforcing effects of other events that maintain behavior.

Initial laboratory studies of drugs as reinforcing events were primarily concerned with determining whether drug injections could maintain behavior in experimental animals. With few exceptions, early studies did well if reinforcement by drug injection was firmly established. The meager amounts of behavior maintained by drugs in those studies distinguished drug-maintained behavior from behavior maintained by more conventionally used reinforcing events, such as food or water presentation, since these latter behaviors were typically maintained at higher rates and with patterns characteristic of the schedule under which the reinforcer was presented. Ironically, the distinguishing features of drug-maintained behavior in laboratory studies were in contradistinction to the excessive features that distinguish human drug-seeking and drug-taking.

An experiment by Pickens and Thompson (1968) on cocaine-reinforced behavior in rats indicated that differences in the manner of scheduling intravenous cocaine injections and more conventional reinforcers accounted for some of the differences between the levels of behavior maintained. Since venous catheters remained patent for relatively short times, drug-maintained responding could be studied only during relatively few experimental sessions. In order to collect more data, those sessions were longer than those used for studying behavior maintained by other events. Performances maintained by cocaine injection were characterized by long pauses and rates of responding that were inversely related to dose of cocaine. In contrast, under schedules of food presentation during shorter experimental sessions, pauses after reinforcement were relatively short and rates of responding were directly related to the amount of food presented. When food-maintained responding was studied in long experimental sessions, however, the rates of responding were, as with cocaine injection, inversely related to the magnitude of reinforcement. Thus, food-maintained behaviors could be made more similar to cocaine-maintained behaviors if conditions of the study were modified to resemble those under which drug-maintained behavior was studied.

Other investigators have modified conditions under which drug-maintained responding was studied so that performances maintained by drug were more similar to those typically maintained by reinforcers such as food presentation. The implications of progress along this line were discussed by Morse (1975). With technical innovations for prolonged catheter life and, importantly, the discovery of procedures and combinations of parameter values that yielded optimal performances, responding maintained by drug injections has recently more closely approximated that maintained by more conventional reinforcing events.

Events that function as reinforcers generally have effects on behavior in addition to reinforcing effects. In most studies responding is maintained by reinforcers presented repeatedly throughout an experimental session according to some schedule. Under these conditions effects of the stimuli other than reinforcing effects can interfere with subsequent responding. Large magnitudes of food as a reinforcer can have satiating effects that interfere with subsequent responding (Goldberg, 1973; Sidman & Stebbins, 1954). Electric-shock presentation can elicit responses that are incompatible with the reinforced response (Smith, Gustavson, & Gregor, 1972). Drugs can have direct pharmacological effects on rates of responding (e.g., Kelleher & Morse, 1968) in addition to their reinforcing effects. For example, Pickens and Thompson (1968) found that within-session intravenous injections of cocaine in rats trained under fixed-ratio schedules of food presentation produced pauses in responding that were similar to those observed after injection in rats self-administering cocaine. Thus, the pauses following cocaine reinforcement were likely due to a direct effect of the drug on subsequent responding.

The conditions under which drugs maintain performances similar to those maintained by other reinforcers often are those that minimize direct pharmacological effects that can interfere with subsequent behavior. One method for minimizing direct pharmacological effects on subsequent responding is to schedule a time-out period following each injection during which stimuli are absent and responses of the subject have no scheduled consequences. Scheduling time-out periods following injections often produces patterns and rates of responding maintained by drug injection that more closely approximate those maintained by other reinforcers (Goldberg, 1973; Kelleher, 1975; Woods & Schuster, 1971).

One function of the time-out following drug injection is that it spaces response-produced injections such that cumulative direct effects of the drugs are lessened. Some schedules have similar effects. Under fixed-interval schedules, for example, there is a minimum time period between successive injections. Although long interval schedules are more effective in minimizing cumulative drug effects, responding may become poorly maintained as the interval is extended. Second-order schedules have been used to maintain extended sequences of responding between scheduled injections. Under one type of second-order schedule, each nth response produces a brief visual stimulus (fixed ratio or FR schedule), and the first FR completed after the lapse of a fixed interval (FI) produces the stimulus accompanied by a drug injection. The entire schedule can be designated FI (FR:S) following the nomenclature of Kelleher (1966).

Second-Order Schedules of Drug Injection

Figure 1 shows a cumulative record of performance of a squirrel monkey under a second-order schedule of cocaine injection where each 30th response produced a 2-second visual stimulus (FR-30:S) and the first FR-30 completed after the lapse of a 5-minute interval produced the stimulus change accompanied by an injection of cocaine. Each presentation of the 2-second visual stimulus is depicted in the record by a slash mark on the cumulative response curve; a 1-minute time-out that followed the injection is depicted by an offset of the lower event line. Each sequence of 30 responses was typically preceded by a pause and the longest pauses occurred early in the interval. Over the entire 5-minute interval, there was a pattern of positive acceleration of responding up to the cocaine injection. This pattern of responding is similar to that obtained with other drugs (Goldberg & Tang, 1977) and other nondrug reinforcing events (Barrett, Katz, & Glowa, 1981; Goldberg, 1973).

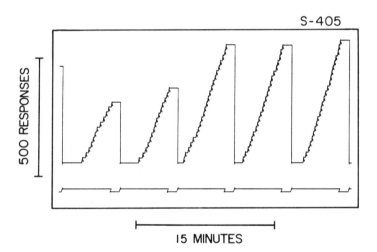

Figure 1: Cumulative record of a performance of a squirrel monkey responding under a second-order schedule of cocaine injection during a portion of one experimental session. Abscissa: time; Ordinate: cumulative responses. Slashes on the cumulative record designate 2-second presentations of the visual stimulus that accompanied cocaine injection at the end of the fixed interval. The offset of the lower event line indicates the 1-minute time-out that followed each cocaine injection. The recording reset to base after each 1-minute time-out. S. R. Goldberg, unpublished data.

Under second-order schedules, the stimuli that ultimately accompany the drug injection can serve to maintain responding themselves as conditioned reinforcers. Kelleher (1958) first suggested that extended sequences of behavior maintained by conditioned reinforcing stimuli might be of practical importance in the study of drugs as reinforcers since the influence of the drug on subsequent behavior could be minimized. In addition to practical utility, second-order schedules have proven to be of use in establishing extended sequences of behavior in experimental animals that are in many ways analogous to extended sequences of behavior in human abusers involving procurement, preparation, and administration of drug. Moreover, the amounts of behavior maintained under second-order schedules are more in accord with observations in human drug abusers of significant portions of their daily activities involving drug-seeking or drug-oriented behavior (Goldberg & Gardner, 1981).

Effects of Drug Dose

Under all schedules of drug injection, the rates of responding maintained are dependent upon the dose of drug administered per injection. Figure 2 shows data from several studies on effects of cocaine dose per injection on response rates maintained under different schedules of cocaine injection. Under the FI 5-minute schedule, the first response after 5 minutes produced a cocaine injection followed by a 1-minute time-out period, and experimental sessions lasted until 15 injections were administered (Goldberg & Kelleher, 1976). Low doses maintained low rates of responding that were comparable to those maintained by vehicle. Higher rates were maintained by higher doses with the maximal rates maintained at a dose of 50 µg/kg/injection. At higher doses, rates of responding were below the maximum rate maintained. The lower response rates at the highest doses are often attributed to direct pharmacological effects of the drug on subsequent responding, since these doses also decrease rates of responding maintained by reinforcers other than drug injection (cf. Spealman & Kelleher, 1979).

Initial studies with second-order schedules (Goldberg, 1973) suggested that a wide range of doses maintained maximal rates of responding. Figure 2 also shows effects of cocaine dose on response rates maintained under an FI 5-minute (FR:S) second-order schedule of cocaine injection with the temporal parameters of the schedule similar to the FI 5-minute schedule. Under the second-order schedule, rates of responding were much higher than those maintained under the FI 5-minute schedule. Additionally, the range of doses that maintained high rates is noteworthy since under the FI 5-minute schedule, rates of responding were decreased below maximum at doses that maintained high rates under the second-order schedule (Goldberg, Kelleher, & Goldberg, 1981a). Possibly, the direct effect on response rate of accumulated cocaine from successive injections was in some manner modulated by the brief stimuli presented under the second-order schedule.

Although spacing injections apart and interposing time-out periods following injections each limit the degree to which direct pharmacological effects alter subsequent responding, with parameters typically employed direct effects are not entirely eliminated. One method of precluding direct effects of the consequent drug injection is to arrange the schedule parameters so that one or several injections are administered, but only at the end of the experimental session. Under schedules such as these, responding is maintained throughout a relatively long interval until a response produces the consequent injection ending the experimental session. Second-order schedules have been particularly useful under these conditions in maintaining responding over long periods of time up to the ultimate injection. In several studies (Goldberg & Tang, 1977; Kelleher & Goldberg, 1977; Goldberg et al., 1981a) in which the injections were administered only at the end of the session, response rates increased with dose of the drug and high rates were maintained at doses that decreased rates under schedules in which injections occurred repeatedly within sessions.

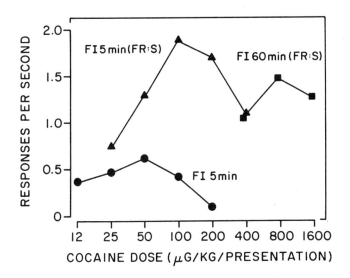

Figure 2: Effects of dose of cocaine per presentation on average rates of responding maintained under different schedules of cocaine injection. Circles: fixed-interval 5-minute schedule with a 1-minute time-out following each injection and 15 injections per experimental session (squirrel monkeys S-467 and S-474). Adapted with permission from Goldberg and Kelleher, 1976. Triangles: second-order schedule, FI 5-minute (FR:S), with a 1-minute time-out following each injection and 15 injections per experimental session. Adapted with permission from Goldberg, Kelleher, and Goldberg, 1981a. Squares: second-order schedule, FI 60-min (FR:S), with 15 injections of cocaine spaced 2 seconds apart following the reinforced response concluding the experimental session. Adapted with permission from Goldberg, Kelleher, and Goldberg, 1981a. Abscissa: dose of cocaine per presentation, log scale. Ordinate: mean overall response rates. See individual studies for details of experimental procedures.

Figure 2 also shows effects of cocaine dose on responding maintained under an FI 60-minute (FR:S) schedule when the experimental session ended after the injection of cocaine. High rates were maintained at a dose of 1.5 mg/kg; higher doses would likely produce convulsions. In contrast under the FI 5-minute (FR:S) schedule when injections occurred throughout the session, response rates were well below the maximum at 0.4 mg/kg/injection (Goldberg et al., 1981a).

Stimulus Functions Under Second-Order Schedules

Functions of brief stimuli presented under second-order schedules of drug injection and food presentation have been extensively reviewed (Goldberg & Gardner, 1981; Gollub, 1977) and here will be summarized only briefly. Figure 3 shows the effects on rates of responding of removing the brief stimuli entirely or of substituting a brief stimulus that is not paired with either cocaine or morphine (Goldberg, Spealman, & Kelleher, 1979). Responding was maintained under second-order schedules in which completion of an FR requirement produced a brief stimulus and the first FR completed after 10 minutes (cocaine) or 60 minutes (morphine) always produced an amber light accompanying the drug injection. For studies of nonpaired brief stimuli, a brief blue light followed completion of each FR, whereas an amber light accompanied the drug injection. For studies on omission of the brief stimuli, the only stimulus change was the brief amber light that accompanied injections. Omissions of the brief stimuli decreased response rates as has been shown in other studies (Goldberg et al., 1981a; Goldberg, Spealman, & Goldberg, 1981b; Goldberg & Tang, 1977; Katz, 1979). Similar results are obtained under second-order schedules with fixed-interval components (Katz, 1979; Kelleher & Goldberg, 1977).

One study (Goldberg et al., 1981a) compared effects of omission of the brief stimuli on responding under second-order schedules of food or cocaine presentation at two different parameter values. Under one schedule food was presented or drug was injected following the first FR unit completed after 5 minutes. Under the other schedule the interval value was 60 minutes and the session ended after food was presented or cocaine was injected. Removing the brief stimuli decreased rates of cocaine-maintained responding under either schedule but only decreased food-maintained responding under the schedule employing the 60-minute interval. These results suggest that the brief stimulus associated with cocaine injection has some properties that are distinct from those of brief stimuli associated with food presentation.

Studies in which nonpaired brief stimuli were substituted for paired brief stimuli have also shown decreases in response rates with nonpaired stimuli (see Figure 3; Goldberg, Spealman, & Kelleher, 1979). The decreases in rates, however, were smaller than those that occurred when the brief stimuli were removed entirely. Similar results were obtained under second-order schedules with fixed-interval components (Katz, 1979). The finding that nonpaired stimuli maintained rates of responding greater than those maintained with stimuli entirely eliminated is not surprising considering the similarity of the paired and nonpaired stimuli.

Comparisons of Drug-Maintained Responding and Food-Maintained Responding

Several studies have compared responding maintained under second-order schedules of drug injection with that maintained under comparable schedules by other reinforcing events. Initial studies indicated that responding maintained under second-order schedules of cocaine injection was maintained at rates higher than those maintained by more conventionally used reinforcing events such as food presentation (Spealman & Goldberg, 1978). Therefore, it was of interest to determine whether the differences in responding maintained by cocaine and other reinforcing events were due to unique properties of cocaine as a reinforcer.

Figure 3: Rates of responding under second-order schedules of intravenous cocaine or morphine injection when the completion of every fixed-ratio component during a fixed interval produced either a paired or nonpaired brief stimulus or when brief stimuli were omitted altogether. Overall rates were calculated by dividing responses by total time elapsed; local rates were calculated by dividing responses by the time elapsed from the first to last response of each fixed-ratio component. Bars show average rates of responding during the last three sessions of each condition for individual monkeys; brackets show ranges. Each condition was studied for 5 to 20 consecutive sessions. Reprinted with permission from Goldberg, Spealman, and Kelleher, 1979. Copyright 1979 by Pergamon Press, Inc.

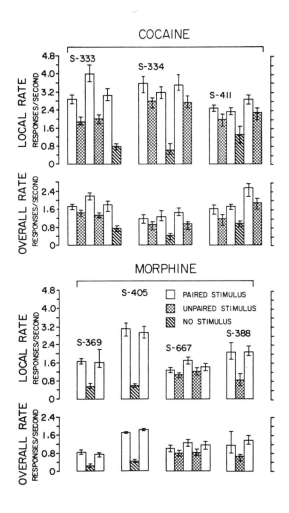

Differences between rates of responding maintained under second-order schedules of cocaine injection and food presentation were found initially in studies where injections were scheduled to recur within experimental sessions. There are a number of effects of repeated presentations of cocaine within sessions which may influence the rates of responding maintained by cocaine. Administration of cocaine can alter subsequent responding due to direct pharmacological effects of the drug on the output of behavior. These effects may become manifest as an increase or a decrease in rates of responding depending on the accumulated dose of cocaine. Additionally, it has been suggested that psychomotor stimulants, such as cocaine, increase the effectiveness of conditioned reinforcing stimuli (e.g., Hill, 1970; Robbins, 1975). Either of these effects of cocaine may better account for differences between cocaine-maintained responding and responding maintained by other events than the postulated unique reinforcing properties of cocaine.

Under second-order schedules in which all drug injections occur at the end of the experimental sessions, the responding maintained is not influenced by direct pharmacological effects of the drug since, with sessions conducted daily, the pharmacological effects have subsided by the next session. In comparisons of food- and cocaine-maintained responding under these schedules, rates of responding maintained by the two events were comparable (Goldberg et al., 1981a; Katz, 1979) suggesting that an effect of cocaine injection within experimental sessions is critical to the differences in rates of responding maintained by cocaine and food presentation. Further, pre-session injection of cocaine in monkeys responding under second-order schedules in which food presentation recurs throughout sessions increases rates of responding to rates comparable to those maintained by cocaine when cocaine injections recur throughout sessions (Goldberg et al., 1981a). Additionally, pre-session injection of cocaine has comparable effects on food- and cocaine-maintained responding when those reinforcing events occur only at the end of experimental sessions (Valentine, Katz, Kandel, & Barrett, 1983). Thus, it appears that the differences in rates of responding maintained by cocaine injection and food presentation under second-order schedules are due to a pharmacological effect of cocaine rather than a unique property of cocaine as a reinforcer. Moreover, the increases in response rates produced by cocaine are comparable regardless of whether responses produce brief stimuli (Goldberg et al., 1981a). Therefore, it appears that the differences in rates of responding maintained by cocaine injection or food presentation are due to the direct effects of cocaine on rates of subsequent responding rather than a potentiation of the reinforcing effectiveness of the brief stimuli.

That under specific schedule conditions behavior maintained by disparate events such as food delivery or drug injection can be similar has several implications for the experimental study of drug abuse and also for psychology in general. In developing performances maintained by drug injections, conditions are arranged that minimize or preclude effects of the injection other than reinforcing effects. A major part of the development of procedures for maintaining behavior with consequent drug injections has been eliminating or minimizing these other effects of drug injections. In studies with more conventional reinforcers, such as food presentation, the procedures that have evolved are those under which other effects of the reinforcer are minimal. For example, the amount of food presented is typically so small that significant changes in the degree of deprivation of the subject do not occur within the experimental session. In general, the conditions under which any event can be suitably used as a reinforcer in laboratory studies depends on eliminating effects other than reinforcing effects that can influence subsequent responding (Morse, 1975). For the most part it is the other effects of a consequent event that make its use as a reinforcer unique. When these other effects are precluded, reinforcing effects of diverse stimuli can be observed to be quite similar. That diverse consequent events can control behavior similarly indicates that the performances maintained have an integrity that transcends the particular reinforcer employed and, moreover, that the schedules under which those events are presented are of critical importance in determining the performances maintained.

Implications of Performances Under Second-Order Schedules for Assessing the Reinforcing Properties of Abused Drugs

The importance of the schedule under which drugs are presented in the behavioral analysis of drug abuse cannot be over emphasized. Under some schedules a drug may be readily self-administered whereas under other schedules it may not be. Thus, questions about the reinforcing strength or efficacy of a particular drug are more profitably couched as questions about the conditions under which that drug will function as a reinforcer. Some investigators have attempted to rank order drugs as to their reinforcing efficacy (e.g., Griffiths, Brady, & Bradford, 1979). However, the rank order of the reinforcing effectiveness of particular drugs would be limited to the conditions studied and of little real applicability.

Some have considered the range of conditions under which a drug will function as a reinforcer as an indication of the reinforcing efficacy of a drug; the assumption being that those drugs that maintain behavior over a more varied range of conditions are more effective reinforcers. Nicotine can both maintain behavior and punish behavior (Goldberg & Spealman, 1982) and, historically, maintenance of behavior by nicotine injection has been difficult to demonstrate in the laboratory (Henningfield & Goldberg, 1983). In contrast, cocaine has been studied as a reinforcer over a wide range of conditions in laboratory studies. However, a conclusion that cocaine is a drug of greater abuse potential than nicotine would stand in marked contrast with epidemiological studies of incidence of use of each of these drugs. Moreover, the rank order of reinforcing efficacy of a drug also has minimal therapeutic significance. A patient abusing a particular drug is given little comfort, and no better prognosis, by the knowledge that the drug is only self-administered under a limited range of conditions in experimental animals. Useful information is provided by studies that determine the conditions under which a drug maintains behavior and how changes in environmental conditions affect the behavior maintained.

The similarity of behaviors controlled by drugs and other consequent events brings into question tacit assumptions that apply to drugs as reinforcers (Morse, 1975). For example, it was noted above that the all-encompassing nature of drug-seeking and drug-oriented behaviors in human drug abusers suggested theories of abuse that emphasized pathology of personality or motivation of the drug abuser. Subsequently, experimental questions of whether drugs were unique as reinforcing stimuli were asked. Extended sequences of behavior under second-order schedules have been established in laboratory animals that are analogous to drug-seeking behaviors of human abusers. These behaviors resemble human drug seeking in that the subject engages in substantial amounts of activity and does virtually nothing else over extended periods of time.

Importantly, these extended sequences of behavior maintained by drug injection also resemble extended sequences of responding maintained by other reinforcers. These similarities emphasize that the all-consuming nature of drug-seeking and drug-taking is not the result of unnatural or pathological features of the drug abuser. Rather, these behaviors are the result of reinforcement by drug in an environment that controls behavior via natural processes such that drug related behavior becomes all but the exclusive activity of the subject. The "compulsive" gambler and overeater are analogous cases under the control of different reinforcing events. Under certain environmental conditions, events such as drug taking, overeating, or gambling may come to control unusual amounts of behavior, possibly because other effects that interfere with continued engagement in those activities are minimized. Under these conditions the normal sources of the "pathological" behavior reside in the unusual environment that creates conditions suitable for the maintenance and control of excessive amounts of behavior.

References

Barrett, J. E., Katz, J. L., & Glowa, J. R. (1981). Effects of d-amphetamine on responding of squirrel monkeys maintained under second-order schedules of food presentation, electric shock presentation or stimulus-shock termination. Journal of Pharmacology and Experimental Therapeutics, **218**, 692-700.

Goldberg, S. R. (1973). Comparable behavior maintained under fixed-ratio and second-order schedules of food presentation, cocaine injection or d-amphetamine injection in the squirrel monkey. Journal of Pharmacology and Experimental Therapeutics, **186**, 18-30.

Goldberg, S. R., & Gardner, M. L. (1981). Second-order schedules: Extended sequences of behavior controlled by brief environmental stimuli associated with drug self-administration. In T. Thompson & C. E. Johanson (Eds.), Behavioral pharmacology of human drug dependence (National Institute on Drug Abuse Research Monograph **37**, pp. 241-270). Washington, DC: U.S. Government Printing Office.

Goldberg, S. R., & Kelleher, R. T. (1976). Behavior controlled by scheduled injections of cocaine in squirrel and rhesus monkeys. Journal of the Experimental Analysis of Behavior, **25**, 93-104.

Goldberg, S. R., Kelleher, R. T., & Goldberg, D. M. (1981a). Fixed ratio responding under second-order schedules of food presentation or cocaine injection. Journal of Pharmacology and Experimental Therapeutics, **218**, 271-281.

Goldberg, S. R., & Spealman, R. D. (1982). Maintenance and suppression of behavior by nicotine injections in squirrel monkeys. Federation Proceedings, **41**, 216-220.

Goldberg, S. R., Spealman, R. D., & Goldberg, D. M. (1981b). Persistent high-rate behavior maintained by intravenous self-administration of nicotine. Science, **214**, 573-575.

Goldberg, S. R., Spealman, R. D., & Kelleher, R. T. (1979). Enhancement of drug-seeking behavior by environmental stimuli associated with cocaine or morphine injections. Neuropharmacology, **18**, 1015-1017.

Goldberg, S. R., & Tang, A. (1977). Behavior maintained under second-order schedules of intravenous morphine injection in squirrel and rhesus monkeys. Psychopharmacology, **51**, 235-242.

Gollub, L. R. (1977). Conditioned reinforcement: Schedule effects. In W. K. Honig & J. E. R. Staddon (Eds.), Handbook of operant behavior (pp. 288-312). Englewood Cliffs, NJ: Prentice-Hall.

Griffiths, R. R., Brady, J. V., & Bradford, L. D. (1979). Predicting the abuse liability of drugs with animal drug self-administration procedures: Psychomotor stimulants and hallucinogens. In T. Thompson & P. B. Dews (Eds.), Advances in behavioral pharmacology (Vol. 2, pp. 163-208). New York: Academic Press.

Henningfield, J. E., & Goldberg, S. R. (1983). Nicotine as a reinforcer in human subjects and laboratory animals. Pharmacology Biochemistry & Behavior, **19**, 989-992.

Hill, R. T. (1970). Facilitation of conditioned reinforcement as a mechanism of psychomotor stimulation. In E. Costa & S. Garattini (Eds.), Amphetamines and related compounds (pp. 781-795). New York: Raven Press.

Katz, J. L. (1979). A comparison of responding maintained under second-order schedules of intramuscular cocaine injection or food presentation in squirrel monkeys. Journal of the Experimental Analysis of Behavior, **32**, 419-431.

Kelleher, R. T. (1958). Fixed-ratio schedules of conditioned reinforcement with chimpanzees. Journal of the Experimental Analysis of Behavior, **1**, 281-289.

Kelleher, R. T. (1966). Chaining and conditioned reinforcement. In W. K. Honig (Ed.), Operant behavior: Areas of research and application (pp. 160-212). New York: Appleton-Century-Crofts.

Kelleher, R. T. (1975). Characteristics of behavior controlled by scheduled injections of drugs. Pharmacological Reviews, 27, 307-323.

Kelleher, R. T., & Goldberg, S. R. (1977). Fixed-interval responding under second-order schedules of food presentation or cocaine injection. Journal of the Experimental Analysis of Behavior, 28, 14-24.

Kelleher, R. T., & Morse, W. H. (1968). Determinants of the specificity of behavioral effects of drugs. Ergebnisse der Physiologie Biologischen Chemie und Experimentellen Pharmakologie, 60, 1-56.

Morse, W. H. (1975). Introduction: The control of behavior by consequent drug injections. Pharmacological Reviews, 27, 301-305.

Pickens, R., & Thompson, T. (1968). Cocaine-reinforced behavior in rats: Effects of reinforcement magnitude and fixed-ratio size. Journal of Pharmacology and Experimental Therapeutics, 161, 122-129.

Robbins, T. W. (1975). The potentiation of conditioned reinforcement by psychomotor stimulant drugs: A test of Hill's hypothesis. Psychopharmacologia, 45, 103-114.

Sidman, M. (1960). Normal sources of pathological behavior. Science, 132, 61-68.

Sidman, M., & Stebbins, W. C. (1954). Satiation effects under fixed-ratio schedules of reinforcement. Journal of Comparative and Physiological Psychology, 47, 114-116.

Smith, R. F., Gustavson, C. R., & Gregor, G. L. (1972). Incompatibility between the pigeon's unconditioned response to shock and the conditioned key-peck response. Journal of the Experimental Analysis of Behavior, 18, 147-153.

Spealman, R. D., & Goldberg, S. R. (1978). Drug self-administration by laboratory animals: Control by schedules of reinforcement. Annual Review of Pharmacology and Toxicology, 18, 313-339.

Spealman, R. D., & Kelleher, R. T. (1979). Behavioral effects of self-administered cocaine: Responding maintained alternately by cocaine and electric shock in squirrel monkeys. Journal of Pharmacology and Experimental Therapeutics, 210, 206-214.

Valentine, J. O., Katz, J. L., Kandel, D. A., & Barrett, J. E. (1983). Effects of cocaine, chlordiazepoxide, and chlorpromazine on responding of squirrel monkeys under second-order schedules of IM cocaine injection or food presentation. Psychopharmacology, 81, 164-169.

Woods, J. H., & Schuster, C. R. (1971). Opiates as reinforcing stimuli. In T. Thompson & R. Pickens (Eds.), Stimulus properties of drugs (pp. 163-175). New York: Appleton-Century-Crofts.

CHAPTER 6

INTRAVENOUS DRUG SELF-ADMINISTRATION: A SPECIAL CASE OF POSITIVE REINFORCEMENT

Roy A. Wise

Center for Studies in Behavioral Neurobiology
Department of Psychology
Concordia University
Montreal, Quebec, Canada H3G 1M8

ABSTRACT

Much has been made of parallels between drug reinforcement and food reinforcement. In several important ways, however, the two differ. Unlike food reinforcement, drug reinforcement has rapid and direct effects in the central nervous system. Where two classes of response--operant and consummatory--are required for food reinforcement, only one--having some of the properties of an operant and some of the properties of a consummatory response--is required for drug reinforcement. Where satiety is delayed by many minutes after food reward, it is immediate with drug reinforcement. These differences must be taken into account when interpreting drug reinforcement studies; in particular, they have important implications for interpreting changes in response and hourly drug intake.

INTRODUCTION

The field of behavioral pharmacology has focused attention over the last two decades on parallels between the behavior supported by drug reinforcement and that supported by more natural reinforcers (Griffiths, Brady, & Bradford, 1979; Johanson, 1978; Kelleher & Goldberg, 1975; Schuster & Johanson, 1981; Schuster & Thompson, 1969). Intravenous drug reinforcement can establish lever-pressing habits similar to the lever pressing established by food pellets, the key-pecking established by kernels of grain, and the coin insertion and lever-pulling established by gambling and arcade devices.

In general, each of the well known characteristics of various schedules of food reinforcement (Ferster & Skinner, 1957) can also be demonstrated with the intravenous drug self-administration paradigm (Johanson, 1978; Spealman & Goldberg, 1978). Habit acquisition is most rapid when one injection is given for each response (FR-1); habit extinction is most protracted when training involves one injection for a varied number of multiple responses. Responding is most regular when reinforcement is given on variable interval (VI) or variable ratio (VR) schedules; response rate varies predictably when reinforcement is given on fixed interval (FI) or fixed ratio (FR) schedules. Important advances in our thinking about drug abuse and in our understanding of its underlying mechanisms have come from exploring these and other parallels between drug reinforcement and food reinforcement.

Just as the early years of drug reinforcement research have involved extensive exploration of the parallels between drugs and "natural" reinforcers, so did much of the work in physiological psychology explore parallels between brain stimulation reinforcement and natural reinforcers. In this case, however, the first impression was that brain stimulation reinforcement was anomalous. Much was made at first of the differences between behavior supported by brain stimulation reinforcement and that supported by food reinforcement. In the case of brain stimulation, partial reinforcement had very weak effects; animals stopped working under partial reinforcement conditions at much higher reinforcement densities than are required to sustain robust lever-pressing for food or water (Deutsch, 1963; Seward, Uyeda, & Olds, 1959). Unlike habits learned for food reinforcement, habits established under partial reinforcement with brain stimulation extinguished more rapidly than did habits established under continuous reinforcement (Sidman, Brady, Conrad, & Schulman, 1955). Massed practice was better than spaced practice in establishing reliable alley running for brain stimulation (Seward, Uyeda, & Olds, 1960). For a time it appeared that brain stimulation did not obey the laws of reinforcement as derived from food reward studies.

Closer analysis revealed that these anomalies were due to fairly obvious differences between brain stimulation reinforcement and food reinforcement paradigms. When steps were taken to make the two paradigms more comparable, the behaviors supported by the two classes of reinforcer became more comparable as well (Trowill, Panksepp, & Gandelman, 1969). One feature that seems to distinguish food reinforcement is that the animal makes two types of response for it--instrumental or operant responses and consummatory or respondent acts. Skinner's (1938) behaviorism draws attention to the operant response, but it turns out (as was appreciated by Skinner, 1935) that the consummatory response is important as well. With brain stimulation, the animal doesn't have to eat the reinforcer but rather has only to earn it (Gibson, Reid, Sakai, & Porter, 1965). When animals are required to earn stimulation by lever-pressing but are further required to "consume" it by licking a dipper to close a circuit which causes current delivery, partial reinforcement and spaced practice become more effective, as is the case with food reinforcement (Gibson et al., 1965).

One of the important consequences of the consummatory response is that it causes a delay between the performance of the operant response and the receipt of its consequence--the reinforcement. When brain stimulation is delayed, the efficacy of partial reinforcement is improved and self-stimulation more closely resembles lever-pressing for food (Gibson et al., 1965; McIntyre & Wright, 1965; Pliskoff, Wright, & Hawkins, 1965). Conversely, when the delay of food reinforcement is decreased (by injecting it directly on the tongue), the efficacy of partial reinforcement is decreased and lever-pressing for food more closely resembles self-stimulation (Gibson et al., 1965).

There are other aspects of brain stimulation reinforcement that contribute further to differences between lever-pressing for food and lever-pressing for stimulation. There is seemingly no deprivation effect in the case of brain stimulation reinforcement; rate of response for brain stimulation reinforcement does not vary as a function of how many hours it has been since the last period of stimulation (Olds, 1956). There is no "hunger" for brain stimulation reinforcement in this sense. Nonetheless, lever-pressing for brain stimulation is potentiated by food deprivation (Hodos & Valenstein, 1960; Hoebel & Teitelbaum, 1962; Olds, 1958a) which is present in most studies of food reinforcement. When animals are reinforced with palatable food under conditions of low hunger, rapid extinction is seen just as is the case with brain stimulation reinforcement (Panksepp & Trowill, 1967); thus it may be that conditions of drive as well as conditions of reinforcement account at least for some of the "anomalies" in brain stimulation reinforcement studies.

A final difference seems unavoidable and it, too, contributes to differences between responding for brain stimulation and responding for food; there is little evidence for satiation in the case of brain stimulation reinforcement (Olds, 1958b). This fact seems unavoidable. While physiological psychologists have found ways to model the effects of hunger with focal brain stimulation (Mendelson, 1966; Wise, 1974), they have, as yet, found no way to mimic satiety such that lever-pressing for brain stimulation would undergo extinction from its own consequences, as is the case with food reinforcement (Morgan, 1974).

Thus experimental and physiological psychologists have arrived at an insight that seems obvious on reflection: There are both similarities and differences between brain stimulation reinforcement and other reinforcers, and there are important lessons to be learned from each. Just as there are both similarities and differences between brain stimulation reinforcement and food reinforcement, so are there both similarities and differences between drug reinforcement and food reinforcement. However, in the case of drug reinforcement, it is the similarities that have received early attention. The present chapter turns to consideration of the differences. In many ways drug reinforcement is more similar to brain stimulation reinforcement than to food reinforcement, and detailed consideration of response chaining, of central delivery, of delay of reinforcement, and of hunger and satiety may prove to be as important for the drug specialist as for the brain stimulation specialist.

SPECIAL FEATURES OF INTRAVENOUS DRUG REINFORCEMENT

Intravenous drug reinforcement shares with brain stimulation reinforcement the facts that it is delivered without a traditional consummatory response, that it interfaces centrally rather than peripherally with the neural mechanism of reinforcement, that it can be varied with quantitative but not qualitative precision, that its central effects are felt with very little delay after the instrumental response, and that, at least in many cases, response rate is not predictable from hours of deprivation. Unlike brain stimulation reinforcement, drug reinforcement does produce satiation; the satiation provided by intravenous drug reinforcers still differs in important ways, however, from the satiation produced by food and water reinforcement. Thus there are several special features that distinguish intravenous drug reinforcement from food or water reinforcement, and each merits careful consideration.

Instrumental-Consummatory Response Chaining

Rats working for water reinforcement typically press a lever to activate a dipper and then lick the dipper to obtain their reinforcement. With food reinforcement the consummatory response is chewing and swallowing. The first response or response series--the "earning" of the reinforcement--is the instrumental or operant response; the ingesting of the reinforcement is the consummatory response. In the case of food and water, the consummatory response is the consumption of the reinforcement, and while these words have a similar root, consummatory in this context is used to designate consummation, not consumption (Woodworth, 1918, p. 40). Intromission and pup retrieval are consummatory responses just like licking, chewing and swallowing. The defining property of a consummatory response is that it terminates or "consummates" a series of instrumental acts. In a chain of goal-directed responses, the consummatory response is the final act in the chain--the one which constitutes achieving the goal. Consummatory acts are usually biologically primitive and species-typical acts; the final acts in an ethologist's <u>fixed</u> <u>action</u> <u>patterns</u> (Moltz, 1965) are good examples.

In the case of lever-pressing for brain stimulation reinforcement or drug reinforcement, the distinction between consummatory and instrumental responses is blurred. The response that earns the reinforcement--usually lever-pressing--is the only response that is required of the animal. In this sense lever-pressing is a consummatory response; it ends the sequence of locomotion, of postural adjustment and of limb or head movement that results in reinforcement and produces, for a time, what has been called a "satisfying state of affairs" (Thorndike, 1911). The lever-pressing response, in the case of brain stimulation reinforcement, shares with biting and swallowing, in the case of food reinforcement, the fact that it consummates a sequence of instrumental acts. On the other hand, the lever-pressing response differs in a number of ways from chewing and swallowing and is, by the definition of the operant psychologist (Skinner, 1935), the same in its <u>essential</u> features to the lever-pressing instrumental response in the food reinforcement situation. Can lever-pressing be considered a consummatory response in the drug reinforcement paradigm and an instrumental response in the food reinforcement paradigm?

There are arguments for rejecting the notion that lever-pressing for drug can be considered an ordinary case of a consummatory act. It lacks the biologically primitive quality of traditional consummatory acts. It is not species-typical and it does not promote individual or species survival. These are not defining criteria of a consummatory response (Woodworth, 1918), but they should nonetheless be considered as having some significance in the analysis of motivated behavior (Glickman & Schiff, 1967). There may be something very special about the neural mechanisms of stereotyped response patterns which have a substantial genetic or early learning component to their topology. One reason for suspecting a fundamental difference between the neural organization of instrumental and consummatory behaviors is that, while neuroleptic drugs disrupt both types of response, the consummatory responses are much more resistant to this disruption than are the instrumental ones (Tombaugh, Tombaugh, & Anisman, 1979; Wise, 1982).

If good parallels are to be expected between lever-pressing for drug and lever-pressing for food, perhaps insights should be gained from physiological psychologists who required their animals to earn brain stimulation by lever-pressing and then required them to "ingest" the stimulation by licking a dipper (Gibson et al., 1965) or by pressing a second lever (Hawkins & Pliskoff, 1964). This chaining of lever-pressing to a second response would most closely approximate the food reinforcement paradigm, making lever-pressing an unambiguous case of an instrumental response.

Delay of Reinforcement

One of the reasons to consider adding a second response to follow lever-pressing in the drug reinforcement paradigm is that such an addition would increase the delay of reinforcement. It is well known that the effectiveness of reinforcement depends on the degree of delay after the instrumental response (Holder, Marx, Holder, & Collier, 1957; Logan, 1952; Peterson, 1956). Immediate positive reinforcers seem to exert stronger control over behavior, at least until the frustration of extinction conditions or partial reinforcement conditions are encountered (Crum, Brown, & Bitterman, 1951; Marx, McCoy, & Tombaugh, 1965). Delay of punishment, on the other hand, seems at least subjectively to increase its impact. Temporal factors are clearly important in behavioral control. In the case of brain stimulation reinforcement, it appears necessary to insert a delay between lever-pressing and the delivery of stimulation if the resulting behavior is to behave like that typical of food and water reinforcement (Gibson et al., 1965; Pliskoff et al., 1965).

In the case of brain stimulation reinforcement, a delay may be particularly important since the switch closure produced by lever-pressing causes almost immediate delivery of stimulation to the brain. Since stimulation is "delivered" centrally, presumably directly in the forebrain circuitry of the reinforcement mechanism (Olds, 1958b), the full benefit of the reinforcement is likely to be felt within milliseconds. The only tangible delay between lever-pressing and the impact of reinforcement should be the time it takes the nerve impulse to travel from the electrode tip to the critical site of the reinforcing event in the brain--presumably a trip of a few millimeters and at most a few synapses (Wise & Bozarth, 1984).

By contrast, food reinforcement is likely to have its significant central effects after a much longer delay, even when delivered directly to the tongue. The food must be dissolved in saliva and perhaps repositioned in the mouth before it reaches the relevant taste buds; it must then depolarize the receptors and generate a nerve impulse; the impulse must then travel several millimeters and cross perhaps several synapses before information of the reinforcing event reaches the central structures directly activated in the case of brain stimulation reinforcement. If food reinforcement and brain stimulation reinforcement do ultimately reach the same critical diencephalic mechanism, as physiological psychologists generally believe (Glickman & Schiff, 1967; Olds, 1958b; Wise, Spindler, & Legault, 1978), food reinforcement must do so after a delay that is many times (perhaps orders of magnitude) longer than the delay of brain stimulation reinforcement. This argument rests on the assumption that it is largely the sensory impact of food that is reinforcing (Pfaffman, 1960); if, as once widely held, it were the post-ingestional reinforcing consequences of food that were most critical for control of behavior, then the delay of reinforcement would be much longer--many orders of magnitude longer for food reinforcement.

The delay of intravenous drug reinforcement is difficult to determine. Different drug injection systems deliver drug with different speeds, usually introduced through the jugular vein, mixing with blood in the heart which is routed through the lungs before proceeding to the brain. There it must cross membranes and diffuse into synaptic spaces. Nerve impulses from the tongue may well reach diencephalic structures as quickly as does blood-borne drug, and this may account for the fact that behavioral pharmacologists have not yet found it necessary to examine the importance of the delay of reinforcement or of response chaining factors that have been studied in relation to brain stimulation reinforcement; drug reinforcement and food reinforcement may turn out to have quite similar delays.

On the other hand, animals do learn about the post-ingestional caloric load of the substances they ingest (Epstein & Teitelbaum, 1962; Le Magnen, 1969), and information regarding that caloric load must reach the brain after very long delays during the digestion of food and its conversion to active metabolites. Whereas sensory information regarding food reaches the brain reasonably quickly, the ingested food itself, unlike injected drug, reaches the brain after considerable delays. Consideration of these delays may become important when comparisons are made between "regulation" of drug intake and "regulation" of food or fluid intake.

Quality of Reinforcement

The fact that drug reaches the brain largely (though not always completely) unchanged from its state in the syringe and activates central receptors in the membranes of neurons of reinforcement circuitry is likely to distinguish drug reinforcement from food reinforcement in an even more fundamental way than simply the speed of its detection. Food reinforcement is said to vary in quality as well as quantity. Drug reinforcement would appear to offer no analogue for what have been termed variations in quality of food reinforcement. In order to understand the implications of this apparent difference, it is necessary to consider carefully just what has been meant by variations in reinforcement quality.

Quality of reinforcement has been defined variously over the years. Usually, differences in quality are inferred from differences in preference for different reinforcers of the same class (different foods or water at different temperatures). Bolles (1975) points out, however, that a true shift in the quality of reinforcement would be a shift from one class (say, food) to another (water). This is not, however, the kind of shift that modern motivational theorists usually discuss under the topic "quality of reinforcement." It is generally food reinforcement that is discussed under this heading, and it is usually variations of the concentration of sweetener that are treated as variations in quality of reinforcement (Beck, 1978; Bolles, 1975).

While studies of this sort were originally considered to be studies of the quantity of reinforcement (e.g., Dufort & Kimble, 1956; Guttman, 1953; Young & Shuford, 1955), they have been reinterpreted as studies of quality of reinforcement (Marx, 1969; Schaeffer & Hanna, 1966; see also Bolles, 1975, p. 425, note 7) on the basis of the fact that it is the sweetness of the substance and not its caloric value that determines preference and operant response rate. Saccharin, which has no caloric value, has varying reinforcing impact as a function of concentration (Collier, 1962; Collier & Myers, 1961; Sheffield & Roby, 1950), just as do glucose and sucrose (Guttman, 1953; Pfaffman, 1960). Moreover, glucose and sucrose are reinforcing in proportion to their relative sweetnesses at various concentrations rather than in proportion to their relative caloric loads (Guttman, 1954). Modern motivation theory defines differences in the sensory impact of food reward as differences in quality and labels differences in nutritional value as differences in quantity (Beck, 1978; Bolles, 1975).

Because of the historical importance of drive reduction theories of reinforcement, it has been important to contrast the nutritional value of food with its sensory value (Pfaffman, 1960). It is unfortunate that the labels for this distinction became "quantity" and "quality," however, since sweetness is also readily measured on quantitative scales. It is not strictly accurate to discuss taste factors as qualitative rather than quantitative. Studies of taste quality have used concentration as a metric, and concentration is certainly a quantitative variable; indeed, the early studies comparing sugar solutions of different concentrations recognized it as such (Young & Shuford, 1955), identifying concentration with magnitude (Collier & Marx, 1959) or with amount (Dufort & Kimble, 1956) of reinforcement. Modern motivational theory might have done better to distinguish sensory and caloric value with different labels than quality and quantity, as concentration of sugar solutions is no less quantitative than calorie counts, and while calorie counts may measure something of relevance, it is questionable that they measure reinforcing impact per se.

It is the fact that food reinforcement is detected peripherally which allowed this modern distinction between quality and quantity to arise. If a simple glucose solution were the reinforcing substance, varying its concentration should logically be treated as varying the quantity, not quality, of reinforcement. The amount (concentration) of a sweetener at the taste receptor determines its sensory impact (Pfaffman, 1960). What if some more complex food substance were sweetened with an additive? Should a sweet 45 mg food pellet be considered to differ qualitatively or quantitatively from a bland 45 mg food pellet? The answer depends on what we define as the _food_ component of the reinforcer. For example, if the 45 mg pellet were composed mostly of cellulose and sweetened with glucose, the _amount_ of food substance would be determined by the amount of glucose (since there is no food value in cellulose). If a pellet of grain were sweetened with saccharin, the grain would represent the food; the sweetener is biologically inert. Here, the caloric value of the grain would probably be treated as _quantity_ of food, and the concentration of the saccharin would probably be treated like the determinant of food quality. Similarly, the volume of water is probably to be treated as the _quantity_ of water reinforcement, and its temperature, despite the fact that it is measured in degrees, is probably to be treated like a quality variable.

These conventions are clearly not well thought out in the reinforcement literature. They are based on the _food_ or _fluid_ value of the reinforcer rather than on its reinforcing impact. They presume the "amount" of reinforcement to be proportional to the biological utility of the goal object. The quantity of food reinforcement is conceded, in this view, to reflect its caloric value; the quantity of water reinforcement is conceded to reflect its hydrational value. These concessions cannot be logically justified. The fact that reinforcement accrues primarily from the sensory impact of the reinforcer means that the true quantity of reinforcement is at best only a correlate of its biological value; biological value is not necessarily well reflected in the sensory impact of a reinforcer. Water reinforcements of different temperature have different impact on behavior (Carlisle, 1977; Gold, Kapatos, Oxford, Prowse, & Quackenbush, 1974; Ramsauer, Freed, & Mendelson, 1974), though they have equal hydrational value. This means that temperature (degree of oral cooling), not volume, is the proper quantitative measure for the reinforcing value of water. Food reinforcements sweetened with saccharin have different behavioral impact though they have equal nutritional value (Sheffield & Roby, 1950). This means that concentration of sweetener, not caloric load, is the proper quantitative measure for the reinforcing value of sweet food. It is likely that the other sensory "qualities" of food, such as concentration of salt, should also be treated as quantitative variables; the power of science comes from the ability to quantify. The critical point here is that it is food's behavioral impact, which is primarily sensory, which determines the strength of a food's reinforcing impact. It is partly the fact that behavior is not governed by the biological utility of a reinforcer which has led to the consideration of quality of reinforcement as being distinct from its amount or quantity. The fact that hungry animals will work for saccharin solutions having no nutritional value (Sheffield & Roby, 1950) and the fact that thirsty animals will work for oral cooling that has no hydrational value (Mendelson & Chillag, 1970) should make it clear that the biological significance of a reinforcing substance need tell us little regarding the reinforcing intensity (quantity of reinforcement) associated with that substance.

However this larger problem is ultimately resolved, it remains the case that there is no real analogue in the study of intravenous drug reinforcement for variations in the sweetness of food or in the temperature of water.

Varying the concentration of drug reinforcers does not so much alter their quality as it alters their intensity and duration of action. Inasmuch as the concentration of a drug is much diluted between its site of injection and its site of interaction with the nervous system, total dose rather than concentration of injected drug solution determines the drug's concentration at the time it reaches its central site of action. The volume of vehicle originally used to dissolve the drug is of minimal importance. By contrast, variations in the concentration of a reinforcing sucrose or saccharin solution are detected at the taste buds before major dilution; both response rates and the firing rates of the taste nerve fibers are tightly correlated with the concentration of sucrose on the tongue (Pfaffman, 1960) rather than with the total dose given. The lack of a peripheral sensor for drug reinforcement thus poses a major difference between drug reinforcement and food or water reinforcement.

It might seem reasonable to think that variations in the molecular structure of a drug should cause a qualitative change in its reinforcing efficacy, particularly if preference measures are used as an index of quality. However, the most straightforward explanation of difference in potency of two agonists for the same receptor would be differences in receptor affinity. The only legitimate qualitative difference between drug reinforcers would seem to be a difference in drug class; drugs are qualitatively different if they act on different anatomical systems or at different receptors. In this case the analogue for differences between two drugs of different quality (say stimulants and narcotics) would be differences between reinforcer category (say food and water). Even stimulants and narcotics might be more fairly viewed as quantitatively different (different in amount) to the degree that their reinforcing effects are mediated by actions in a common neural circuit (Bozarth & Wise, 1981; Wise & Bozarth, 1984). True differences in quality in this case would be attributed to differences in "side effects" rather than to differences in reinforcing effect per se.

Quantity of Reinforcement

As should be apparent from the discussion of quality of reinforcement, quantity of reinforcement is not yet satisfactorily defined in the case of either food or water. The phrases "quantity of reinforcement" and "amount of reinforcement" do not have agreed meanings (Schaffer & Hanna, 1966). They have been used variously by different authors to reflect the total number of food pellets in training, the number of food pellets per trial, the number of licks or pellets per reinforcement, the weight of the pellet, or the volume of the dipper or food cup. Only the weight or volume dimensions are of interest here, where quantity of reinforcement is defined, for drug reinforcement, as the dose per injection or unit dose.

Where measures of quantity of food reinforcement are poorly defined, quantity of brain stimulation reinforcement is well defined. Here, the quantity of reinforcement is varied by changing the intensity, frequency, or duration of stimulation. Over the interesting ranges of these variables, there seems to be a reasonably linear trade-off between intensity and frequency (Gallistel, Shizgal, & Yeomans, 1981); the reinforcement mechanism seems reasonably indifferent to whether stimulation intensity is increased (increasing the number of fibers activated by each pulse) or stimulation frequency is increased (increasing the number of times a fixed set of fibers fire during each stimulation train). Whether intensity is varied (with frequency held constant) or frequency is varied (with intensity held constant), increases in the amount of reinforcement cause increased rates of responding to a point. With high levels of stimulation responding approaches an asymptote; in some cases response levels can even fall with further increases in stimulation intensity. The interesting range of reinforcement parameters is the range between threshold levels and the levels producing maximal behavioral output. Within that range there is a monotonic increase in response rate associated with increases in reinforcement magnitude. It is relatively easy to define quantity of reinforcement in the case of brain stimulation because we have reasonably good evidence of the effects of brain stimulation reinforcement on the firing patterns of the neurons that constitute the reinforcement mechanism of the brain (Gallistel et al., 1981).

A similar picture emerges with food reinforcement if we consider magnitude of reinforcement to vary with glucose, sucrose, or saccharin concentration in the tradition of the 1940s and 1950s. Rate of responding in simple FR-1 tasks increases monotonically over the interesting range of concentrations, starting at concentrations near the detection threshold and leveling off at concentrations that produce maximal response rates. At higher concentrations response rate can fall, particularly if long sessions are involved. The decrease seems largely due to post-ingestional (satiety) factors associated with sugars (Collier, 1962; Collier & Myers, 1961) and with bitter taste associated with high concentrations of saccharin (Pfaffman, 1960) rather than to variations in the factor of reinforcement magnitude itself. At the high concentrations where response rate levels off, so does the elicited rate of firing of the fibers of the taste nerve (Pfaffman, 1960); this, again, serves to delimit the range of interesting concentrations. Thus when concentration at the taste bud is viewed as a measure of the quantity of reinforcement, the relation between response rate and quantity of food reinforcement resembles the relation between response rate and quantity of brain stimulation reinforcement.

The case of drug reinforcement appears to be distinctly different. The general relation of response rate to quantity of drug reinforcement is suggested to be biphasic over the range of interesting unit doses with an ascending limb of increasing response rates associated with lower doses and a descending limb of decreasing response rates associated with higher doses. The range of doses associated with the ascending limb does not represent doses which produce reliably spaced responding, however. This dose range is associated with both within-subject and between-subject variability, with alternations between periods of very high response rates and periods of no responding. Thus most investigators do not report graded changes in responding across this portion of the dose range. Rather, when magnitude of reinforcement is systematically varied, most investigators vary it over the range of unit doses that are inversely related to response rate (Downs & Woods, 1974; Glick, Cox, & Crane, 1975; Pickens & Thompson, 1968; Woods & Schuster, 1968; Yokel & Pickens, 1973). When the ascending limb is represented in FR-1 studies, it is usually not really determined across a graded range of effective doses. Rather it is inferred from one to two low doses that fail to sustain responding at all and the first dose that does sustain responding--usually at the highest rate observed in the study (e.g., Glick & Cox, 1977, 1978; Glick, Cox, & Crane, 1975). In such cases the "ascending limb" is defined by drawing a line between points representing the effects of non-reinforcing doses and the point representing the first dose of the descending limb. This is really a trivial case of function which is truly well-defined as "biphasic" only when animals are required to respond on partial reinforcement schedules. When animals are required to make several responses for each injection, then there truly is an ascending limb to the dose-response curve (Balster & Schuster, 1973; Goldberg & Kelleher, 1976; Kelleher, 1976), though, even here, it is likely to include a small range of doses (see, e.g., Goldberg, 1973).

In the case of drug reinforcement, it is the descending limb, not the ascending limb, that is most interesting. Responding in the descending limb of the function has been widely examined, even in the case of FR-1 responding. Here response rates are reliable both within and across subjects, and graded changes in response rate reliably accompany graded changes in injection dose (Yokel & Pickens, 1973, 1974). Thus, at least in the case of the widely studied and well-defined ranges of their effectiveness, increases in magnitude of food reinforcement (also brain stimulation reinforcement) cause increases in response rate, whereas increases in drug reinforcement cause decreases in response rate.

Does this signal a fundamental difference between drug reinforcement and other reinforcements, or is it merely an artifact of focusing on different portions of the function relating reinforcement magnitude to response rate? Perhaps the descending limb of the dose response curve in drug self-administration is analogous to the descending limb of the function relating reinforcement magnitude to response rate in saccharin or brain stimulation studies. This is a possibility which cannot be completely ruled out on the basis of present data. The "interesting" portions of the rate-concentration functions for food reinforcement and the rate-intensity and rate-frequency functions for brain stimulation reinforcement are anchored at the lower extreme by reinforcement thresholds. The threshold for drug reinforcement is not so readily determined, however. While some might argue that thresholds anchor the lower end of the ascending limb of the dose-response curves, my feeling is that threshold anchors the descending, not the ascending, limb. In our experience the lowest drug dose that maintains reliable responding does so at the highest observed response rate. Thus I would argue that the dose-response curve for drug self-administration is fundamentally different from the concentration-response curve for sucrose reinforcement; the one is a monotonically decreasing function across its interesting range, while the other is a monotonically increasing function across its interesting range. I would not, however, argue that this reveals a fundamental difference in the effects of magnitude of reinforcement for drug and food. Differences in the ability of drugs and foods to produce satiety are confounded with their magnitude of reinforcement in the usual paradigms, and it is satiety, more than reinforcement, that controls rate of responding for drug in most paradigms.

Satiating Bolus

In the case of brain stimulation reinforcement, the most probable explanation for the descending limb of the rate-intensity function is that stimulation spreads to adjacent systems, producing motoric artifacts or aversive side effects. It is not the case that high intensities satiate the animal. In the case of sugars and saccharin, the descending limb of the concentration-response curve has been related to bitter taste and post-ingestional factors, but, again, not to what is normally termed satiety (Collier & Myers, 1961). The descending limb of the dose-response curve for drug reinforcement, on the other hand, reflects the fact that drug, unlike food and brain stimulation, is usually given in immediately satiating doses. This point requires some elaboration.

In a typical FR-1 food reinforcement study, 22-hour deprived rats lever-press about 200 or 250 times without pausing except to eat their earned 45 mg food pellets (e.g., Wise, de Wit, Gerber, & Spindler, 1978). This number of pellets is earned and eaten in about 20 minutes, and at the end of this time the animals generally turn to grooming and then to sleeping. By contrast, in a typical FR-1 drug reinforcement study, rats lever-press much less frequently with relatively uniform pauses between responses (e.g., Yokel & Pickens, 1973). The pauses between responses can be extended by giving free infusions of drug (Pickens & Thompson, 1971), just as the intervals between meals can be extended by infusions of sugars (Nikolaidis & Rowland, 1976). Thus, "typical" food reinforcement and drug reinforcement paradigms differ critically in that each drug reinforcement is sufficient to cause a satiety period, while each food reinforcement constitutes less than 1% of a satiating meal.

This is not merely due to the fact that small amounts of food reinforcement and large amounts of drug reinforcement are given. In part, the difference in the satiating capacities of food pellets and drug injections is due to the different access that food and drug have to the brain and hormonal mechanisms that regulate satiety; in addition to the differences in delay of reinforcement already discussed, there is a difference in the delay of satiation between food reinforcement and drug reinforcement. Whereas intravenous drug reaches the mechanism of both its reinforcing and its satiating actions in seconds, ingested food reaches the peripheral site of reinforcing action in seconds but does not reach the central mechanism underlying satiety for a much longer time. Thus food which might be sufficient, after absorption and partial metabolism, to establish a substantial period of satiety has no such behavioral impact until long after additional food has usually been ingested (Davis, Gallagher, Ladlove, & Turausky, 1969). While there is a sensory component to food-related satiety (Mook, 1963), it is not analogous to the satiety produced by drug reaching and occupying its ultimate site of satiating action.

As mentioned earlier, mean rate of responding for drug varies inversely with dose per injection; the larger the injection the longer the period of satiety (Weeks & Collins, 1964; Yokel & Pickens, 1973, 1974). This is not so much an explanation of behavior as a definition of the term "satiety." Over the lower range of doses where mean response rate seems to increase with injection dose, drug is, by definition, non-satiating; animals respond immediately after each injection (or they do not respond at all).

One way to view the fact that increased magnitude of reinforcement causes increased rates of responding for brain stimulation and for food, while it causes decreased rates of responding for drugs, involves consideration of the brain mechanisms of reinforcement and the relative impact of food, stimulation, and drugs upon those mechanisms. Variations in concentration of sweet solutions or in the frequency of brain stimulation seem to alter the intensity of reinforcement. Thus animals prefer in choice tests the high currents (Hodos & Valenstein, 1962) and concentrations (Pfaffman, 1960) associated with high response rates in lever-press tasks. With food reinforcement and brain stimulation reinforcement, high response rates are associated with preferred magnitudes of reinforcement. With drug reinforcement such preferences are not necessarily seen (Yokel, this volume; but see Iglauer & Woods, 1974). Here increased magnitude of reinforcement seems not so much to alter the intensity of reinforcement as to alter its duration. The fact that animals have a good deal of opportunity to lever-press for more drugs suggests the same conclusion; if higher blood levels of drug were to increase the intensity of reinforcement, why would animals not merely respond more frequently?

It was once thought that more frequent responding might be prohibited by high-dose drug effects--either by aversive side effects or by incapacitating side effects (Wilson & Schuster, 1972). These hypotheses can now be ruled out. If high blood concentrations were aversive, then animals would prefer lower doses to larger ones, but such preferences are not seen. Rats seem to have no particular preference for low or high doses (Yokel, this volume), and monkeys prefer higher doses (Iglauer & Woods, 1974: Note that preference for high doses may not reflect greater intensity of reinforcement; monkeys may prefer higher doses for their longer duration, a property rats may not have the capacity to appreciate.). Thus it seems unlikely that aversive side effects limit drug intake significantly. It is also clear that motoric side effects do not constitute a limiting factor. Rats will lever-press several hundred times for brain stimulation in the interval between normal responses for drug when it is available on a concurrent schedule (Bozarth, Gerber, & Wise, 1980; Wise, Yokel, Gerber, & Hansson, 1977). It would thus appear that responding for drug is not limited actively by either aversive side effects or motoric incapacitation.

The fact that drug is given in an immediately satiating bolus while brain stimulation, food, and water are given in quanta that are not satiating (or at least not immediately satiating) seems to account for differences in the control of response rate by changes in unit dose. What, then, is the nature of this control in the unusual condition of drug reinforcement? Where an increase in the amount of brain stimulation per reinforcement leads to an increase in the number of responses per hour (Gallistel et al., 1981), an increase in the amount of drug reinforcement has the opposite effect. Rats generally compensate rather accurately for increased drug per injection, for alterations in drug isomer, or for changes in work requirements (Pickens, 1968; Pickens & Thompson, 1968; Yokel, this volume; Yokel & Pickens, 1973, 1974). Over a wide range of these variables, rats maintain a relatively constant hourly drug intake.

The dynamics of hourly drug intake have been particularly well studied in the stimulant self-administration paradigm. In this case response rate is governed largely by rate of metabolism of the drugs; the mean time between responses for different doses can be predicted from the metabolic kinetics of the drugs (Yokel & Pickens, 1974). Moreover, if drug is sampled at the time of each injection, blood concentrations reliably fall to the same threshold level--0.2 µg/ml of blood in the case of d-amphetamine--regardless of whether high or low doses are being earned (Yokel & Pickens, 1974). The rate of responding is accelerated or decelerated by treatments which accelerate or decelerate amphetamine metabolism, respectively (Dougherty & Pickens, 1974). Thus the factor which appears to limit drug intake is satiety; intake is limited passively when blood concentrations exceed satiating levels.

OVERVIEW

Rate of responding for drug reinforcement is under a seemingly unique control of magnitude of reinforcement. Whereas dose per injection is, over the interesting range of doses, inversely related to response rate for drug reinforcement, intensity and frequency per stimulation train and concentration of sweet solutions are, over the interesting ranges of these parameters, directly related to response rate for brain stimulation and sweet solutions, respectively. The unique dynamics of control of response rate for drug reinforcement may derive from a number of facts which distinguish drug reinforcement from food reinforcement. The most salient of these is that rate of responding for intravenous drug reinforcement is controlled by the duration of satiating action of the drug, which is felt immediately, while rate of responding for food or brain stimulation reward is controlled by some aspect of the intensity or quality of reinforcement which occurs either in the absence of satiety (in the case of brain stimulation) or occurs before the satiating consequences of ingestion are detected (in the case of food). There is no obvious analogue for graded intensity or quality in the case of drug reinforcement, perhaps because the reinforcing event is not sensed peripherally as in the case of food (Pfaffman, 1960) or trans-synaptically as in the case of brain stimulation (Gallistel et al., 1981). Whatever the explanation, changes in rate of responding for drug must be carefully interpreted, and this will be illustrated in subsequent sections. Care must also be taken in drawing parallels between drug-reinforced responding and responding maintained by more natural reinforcers. Just as differences in response chaining and delay of reinforcement must contribute to the differences between responding for brain stimulation and responding for food, so may similar factors contribute to unappreciated differences between responding for drugs and responding for food.

CENTRAL MANIPULATIONS THAT INFLUENCE RESPONSE RATE

Psychomotor stimulant self-administration in the rat is marked by many characteristics also found in brain stimulation reinforcement studies (Pickens & Harris, 1968). Both intravenous stimulants and intracranial electrical stimulation can be powerfully reinforcing, dominating rat behavior even in conflict situations. Rate of responding is regular in both cases, and responding is in both cases sustained for long periods without interruption. In both cases the rate of responding is independent of previous abstinence periods, and in both cases spontaneous abstinence periods occur with unpredictable onset and duration (Pickens & Harris, 1968).

Much has been made of the fact that stimulant self-administration increases when dopaminergic synapses are blocked with pimozide, butaclamol or other neuroleptics (de Wit & Wise, 1977; Yokel & Wise, 1975, 1976). There are two reasons for the attention to this finding. First, it clearly tells us something neuroleptics are not doing; they are not rendering the animals incapable of initiating voluntary movement or of organizing complex goal-directed behavior. They are not simply causing the catalepsy that can be seen in certain testing conditions (Janssen, Dresse, Lenaerts, Niemegeers, Pinchard, Schaper, Schellekens, Van Nueten, & Verbruggen, 1968). They are not impairing the animals such that they cannot perform at their normal response levels. Similar response increases are not seen with other reinforcers such as brain stimulation (Fouriezos & Wise, 1976) or food (Wise et al., 1978a, 1978b), and in these cases the possibility of motoric impairment has been a major issue (Wise, 1982). The fact that this issue could be readily resolved in the case of stimulant self-administration was thus one important reason for the attention to neuroleptic-induced response accelerations.

The second reason that the response accelerations have received so much consideration is that they appear (with somewhat less certainty) to suggest something about the nature of what is occurring. The response accelerations parallel the effects of reinforcement reductions, and they thus suggest that neuroleptics cause such reductions in the stimulant self-administration paradigm. While this conclusion cannot be drawn with complete certainty--it is much more clear that the animals are free of motor deficits than they are impaired by reinforcement deficit--nonetheless it has been generally accepted (see, e.g., Ettenberg, Bloom, Koob, & Pettit, 1982; Lyness, Friedle, & Moore, 1979; Roberts, Corcoran, & Fibiger, 1977; Roberts & Koob, 1982; Roberts, Koob, Klonoff, & Fibiger, 1980). Indeed, the view that increased (compensatory) responding must reflect a decrease in reinforcing stimulant impact has been accepted so globally that it has seemingly become the sine qua non of the paradigm. Some workers (e.g., Ettenberg et al., 1982) seem to hold that rate increases are not only a sufficient condition for inferring a decrease in the reinforcing impact of intravenous drug but that they are also a necessary condition for such a conclusion. This position will be examined more closely in the next section.

The rate increases that are sometimes seen when stimulant self-administration is challenged with neuroleptics (de Wit & Wise, 1977; Yokel & Wise, 1975, 1976) or with lesions of dopaminergic reinforcement mechanisms (Roberts et al., 1980) take two forms. With minimal challenges (low doses of neuroleptics), there is a sustained increase in drug intake which lasts in proportion to the dose of the challenge drug. Here the animal behaves as if the neuroleptic were a competitive antagonist at the critical receptor; the animal maintains a higher than normal concentration of stimulant in the blood, as would be required to displace neuroleptic molecules from dopamine receptors in the CNS. The rat normally responds for d-amphetamine whenever blood concentration falls to about 0.2 μg/ml (Yokel & Pickens, 1974); under low doses of neuroleptics, rats respond more frequently (Yokel & Wise, 1975, 1976), thus initiating responses when a higher concentration threshold is crossed. Because amphetamine is metabolized by first order kinetics--the higher the blood level the faster the metabolism--the animals must not only respond more in order to initially elevate blood concentration above 0.2 μg/ml, but they must also continue to respond faster to maintain concentration above this level.

When higher doses of neuroleptic are given (Yokel & Wise, 1975, 1976), or in some cases when dopamine systems are lesioned (Roberts et al., 1980), responding is biphasic. The initial phase is a period of accelerated responding; it is followed by a period of non-responding. This parallels what is seen when reinforcing injections are terminated. The interpretation is that the animal is unable to earn sufficient drug, during the period of accelerated responding, to counteract the high dose neuroleptic treatment; thus responding ceases. The early phase of accelerated responding is not simply a period when the neuroleptic is only partially absorbed (and thus acting like a low dose); since when stimulant access is delayed until after peak central neuroleptic action has been reached, the same period of initial acceleration is still seen in a significant portion of cases (Yokel & Wise, 1976).

Interpreting Monophasic Decreases in Rate of Self-Administration

Much has been made of compensatory increases in drug intake that are seen when psychomotor stimulant self-administration is challenged with drugs that impair dopaminergic function (Ettenberg et al., 1982; Pickens, Meisch, & Dougherty, 1968; Wilson & Schuster, 1972; de Wit & Wise, 1977; Yokel & Wise, 1975, 1976). It is a great help to interpretation when rate increases are observed in response to a pharmacological challenge or experimental lesion that might otherwise be suspected to impair performance capacity in some way. It is dangerous, however, to draw any firm conclusion when there is a failure to see compensatory rate increases; failure to see rate increases might be caused by any number of factors and cannot, by itself, be interpreted. This might be argued on purely logical grounds, but there are good data to illustrate the point.

Specialists are agreed that psychomotor stimulant reinforcement depends on stimulant actions at one or more sets of dopaminergic synapses in the forebrain (Baxter et al., 1974, 1976; Davis & Smith, 1975; Ettenberg et al., 1982; Lyness et al., 1979; Risner & Jones, 1976, 1980; Roberts et al., 1977, 1980; Roberts & Koob, 1982; Roberts & Zito, this volume; Spyraki, Fibiger, & Phillips, 1982; de Wit & Wise, 1977; Yokel, this volume; Yokel & Wise, 1975, 1976, 1978). The accelerated responding for amphetamine which is caused by neuroleptics is one cornerstone of this conclusion, but there are others. One critical corroborative fact is that humans report decreased amphetamine euphoria after neuroleptics (Gunne, Anggard, & Jonsson, 1972). Another is that rats no longer work for amphetamine or cocaine when dopamine systems are lesioned (Lyness et al., 1979; Roberts et al., 1977, 1980; Roberts & Koob, 1982) or when neuroleptics are injected into dopamine terminal fields in the brain (Phillips & Broekkamp, 1980). Finally, apomorphine and piribedil, selective dopamine receptor agonists, have amphetamine-like reinforcing effects of their own (Baxter et al., 1974; Davis & Smith, 1977; Yokel & Wise, 1978). Had we required that dopamine antagonism or dopaminergic lesions cause compensatory increases in stimulant intake, however, these last two lines of evidence might not have been interpreted correctly.

First, lesions of the nucleus accumbens did not, at least in the first experiments (Lyness et al., 1979; Roberts et al., 1977), cause compensatory increases in amphetamine or cocaine intake. They simply blocked acquisition of the lever-pressing habit in naive animals (Lyness et al., 1979) and caused such responding to decrease in trained animals (Roberts et al., 1977). What does the lack of compensatory increases in responding reflect? In the case of naive animals, the lack of compensatory increases obviously means nothing; responding is expected to show compensatory increases only in well-trained animals. But what about the trained animals? If one were predisposed to link response increases in one-to-one fashion with reinforcement reduction, one might conclude that the lesion failed to reduce the reinforcing impact of the drug. If, on the other hand, one did not have such a predisposition, one might reasonably infer that the lesion had perhaps blocked the reinforcing drug effect. In point of fact, Roberts, who did the initial lesion study, was tenacious enough to try variations on the paradigm until compensatory increases were demonstrated in a number of animals (Roberts et al., 1980). Response increases in these cases rule out the possibility that the lesions merely impair response capability; note that this conclusion does not require response increases in all animals under all testing conditions.

The second informative case involves apomorphine self-administration. Apomorphine is self-administered in much the same way as is amphetamine (Baxter et al., 1974; Davis & Smith, 1977; Yokel & Wise, 1978; Wise et al., 1976). Apomorphine is a selective dopaminergic agonist, so it would be surprising if its reinforcing action were mediated somewhere other than the dopaminergic synapse. If its reinforcing action were mediated at the dopaminergic synapse, then the reinforcing effects should be blocked by neuroleptics (which block post-synaptic receptors) and not by alpha-methyltyrosine (which blocks dopamine synthesis). Indeed, dopamine synthesis blockade has no effect on apomorphine self-administration (Baxter, Gluckman, & Scerni, 1976), and neuroleptics block apomorphine self-administration (Yokel & Wise, 1978). However, once again acceleration of apomorphine self-administration is not seen (Yokel & Wise, 1978). Low doses of neuroleptics (which cause accelerated amphetamine self-administration; Yokel & Wise, 1976) have no effect on apomorphine self-administration, while high doses cause responding to drop out without an early phase of accelerated responding. The reasons for the lack of accelerated responding are not clear, but no one has suggested this fact to imply that the mechanism of apomorphine reinforcement involves a non-dopaminergic action of the drug.

How, then, should one interpret the findings of Ettenberg et al. (1982) that flupenthixol did not cause sustained increases in heroin self-administration at moderate doses (which did cause increases in cocaine self-administration) and did not cause complete cessation of responding for heroin at a high dose (that did cause cessation of cocaine self-administration)? How should one interpret the fact that naltrexone, on the other hand, caused increased responding for heroin but not for cocaine? Ettenberg et al. conclude from these findings that two independent reinforcement mechanisms are activated, one by heroin and another by cocaine; they take their data to refute the view (Bozarth & Wise, 1981; Wise & Bozarth, 1984) that opiates and stimulants act at serial elements in a common reinforcement substrate. Their conclusion rests primarily on the interpretation of the effects of flupenthixol on heroin self-administration, since naltrexone would not be expected to alter cocaine intake by either theory (It acts "upstream" from the site of stimulant action in the proposed circuit.).

While the effects of naltrexone on heroin self-administration, the lack of effect of naltrexone on cocaine self-administration, and the effects of flupenthixol on cocaine self-administration are all compatible with the notion that cocaine acts downstream from the site of heroin action in a common reinforcement circuit (Wise & Bozarth, 1984), such a view demands that neuroleptics, which act at the postulated final common path, block the reinforcing affects of both drugs. Ettenberg et al. (1982) saw reduced heroin self-administration with their highest doses of flupenthixol; thus the Ettenberg et al. argument that flupenthixol fails to block the reinforcing effects of heroin rests largely on the fact that flupenthixol failed to increase heroin self-administration in the way that it increased cocaine self-administration. Is such a conclusion justified?

If it is granted that a rate increase proves a reinforcement reduction (a vulnerable assumption, but one that Ettenberg et al. seem prepared to make), it nonetheless fails to follow logically that the absence of a rate increase proves the absence of a reinforcement reduction. There are several alternative explanations of the absence of rate increases in lesioned or neuroleptic-treated animals, one of which is that flupenthixol causes (in addition to any effect on reinforcement mechanisms) response debilitation, as Ettenberg, Bloom, and Koob (1981) argue elsewhere. One might ask why flupenthixol would impair heroin self-administration at the same doses that increased cocaine self-administration; one possibility is mentioned elsewhere in the Ettenberg et al. (1982) paper: Cocaine antagonizes the effects of flupenthixol (but not naltrexone) by increasing dopamine concentrations at its receptor. Cocaine, a stimulant, would thus be expected to antagonize the sedative side effects of the neuroleptic, while heroin, a depressant, would be expected to augment them. Whether or not this particular alternative explanation is valid, it is important to remember that failure to find evidence for a hypothesis is not necessarily evidence against that hypothesis. Failure to find a smoking gun is not proof of innocence.

The question of whether reinforcement impairment is necessarily reflected in response acceleration is an empirical question, and there are data of relevance available. There are clear cases where neuroleptics fail to cause response acceleration but are nonetheless thought to attenuate intravenous drug reinforcement. The first has been mentioned; pimozide at low doses fails to accelerate responding for apomorphine, though it does, at high doses, cause apomorphine self-administration to cease (without an "extinction burst" of initial high-rate responding; Yokel & Wise, 1978). A second example is evident in Ettenberg et al.'s data; the high dose of flupenthixol caused cessation of cocaine self-administration without any "extinction burst" of accelerated responding such as is seen when pimozide, rather than flupenthixol, is used (de Wit & Wise, 1977). Ettenberg et al. (1982) do not suggest that the failure of flupenthixol to cause acceleration prior to cessation raises any question about the ability of flupenthixol to block cocaine reinforcement. A third comes from our experience with opiate antagonists; many of our animals cease responding for heroin without any response acceleration after naloxone or naltrexone (Bozarth & Wise, unpublished observations). Moreover, while Roberts et al. (1980) were able to find instances of response acceleration in their lesioned animals (when time for recovery was given before testing), they did not see such acceleration in all of their animals.

Thus it seems unwarranted to take the absence of response acceleration as evidence that neuroleptics fail to attenuate intravenous drug reinforcement. As shown by the case of apomorphine, neuroleptics can block drug reinforcement with neither sustained response increase at low neuroleptic doses nor early acceleration before extinction at high neuroleptic doses. Lesions can similarly block stimulant reinforcement without compensatory increases. The presence of compensatory increases in drug intake should probably not be treated as a sufficient condition for inferring a decrease in reinforcing impact; such increases should certainly not be treated as a necessary condition for such inferences. Monotonic decreases in drug intake--decreases without initial accelerations and without associated increases when lower doses are tested--must then be treated as inconclusive evidence by themselves. It is for this reason that our inference of decreased opiate reward under conditions of neuroleptic challenge was not based on intravenous self-administration evidence but on evidence from the conditioned place preference paradigm. It is the fact that neuroleptics block opiate-conditioned place preference (Bozarth & Wise, 1981; Spyraki, Fibiger, & Phillips, 1983), taken with the fact that neuroleptics in sufficient dose cause rats to stop lever-pressing for intravenous heroin (Bozarth & Wise, unpublished observations), that led us to believe that dopaminergic systems play a critical role in opiate reinforcement.

Interpreting Shifts in Biphasic Dose-Response Curves

Changes in drug intake following brain lesions are difficult to interpret (see Roberts & Zito, this volume). Even when changes are not monotonic--even when drug intake increases at some unit doses and decreases at others--there is no simple rule for deciding whether decreased intake means stronger or weaker reinforcement. Interpretation of lesion effects cannot rest simply on parallels with other challenges or with other reinforcers.

Glick et al. (1975) have shown that rats take less intravenous morphine after lesions of the caudate nucleus. They see a shift in the entire dose-response curve over a range of effective doses which span the descending limb of the dose effect curve and which include one low dose that sustained responding before but not after the lesions. They have interpreted these data to mean that caudate lesions "increase sensitivity to the rewarding effect of morphine" (p. 222). Here is another case where interpretation of changes in response rate is complicated. As pointed out by Glick et al., there are several viable hypotheses as to the significance of their data; one possibility suggested by consideration of the mechanism of opiate reinforcement is almost opposite to the conclusion of Glick et al.

Opiates act at receptor sites embedded in neural membranes. The action of opiates at their receptors seems complex (Barker, Macdonald, Neale, & Smith, 1978), but ultimately their effect is to enhance or to inhibit activity in neural circuits. When receptors are blocked by an opiate antagonist, increased opiate intake might be expected; such intake would increase the opiate concentration and compensate for a fixed concentration of a competitive antagonist by displacing the antagonist from the opiate receptors. One of the findings which lends credence to the assumption that reduced sensitivity to the reinforcing effect of morphine results in an increase in self-administration rate is the finding that opiate antagonists do, at low and moderate doses, often cause increased responding for opiates (Ettenberg et al., 1982; Goldberg, Schuster, & Woods, 1971).

Can the opposite effect (decreased responding) be taken as reflecting the opposite condition (increased sensitivity to reinforcing opiates)? It would seem logical to assume so if the decreased responding were caused by some treatment known to produce increased receptor number or affinity. Chronic naloxone or naltrexone might be expected to cause opiate supersensitivity by increasing receptor affinity or number (Tang & Collins, 1978); release from such treatment might be expected to produce a decrease in the normal hourly intake of morphine in a self-administered paradigm. What about the case where some of the target neurons are destroyed by an electrolytic lesion? Is it reasonable to expect such a treatment to produce an analogous state? The lesion would decrease the number of available receptors by killing the cells on which the receptors are localized. How could such a manipulation cause an increase in sensitivity to morphine? Glick and his colleagues presumed (Glick & Cox, 1975; Glick et al., 1975) morphine to be a dopamine antagonist, and they suggested the interpretation that the lesion increases morphine sensitivity by decreasing the number of dopaminergic terminals where morphine must have inhibitory effects in order to produce a reinforcing state of affairs. Such an interpretation is not as straightforward as it might seem, however, since decreasing the number of neurons that morphine inhibits would not alter the critical concentration of drug at the receptors of the remaining neurons; nor would it seem likely to alter the receptor number or receptor affinity on those neurons. Thus, thinning the receptor population by lesioning the receptor substrate is not directly analogous to the effects of chronic receptor blockade. It is difficult to imagine how thinning the neural population containing the receptors for a given drug might increase the sensitivity for that drug. It is also difficult to understand how morphine would create a reinforcing state of affairs by inhibiting dopaminergic function when amphetamine, cocaine, and apomorphine seem to create a reinforcing state of affairs by stimulating dopaminergic function (Baxter et al., 1974, 1976; Davis & Smith, 1975, 1977; Ettenberg et al., 1982; Lyness et al., 1979; Risner & Jones, 1976, 1980; Roberts & Koob, 1982; Roberts et al., 1977, 1980; de Wit & Wise, 1977; Yokel & Wise, 1975, 1976, 1978).

Is there any more attractive explanation for the decrease in response rate seen when the presumed mechanism of drug reinforcement is thinned by lesioning? One possibility comes from comparing drug reinforcement with brain stimulation reinforcement. When the number of reward fibers activated by reinforcing stimulation is decreased (This is the main consequence of reducing the stimulation current or of making a lesion at the tip of the stimulating electrode.), the animals show decreased responding for stimulation (Hawkins & Pliskoff, 1964; van Sommers & Teitelbaum, 1974). Changing stimulation current, like lesioning the reward substrate, decreases the number of fibers activated in the reinforcement mechanism. This is believed to cause a decrease in the intensity of reinforcement, since it decreases the contribution of spatial summation at the next synapse in the circuit (Gallistel et al., 1981). One might ask why animals do not compensate by increasing their rate of responding just as they compensate for decreased drug reinforcement in the self-administration paradigm. The answer can perhaps never be known, but in the case of brain stimulation reinforcement, as in the case of reduced concentration of food reinforcement, they do not.

Perhaps animals take less morphine after caudate lesions because, as in the case of reduced current in the brain stimulation paradigm, lesions reduce the intensity of reinforcement. Whereas neuroleptics or reduced unit doses cause reduced reinforcement duration--which can be counteracted by taking drug more frequently--lesions reduce the intensity of drug reinforcement by reducing the number of neurons influenced by the reinforcer. Changes in the number of neurons influenced by the reinforcing drug would change the impact of the drug in a way that cannot be reversed by compensatory responding. Suppose 50% of the opiate reward mechanism were eliminated; could doubling the opiate concentration restore the full drug effect? Suppose only 5% of the opiate reward mechanism were left intact; could any amount of drug restore full drug impact? To suggest that increased frequency of injection can offset less drug per injection is to state the obvious. To suggest that increased frequency of injection and the resulting increase in drug concentration in the body can offset the effects of a competitive antagonist seems almost equally obvious. It seems quite unlikely, on the other hand, that increased frequency of injection could offset damage to the population of neurons influenced by the reinforcing drug. In a situation where there is no plausible mechanism for the ability of increased response frequency to compensate for an experimental manipulation, changes in drug intake should probably not be inferred to reflect compensatory mechanisms.

Thus, in the case of caudate lesions, it seems unlikely that decreased drug intake means an increase in drug impact. Decreased drug intake reflects increased drug impact in cases where impact can be equated with duration of effective action. In a case where decreased intake cannot be attributed to increased duration of effective action, the possibility of decreased intensity of drug effect must be considered. In the case of damage to the substrate of the drug effect, decreased intensity of drug effect is much more likely than increased duration of drug effect. Thus, once again, it is clear that changes in response rate require careful interpretation. It cannot be assumed that all biphasic decreases in response rate reflect increased drug sensitivity, just as it cannot be assumed that all monophasic decreases in response rate reflect performance debilitation.

SUMMARY AND CONCLUSIONS

There are several ways that drugs behave like other reinforcers. When a series of chained responses is required to earn drug and when the intake of drug lags appreciably behind such chained responses, responding for drug is likely to resemble responding for food. Habits learned under partial reinforcement are likely to be more difficult to break than those learned under continuous reinforcement; responding under regular reinforcement is likely to be cyclic in rate whereas responding under irregular reinforcement is likely to be regular in rate. Secondary reinforcers are likely to sustain responding in the absence of primary reinforcement and drug-associated cues are likely to reinstate responding when it has been extinguished.

There are other ways that drug reinforcement differs from food reinforcement and brain stimulation reinforcement. When satiating doses of drug are given, each is more like a meal than like a food morsel, and the pauses between injections are more likely to resemble the pauses between meals than the pauses between bites. Response rate varies inversely with drug dose in this case, and antagonists of the drug in question are likely to produce response increases though they will not always do so. When they do, the behavior sustained by drug reinforcement will respond in a manner opposite to that sustained by food reinforcement or brain stimulation reinforcement. When the response mechanism is thinned by a lesion, on the other hand, the behavior of drug-reinforced animals is likely to shift in the opposite direction--now in parallel with the effects of lesions or antagonist challenge of brain stimulation reinforcement or of food reinforcement.

Because rate of drug self-administration can sometimes be increased and sometimes be decreased by pharmacological or surgical intervention, one cannot determine simply from a change in response rate whether drug reinforcement has been enhanced or attenuated. Food reinforcement and brain reinforcement are each inadequate models for interpreting some challenges of drug self-administration, and neither can be applied without careful consideration. It is not prudent to draw inferences about the impact of central manipulations on drug reinforcement without considering both similarities and differences between drug reinforcement and other forms of reinforcement. Only with converging evidence from independent sources can changes in drug self-administration rate be safely interpreted. It seems generally more reasonable to infer a decrease in reinforcing drug impact from an increase in self-administration rate than to infer an increase in drug impact from a decrease in self-administration rate; indeed, the interpretation of decreases in response rate is a difficult undertaking regardless of the reinforcer. Parallels from one class of reinforcer to another are not likely to be useful unless they are buttressed with very careful analysis.

REFERENCES

Balster, R. L., & Schuster, C. R. (1973). Fixed-interval schedule of cocaine reinforcement: Effect of dose and infusion duration. Journal of the Experimental Analysis of Behavior, 20, 119-129.

Barker, J. L., Macdonald, R. L., Neale, J. H., & Smith, T. G. (1978). Opiate peptide modulation of amino acid responses suggests novel form of neuronal communication. Science, 199, 1451-1453.

Baxter, B. L., Gluckman, M. I., & Scerni, R. A. (1976). Apomorphine self-injection is not affected by alpha-methylparatyrosine treatment: Support for dopaminergic reward. Physiology & Behavior, 4, 611-612.

Baxter, B. L., Gluckman, M. I., Scerni, R. A., & Stein, L. (1974). Self-injection of apomorphine in the rat: Positive reinforcement by a dopamine receptor stimulant. Pharmacology Biochemistry & Behavior, 2, 387-391.

Beck, R. C. (1978). Motivation. New York: Prentice-Hall.

Bolles, R. C. (1975). Theory of motivation, 2nd Edition. New York: Harper & Row.

Bozarth, M. A., Gerber, G. J., & Wise, R. A. (1980). Intracranial self-stimulation as a technique to study the reward properties of drugs of abuse. Pharmacology Biochemistry & Behavior, 13(Suppl. 1), 245-247.

Bozarth, M. A., & Wise, R. A. (1981). Heroin reward is dependent on a dopaminergic substrate. Life Sciences, 29, 1881-1886.

Carlisle, H. J. (1977). Temperature effects on thirst: Cutaneous or oral receptors? Physiological Psychology, 5, 247-249.

Collier, G. (1962). Some properties of saccharin as a reinforcer. Journal of Experimental Psychology, 64, 184-191.

Collier, G., & Marx, M. H. (1959). Changes in performance as a function of shifts in the magnitude of reinforcement. Journal of Experimental Psychology, 57, 305-309.

Crum, J., Brown, W. L., & Bitterman, M. E. (1951). The effect of partial and delayed reinforcement on resistance to extinction. American Journal of Psychology, 64, 228-237.

Davis, J. D., Gallagher, R. J., Ladlove, R. F., & Turausky, A. J. (1969). Inhibition of food intake by a humoral factor. Journal of Comparative and Physiological Psychology, 67, 407-414.

Davis, W. M., & Smith, S. G. (1977). Catecholaminergic mechanisms of reinforcement: Direct assessment by drug self-administration. Life Sciences, 20, 483-492.

Deutsch, J. A. (1963). Learning and electrical self-stimulation of the brain. Journal of Theoretical Biology, 4, 193-214.

de Wit, H., & Wise, R. A. (1977). Blockade of cocaine reinforcement in rats with the dopamine receptor blocker pimozide, but not with the noradrenergic blockers phentolamine or phenoxybenzamine. Canadian Journal of Psychology, 31, 195-203.

Dougherty, J., & Pickens, R. (1974). Effects of phenobarbital and SKF 525A on cocaine self-administration in rats. Drug Addiction, 3, 135-143.

Downs, D. A., & Woods, J. H. (1974). Codeine- and cocaine-reinforced responding in rhesus monkeys: Effects of dose on response rates under a fixed ratio schedule. Journal of Pharmacology and Experimental Therapeutics, 191, 179-188.

Dufort, R. H., & Kimble, G. A. (1956). Changes in response strength with changes in the amount of reinforcement. Journal of Experimental Psychology, 51, 185-191.

Epstein, A. N., & Teitelbaum, P. (1962). Regulation of food intake in the absence of smell, taste, and other oropharyngeal sensations. Journal of Comparative and Physiological Psychology, 55, 753-759.

Ettenberg, A., Bloom, F. E., & Koob, G. F. (1981). Response artifact in the measurement of neuroleptic-induced anhedonia. Science, 213, 357-359.

Ettenberg, A., Bloom, F. E., Koob, G. F., & Pettit, H. O. (1982). Heroin and cocaine intravenous self-administration in rats: Mediation by separate neural systems. Psychopharmacology, 78, 204-209.

Ferster, C. B., & Skinner, B. F. (1957). Schedules of reinforcement. New York: Appleton-Century-Crofts.

Fouriezos, G., & Wise, R. A. (1976). Pimozide-induced extinction of intracranial self-stimulation: Response patterns rule out motor or performance deficits. Brain Research, 103, 377-380.

Gallistel, C. R., Shizgal, P., & Yeomans, J. S. (1981). A portrait of the substrates for self-stimulation. Psychological Review, 88, 228-273.

Gibson, W. E., Reid, L. D., Sakai, M., & Porter, P. B. (1965). Intracranial reinforcement compared with sugar-water reinforcement. Science, 148, 1357-1358.

Glick, S. D., & Cox, R. D. (1975). Self-administration of haloperidol in rats. Life Sciences, 16, 1041-1046.

Glick, S. D., & Cox, R. D. (1977). Changes in morphine self-administration after brain-stem lesions in rats. Psychopharmacology, 52, 151-156.

Glick, S. D., & Cox, R. D. (1978). Changes in morphine self-administration after tel-diencephalic lesions in rats. Psychopharmacology, 57, 283-288.

Glick, S. D., Cox, R. D., & Crane, A. M. (1975). Changes in morphine self-administration and morphine dependence after lesions of the caudate nucleus. Psychopharmacologia, 41, 219-224.

Glickman, S. E., & Schiff, B. B. (1967). A biological theory of reinforcement. Psychological Review, 74, 81-109.

Gold, R. M., Kapatos, G., Oxford, T. W., Prowse, J., & Quackenbush, P. M. (1973). Role of water temperature in the regulation of water intake. Journal of Comparative and Physiological Psychology, 85, 52-63.

Goldberg, S. R. (1973). Comparable behavior maintained under fixed-ratio and second-order schedules of food presentation, cocaine injections of or d-amphetamine injection in the squirrel monkey. Journal of Pharmacology and Experimental Therapeutics, 186, 18-30.

Goldberg, S. R., & Kelleher, R. T. (1976). Behavior controlled by scheduled injections of cocaine in squirrel and rhesus monkeys. Journal of the Experimental Analysis of Behavior, 25, 93-104.

Griffiths, R. R., Brady, J. V., & Bradford, L. D. (1979). Predicting the abuse liability of drugs with animal self-administration procedures. In T. Thompson & P. E. Dews (Eds.), Advances in behavioral pharmacology (Vol. 2, pp. 39-73). New York: Academic Press.

Gunne, L. M., Anggard, E., & Jonsson, L. E. (1972). Clinical trials with amphetamine-blocking drugs. Psychiatria, Neurologia, Neurochirurgia, 75, 225-226.

Guttman, N. (1953). Operant conditioning, extinction, and periodic reinforcement in relation to concentration of sucrose used as reinforcing agent. Journal of Experimental Psychology, 46, 213-224.

Guttman, N. (1954). Equal-reinforcement values for sucrose and glucose solutions compared with equal sweetness values. Journal of Comparative and Physiological Psychology, 47, 358-361.

Hawkins, T. D., & Pliskoff, S. S. (1964). Brain stimulation intensity, rate of self-stimulation, and reinforcement strength: An analysis through chaining. Journal of the Experimental Analysis of Behavior, 7, 285-288.

Hodos, W., & Valenstein, E. S. (1960). Motivational variables affecting the rate of behavior maintained by intracranial stimulation. Journal of Comparative and Physiological Psychology, 53, 502-508.

Hoebel, B. G., & Teitelbaum, P. (1962). Hypothalamic control of feeding and self-stimulation. Science, 135, 375-377.

Holder, W. B., Marx, M. H., Holder, E. E., & Collier, G. (1957). Response strength as a function of delay in a runway. Journal of Experimental Psychology, 53, 316-323.

Iglauer, C., & Woods, J. H. (1974). Concurrent performances: Reinforcement by different doses of intravenous cocaine in rhesus monkeys. Journal of Experimental Analysis of Behavior, 22, 179-196.

Janssen, P. A. J., Dresse, A., Lenaerts, F. M., Niemegeers, C. J. E., Pinchard, A., Schaper, W. K. A., Schellekens, K. H., Van Nueten, J. M., & Verbruggen, F. J. (1968). Pimozide, a chemically novel, highly potent and orally long-acting neuroleptic drug. Arzneimittel-Forschung, 18, 261-279.

Johanson, C. E. (1978). Drugs as reinforcers. In D. E. Blackman & D. J. Sanger (Eds.), Contemporary research in behavioral pharmacology (pp. 325-390). New York: Plenum Press.

Kelleher, R. T. (1976). Characteristics of behavior controlled by scheduled injections of drugs. Pharmacological Reviews, 27, 307-323.

Kelleher, R. T., & Goldberg, S. R. (1975). Control of drug-taking by schedules of reinforcement. Pharmacological Reviews, 27, 291-299.

Le Magnen, J. (1969). Peripheral and systemic actions of food in the caloric regulation of intake. Annals of the New York Academy of Sciences, 57, 1126-1156.

Logan, F. (1952). The role of delay of reinforcement in determining reaction potential. Journal of Experimental Psychology, 43, 393-399.

Lyness, W. H., Friedle, N. M., & Moore, K. E. (1977). Destruction of dopaminergic nerve terminals in nucleus accumbens: Effect on d-amphetamine self-administration. Pharmacology Biochemistry & Behavior, 11, 553-556.

Marx, M. H. (1969). Positive contrast in instrumental learning from qualitative shift in incentive. Psychonomic Science, 16, 254-255.

Marx, M. H., McCoy, D. F., & Tombaugh, J. W. (1965). Resistance to extinction as a function of constant delay of reinforcement. Psychomonic Science, 2, 333-334.

McIntyre, R. W., & Wright, J. E. (1965). Differences in extinction in electrical brain-stimulation under traditional procedures of reward presentation. Psychological Reports, 16, 909-913.

Mendelson, J. (1966). The role of hunger in T-maze learning for food by rats. Journal of Comparative and Physiological Psychology, 62, 341-349.

Mendelson, J., & Chillag, D. (1970). Tongue cooling: A new reward for thirsty rodents. Science, 170, 1418-1420.

Moltz, H. (1965). Contemporary instinct theory and the fixed action pattern. Psychological Review, 72, 27-47.

Mook, D. G. (1963). Oral and post-ingestional determinants of the intake of various solutions in rats with esophageal fistulas. Journal of Comparative and Physiological Psychology, 56, 645-659.

Morgan, M. (1974). Resistance to satiation. Animal Behavior, 22, 449-466.

Nikolaidis, S., & Rowland, N. (1976). Metering of intravenous versus oral nutrients and regulation of energy balance. American Journal of Physiology, 231, 661-668.

Olds, J. (1956). Runway and maze behavior controlled by basomedial forebrain stimulation in the rat. Journal of Comparative and Physiological Psychology, 49, 507-512.

Olds, J. (1958a). Effects of hunger and male sex hormones on self-stimulation of the brain. Journal of Comparative and Physiological Psychology, 51, 320-324.

Olds, J. (1958b). Satiation effects in self-stimulation of the brain. Journal of Comparative and Physiological Psychology, 51, 675-678.

Panksepp, J., & Trowill, J. A. (1967). Intraoral self injection: Effects of delay of reinforcement on resistance to extinction and implications for self-stimulation. Psychonomic Science, 9, 405-406.

Peterson, L. R. (1956). Variable delayed reinforcement. Journal of Comparative and Physiological Psychology, 49, 232-234.

Pfaffman, C. (1960). The pleasures of sensation. Psychological Review, 67, 253-268.

Phillips, A. G., & Broekkamp, C. L. (1980). Inhibition of intravenous cocaine self-administration by rats after microinjections of spiroperidol into the nucleus accumbens. Society for Neuroscience Abstracts, 6, 105.

Pickens, R. (1968). Self-administration of stimulants by rats. International Journal of the Addictions, 3, 215-221.

Pickens, R., & Harris, W. (1968). Self-administration of d-amphetamine by rats. Psychopharmacology, 12, 158-163.

Pickens, R., Meisch, R. A., & Dougherty, J. A. (1968). Chemical interactions in methamphetamine reinforcement. Psychological Reports, 23, 1267-1270.

Pickens, R., & Thompson, T. (1968). Cocaine-reinforced behavior in rats: Effects of reinforcement magnitude and fixed-ratio size. Journal of Pharmacology and Experimental Therapeutics, 161, 122-129.

Pickens, R. & Thompson, T. (1971). Characteristics of stimulant drug reinforcement. In T. Thompson & R. Pickens (Eds.), Stimulus properties of drugs (pp. 177-192). New York: Appleton, Century, Crofts.

Pliskoff, S. S., Wright, G. E., & Hawkins, D. T. (1965). Brain stimulation as a reinforcer: Intermittent schedules. Journal of the Experimental Analysis of Behavior, 8, 75-80.

Ramsauer, S., Freed, W. J., & Mendelson, J. (1974). Effects of water temperature on the reward value and satiating capacity of water in water-deprived rats. Behavioral Biology, 11, 381-393.

Risner, M. E., & Jones, B. E. (1976). Role of noradrenergic and dopaminergic processes in amphetamine self-administration. Pharmacology Biochemistry & Behavior, 5, 477-482.

Risner, M. E., & Jones, B. E. (1980). Intravenous administration of cocaine and norcocaine by dogs. Psychopharmacology, 71, 83-89.

Roberts, D. C. S., Corcoran, M. E., & Fibiger, H. C. (1977). On the role of ascending catecholamine systems in intravenous self-administration of cocaine. Pharmacology Biochemistry & Behavior, 6, 615-620.

Roberts, D. C. S., & Koob, G. F. (1980). Disruption of cocaine self-administration following 6-hydroxydopamine lesions of the ventral tegmental area in rats. Pharmacology Biochemistry & Behavior, 17, 901-904.

Roberts, D. C. S., Koob, G. F., Klonoff, P., & Fibiger, H. C. (1980). Extinction and recovery of cocaine self-administration following 6-OHDA lesions of the nucleus accumbens. Pharmacology Biochemistry & Behavior, 12, 781-787.

Schaeffer, R. W., & Hanna, B. (1966). Effects of quality and quantity of reinforcement upon response rate in acquisition and extinction. Psychological Reports, 18, 819-829.

Schuster, C. R. (1970). Psychological approach to opiate dependence and self-administration by laboratory animals. Federation Proceedings, 29, 2-5.

Schuster, C. R., & Balster, R. L. (1973). Self-administration of agonists. In H. W. Kosterlitz, H. O. J. Collier, & J. E. Villarreal (Eds.), Agonist and antagonist actions of narcotic analgesic drugs. Baltimore: University Park Press.

Schuster, C. R., & Johanson, C. E. (1981). An analysis of drug-seeking behavior in animals. Neuroscience & Biobehavioral Reviews, 5, 315-323.

Schuster, C. R., & Thompson, T. (1969). Self-administration of and behavioral dependence on drugs. Annual Review of Pharmacology, 9, 483-502.

Seward, J. P., Uyeda, A. A., & Olds, J. (1959). Resistance to extinction following intracranial self-stimulation. Journal of Comparative and Physiological Psychology, 52, 294-299.

Seward, J. P., Uyeda, A. A., & Olds, J. (1960). Reinforcing effect of brain stimulation on runway performance as a function of interval between trials. Journal of Comparative and Physiological Psychology, 53, 224-227.

Sheffield, F. D., & Roby, T. B. (1950). Reward value of a non-nutritive sweet taste. Journal of Comparative and Physiological Psychology, 43, 471-481.

Sidman, M., Brady, J. V., Conrad, D. G., & Schulman, A. (1955). Reward schedules and behavior maintained by intracranial self-stimulation. Science, 122, 830-831.

Skinner, B. F. (1935). The generic nature of the concepts of stimulus and response. Journal of General Psychology, 12, 40-65.

Skinner, B. F. (1938). The behavior of organisms. New York: Appleton.

van Sommers, P., & Teitelbaum, P. (1974). Spread of damage produced by electrolytic lesions in the hypothalamus. Journal of Comparative and Physiological Psychology, 86, 288-299.

Spealman, R. D., & Goldberg, S. R. (1978). Drug self-administration by laboratory animals: Control by schedules of reinforcement. Annual Review of Pharmacology and Toxicology, 18, 313-339.

Spyraki, C., Fibiger, H. C., & Phillips, A. G. (1982). Dopaminergic substrates of amphetamine-induced place preference conditioning. Brain Research, 253, 185-193.

Spyraki, C., Fibiger, H. C., & Phillips, A. G. (1983). Attenuation of heroin reward in rats by disruption of the mesolimbic dopamine system. Psychopharmacology, 79, 278-283.

Tang, A. H., & Collins, R. J. (1978). Enhanced analgesic effects of morphine after chronic administration of naloxone in the rat. European Journal of Pharmacology, 47, 473-474.

Thorndike, E. L. (1911). Animal intelligence. New York: Macmillan.

Tombaugh, T. N., Tombaugh, J., & Anisman, H. (1979). Effects of dopamine receptor blockade on alimentary behaviors: Home cage food consumption, magazine training, operant acquisition, and performance. Psychopharmacology, 66, 219-225.

Trowill, J. A., Panksepp, J., & Gandelman, R. (1969). An incentive model of rewarding brain stimulation. Psychological Review, 76, 264-281.

Weeks, J. R., & Collins, R. J. (1964). Factors affecting voluntary morphine intake in self-maintained addicted rats. Psychopharmacologia, 6, 267-279.

Wilson, M. C., & Schuster, C. R. (1972). The effects of chlorpromazine on psychomotor stimulant self-administration in the rhesus monkey. Psychopharmacologia, 26, 115-126.

Wise, R. A. (1974). Lateral hypothalamic electrical stimulation: Does it make animals hungry? Brain Research, 67, 187-209.

Wise, R. A. (1982). Neuroleptics and operant behavior: The anhedonia hypothesis. Behavioral and Brain Sciences, 5, 39-87.

Wise, R. A., & Bozarth, M. A. (1984). Brain reward circuitry: Four circuit elements "wired" in apparent series. Brain Research Bulletin, 12, 203-208.

Wise, R. A., de Wit, H., Gerber, G. J., & Spindler, J. (1978). Neuroleptic-induced "anhedonia" in rats: Pimozide blocks the reward quality of food. Science, 201, 262-264.

Wise, R. A., Spindler, J., & Legault, L. (1978). Major attenuation of food reward with performance-sparing doses of pimozide in the rat. Canadian Journal of Psychology, 32, 77-85.

Wise, R. A., Yokel, R. A., & de Wit, H. (1976). Both positive reinforcement and conditioned taste aversion from amphetamine and apomorphine in rats. Science, 191, 1273-1275.

Wise, R. A., Yokel, R. A., Gerber, G. J., & Hansson, P. (1977). Concurrent intracranial self-stimulation and intravenous amphetamine self-administration in rats. Pharmacology Biochemistry & Behavior, 7, 459-461.

Woods, J. H., & Schuster, C. R. (1968). Reinforcement properties of morphine, cocaine, and SPA as a function of unit dose. International Journal of the Addictions, 3, 231-237.

Woodworth, R. S. (1918). Dynamic psychology. New York: Columbia University Press.

Yokel, R. A., & Pickens, R. (1973). Self-administration of optical isomers of amphetamine and methylamphetamine by rats. Journal of Pharmacology and Experimental Therapeutics, 187, 27-33.

Yokel, R. A., & Pickens, R. (1974). Drug level of d- and l-amphetamine during intravenous self-administration. Psychopharmacologia, 34, 255-264.

Yokel, R. A., & Wise, R. A. (1975). Increased lever pressing for amphetamine after pimozide in rats: Implications for a dopamine theory of reward. Science, 187, 547-549.

Yokel, R. A., & Wise, R. A. (1976). Attenuation of intravenous amphetamine reinforcement by central dopaminergic blockade in rats. Psychopharmacology, 48, 311-318.

Yokel, R. A., & Wise, R. A. (1978). Amphetamine-type reinforcement by dopamine agonists in the rat. Psychopharmacology, 58, 289-296.

Young, P. T., & Shuford, E. H. (1955). Quantitative control of motivation through sucrose solutions of different concentrations. Journal of Comparative and Physiological Psychology, 48, 114-118.

CHAPTER 7

ORAL DRUG SELF-ADMINISTRATION: DRUGS AS REINFORCERS

Richard A. Meisch and Marilyn E. Carroll

Department of Psychiatry
University of Minnesota
Minneapolis, Minnesota 55455

ABSTRACT

Drugs from the four major classes of abused drugs can serve as reinforcers when taken orally. In studies from several laboratories rats, rhesus monkeys, and baboons have served as subjects. Surprisingly, behavior reinforced by orally delivered drugs appears quite strong despite the long delay between ingestion and onset of drug effects. Drug delivery, if appropriately scheduled, can maintain high rates of responding over long periods of time. The rate and pattern of drug reinforced behavior vary in an orderly way according to a number of variables such as drug concentration, reinforcement schedule, and feeding conditions (e.g., food deprivation vs. food satiation). The significance of these findings is that an animal model of oral drug (including alcohol) abuse now exists. This is important because the oral route is the most common route of drug abuse in humans. Furthermore, unlike the intravenous route where short catheter life limits experiments, the oral route permits complex sequential experiments that span many years.

INTRODUCTION

In the 1960s techniques were developed so that animals could inject themselves with drugs (Deneau, Yanagita, & Seevers, 1969; Thompson & Schuster, 1964; Weeks, 1962). These techniques have now been used in many studies (for reviews see Griffiths, Bigelow, & Henningfield, 1980; Johanson, 1978; Johanson & Schuster, 1981; Pickens, Meisch, & Thompson, 1978; Spealman & Goldberg, 1978). Two major conclusions emerging from these studies are that the drugs that serve as reinforcers for animals are the same drugs that humans abuse (Griffiths & Balster, 1979; Johanson & Balster, 1978) and that drug taking behavior is a specific instance of operant behavior--behavior controlled by its consequences.

SELF-ADMINISTRATION OF ORALLY DELIVERED DRUGS VS. BEHAVIOR REINFORCED BY ORALLY DELIVERED DRUGS

There are many ways to obtain drug self-administration. Animals can be restricted to a liquid solution containing the drug. Extrinsic reinforcement can be used, such as making food pellet delivery or escape from electric shock contingent upon drinking. If one's objective is simply to get the animal to self-dose, then these are good methods. However, oral drug self-administration must not be confused with behavior reinforced by orally delivered drugs. This paper is concerned with the latter topic. With drug reinforced behavior, intake of the drug is not secondary to induced intake of the vehicle or to extrinsic reinforcement of drinking. To demonstrate that a drug is serving as a positive reinforcer, it is generally accepted that one should document three findings. First, drug presentation must be shown to maintain characteristic patterns of intermittently reinforced behavior. Second, rates of drug maintained behavior must exceed rates of vehicle maintained behavior when the vehicle is presented either sequentially or concurrently with the drug. Finally, orderly concentration response curves must be demonstrated.

Techniques are now available so that drug-reinforced behavior can be studied when drugs serve as reinforcers under conditions where they are taken intragastrically (Altshuler, Weaver, & Phillips, 1975; Yanagita & Takahashi, 1973), intramuscularly (Goldberg, Morse, & Goldberg, 1976; Katz, 1979), and by inhalation (Wood, Grubman, & Weiss, 1977; Yanagita, Takahashi, Ishida, & Funamoto, 1970).

ESTABLISHMENT OF ORALLY DELIVERED DRUGS AS REINFORCERS

Over the last 15 years, techniques have been developed at the University of Minnesota that permit the establishment of orally delivered drugs as reinforcers for both rats and rhesus monkeys. The general strategy is to food deprive the animals and then to give them their ration of food during daily 3-hour sessions. Water drinking reliably follows eating. Next, low drug concentrations are substituted for water, and across sessions the drug concentration is gradually increased. Once an intermediate concentration is reached, the time of feeding is shifted from within the session to after the session so that drinking is no longer induced by presentation of food. If the drug has come to function as a reinforcer, then drinking persists even when it is no longer induced by food. To confirm that the drug is functioning as a reinforcer, several tests are performed. Delivery of the drug is intermittently scheduled, and response rates maintained by the drug and the vehicle are compared. Often a concentration response function is obtained. These steps are illustrated below by results of a study done with rhesus monkeys and ethanol (Henningfield & Meisch, 1977).

In this study ethanol was established as a reinforcer for four ethanol-naive rhesus monkeys. The monkeys lived in their experimental chambers. Sessions were 3 hours in duration and were conducted daily at a regular starting time. Each session was preceded and followed by a 1-hour time-out when responding had no consequences and data were recorded and solutions changed. Water was continuously available during the 19-hour intersession periods.

The monkeys were reduced to and maintained at 80% of their free-feeding weights. Liquids were delivered through a spout that had an electronic sensing device for detecting lip-contacts. Each lip contact resulted in an illumination of a feed-back light above the spout and operation of a solenoid-controlled valve that permitted the delivery of 0.5 ml of liquid. Details of the apparatus and drinking device have been reported (Henningfield & Meisch, 1976a; Meisch & Henningfield, 1977).

During the initial phase, the baseline rate of water drinking was determined. Figure 1 shows that in general little drinking occurred. An

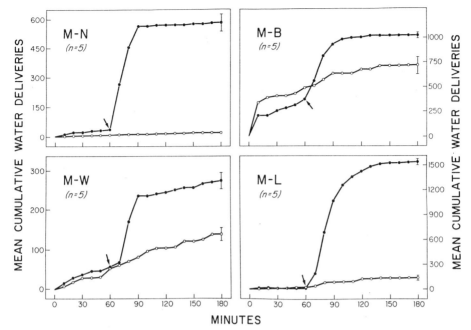

Figure 1: Cumulative means (n = 5) of liquid deliveries at 10-minute intervals during 3-hour sessions. Filled circles indicate water deliveries during sessions when food pellets were available. Unfilled circles indicate water deliveries during sessions when food was not concurrently available. Brackets show the standard error of the mean. Absence of brackets indicates that the standard error value fell within the area occupied by the plotted point. Arrows mark the first interval when food pellets were available. Reprinted with permission from Henningfield and Meisch, 1977.

exception was monkey M-B who showed a high rate of water intake. In the next phase drinking was induced by giving the monkeys access to their daily ration of food within instead of after the session. Food access began at the second hour of the 3-hour session. Figure 1 shows that a high rate of water drinking promptly followed eating.

In the next phase a series of increasing ethanol concentrations (0.5, 1, 2, 4, 5.6, and 8% w/v) was substituted for water. Each concentration was present for at least five sessions and until behavior stabilized. Figure 2 shows that during this induced drinking phase the number of liquid deliveries was an inverted U-shaped function of ethanol concentration. Although the number of deliveries decreased at the higher concentrations, the quantity of ethanol consumed (g per kg of body weight) went up with increases in the concentration. At concentrations of 0.5, 1, 2, 4, 5.6, and 8%, the monkeys drank 0.31, 0.74, 1.42, 2.18, 2.84, and 3.14 g/kg/3-hour session, respectively.

Once behavior was stable at 8%, the time of feeding was permanently switched from within the session to 1 hour after the end of the session.

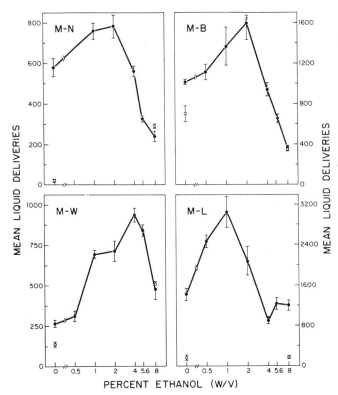

Figure 2: Mean liquid deliveries (n = 5) per 3-hour session as a function of ethanol concentration. Filled circles indicate that food was available during the sessions (food-induced drinking procedure). Open circles indicate that food was available after the termination of the session, and only liquid was available during the session. Brackets show the standard error of the mean. Note the different scales of the ordinates. Reprinted with permission from Henningfield and Meisch, 1977.

Figure 2 shows that for three of the four monkeys ethanol drinking persisted at levels close to the induced drinking levels. The fourth monkey, M-L, showed the highest intake during the induced drinking phase, 5.76 g/kg/3-hour session. This monkey's drinking declined the most and reached a level of 0.99 g/kg/3-hour session. Nevertheless, he continued to consume the ethanol solution and as subsequent tests showed, ethanol had been established as a reinforcer for all monkeys.

In the next phase the number of responses required per ethanol delivery, that is the fixed-ratio (FR) schedule of reinforcement, was increased in the following steps: 1, 2, 4, 8, 16. Figure 3 shows that as the response requirement was increased, the number of responses increased directly with the response requirement, whereas the number of liquid deliveries remained relatively constant. At FR-16 the mean intake was 1.96 g/kg/3-hour session. Liquid deliveries were distributed in a negatively accelerated pattern; that is, the highest rate was at the beginning of the session. The large initial burst was followed by a pause and then by smaller bouts in the latter part of the session. Responding, when it occurred, was characteristic of FR responding maintained by other reinforcers.

In the last phase water was substituted for 8% ethanol. After behavior was stable for five sessions, the ethanol was reintroduced. Responding was maintained at substantially higher rates by the ethanol solution than by water

Figure 3: Mean responses and 8% ethanol deliveries (n = 5) as a function of fixed-ratio size. Brackets show the standard error of the mean. Absence of brackets indicates that standard error values fell within an area occupied by the plotted point. Reprinted with permission from Henningfield and Meisch, 1977.

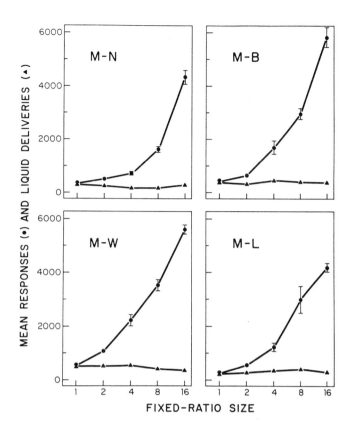

(see Figure 4). Thus, ethanol was serving as a positive reinforcer. Note that the data for monkey M-B are from sessions at FR-32 rather than at FR-16. For this monkey when water was substituted for 8% ethanol at FR-16, his response rate increased in the presence of water; thus, the FR value was increased to FR-32. With other monkeys it has been occasionally noted that at low FR values, vehicle maintained responding may equal or exceed that maintained by drug (Henningfield & Meisch, 1976b). However, clear differences in response rates emerged when the magnitude of the response requirement was increased.

PROCEDURES USED TO ESTABLISH ORALLY DELIVERED DRUGS AS REINFORCERS

A number of techniques have been used to establish orally delivered drugs as reinforcers. In one study several of these techniques were compared. With rats three different strategies were successfully used to obtain ethanol reinforced responding (Meisch, 1975). In the first procedure food-induced drinking was used in a manner similar to that described above for rhesus monkeys. In the second procedure schedule-induced polydipsia was used to generate high levels of water drinking; and once water intake was stable, the water was replaced by 8% (w/v) ethanol. Schedule-induced polydipsia refers to the excessive water intake that occurs when food deprived animals receive small pellets of food at the rate of approximately one pellet per minute (Falk, 1961,

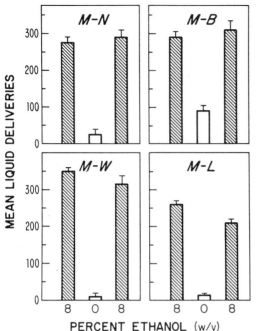

Figure 4: Mean liquid deliveries (n = 5) per 3-hour session when either 8% ethanol (striped bars) or water (open bars) was present. Brackets show the standard error of the mean. Liquid deliveries for monkey M-B were contingent on FR-32 whereas liquid deliveries for the other three monkeys were contingent on FR-16. Reprinted with permission from Henningfield and Meisch, 1977.

1971). After five sessions of schedule-induced ethanol drinking, the food schedule was terminated, and water drinking dropped to low values; whereas, ethanol drinking persisted at values significantly greater than water values. Schedule-induced polydipsia has also been used to establish etonitazene as a reinforcer for rats (Leander & McMillan, 1975; McMillan & Leander, 1976; Meisch & Stark, 1977a), and it has been used to establish ethanol (Meisch, Henningfield, & Thompson, 1975), phencyclidine (Carroll & Meisch, 1980b), and etonitazene (Carroll & Meisch, 1978) as reinforcers for rhesus monkeys. With the third procedure rats were food deprived and ethanol was simply made available in the liquid reservoir (Meisch, 1975). This procedure was also effective. Importantly, once ethanol reinforced responding was stable and no longer induced, the pattern of responding was similar regardless of the acquisition procedure used.

Two additional procedures have been used in recent studies to establish orally delivered drugs as reinforcers for rhesus monkeys. With the first procedure the drug solution was simply made available to food-satiated rhesus monkeys for 3 hours daily (Carroll, 1982b). Another group received the same treatment but was food deprived. Phencyclidine was rapidly established as a reinforcer in both groups. A second procedure, that has been tested recently, involves drug substitution. This procedure parallels intravenous drug self-administration research (cf. Johanson & Balster, 1978). d-Amphetamine, ketamine (Carroll & Stotz, 1983), methohexital (Carroll, Stotz, Kliner, & Meisch, 1984) and phencyclidine analogs (Carroll, 1982a) have been established as reinforcers for rhesus monkeys by substituting these drugs for pentobarbital or phencyclidine. Drug history appears to be an important determinant of the success of these substitution procedures (Carroll et al., 1984). Despite the existence of these and other procedures for establishing orally delivered drugs

Table 1

Establishment of Orally Delivered Drugs as Reinforcers

Rats

codeine	Suzuki et al., 1982
ethanol	Marcucella et al., 1984; Meisch, 1969, 1975; Meisch & Thompson, 1971, 1974b; Poling & Thompson, 1977a; Roehrs & Samson, 1981; Samson & Falk, 1974
etonitazene	Beardsley & Meisch, 1981; Carroll & Meisch, 1979a, 1979b; Leander & McMillan, 1975; Lewis et al., 1975; McMillan & Leander, 1976; Meisch & Kliner, 1979; Meisch & Stark, 1977a
fentanyl	Carroll & Meisch, 1984
morphine	Suzuki et al., 1982

Rhesus monkeys

d-amphetamine	Carroll & Stotz, 1983
ethanol	Henningfield & Meisch, 1977; Meisch et al., 1975; Meisch & Henningfield, 1977
etonitazene	Carroll & Meisch, 1978
ketamine	Carroll & Stotz, 1983
methohexital	Carroll et al., 1984
PCE (N-ethyl-1-phencyclohexylamine)	Carroll, 1982a
pentobarbital	DeNoble et al., 1982; Meisch et al.,1981
phencyclidine	Carroll, 1982a, 1982b, 1982c, 1984a, 1984b, 1985a, 1985b; Carroll & Meisch, 1980b
TCP {1-[1-(2-thienyl) cyclohexyl] piperidine}	Carroll, 1982a

Baboons

ethanol	Henningfield et al., 1981
methohexital	Ator & Griffiths, 1983

----

as reinforcers, there is still no standard procedure that is uniformly effective with all drugs. Table 1 lists drugs that have been established as reinforcers when taken orally, and the reader is referred to the references listed for details of how particular drugs came to function as reinforcers. Note that more drugs have been established as reinforcers for rhesus monkeys than for rats.

FACTORS CONTROLLING BEHAVIOR REINFORCED BY ORALLY DELIVERED DRUGS

Drug Concentration

Generally, drug-reinforced responding is an inverted U-shaped function of drug concentration (e.g., Figure 5). Table 2 lists studies in which concentration was varied. In contrast to rate of responding, drug intake (mg of drug/kg of body weight/session) increases as drug concentration is increased (see Figure 5). Varying drug concentration is one way to vary amount of drug per response sequence. Another way is to hold concentration constant but vary the volume delivered. This procedure has been used in one study (Henningfield & Meisch, 1975), and the results were consistent with those obtained when concentration was varied.

Schedules of Reinforcement

Orally delivered drugs can maintain responding that is intermittently reinforced. The most frequently studied schedule in both oral and intravenous studies is the fixed-ratio (FR) schedule (Spealman & Goldberg, 1978). Under such a schedule delivery of the drug is contingent upon emission of a fixed number of responses. Two results are reliably observed when FR size is increased: (1) response rate first increases and then decreases and (2) liquid deliveries initially remain constant and then systematically decrease (Meisch & Thompson, 1973). Figure 3 shows these functions for FRs of 16 and lower. Table 3 lists studies of FR responding maintained by oral drug delivery. In intravenous studies as animals become more experienced, responding can be maintained at lower drug doses and at higher FRs (Goldberg, 1973). It is our impression that when the oral route is used behavior can be maintained under a broader range of conditions as the animals become more experienced.

Orally delivered drugs can also maintain behavior reinforced under interval schedules (Anderson & Thompson, 1974; Beardsley, Lemaire, & Meisch, 1983; Carroll, 1985b; Treibergs & Meisch, 1979). A special case of interval schedules occurs when drugs are delivered only at the end of the session (Carroll, 1984b; 1985b; Meisch & Thompson, 1974a). This method of scheduling drug delivery permits the antecedent behavior to be reinforced by drug delivery, but responding is not disrupted by the effects (e.g., intoxication) that follow drug intake (Goldberg et al., 1976; see also Katz & Goldberg, this volume).

SECOND ORDER SCHEDULES AS A MEANS OF REDUCING THE EFFECTS OF DRUG INTAKE ON DRUG-REINFORCED BEHAVIOR

Second-order schedules have been extensively used to study behavior maintained by intravenously delivered drugs (e.g., Goldberg, Kelleher, & Morse, 1975; Katz & Goldberg, this volume), and they have recently been applied to behavior maintained by orally delivered drugs (Carroll, 1984b, 1985b). Under a second-order schedule, behavioral requirements specified by one schedule are considered as a unitary response that is reinforced according to a second schedule (Kelleher, 1966a, 1966b). These schedules can be used to generate

Table 2

Studies of Drug Concentration on Behavior Reinforced by Oral Delivery of Drugs

----

Rats

ethanol	Beardsley et al., 1978; Meisch, 1975; Meisch & Beardsley, 1975; Meisch & Thompson, 1971, 1974b, 1974c; Poling & Thompson, 1977b
etonitazene	Carroll & Meisch, 1979a; Meisch & Stark, 1977a

Rhesus monkeys

d-amphetamine	Carroll & Stotz, 1983
ethanol	Henningfield & Meisch, 1977, 1978, 1979; Meisch et al., 1975; Meisch & Henningfield, 1977
etonitazene	Carroll & Meisch, 1978
ketamine	Carroll & Stotz, 1983
methohexital	Carroll et al., 1984
PCE (N-ethyl-1-phencyclohexylamine)	Carroll, 1982a
pentobarbital	DeNoble et al., 1982; Lemaire & Meisch, 1984; Meisch et al., 1981
phencyclidine	Carroll, 1984a, 1985a; Carroll & Meisch, 1980b; Carroll & Stotz, 1983
TCP {1-[1-(2-thienyl) cyclohexyl] piperidine}	Carroll, 1982a

Baboons

ethanol	Henningfield et al., 1981
methohexital	Ator & Griffiths, 1983

----

high rates and long sequences of behavior, to increase low rates of responding for certain drugs such as nicotine (Goldberg, Spealman, & Goldberg, 1981), to provide a complex behavioral baseline upon which to compare reinforcers, and to prevent intoxication or overdose by scheduling long intervals between drug infusions or by providing all drug at the end of the session.

A recent study was conducted in our laboratory to compare the effects of food satiation and food deprivation on behavior maintained by a second-order schedule. In one study three rhesus monkeys responded under a second-order fixed interval (FI) 60-minute (FR-16:S) schedule for either 300 or an unlimited

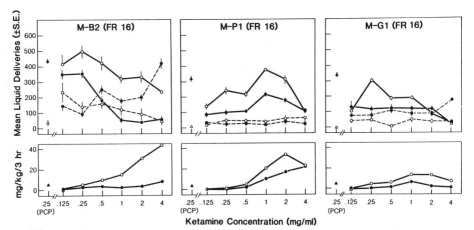

Figure 5: Mean liquid deliveries and drug intake (mg/kg) are presented as a function of phencyclidine (PCP) or ketamine concentration for monkeys M-B2, M-P1, and M-G1. Concentrations were presented in the following order--PCP: 0.25, 0.5, 1, 2, 4, and 0.5 mg/ml; ketamine: 0.25, 0.125, and 0.5 mg/ml. The FR schedule parameters for liquid deliveries are indicated in parentheses. **Upper frames:** filled triangles, PCP deliveries, and open triangles, water deliveries under a concurrent FR-16 schedule. Open circles, food deprivation sessions; filled circles, food satiation sessions; solid lines, ketamine deliveries; dashed lines, concurrent water deliveries. **Lower frames:** PCP intake (mg/kg) is indicated by triangles. Open circles, ketamine intake during food deprivation sessions; filled circles, ketamine intake during food satiation sessions. Each point refers to a mean (±SEM) of the last five sessions of stable behavior at each condition. Reprinted with permission from Carroll and Stotz, 1983. Copyright 1983 by the American Society for Pharmacology and Experimental Therapeutics.

number of phencyclidine (0.25 mg/ml) deliveries (0.55 ml each) while food satiated or food deprived (Carroll, 1985b). The stimulus (S) presented after each 16 responses was a brief auditory and visual stimulus and delivery of a small amount of water (0.02 ml) for 20 milliseconds. During food deprivation the second-order schedule produced high, steady rates of responding (e.g., 74.4 to 156.6 responses/minute) throughout the 60-minute interval. However, during food satiation, response rates declined to a range of 21 to 67.8, and the pattern of responding became more sporadic. Schedule-maintained responding during the 60-minute interval was not altered by the number of liquid deliveries available at the end of the session (300 vs. an unlimited number, approximately 750 to 1350). To evaluate the importance of brief stimulus presentations to the persistence of high rates of responding, brief stimulus presentations were removed; thus, the schedule was a tandem FI 60-minute/FR-16. The monkeys were also tested under a simple FI 60-minute schedule. Response rates decreased to a maximum of 33.6 and 7.8 responses/minute under the tandem and FI schedules, respectively, and these response rates decreased again by about one half when the monkeys were food satiated. These results showed that long sequences of behavior could be maintained by time-based schedules with all drug delivered orally at the end of the session. Response rates were markedly increased by food deprivation even when the amount of drug delivered at the end

Table 3

Studies of Fixed-Ratio Responding Maintained by Oral Drug Delivery

---

Rats

codeine	Suzuki et al., 1982
ethanol	Meisch & Thompson, 1973; Roehrs & Samson, 1981
etonitazene	Meisch & Stark, 1977a, 1977b
morphine	Suzuki et al., 1982

Rhesus monkeys

ethanol	Henningfield & Meisch, 1976b; Henningfield & Meisch, 1977
etonitazene	Carroll & Meisch, 1978
pentobarbital	DeNoble et al., 1982; Lemaire & Meisch, 1984; Meisch et al., 1981
phencyclidine	Carroll, 1982b; Carroll & Meisch, 1980b

---

of the session was fixed at 300 deliveries indicating that increases in response rate due to food deprivation can occur independently of increases in drug intake.

In another study with six monkeys, a second-order FR-240 (FR-20:S) schedule was used to generate high rates of responding in monkeys that had been performing under concurrent FR-16 schedules for 300 deliveries of phencyclidine 0.25 mg/ml (Carroll, 1984b). According to this schedule a brief stimulus was presented each time 20 lip-contact responses were completed. The stimulus consisted of a brief auditory and visual signal and the delivery of 0.02 ml of liquid. After 240 brief stimuli had been delivered, 300 phencyclidine deliveries were available from another drinking spout under an FR-1 schedule. After 10 sessions under the second-order schedule, the monkeys were returned to the concurrent FR-16 schedules. Phencyclidine-maintained responding increased by 42% after second-order schedule training, and this increase appeared to be irreversible. A control group received the same second-order schedule training with a saccharin solution rather than phencyclidine, and another control group received the same amount of phencyclidine (under an FR-1 schedule) as the initial group did during training, except they were not trained under a second-order schedule. Neither of these groups showed a change in concurrent FR-16 performance. Thus, drug-reinforced behavior was markedly influenced by a combination of brief behavioral and drug histories.

FOOD DEPRIVATION EFFECTS ON DRUG-REINFORCED BEHAVIOR

Food deprivation increases drug intake and drug reinforced behavior (for a review see Carroll & Meisch, 1984). The increases occur with drugs from four pharmacological classes: general depressants, opioids, psychomotor stimulants, and the dissociative anesthetics. These increases are found with both the oral

and intravenous routes and with both rats and rhesus monkeys. Figure 5
illustrates that over a range of ketamine concentrations, more ketamine
deliveries were obtained when monkeys were food deprived than when they were
food satiated (Carroll & Stotz, 1983). Figure 6 shows results from another
experiment (Kliner & Meisch, 1982a). Food satiation produced an abrupt
decrease in pentobarbital deliveries for four monkeys that had been maintained
at 70 to 75% of their free-feeding body weights. These decreases lasted
throughout the entire 30-day food satiation phase. When the monkeys were again
food deprived, pentobarbital deliveries gradually increased to their former
levels. Table 4 lists studies published since 1970 that have reported such
increases when the oral route is used. Prior to 1970 many investigators noted
that food deprivation increases ethanol intake, and these increases were
attributed to the caloric property of ethanol (for a review see Meisch, 1977).
Some possible explanations for the increased drug intake have been ruled out.
For example, the greater drug intake during food deprivation is not due to a
nonspecific increase in activity or to increased intake of the vehicle. Food
deprivation appears to act by enhancing the reinforcing efficacy of the drugs,
but the mechanism is not known. The increases in drug intake due to food

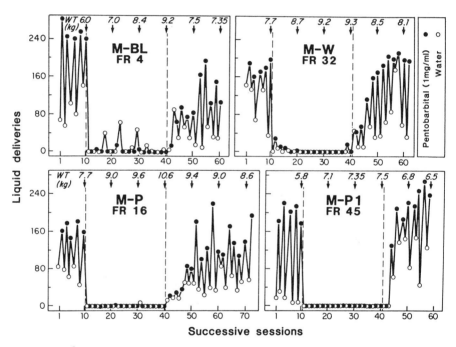

Figure 6: Liquid deliveries of 1 mg/ml pentobarbital (filled points)
or water (open points) are plotted as a function of food condition:
deprivation (sessions 1 to 10), satiation (sessions 11 to 40), and
redeprivation (sessions > 41). Numbers and arrows above data points
refer to the body weights of monkeys (in kilograms) and the
respective days on which they were obtained. Note that the FR size
differed for each of the four monkeys tested. Reprinted with
permission from Kliner and Meisch, 1982a. Copyright 1982 by Ankho
International, Inc.

Table 4

Studies of Food Deprivation and Food Satiation
on Behavior Reinforced by Oral Drug Delivery

Rats

ethanol	Beardsley et al., 1978; Meisch & Thompson, 1973, 1974b; Roehrs & Samson, 1982
etonitazene	Carroll et al., 1979; Carroll & Meisch, 1979b, 1980a, 1981; Meisch & Kliner, 1979; Meisch & Stark, 1977b
fentanyl	Carroll & Meisch, 1984

Rhesus monkeys

d-amphetamine	Carroll & Stotz, 1983
ethanol	Kliner & Meisch, unpublished data
ketamine	Carroll & Stotz, 1983
methohexital	Carroll et al., 1984
pentobarbital	Kliner & Meisch, 1982a, 1982b
phencyclidine	Carroll, 1982b, 1985b; Carroll & Meisch, 1980b; Carroll & Stotz, 1983

----

deprivation may be a specific case of a more general phenomenon, for increased intravenous drug self-administration has been reported to occur during water deprivation (Carroll & Boe, 1982).

CONCLUSIONS

Drugs from the four major classes of abused drugs--opioids, psychomotor stimulants, dissociative anesthetics, and general depressants--can function as effective reinforcers when taken by mouth. The subjects used in these studies have included rats, rhesus monkeys, and baboons. Several different procedures can be used to establish drugs as reinforcers. Work in our laboratory has shown that some acquisition procedures can effectively establish some drugs as reinforcers in only a few weeks. However, no one procedure is uniformly effective for all drugs and subjects.

There are many advantages to using the oral route. Long sequential experiments can be conducted, and invasive surgical procedures and sterile conditions are not necessary. Importantly, the oral route is the most common route of drug abuse in humans. However, there are several limitations to the oral procedure. For example, the aversive taste of drug solutions may limit the range of concentrations that can be tested, and it often takes longer with the oral route than with the intravenous route to establish drugs as reinforcers. It appears to be more difficult to establish orally delivered drugs as reinforcers for rats than it is for rhesus monkeys. Monkeys are more expensive than rats, but their experimental life is longer than that of rats.

Acquisition procedures and their results vary considerably with drugs and species, but once drug reinforced behavior has been established, the amount and pattern of responding seem to be independent of the particular training procedure used. The stabilized pattern of responding is characterized by a negatively accelerated time course; that is, the highest rate of responding is at the beginning of the session. Number of drug deliveries is an inverted U-shaped function of drug concentration; whereas, drug intake (mg of drug/kg of body weight/hour) is a direct function of drug concentration. High persistent rates of responding can be maintained under intermittent schedules of reinforcement. Under many conditions food deprivation increases drug reinforced behavior. Findings obtained with the oral route confirm and extend findings obtained with the intravenous route. These findings also demonstrate the feasibility of using the oral route in studies of drug reinforced behavior.

ACKNOWLEDGMENTS

Preparation of this manuscript was supported by NIAAA Grant AA 00299, NIDA Grant DA 00944, and Research Scientist Development Award DA 00007 to R. A. M. and by Grants DA 02486 and DA 03240 to M. E. C.

REFERENCES

Altshuler, H. L., Weaver, S., & Phillips, P. (1975). Intragastric self-administration of psychoactive drugs by the rhesus monkey. Life Sciences, 17, 883-890.

Anderson, W. W., & Thompson, T. (1974). Ethanol self-administration in water satiated rats. Pharmacology Biochemistry & Behavior, 2, 447-454.

Ator, N. A., & Griffiths, R. R. (1983). Oral self-administration of methohexital in baboons. Psychopharmacology, 79, 120-125.

Beardsley, P. M., Lemaire, G. A., & Meisch, R. A. (1983). Effects of minimum-interreinforcer interval on ethanol-maintained performance in rats. Pharmacology Biochemistry & Behavior, 19, 843-847.

Beardsley, P. M., & Meisch, R. A. (1981). A precision drinking device for rats tested with water, etonitazene, and ethanol. Pharmacology Biochemistry & Behavior, 14, 871-876.

Carroll, M. E. (1982a). Oral self-administration of phencyclidine analogs by rhesus monkeys: Conditioned taste and visual reinforcers. Psychopharmacology, 78, 116-120.

Carroll, M. E. (1982b). Rapid acquisition of oral phencyclidine self-administration in food-deprived and food-satiated rhesus monkeys: Concurrent phencyclidine and water choice. Pharmacology Biochemistry & Behavior, 17, 341-346.

Carroll, M. E. (1982c). Tolerance to the behavioral effects of orally self-administered phencyclidine. Drug and Alcohol Dependence, 9, 213-224.

Carroll, M. E. (1984a). Effects of d-amphetamine and pentobarbital on self-administration of orally-delivered phencyclidine in rhesus monkeys. Pharmacology Biochemistry & Behavior, 20, 137-143.

Carroll, M. E. (1984b). The effect of second-order schedule history on fixed-ratio performance maintained by orally-delivered phencyclidine in rhesus monkeys. Pharmacology Biochemistry & Behavior, 2, 779-787.

Carroll, M. E. (1985a). Concurrent phencyclidine and saccharin access: Presentation of an alternative reinforcer reduces drug intake. Journal of the Experimental Analysis of Behavior, 43, 131-144.

Carroll, M. E. (1985b). Performance maintained by orally-delivered phencyclidine under second-order, tandem and fixed interval schedules in food-satiated and food-deprived rhesus monkeys. Journal of Pharmacology and Experimental Therapeutics, 232, 351-359.

Carroll, M. E., & Boe, I. N. (1982). Increased intravenous drug self-administration during deprivation of other reinforcers. Pharmacology Biochemistry & Behavior, 17, 563-567.

Carroll, M. E., France, C. P., & Meisch, R. A. (1979). Food deprivation increases oral and intravenous drug intake in rats. Science, 205, 319-321.

Carroll, M. E., & Meisch, R. A. (1978). Etonitazene as a reinforcer: Oral intake of etonitazene by rhesus monkeys. Psychopharmacology, 59, 225-229.

Carroll, M. E., & Meisch, R. A. (1979a). Concurrent etonitazene and water intake in rats: Role of taste, olfaction and auditory stimuli. Psychopharmacology, 64, 1-7.

Carroll, M. E., & Meisch, R. A. (1979b). Effects of food deprivation on etonitazene consumption in rats. Pharmacology Biochemistry & Behavior, 10, 155-159.

Carroll, M. E., & Meisch, R. A. (1980a). Effects of feeding conditions on drug-reinforced behavior: Maintenance at reduced body weights vs. availability of food. Psychopharmacology, 68, 121-124.

Carroll, M. E., & Meisch, R. A. (1980b). Oral phencyclidine (PCP) self-administration in rhesus monkeys: Effects of feeding conditions. Journal of Pharmacology and Experimental Therapeutics, 214, 339-346.

Carroll, M. E., & Meisch, R. A. (1981). Determinants of increased drug self-administration due to food deprivation. Psychopharmacology, 74, 197-200.

Carroll, M. E., & Meisch, R. A. (1984). Increased drug-reinforced behavior due to food deprivation. In T. Thompson, P. B. Dews, & J. E. Barrett (Eds.), Advances in behavioral pharmacology (Vol. 4, pp. 47-88). New York: Academic Press.

Carroll, M. E., & Stotz, D. C. (1983). Oral d-amphetamine and ketamine self-administration by rhesus monkeys: Effects of food deprivation. Journal of Pharmacology and Experimental Therapeutics, 227, 28-34.

Carroll, M. E., Stotz, D. C., Kliner, D. J., & Meisch, R. A. (1984). Self-administration of orally-delivered methohexital in rhesus monkeys with phencyclidine or pentobarbital histories: Effects of food deprivation and satiation. Pharmacology Biochemistry & Behavior, 20, 145-151.

Deneau, G., Yanagita, T., & Seevers, M. H. (1969). Self-administration of psychoactive substances by the monkey: A measure of psychological dependence. Psychopharmacologia, 16, 30-48.

DeNoble, V. J., Svikis, D. S., & Meisch, R. A. (1982). Orally delivered pentobarbital as a reinforcer for rhesus monkeys with concurrent access to water: Effects of concentration, fixed-ratio size, and liquid position. Pharmacology Biochemistry & Behavior, 16, 113-117.

Falk, J. L. (1961). Production of polydipsia in normal rats by an intermittent food schedule. Science, 133, 195-196.

Falk, J. L. (1971). The nature and determinants of adjunctive behavior. Physiology & Behavior, 6, 577-588.

Goldberg, S. R. (1973). Comparable behavior maintained under fixed-ratio and second-order schedules of food presentation, cocaine injection or d-amphetamine injection in the squirrel monkey. Journal of Pharmacology and Experimental Therapeutics, 186, 18-30.

Goldberg, S. R., Kelleher, R. T., & Morse, W. H. (1975). Second-order schedules of drug injection. Federation Proceedings, 34, 1771-1776.

Goldberg, S. R., Morse, W. H., & Goldberg, D. M. (1976). Behavior maintained under a second-order schedule by intramuscular injection of morphine or cocaine in rhesus monkeys. Journal of Pharmacology and Experimental Therapeutics, 199, 278-286.

Goldberg, S. R., Spealman, R. D., & Goldberg, D. M. (1981). Persistent behavior at high rates maintained by intravenous self-administration of nicotine. Science, 214, 573-575.

Griffiths, R. R., & Balster, R. L. (1979). Opioids: Similarities between evaluations of subjective effects and animal self-administration results. Clinical Pharmacology and Therapeutics, 25, 611-617.

Griffiths, R. R., Bigelow, G. E., & Henningfield, J. E. (1980). Similarities in animal and human drug taking behavior. In N. K. Mello (Ed.), Advances in substance abuse: Behavioral and biological research (Vol. 1, pp. 1-90). Greenwich, CT: JAI Press.

Henningfield, J. E., Ator, N. A., & Griffiths, R. R. (1981). Establishment and maintenance of oral ethanol self-administration in the baboon. Drug and Alcohol Dependence, 7, 113-124.

Henningfield, J. E., & Meisch, R. A. (1975). Ethanol-reinforced responding and intake as a function of volume per reinforcement. Pharmacology Biochemistry & Behavior, 59, 323-342.

Henningfield, J. E., & Meisch, R. A. (1976a). Drinking device for rhesus monkeys. Pharmacology Biochemistry & Behavior, 4, 609-610.

Henningfield, J. E., & Meisch, R. A. (1976b). Ethanol as a positive reinforcer via the oral route for rhesus monkeys: Maintenance of fixed-ratio responding. Pharmacology Biochemistry & Behavior, 4, 473-475.

Henningfield, J. E., & Meisch, R. A. (1977). Establishment of orally delivered ethanol as a positive reinforcer for rhesus monkeys. Reports from the research laboratories of the Department of Psychiatry (No. PR-77-4). Minneapolis: University of Minnesota.

Henningfield, J. E., & Meisch, R. A. (1978). Ethanol drinking by rhesus monkeys as a function of concentration. Psychopharmacology, 57, 133-136.

Henningfield, J. E., & Meisch, R. A. (1979). Ethanol drinking by rhesus monkeys with concurrent access to water. Pharmacology Biochemistry & Behavior, 10, 777-782.

Johanson, C. E. (1978). Drugs as reinforcers. In D. E. Blackman & D. J. Sanger (Eds.), Contemporary research in behavioral pharmacology, (pp. 325-390). New York: Plenum Press.

Johanson, C. E., & Balster, R. L. (1978). A summary of the results of a drug self-administration study using substitution procedures in rhesus monkeys. Bulletin on Narcotics, 30, 43-54.

Johanson, C. E., & Schuster, C. R. (1981). Animal models of drug self-administration. In N. K. Mello (Ed.), Advances in substance abuse (Vol. 2, pp. 219-297). Greenwich, CT: JAI Press.

Katz, J. L. (1979). A comparison of responding maintained under second-order schedules of intramuscular cocaine injection or food presentation in squirrel monkeys. Journal of the Experimental Analysis of Behavior, 32, 419-431.

Kelleher, R. T. (1966a). Chaining and conditioned reinforcement. In W. K. Honig (Ed.), Operant behavior: Areas of research and application (pp. 160-212). New York: Appleton-Century-Crofts.

Kelleher, R. T. (1966b). Conditioned reinforcement in second-order schedules. Journal of the Experimental Analysis of Behavior, 9, 475-485.

Kliner, D. J., & Meisch, R. A. (1982a). The effects of food deprivation and satiation on oral pentobarbital self-administration in rhesus monkeys. Pharmacology Biochemistry & Behavior, 16, 579-584.

Kliner, D. J., & Meisch, R. A. (1982b). The effects of food deprivation and fixed-ratio size on pentobarbital-maintained behavior in rhesus monkeys. Reports from the research laboratories of the Department of Psychiatry (No. PR-82-2). Minneapolis: University of Minnesota.

Leander, J. D., & McMillan, D. E. (1975). Schedule-induced narcotic ingestion. Pharmacological Reviews, 27, 475-487.

Lemaire, G. A., & Meisch, R. A. (1984). Pentobarbital self-administration in rhesus monkeys: Drug concentration and fixed-ratio size interactions. Journal of the Experimental Analysis of Behavior, 42, 37-49.

Lewis, M. J., Margules, D. L., & Ward, O. B., Jr. (1975). Opioid-reinforced operant behavior: Selective suppression by alpha-methyl-para-tyrosine. Journal of Comparative and Physiological Psychology, 88, 519-527.

Marcucella, H., Monroe, I., & MacDonall, J. S. (1984). Periodic ethanol availability and drinking bouts. Journal of Pharmacology and Experimental Therapeutics, 230, 658-664.

McMillan, D. E., & Leander, J. D. (1976). Schedule-induced oral self-administration of etonitazene. Pharmacology Biochemistry & Behavior, 4, 137-141.

Meisch, R. A. (1969). Increased rate of ethanol self-administration as a function of experience. Reports from the research laboratories of the Department of Psychiatry (No. PR-69-3). Minneapolis: University of Minnesota.

Meisch, R. A. (1975). The function of schedule-induced polydipsia in establishing ethanol as a positive reinforcer. Pharmacological Reviews, 27, 465-473.

Meisch, R. A. (1977). Ethanol self-administration: Infrahuman studies. In T. Thompson & P. B. Dews (Eds.), Advances in behavioral pharmacology (Vol. 1, pp. 35-84). New York: Academic Press.

Meisch, R. A., & Beardsley, P. (1975). Ethanol as a reinforcer for rats: Effects of concurrent access to water and alternate positions of water and ethanol. Psychopharmacologia, 43, 19-23.

Meisch, R. A., & Carroll, M. E. (1981). Establishment of orally delivered drugs as reinforcers for rhesus monkeys: Some relations to human drug dependence. In T. Thompson & C. E. Johanson (Eds.), Behavioral pharmacology of human drug dependence, (National Institute on Drug Abuse Research Monograph 37, pp. 197-209). Washington, DC: U.S. Government Printing Office.

Meisch, R. A., & Henningfield, J. E. (1977). Drinking of ethanol by rhesus monkeys: Experimental strategies for establishing ethanol as a reinforcer. Advances in Experimental Medicine and Biology, 85-B, 443-463.

Meisch, R. A., Henningfield, J. E., & Thompson, T. (1975). Establishment of ethanol as a reinforcer for rhesus monkeys via the oral route: Initial results. Advances in Experimental Medicine and Biology, 59, 323-342.

Meisch, R. A., & Kliner, D. J. (1979). Etonitazene as a reinforcer for rats: Increased etonitazene-reinforced behavior due to food deprivation. Psychopharmacology, 63, 97-98.

Meisch, R. A., Kliner, D. J., & Henningfield, J. E. (1981). Pentobarbital drinking by rhesus monkeys: Establishment and maintenance of pentobarbital-reinforced behavior. Journal of Pharmacology and Experimental Therapeutics, 217, 114-120.

Meisch, R. A., & Stark, L. J. (1977a). Establishment of etonitazene as a reinforcer for rats by use of schedule-induced drinking. Pharmacology Biochemistry & Behavior, 7, 195-203.

Meisch, R. A., & Stark, L. J. (1977b). Etonitazene as a reinforcer via the oral route for rats: Effects of etonitazene concentration and food intake on etonitazene-reinforced behavior. Reports from the research laboratories of the Department of Psychiatry (No. PR-77-3). Minneapolis: University of Minnesota.

Meisch, R. A., & Thompson, T. (1971). Ethanol intake in the absence of concurrent food reinforcement. Psychopharmacologia, 22, 72-79.

Meisch, R. A., & Thompson, T. (1973). Ethanol as a reinforcer: Effects of fixed-ratio size and food deprivation. Psychopharmacologia, 28, 171-183.

Meisch, R. A., & Thompson, T. (1974a). Ethanol as a reinforcer: An operant analysis of ethanol dependence. In J. M. Singh & H. Lal (Eds.), Drug addiction, Vol. 3: Neurobiology and influences on behavior (pp. 117-133). Miami: Symposia Specialists.

Meisch, R. A., & Thompson, T. (1974b). Rapid establishment of ethanol as a reinforcer for rats. Psychopharmacologia, 37, 311-321.

Meisch, R. A., & Thompson T. (1974c). Ethanol intake as a function of concentration during food deprivation and satiation. Pharmacology Biochemistry & Behavior, 2, 589-596.

Pickens, R., Meisch, R. A., & Thompson, T. (1978). Drug self-administration: An analysis of the reinforcing effects of drugs. In L. L. Iversen, S. D. Iversen, & S. H. Snyder (Eds.), Handbook of psychopharmacology (Vol. 12, pp. 1-37). New York: Plenum Press.

Poling, A., & Thompson, T. (1977a). Suppression of ethanol-reinforced lever pressing by delaying food availability. Journal of the Experimental Analysis of Behavior, 28, 271-283.

Poling, A., & Thompson, T. (1977b). Effects of delaying food availability contingent on ethanol-maintained lever pressing. Psychopharmacology, 51, 289-291.

Roehrs, T. A., & Samson, H. H. (1981). Ethanol reinforced behavior assessed with a concurrent schedule. Pharmacology Biochemistry & Behavior, 15, 539-544.

Roehrs, T. A., & Samson, H. H. (1982). Relative responding on concurrent schedules: Indexing ethanol's reinforcing efficacy. Pharmacology Biochemistry & Behavior, 22, 393-396.

Samson, H. H., & Falk, J. L. (1974). Alteration of fluid preference in ethanol-dependent animals. Journal of Pharmacology and Experimental Therapeutics, 190, 365-376.

Spealman, R. D., & Goldberg, S. R. (1978). Drug self-administration by laboratory animals: Control by schedules of reinforcement. Annual Review of Pharmacology and Toxicology, 18, 313-339.

Suzuki, T., Uesugi, J., Yoshii, T., Yanaura, S., & Kawai, T. (1982). Preference for and oral self-administration of morphine and codeine in rats. In S. Saito & T. Yanagita (Eds.), Learning and memory drugs as reinforcer (pp. 202-220). Amsterdam: Excerpta Medica.

Thompson, T., & Schuster, C. R. (1964). Morphine self-administration, food-reinforced, and avoidance behaviors in rhesus monkeys. Psychopharmacologia, 5, 87-94.

Treibergs, J. E., & Meisch, R. A. (1979). Ethanol-reinforced performance of rats: Effects of brief stimuli and food deprivation and satiation. Reports from the research laboratories of the Department of Psychiatry (No. PR-79-2). Minneapolis: University of Minnesota.

Weeks, J. R. (1962). Experimental morphine addiction: Method for automatic intravenous injections in unrestrained rats. Science, 138, 143-144.

Wood, R. W., Grubman, J., & Weiss, B. (1977). Nitrous oxide self-administration by the squirrel monkey. Journal of Pharmacology and Experimental Therapeutics, 202, 491-499.

Yanagita, T., & Takahashi, S. (1973). Dependence liability of several sedative-hypnotic agents evaluated in monkeys. Journal of Pharmacology and Experimental Therapeutics, 185, 307-316.

Yanagita, T., Takahashi, S., Ishida, K., & Funamoto, H. (1970). Voluntary inhalation of volatile anesthetics and organic solvents by monkeys. Japanese Journal of Clinical Pharmacology, 1, 13-16.

CHAPTER 8

ORAL SELF-ADMINISTRATION OF ALCOHOL:
A VALID APPROACH TO THE STUDY OF
DRUG SELF-ADMINISTRATION AND HUMAN ALCOHOLISM

Z. Amit, B. R. Smith, and E. A. Sutherland

Center for Studies in Behavioral Neurobiology
Department of Psychology
Concordia University
Montreal, Quebec, Canada H3G 1M8

Abstract

The purpose of the present paper is to examine the use of animal models in psychopharmacology with particular emphasis on oral self-administration of drugs. As most of the studies in this area involve alcohol, the bulk of this paper will deal with questions related to this abused drug. Various techniques of oral self-administration are reviewed and their utility as methods of investigation in the area of psychopharmacology are examined. It is concluded that the question under investigation is critical in determining the validity of any animal model and that the use of oral paradigms may be the most appropriate method to examine the question of alcohol self-administration.

Many methods of drug administration can be used in the study of drug action, and the choice of one technique over another should be determined exclusively by the specific question under examination. This is particularly the case in the area of drug self-administration. Numerous procedures have been used in humans to elucidate the mechanisms mediating the self-administration of various substances; however, obvious ethical, methodological and practical considerations place limits on the kinds of information that can be gained from these studies. in general, these studies utilize clinical populations with long histories of drug intake and use relatively non-invasive procedures of drug administration.

In order to investigate more basic internal, biobehavioral mechanisms underlying drug intake, it became necessary to develop appropriate animal models. While many criteria have been suggested in order for an animal model to qualify as adequate, one criterion seems to be immutable--the data gathered in animal studies must have predictive validity to human voluntary drug intake.

As with other areas of psychopharmacology, many animal models of drug self-administration exist, and the suitability of each should be (but has not always been) determined by the question and the drug under study. One important consideration in the selection of a particular methodology is the route of administration employed for the drug. Many drugs are taken by humans via the oral route: In fact, the oral route of drug intake is by far the most common. This is evidenced by the exclusive utilization of this route for alcohol intake, cannabis intake and the ingestion of minor tranquilizers, barbiturates and hallucinogens. In addition, opium, cocaine and some psychomotor stimulants are frequently taken through the oropharyngeal route. Nevertheless, the validity of the oral route in animal studies of drug self-administration does not enjoy a broad consensus. For example, animal studies using oral self-administration of ethanol as a model of human alcohol intake have been the subject of an ongoing controversy (Amit & Sutherland, 1976; Amit, Sutherland & White, 1976; Cicero, 1980; Lester & Freed, 1973; Mello, 1973). Many criticisms have been leveled against the appropriateness of animal models of human alcohol use and this whole issue has produced its fair share of extreme antagonists and protagonists.

The purpose of the present review is to examine this technique with regard to its suitability as a model of human drug administration. Since the choice of this route has been particularly prevalent in animal studies of ethanol intake, this paper will focus on work in this area as an example to illustrate issues relating to the oral route in the field of drug self-administration in general.

It has been shown that animals will preferentially consume large quantities of ethanol when it is presented in a free choice with water (Kahn & Steller, 1960; Richter & Campbell, 1940; Wilson, 1972). This observation, however, is most commonly seen when the ethanol concentrations are below 6% since rats display a natural aversion to solutions of higher concentrations (Eriksson, 1968; Meisch, 1977; Myers, 1968). However it is important to note that preferences for ethanol solutions in concentrations exceeding 20% have also been reported (Mendelson & Mello, 1964). A related problem is the fact that animals under conditions of voluntary consumption do not seem to consume sufficient amounts of ethanol to result in intoxication. Furthermore, signs of physical dependence are not normally observed in this paradigm. These two factors (i.e., the inability to produce drinking to intoxication and the absence of the development of physical dependence) which were linked to the reluctance of animals to drink sufficient amounts of ethanol have been suggested as necessary conditions in any animal model of alcohol intake (Lester & Freed, 1973).

As a result of this suggestion and despite the fact that the importance of these factors in determining the adequacy of animal models of alcoholism has been seriously challenged (e.g., Amit et al., 1976; Eriksson, 1968), many investigators have focused on the development of techniques to induce animals to consume larger amounts of ethanol. One such method has been to restrict all drinking liquids to ethanol solutions. It was shown that animals drank more ethanol during forced-choice periods than when they had the option of a free choice with water (Carey, 1972; Eimer & Senter, 1968; Ratcliffe, 1972; Rick & Wilson, 1966; Wise, 1973). This method has produced equivocal results when animals are subsequently given a free-choice test, as this procedure has been reported to lead to increased ethanol intake (Campbell, Taylor, & Haslett, 1967; Mirone, 1952, 1957; Myers, 1961; Parisella & Pritham, 1964; Powell, Kamano & Martin, 1966; Wallgren & Forsander, 1963) as well as decreased or no change in intake (Eimer & Senter, 1968; Rodgers & McClearn, 1962; Rodgers, Ward, Thiessen, & Whitworth, 1967). Ethanol has also been offered in a liquid diet as the only source of nutrients and while intake increased sufficiently to produce dependence, a free-choice test revealed that the animals maintained an aversion to ethanol despite the presence of withdrawal symptoms (Hunter, Walker, & Riley, 1974).

A number of studies have attempted to provide response contingent reinforcement in an attempt to induce increased ethanol drinking. Lick-contingent hypothalamic stimulation (Martin & Myers, 1972) and reinforcement with milk (Mello & Mendelson, 1965a) or food (Black & Martin, 1972; Coulson, Koffer, & Coulson, 1971; Keehn, 1969; Keehn & Coulson, 1970; Perensky, Senter, & Jones, 1968; Senter, Smith, & Lewin, 1967) have been used to induce consumption of intoxicating amounts of ethanol. While this criterion was achieved, discontinuation of the response contingencies resulted in decreased ethanol intake (Black & Martin, 1972; Martin & Myers, 1972; Mello & Mendelson, 1965a). The use of electric shock and escape contingencies has also failed to produce continued elevated ethanol intake since termination of the shock caused ethanol consumption to return to baseline levels (Kamback, 1973; Ramsey & Van Dis, 1967; Senter et al., 1967).

One procedure which has been relatively successful in achieving ethanol intake leading to dependence has been the use of schedule-induced polydipsia. It was demonstrated that food-deprived rats receiving small pellets of food spaced over time would consume larger quantities of fluid (Falk, 1961). When ethanol was substituted for water, rats consumed intoxicating quantities of ethanol (Everett & King, 1970; Falk, Samson, & Winger, 1972; Freed, 1972; Lester, 1961; Meisch & Thompson, 1972; Ogata, Ogata, Mendelson, & Mello, 1972; Samson & Falk, 1974; Senter & Sinclair, 1967) and physical dependence was observed following several ethanol polydipsia sessions per day (Falk et al., 1972). The termination of the concurrent food reinforcement does not result in a decrease in ethanol intake as a preference for ethanol over water remains (Falk et al., 1972; Freed, Carpenter, & Hymowitz, 1970; Freed & Lester, 1970; Meisch & Thompson, 1971, 1974). However, it is important to note that the concentration of ethanol solutions in Falk's studies was low (5.6%) and, therefore, in the range that animals prefer normally. When the concentration of ethanol solutions was increased to 20%, preference was not maintained after polydipsia sessions were discontinued (Meisch & Thompson, 1972).

Electrical brain stimulation has also been used to elevate ethanol drinking and has been reported to produce a voluntary preference for relatively concentrated solutions of ethanol (Amir & Stern, 1978; Amit, Stern, & Wise, 1970; Corcoran & Amit, 1974). This preference persisted long after the stimulation was discontinued (Amit & Stern, 1971; Amit et al., 1970; Wayner, Gawronski, Roubie, & Greenberg, 1971; Wayner & Greenberg, 1972). Signs of physical dependence, however, were not reported.

Each of the techniques described above produces an increased intake of alcohol; however, in most cases a prolonged voluntary preference for ethanol is not established and intake during each manipulation can hardly be described as "voluntary." With this in mind investigators developed a procedure which relied on voluntary consumption with a specific schedule of presentation to induce animals to obtain a preference for high concentrations of ethanol. This technique utilizes a phenomenon known as the "alcohol deprivation effect," first described by Sinclair and Senter (1968). It was shown that periodic availability of ethanol, presented in a free choice with water, resulted in increased ethanol consumption of solutions which would otherwise be avoided. This method was first described by Amit and Stern (1971) and later confirmed by others (Pinel, Mucha, & Rovner, 1976; Sinclair & Senter, 1968; Wayner & Greenberg, 1972; Wise, 1973). As a result of this technique, a prolonged preference for the ethanol solutions was maintained.

The examination of the procedures to increase voluntary consumption of ethanol in animals as described above, which attempted to meet Lester and Freed's postulated criteria for an animal model of human alcoholism (Lester & Freed, 1973), may have combined two unrelated issues. The present authors (Amit et al., 1976) and others (Meisch, 1980; Sinclair, 1980) have argued that the phenomena of alcohol intoxication and physical dependence, on the one hand, and voluntary consumption of ethanol, on the other hand, may be unrelated. (For a detailed discussion of this issue, see Amit et al., 1976.)

If this is in fact the case, as the bulk of animal data as well as some of the human data seem to suggest, then the inclusion of both requirements in the same model produces an unnecessary confusion. Thus, as mentioned earlier, the adequacy of an experimental procedure must be determined by the question it attempts to study. In other words, if the research is attempting to focus on mechanisms underlying intoxication and physical dependence, then techniques to produce these states are relevant and necessary. If, on the other hand, the focus of the research is ethanol self-administration, then a well-controlled preference paradigm is the necessary and sufficient condition.

There has recently been growing acceptance for the notion that alcohol self-administration in humans is a distinct set of responses governed primarily by its reinforcing properties (Amit & Sutherland, 1976; Bigelow & Liebson, 1972; Mello & Mendelson, 1965b, 1972; Sanders, Nathan, & O'Brien, 1976). In a similar fashion it has been demonstrated that ethanol drinking in animals is also an operant response which can be modified by the same manipulations as any other operant response (Amit & Stern, 1969; Meisch, 1977, 1980; Sinclair, 1974). Lester and Freed (1972) challenged that view and suggested that animals consume ethanol for its caloric value and not for its reinforcing, psychopharmacological effects. While this is a relevant argument, it does not seem to be defensible since it has been demonstrated that food-satiated animals will drink ethanol solutions greater than 8% concentration in preference to water (Beardsley, Lemaire, & Meisch, 1978; Meisch & Thompson, 1973; 1974). In addition, animals have been shown to work for ethanol despite free access to food and water (Penn, McBride, Lumeng, Gaff, & Li, 1978; Sinclair, 1974). Also, merely depriving animals of food did not result in increased ethanol intake (Amit & Stern, 1969). Animals drinking more ethanol than water in situations where food and competing fluids are continuously available seem likely to be doing so for reasons other than thirst and hunger. Furthermore, the fact that hungry animals will not increase their ethanol consumption relative to satiated controls argues quite strongly against the "drinking for calories" hypothesis.

Even among those who adhere to the notion that drug self-administration is governed primarily by its reinforcing properties, there has been some doubt as to the appropriateness of the oral route of intake for studying the reinforcing properties of ethanol (Wise & Bozarth, 1982). Wise's main argument is that under conditions of free choice one cannot observe the willingness of animals to work for alcohol. Since the ability of animals to work or to perform a distinct operant is purported to be a prerequisite for demonstrating reinforcement bound behavior, the clarification of this issue becomes critical. This position, once again, is not defensible since it has been shown that animals will learn to perform a task in order to drink ethanol (Anderson & Thompson, 1974; Meisch, 1980, this volume; Meisch & Beardsley, 1975; Penn et al., 1978) and will learn a new response to obtain drops of ethanol through the oral route (Sinclair, 1974). It would appear then that animals will orally consume ethanol for its pharmacologically reinforcing effects. In this context it is interesting to note that the behavioral responses of the animals to ethanol consumed through this route are strikingly similar to those displayed with other reinforcing drugs or substances (e.g., food and water). Furthermore, humans can also be observed to perform similar behaviors in a laboratory setting in order to obtain alcohol (Ludwig, Wikler, & Stark, 1974; Mello & Mendelson, 1972; Sanders et al., 1976).

Finally, it has been shown that the same neurochemical manipulation that will block oral self-administration of ethanol (Amit, Brown, Levitan, & Ogren, 1977) will also block intragastric self-administration of ethanol (Davis, Werner, & Smith, 1979). Davis et al. (1979) have also demonstrated that this neurochemical manipulation will also block second order conditioning of a stimulus previously paired with ethanol. This set of observations argues strongly for the fact that alcohol is a substance endowed with primary reinforcing properties which seem to underlie alcohol self-administration through any route of administration.

As mentioned in the opening section of this paper, the ultimate test of the viability of an animal model must be its ability to generate inferences to the human condition it was set up to model. The question remains: Does the oral self-administration of ethanol in animals allow us to draw inferences to human voluntary consumption of alcohol? As we have argued in preceding sections of this review, until fairly recently such data was generally unavailable. The attempts to validate such an animal model were therefore often based on tenets which were derived from more or less relevant theoretical considerations. As new data emerged, many of the earlier theoretical assumptions proved to be less critical or even irrelevant.

More recently, several lines of alcohol research have provided empirical evidence suggesting that an oral preference model of ethanol intake in animals may be predictive of alcohol self-administration in humans. One area of alcohol research which has shown concordance between animal and human data is the investigation of a genetic component of alcohol intake which has been studied exclusively through the oral self-administration paradigm.

An increasing body of evidence suggests than an inherited predisposition towards alcoholism may exist in humans (for a review, see Goodwin, 1979). In this context it is interesting to note that Schuckit and Rayses (1979) reported that human populations with high risk for alcoholism have high levels of acetaldehyde. In animals it has been demonstrated (Brown, Amit, & Smith, 1980) that self-administration of acetaldehyde is correlated with oral self-administration of ethanol. Recent data seem to point to an alteration in the alcohol metabolizing enzymes, specifically those enzymes responsible for the metabolism of ethanol's primary metabolite acetaldehyde as the critical factor in this predisposition (Ewing, Rouse, & Pellizzari, 1974; Haranda, Agarwal, Goedde, & Ishikawa, 1983; Mizoi, Ijiri, Tatsumo, Kijima, Fujiwara, Adachi, & Hishida, 1979; Mizoi, Tatsumo, Adachi, Kogame, Fukunasa, Fujiwara, Hishida, & Ijiri, 1983; Reed, Kalant, Gibbons, Kapur, & Rankin, 1976; Zeiner, Paredes, & Christianson, 1979).

Research has also demonstrated that alcohol consumption can be selectively bred in rats (e.g., Eriksson, 1968; Li & Lumeng, 1977; Lumeng, Hawkins, & Li, 1977) and in mice (e.g., Rodgers & McClearn, 1962) suggesting that ethanol consumption in both humans and animals may be genetically determined. Furthermore, it has been shown that the activity of aldehyde dehydrogenase, the primary enzyme responsible for acetaldehyde metabolism, is highly correlated with voluntary ethanol consumption in several strains of rats and mice (Amir, 1977, 1978; Schlesinger, Kakihana, & Bennett, 1966; Sheppard, Albersheim, & McClearn, 1968; Socaransky, Aragon, Amit, & Blander, 1984). These reports are indicative of a concordance in the results of studies using an oral route of administration between human and animal experiments examining the genetic determinants of alcohol consumption.

While these results are an example of indirect evidence supporting the predictive value of animal consumption studies, a direct comparison involving identical manipulations in animals and man is necessary in order to properly evaluate the utility of this experimental procedure. Recently, this approach was used in an attempt to compare the mediators of alcohol self-administration in rats and man. It was observed that the administration of zimelidine, a serotonin re-uptake inhibitor, attenuated voluntary ethanol consumption in rats as measured in an oral preference paradigm (Lawrin, Naranjo, & Sellers, 1983; Rockman, Amit, Carr, Brown, & Ogren, 1979). This finding led two independent laboratories to test zimelidine's effect on alcohol consumption in humans. Both groups reported similar findings with zimelidine treatment resulting in a decreased alcohol intake (Sutherland, Amit, Sossanpour, & Selvaggi, 1983) and an increased number of abstinent days (Narnajo, Lawrin, Addison, Roach, Harrison, Sanchez-Craig, & Sellers, 1983; Narnajo, Sellers, Roach, Woodley, Sanchez-Craig, & Sykora, 1983). While additional studies are necessary in order to elucidate the mechanisms of this observation and also to determine the significance of the drug effect, it is nevertheless the case that these results suggest, independent of the specific mechanism involved, that animal oral consumption studies may serve as a predictor of human self-administration of alcohol.

The purpose of the present review was to evaluate the oral self-administration model of ethanol intake in animals as a viable procedure to study human voluntary consumption of alcohol in particular and also to assess the model's usefulness for the study of oral self-administration of psychoactive drugs in general. We presented evidence demonstrating that the oral self-administration paradigm is endowed with all the properties required of other "valid" self-administration paradigms--animals will work and will perform an operant to obtain ethanol through the oral route, they will also respond to a second order conditioned stimulus previously paired with alcohol and, finally, the same neuropharmacological manipulations will block both oral and intragastric self-administration of ethanol. We also argued that the objections raised against the animal model as a tool for studying human alcohol consumption have become either noncritical or irrelevant in that the reluctance of animals to drink to intoxication and the absence of withdrawal signs were shown to be either incorrect or unimportant in the context of a paradigm which perceives reinforcement to be the primary factor mediating voluntary consumption of alcohol.

Finally, we presented evidence, unique in the field of drug self-administration, that the predictive validity of the animal model of oral alcohol intake was tested directly in human populations and found to be defensible. We therefore conclude that oral self-administration of ethanol in animals is a valid procedure to study mechanisms of drug self-administration and a uniquely suitable approach to investigate human consumption of alcohol.

References

Amir, S. (1977). Brain and liver aldehyde dehydrogenase. Relations to ethanol consumption in Wistar rats. Neuropharmacology, **16**, 781-784.
Amir, S. (1978). Brain aldehyde dehydrogenase: Adaptive increase following prolonged ethanol administration in rats. Neuropharmacology, **17**, 463-467.
Amir, S., & Stern, M. H. (1978). Electrical stimulation and lesions of the medial forebrain bundle in the rat: Changes in voluntary ethanol consumption and brain aldehyde dehydrogenase activity. Psychopharmacology, **57**, 167-174.

Amit, Z., Brown, Z. W., Levitan, D. E., & Ogren, S-O. (1977). Noradrenergic mediation of the positive reinforcing properties of ethanol: I. Suppression of ethanol consumption in laboratory rats following dopamine-beta-hydroxylase inhibition. Archives Internationale de Pharmacodynamie et de Therapie, 230, 65-75.

Amit, Z., & Stern, M. H. (1969). Alcohol ingestion without oropharyngeal sensations. Psychonomic Science, 15, 162-163.

Amit, Z., & Stern, M. H. (1971). A further investigation of alcohol preference in the laboratory rat induced by hypothalamic stimulation. Psychopharmacology, 21, 317-327.

Amit, Z., Stern, M. H., & Wise, R. A. (1970). Alcohol preference in the laboratory rat induced by hypothalamic stimulation. Psychopharmacology, 17, 367-377.

Amit, Z., & Sutherland, E. A. (1976). The relevance of recent animal studies for the development of treatment procedures for alcoholics. Drug and Alcohol Dependence, 1, 3-13.

Amit, Z., Sutherland, E. A., & White, N. (1976). The role of physical dependence in animal models of human alcoholism. Drug and Alcohol Dependence, 1, 435-440.

Anderson, W. W., & Thompson, T. (1974). Ethanol self-administration in water satiated rats. Pharmacology Biochemistry & Behavior, 2, 367-377.

Beardsley, P. M., Lemaire, G. A., & Meisch, R. A. (1978). Ethanol reinforced behavior of rats with concurrent access to food and water. Psychopharmacology, 59, 7-11.

Bigelow, G., & Liebson, I. (1972). Cost factors controlling alcoholic drinking. Psychological Record, 22, 305-314.

Black, E. L., & Martin, G. L. (1972). Extinction of alcohol drinking in rats following acquisition on a fixed-ratio schedule of reinforcement. Psychonomic Science, 29, 152-154.

Brown, Z. W., Amit, Z., & Smith, B. (1980). Intraventricular self-administration of acetaldehyde and voluntary consumption of ethanol in rats. Behavioral and Neural Biology, 28, 150-155.

Campbell, B., Taylor, J. T., & Haslett, W. L. (1967). Anti-alcohol properties of metronidazole in rats. Proceedings of the Society for Experimental Biology and Medicine, 124, 191-195.

Carey, R. J. (1972). A decrease in ethanol preference in rats resulting from forced ethanol drinking under fluid deprivation. Physiology & Behavior, 8, 373-375.

Cicero, T. J. (1980). Animal models of alcoholism? In K. Eriksson, J. D. Sinclair, & K. Kiianmaa (Eds.), Animal models in alcohol research (pp. 99-117). New York: Academic Press.

Corcoran, M. E., & Amit, Z. (1974). Reluctance of rats to drink hashish suspensions: Free-choice and forced consumption and the effects of hypothalamic stimulation. Psychopharmacology, 35, 129-147.

Coulson, G. E., Koffer, K. B., & Coulson, U. (1971). Reinforcement of ethanol consumption in rats by an increase in the frequency of food pellet delivery. Psychonomic Science, 23, 103-104.

Davis, W. M., Werner, T. E., & Smith, S. G. (1979). Reinforcement with intragastric infusions of ethanol: Blocking effect of FLA-57. Pharmacology Biochemistry & Behavior, 11, 545-548.

Eimer, E. O., & Senter, R. J. (1968). Alcohol consumption in domestic and wild rats. Psychonomic Science, 10, 319-320.

Eriksson, K. (1968). Genetic selection for voluntary alcohol consumption in the albino rat. Science, 159, 739-741.

Everett, P. B., & King, R. A. (1970). Schedule-induced alcohol ingestion. Psychonomic Science, 18, 278-279.

Ewing, J. A., Rouse, B. A., & Pellizzari, E. D. (1974). Alcohol sensitivity and ethnic background. American Journal of Psychiatry, 131, 206-210.

Falk, J. L. (1961). Production of polydipsia in normal rats by an intermittent food schedule. Science, 133, 195-196.

Falk, J. L., Samson, H. H., & Winger, G. (1972). Behavioral maintenance of high concentration of blood ethanol and physical dependence in the rat. Science, 177, 811-813.

Freed, E. X. (1972). Alcohol polydipsia in the rat as a function of caloric need. Quarterly Journal of Studies on Alcohol, 33, 504-507.

Freed, E. X., Carpenter, J. A., & Hymowitz, N. (1970). Acquisition and extinction of schedule-induced polydipsia consumption of alcohol and water. Psychological Reports, 26, 915-922.

Freed, E. X., & Lester, D. (1970). Schedule-induced consumption of ethanol: Calories or chemotherapy? Physiology & Behavior, 5, 555-560.

Goodwin, D. W. (1979). Alcoholism & heredity: A review and a hypothesis. Archives of General Psychiatry, 36, 57-61.

Haranda, S., Agarwal, D. P., Goedde, H. W., & Ishikawa, B. (1983). Aldehyde dehydrogenase isoenzyme variation and alcoholism in Japanese. Pharmacology Biochemistry & Behavior, 18(Suppl. 1), 151-154.

Hunter, B. E., Walker, D. W., & Riley, J. N. (1974). Dissociation between physical dependence and volitional ethanol consumption: Role of multiple withdrawal episodes. Pharmacology Biochemistry & Behavior, 2, 523-529.

Kahn, M., & Stellar, E. (1960). Alcohol preference in normal and anosmic rats. Journal of Comparative and Physiological Psychology, 53, 571-575.

Kamback, M. C. (1973). Drinking as an avoidance response by pigtail monkey (Macac nemistrina). Quarterly Journal of Studies on Alcohol, 34, 943-946.

Keehn, J. D. (1969). "Voluntary" consumption of alcohol by rats. Quarterly Journal of Studies on Alcohol, 30, 320-329.

Keehn, J. D., & Coulson, G. E. (1970). Ethanol consumption by rats on a differential probability of reinforcement schedule. Psychonomic Society, 19, 283-284.

Lawrin, M., Naranjo, C. A., & Sellers, E. M. (1983). Studies on the mechanism of zimelidine-induced decrease in alcohol consumption in rats. Proceedings Canadian Federation of Biological Societies, 26, 116.

Lester, D. (1961). Self-maintenance of intoxication in the rat. Quarterly Journal of Studies on Alcohol, 22, 223-231.

Lester, D., & Freed, E. (1972). The rat views alcohol--nutrition or nirvana? In O. Forsander & K. Eriksson (Eds.), Biological aspects of alcohol consumption (pp. 51-57). Helsinki: Finnish Foundation for Alcohol Studies.

Lester, D., & Freed, E. X. (1973). Criteria for an animal model of alcoholism. Pharmacology Biochemistry & Behavior, 1, 103-107.

Li, T. K., & Lumeng, L. (1977). Alcohol metabolism of inbred strains of rats with alcohol preference and non-preference. In R. G. Thurman, J. R. Williamson, H. Drott, & B. Chance (Eds.), Alcohol and aldehyde metabolizing systems (pp. 625-633). New York: Academic Press.

Ludwig, A. M., Wikler, A., & Stark, L. H. (1974). The first drink: Psychological aspects of craving. Archives of General Psychiatry, 30, 539-547.

Lumeng, L., Hawkins, T. C., & Li, T. K. (1977). New strains of rats with alcohol preference and non-preference. In R. G. Thurman, J. R. Williamson, H. Drott, & B. Chance (Eds.), Alcohol and aldehyde metabolizing systems, (pp. 537-544). New York: Academic Press.

Martin, G. E., & Myers, R. D. (1972). Ethanol ingestion in the rat induced by rewarding brain stimulation. Physiology & Behavior, 8, 1151-1160.

Meisch, R. A. (1977). Ethanol self-administration: Infrahuman studies. In T. Thompson & P. B. Dews (Eds.), Advances in behavioral pharmacology (Vol. I, pp. 35-84). New York: Academic Press.

Meisch, R. A. (1980). Ethanol as a reinforcer for rats, monkeys and humans. In K.Eriksson, J. D. Sinclair & K. Kiianmaa (Eds.), Animal models in alcohol research (pp. 153-158). New York: Academic Press.

Meisch, R. A., & Beardsley, P. (1975). Ethanol as a reinforcer for rats: Effects of concurrent access to water and alternate positions of water and ethanol. Psychopharmacology, 43, 19-23.

Meisch, R. A., & Thompson, T. (1971). Ethanol intake in the absence of concurrent food reinforcement. Psychopharmacology, 22, 72-79.

Meisch, R. A., & Thompson, T. (1972). Ethanol intake during schedule-induced polydipsia. Physiology & Behavior, 8, 471-475.

Meisch, R. A., & Thompson, T. (1973). Ethanol as a reinforcer: Effects of fixed-ratio size and food deprivation. Psychopharmacology, 28, 171-183.

Meisch, R. A., & Thompson, T. (1974). Rapid establishment of ethanol as a reinforcer for rats. Psychopharmacology, 37, 311-321.

Mello, N. K. (1973). A review of methods to induce alcohol addiction in animals. Pharmacology Biochemistry & Behavior, 1, 89-101.

Mello, N. K., & Mendelson, J. H. (1965a). Operant drinking of alcohol on a rate-contingent ration schedule of reinforcement. Journal of Psychiatric Research, 3, 145-152.

Mello, N. K., & Mendelson, J. H. (1965b). Operant analysis of drinking patterns of chronic alcoholics. Nature, 206, 43-46.

Mello, N. K., & Mendelson, J. H. (1972). Drinking patterns during work-contingent alcohol acquisition. Psychosomatic Medicine, 34, 139-164.

Mendelson, J. H., & Mello, N. K. (1964). Ethanol and whiskey drinking patterns in rats under free-choice and forced-choice conditions. Quarterly Journal of Studies on Alcohol, 25, 1-25.

Mirone, L. (1952). The effect of ethyl alcohol on growth, fecundity and voluntary consumption of alcohol by mice. Quarterly Journal of Studies on Alcohol, 13, 365-369.

Mirone, L. (1957). Dietary deficiency in mice in relation to voluntary alcohol consumption. Quarterly Journal of Studies on Alcohol, 18, 552-560.

Mizoi, Y., Ijiri, I., Tatsumo, Y., Kijima, T., Fujiwara, S., Adachi, J., & Hishida, S. (1979). Relationship between facial flushing and blood acetaldehyde levels after alcohol intake. Pharmacology Biochemistry & Behavior, 10, 303-311.

Mizoi, Y., Tatsumo, Y., Adachi, J., Kogame, M., Fukunasa, T., Fujiwara, S., Hishida, S., & Ijiri, I. (1983). Alcohol sensitivity related to polymorphism of alcohol-metabolizing enzymes in Japanese. Pharmacology Biochemistry & Behavior, 18(Suppl. 1), 127-134.

Myers, R. D. (1961). Changes in learning, extinction and fluid preferences as a function of alcohol consumption in rats. Journal of Comparative and Physiological Psychology, 54, 510-516.

Myers, R. D. (1968). Ethyl alcohol consumption: Valid measurement in albino rats. Science, 161, 76.

Naranjo, C. A., Lawrin, M., Addison, D., Roach, C. A., Harrison, M., Sanchez-Craig, M., & Sellers, E. M. (1983). Zimelidine (Z) decreases alcohol consumption (AC) in non-depressed heavy drinkers. Clinical Pharmacology and Therapeutics, 33, 241.

Naranjo, C. A., Sellers, E. M., Roach, C. A., Woodley, D. V., Sanchez-Craig, M., & Sykora, K. (1983). Zimelidine induced variations in ethanol intake in non-depressed heavy drinkers. Clinical Pharmacology and Therapeutics, 35, 374-381.

Ogata, H., Ogata, F., Mendelson, J. H., & Mello, N. K. (1972). A comparison of techniques to induce alcohol dependence and tolerance in the mouse. Journal of Pharmacology and Experimental Therapeutics, 180, 216-230.

Parisella, R. M., & Pritham, G. H. (1964). Effect of age on alcohol preference by rats. Quarterly Journal of Studies on Alcohol, 25, 248-252.

Penn, D. E., McBride, W. S., Lumeng, L., Gaff, T. M., & Li, T. K. (1978). Neurochemical and operant behavioral studies of a strain of alcohol preferring rats. Pharmacology Biochemistry & Behavior, 8, 475-481.

Perensky, J. J., Senter, R. J., & Jones, R. B. (1968). Induced alcohol consumption through positive reinforcement. Psychonomic Science, 11, 109-110.

Pinel, J. P. J., Mucha, R. F., & Rovner, L. I. (1976). Temporary effects of periodic alcohol availability. Behavioral Biology, 16, 227-232.

Powell, B. J., Kamano, D. K., & Martin, L. K. (1966). Multiple factors affecting volitional consumption of alcohol in the Abrams Wistar rat. Quarterly Journal of Studies on Alcohol, 27, 7-15.

Ramsey, R. W., & Van Dis, H. (1967). The role of punishment in the aetiology and continuance of alcohol drinking in rats. Behavioral Research and Therapy, 5, 229-235.

Ratcliffe, F. (1972). Ethanol dependence in the rat: Its production and characteristics. Archives Internationale de Pharmacodynamie et de Therapie, 196, 146-156.

Reed, T. E., Kalant, H., Gibbons, R. J., Kapur, B. M., & Rankin, J. C. (1976). Alcohol and acetaldehyde metabolism in Caucasians, Chinese and Amerinds. Canadian Medical Association Journal, 115, 851-855.

Richter, C. P., & Campbell, K. (1940). Alcohol taste thresholds and concentration of solution preferred by rats. Science, 91, 507-508.

Rick, J. T., & Wilson, C. W. M. (1966). Alcohol preference in the rat: Its relationship to total fluid consumption. Quarterly Journal of Studies on Alcohol, 27, 447-458.

Rockman, G. E., Amit, Z., Carr, G., Brown, Z. W., & Ogren, S-O. (1979). Attenuation of ethanol intake by 5-hydroxytryptamine uptake blockade in laboratory rats: I. Involvement of brain 5-hydroxytryptamine in the mediation of the positive reinforcing properties of ethanol. Archives Internationale de Pharmacodynamie et de Therapie, 241, 245-259.

Rodgers, D. A., & McClearn, G. E. (1962). Alcohol preference of mice. In E. L. Bliss (Ed.), Roots of behavior (pp. 68-95). New York: Harper.

Rodgers, D. A., Ward, P. A., Thiessen, D. D., & Whitworth, N. S. (1967). Pathological effects of prolonged voluntary consumption of alcohol by mice. Quarterly Journal of Studies on Alcohol, 28, 618-630.

Samson, H. H., & Falk, J. L. (1974). Alteration of fluid preference in ethanol-dependent animals. Journal of Pharmacology and Experimental Therapeutics, 190, 365-376.

Sanders, R. M., Nathan, P. E., & O'Brien, J. S. (1976). The performance of adult alcoholics working for alcohol: A detailed operant analysis. British Journal of Addiction, 71, 307-319.

Schlesinger, K., Kakihana, R., & Bennett, E. L. (1966). Effects of tetraethylthiuram disulfide (Antabuse) on the metabolism and consumption of ethanol in mice. Psychonomic Science, 28, 514-520.

Schuckit, M. A., & Rayses, V. (1979). Ethanol ingestion: Differences in blood acetaldehyde concentrations in relatives of alcoholics and controls. Science, 203, 54-55.

Senter, R. J., & Sinclair, J. D. (1967). Self-maintenance of intoxication in the rat: A modified replication. Psychonomic Science, 9, 291-292.

Senter, R. J., Smith, F. W., & Lewin, S. (1967). Ethanol ingestion as an operant response. Psychonomic Science, 8, 291-292.

Sheppard, J. E., Albersheim, P., & McClearn, G. E. (1968). Enzyme activities and ethanol preference in mice. Biochemical Genetics, 2, 205-212.

Sinclair, J. D. (1980). Comparison of the factors which influence voluntary drinking in humans and animals. In K. Eriksson, J. D. Sinclair, & K. Kiianmaa (Eds.), Animal models in alcohol research (pp. 119-137). New York: Academic Press.

Sinclair, J. D., & Senter, R. J. (1968). Development of an alcohol deprivation effect in rats. Quarterly Journal of Studies on Alcohol, 29, 863-867.

Sinclair, J. E. (1974). Rats learning to work for alcohol. Nature, 244, 590-592.

Socaransky, S. M., Aragon, C. M. G., Amit, Z., & Blander, A. (1984). Higher correlation of ethanol consumption with brain than liver ALDH in three strains of rats. Psychopharmacology, 84, 250-253.

Sutherland, E. A., Amit, Z., Sossanpour, M., & Selvaggi, N. (1983). A new psychopharmacological approach to treatment of alcoholism: Blockade of positive reinforcement with zimelidine. Alcoholism: Clinical and Experimental Research, 7, 123.

Wallgren, H., & Forsander, O. (1963). Effect of adaptation to alcohol and of age on voluntary consumption of alcohol by rats. British Journal of Nutrition, 17, 453-457.

Wayner, M. J., Gawronski, D., Roubie, C., & Greenberg, I. (1971). Effect of ethyl alcohol on lateral hypothalamic neurons. In N. K. Mello & J. H. Mendelson (Eds.), Recent advances in studies of alcoholism (pp. 219-273). Washington, DC: U.S. Government Printing Office.

Wayner, M. J., & Greenberg, I. (1972). Effects of hypothalamic stimulation, acclimation and periodic withdrawal on ethanol consumption. Physiology & Behavior, 9, 737-740.

Wilson, C. W. M. (1972). The limiting factors in alcohol consumption. In O. Forsander & E. K. Eriksson (Eds.), Biological aspects of alcoholism (pp. 207-215). Helsinki: Finnish Foundation for Alcohol Studies.

Wise, R. A. (1973). Voluntary ethanol intake in rats following exposure to ethanol on various schedules. Psychopharmacology, 29, 203-210.

Wise, R. A., & Bozarth, M. A. (1982). Action of drugs of abuse on brain reward systems: An update with specific attention to opiates. Pharmacology Biochemistry & Behavior, 17, 239-243.

Zeiner, A. R., Paredes, A., & Christianson, H. D. (1979). The role of acetaldehyde in mediating reactivity to an acute dose of ethanol among different racial groups. Alcoholism: Clinical and Experimental Research, 3, 11-18.

CHAPTER 9

INTRACRANIAL SELF-ADMINISTRATION PROCEDURES FOR THE ASSESSMENT OF DRUG REINFORCEMENT

Michael A. Bozarth

Center for Studies in Behavioral Neurobiology
Department of Psychology
Concordia University
Montreal, Quebec, Canada   H3G 1M8

ABSTRACT

Procedures used for intracranial drug self-administration are described. The experimental approach uses lever-pressing and is a direct extension of methods used in intravenous drug self-administration studies. Some of the important factors that must be considered when conducting these experiments are discussed. Although intracranial self-administration potentially offers several advantages for the study of drug reinforcement, methodological difficulties have severely limited the routine application of this technique.

INTRODUCTION

The general procedures that have been developed for intravenous self-administration can be adapted to study reinforcement from drug injections directly into the brain. These injections may be into the cerebral ventricles (i.e., intraventricular) or directly into brain tissue (i.e., intracranial). The operant response requirements are usually the same as those used with intravenous drug self-administration (i.e., lever pressing). Many of the control procedures necessary to assure the validity of the conclusions drawn from these studies are also comparable, although several new types of controls must also be tested during intracranial self-administration.

There are a number of potential advantages to studying reinforcement from microinjections directly into the brain. First, injection sites are proximal (at least in theory) to their site of action; this minimizes the influence of diffusion barriers such as the blood-brain barrier and circumvents both first pass and local metabolism of the test compound that can accompany systemic drug administration. Also, drug loss to irrelevant pharmacokinetic compartments is decreased because the drug is administered directly to the biophase (i.e., site of action). Thus, drugs that penetrate the blood-brain barrier with great difficulty, that are rapidly metabolized, or that are available only in limited quantities can be tested for their reinforcing effects by direct cerebral microinjections.

Second, the site of action for a drug's reinforcing effect may be localized with intracranial self-administration. Brain regions where a drug is self-administered are likely to be close to the target of drug action. This approach has several advantages over the more commonly used technique of assessing brain lesion effects on systemic drug self-administration. The latter method suffers from nonspecific lesion effects, from changes in the sensitivity of the lesioned neurons, and from the inherent limitation that lesions identify, at best, systems involved in a drug's action but do not determine whether the drug is acting directly at that system (i.e., do not identify the area where the drug effect is initiated; see Bozarth, 1983). If appropriate control procedures are used, intracranial self-administration offers the most direct method of identifying the brain region where a drug initiates its rewarding action.

Third, if different receptor fields mediate different effects from a drug, it should be possible to minimize the influence of secondary effects on measures of drug reinforcement. For example, the peripheral sympathetic excitatory effects of psychomotor stimulants at the level of the autonomic ganglia should not be present during central microinjections of these compounds. This permits the study of stimulant reinforcement without the concomitant autonomic effects usually associated with their administration. Similarly, if the sedative or analgesic actions of opioids are due to a drug effect at brain sites that are different from those involved in their reinforcing effects, then it would be possible to study opioid reinforcement without the potentially confounding influence of sedation and analgesia (see Bozarth, 1983).

EARLY STUDIES

There were several early reports of intracranial self-administration. Cholinergic substances (Morgane, 1962; Myers, 1963) were reported to be self-administered into the hypothalamus and the septum by laboratory rats. The published reports of this work, however, gave few details of the experimental procedures. One full paper was published by Olds and Olds (1958) describing the self-administration of a monoamine oxidase inhibitor (i.e., iproniazid) into the hypothalamic area. Shortly after this promising report, a review of this work and of research involving the intracranial self-administration of other substances was published suggesting that the self-administration of these compounds resulted from nonspecific physico-chemical drug actions (J. Olds, 1962). Although this synopsis was seemingly discouraging, it laid the foundation for both the methodological requirements and some necessary control procedures for establishing the validity of intracranial self-administration experiments.

A detailed report by Olds, Yuwiler, Olds, and Yun (1964) summarized studies with 1,327 rats tested for intracranial self-administration of a wide variety of compounds. This paper emphasized basic ionic effects involved in self-administration and further illustrated the importance of controls for nonspecific physico-chemical effects following intracranial drug injections. Data showing the intracranial self-administration of cholinergic substances into the lateral hypothalamus were presented as evidence for an involvement of acetylcholine in reward processes, but even this effect was attributed to a physico-chemical action on neuronal fibers and not a direct synaptic action. During the next decade and a half, only one report was published involving intracranial self-administration. In an abstract E. Stein and J. Olds (1976) reported that morphine was intracranially self-administered at various brain sites also supporting electrical brain stimulation reward. A full report of this work was never published, but M. Olds (1979) later published a paper describing intracranial morphine self-administration into the lateral hypothalamus using the same experimental procedure.

CONTROL PROCEDURES

There are a several important factors to consider when studying the effects of central drug injections on behavior. These considerations demand that certain control conditions are tested to eliminate alternative explanations of the drug-taking behavior. The main factors can be conveniently divided into three broad categories: tests for behavioral, pharmacological, and anatomical specificity. Each topic addresses specific issues concerned with the interpretation of data from intracranial self-administration experiments and each suggests specific tests of the validity of such data. Although these factors have been previously described (see Bozarth, 1983), a brief summary of the basic principles involved in the assessment of intracranial self-administration studies is appropriate here.

Behavioral Specificity

The first requirement of any self-administration study is the demonstration that the animals are working for the rewarding effects of the drug injections. Both systemic and central drug injections can produce increases in locomotor activity, and such increased activity could lead to accidental lever-contacts that are mistakenly interpreted as evidence for self-administration. In particular, morphine applied to the ventral tegmental area produces increases in exploratory and locomotor activity (Joyce & Iversen, 1979) that must be considered when evaluating lever-pressing behavior. There are two primary methods that have been used to determine the relative contribution of nonspecific behavioral arousal to the lever-counts obtained during self-administration testing. The first method uses each subject as its own control, while the second method requires that two subjects be tested concurrently, one serving as the experimental subject and the other as the control subject.

The first method compares lever-press rates on two levers: one lever produces response-contingent drug injections while the other has no scheduled effect; lever-pressing on the second lever is interpreted as an indication of nonspecific lever-depressions. Although this method has been successfully used to demonstrate behavioral specificity during intracranial drug self-administration (e.g., Goeders & Smith, 1983; Monaco, Hernadez, & Hoebel, 1981), the results of this test can be variable. With behaviorally activating drug injections, the subject may depress both the active lever and depress the inactive lever during the rewarding drug injection. Thus, the rewarding effect of the drug injection would actually be paired with both levers. Because there is no penalty for pressing the inactive control lever, the discrimination learning may not be very strong. Animals may show response generalization to the inactive lever and thus increase response rates on both levers. Two-lever choice testing with intravenous heroin self-administration frequently shows excellent discrimination between active and inactive levers, but some animals show high levels of responding on the inactive lever (Bozarth, unpublished observations). When this occurs, certain subjects demonstrate behavioral specificity (i.e., preferential lever-pressing on the lever associated with drug injections), but others do not. A simple averaging of response rates on the two levers across different subjects can result in a failure to demonstrate an overall preference for the active lever. Furthermore, if a subject shows stereotypic responding on an inactive lever, the response rate on that lever can be several times the response rate on the drug-contingent lever. Averaging inflates the number of inactive lever responses obscuring the fact that other subjects may show good two-lever discrimination. The alternative procedure of using selected subjects to demonstrate two-lever choice responding can dangerously bias the experimental interpretation, although the exclusion of a small percentage of subjects stereotyping on the inactive lever is probably justified. In either case it is important that all data be presented so that the reader is free to draw his own conclusion regarding the behavioral specificity of the response.

A second method of determining if the lever-pressing is a consequence of the rewarding action of the drug is to use a yoked control procedure. With this method two animals are tested concurrently. One animal is allowed to lever press for response-contingent drug injections while the other subject is tested with an inactive lever. The lever presses of the first animal produce concurrent injections in both subjects, and the lever pressing of the second subject is simply measured as an indication of nonspecific behavioral arousal. This procedure has proven effective in studies of ventral tegmental morphine self-administration (Bozarth & Wise, 1981) as well as in studies of intravenous drug self-administration. A potential problem is that cues (e.g., activation of a cue light) accompanying the rewarding drug effect may become associated with drug reward (see Smith & Davis, this volume; Stewart & de Wit, this volume) in both subjects, and the yoked control animal may also approach these cues. This can be a problem if a cue light is illuminated directly above the lever and the control animals are repeatedly tested. Arousal and approach behavior associated with the illumination of the cue light may lead to an increase in contacts with the inactive lever. This potential problem might be eliminated by using an auditory cue associated with drug delivery. Even then, however, conditioned increases in locomotor activity may lead to increased accidental lever contacts.

Either approach to assessing the behavioral specificity of intracranial self-administration is valid. The two-lever choice test has the advantage of minimizing the number of subjects that must be tested because each subject serves as its own control. It is probably more difficult to obtain clear evidence of behavioral specificity with this method, and presentation of selected subjects demonstrating differential response rates on the two levers may bias the experimental conclusion. The yoked control procedure may provide evidence for behavioral specificity which is more easily obtainable (e.g., less likely to be influenced by response generalization producing elevated response rates on the inactive lever), but additional subjects must be tested and it may be influenced by conditioning effects. Nonetheless, reliable data from either procedure is an adequate demonstration of behavioral specificity.

Pharmacological Specificity

After the clear demonstration of behavioral specificity, the next issue of importance is the demonstration that the observed rewarding effect of the central drug injections is not the result of some nonspecific action of the compound. Microinjection of drugs into brain tissue can cause a number of nonspecific changes in the cell environment. Changes in pH, osmolarity, and regional ion balance can all occur and any of these effects might cause nonspecific activation of cells proximal to the injection site. In addition, for drugs that have rewarding effects from systemic injections, it may be important to show that the same mechanisms are involved in reward from both systemic and central drug administration.

For compounds that act at specific receptors, tests of pharmacological specificity can be conducted using receptor antagonists. In the case of opiates, these tests are particularly easy because opiate reward involves the activation of opiate receptors and because specific antagonists are available for these receptors. For example, pretreatment with an opiate antagonist such as naloxone should block the rewarding effect of central morphine if the rewarding action depends on activation of opiate receptors. Substances not having specific receptors or identified mechanisms of action (e.g., barbiturates) and substances with potent local anesthetic effects (e.g., cocaine) are more problematic. The use of active and inactive stereoisomers should reveal if the rewarding action of these compounds involves specific mechanisms or nonspecific physico-chemical actions of these substances.

When receptor antagonist or inactive stereoisomers are not available (e.g., ethanol), an alternative method of assessing pharmacological specificity must be used. If the neurochemical effect of a compound that is critically involved in its reinforcing action has been identified, then pharmacological treatments that block this neurochemical effect might be used to test the importance of this process in reward from central drug. For example, the rewarding effects of intravenous cocaine have been shown to depend on the activation of dopaminergic mechanisms, and the disruption of dopaminergic neurotransmission has been used as a test of the pharmacological specificity of reward from centrally administered cocaine. Treatment with a drug that blocks dopamine receptors attenuates intracranial cocaine self-administration into the frontal cortex (Goeders & Smith, 1983). This has been interpreted as showing that central cocaine is rewarding by the same mechanism as that involved in systemic cocaine self-administration. Caution should be exercised, however, when drawing such conclusions. Dopamine-receptor blockade has been associated with decreased locomotor activity, and the decrease in intracranial cocaine self-administration could result from a simple sedative action of the neuroleptic. Tests of active vs. inactive stereoisomers of cocaine would clearly be the preferred method of determining pharmacological specificity.

Anatomical Specificity

Anatomical specificity can be divided into two general questions: Is the rewarding drug effect due to an activation of neural mechanisms proximal to the site of injection, and how many other brain regions support the intracranial self-administration of a given compound? The first question addresses issues related to the spread of drug from the site of injection and is designed to determine if drug diffusion to a distal site of action is involved in the observed response. The second question involves anatomical mapping of the brain to determine if the observed behavior is related to a drug action in a single brain region or whether multiple brain sites can support the same response.

Physical Tests of Drug Diffusion

The diffusion of drug following intracranial injections can be assessed using methods that physically measure the quantity of drug present at different locations around the microinjection site. Radiolabeled drug can be injected and the drug spread determined with autoradiography. Serial brain sections both anterior and posterior to the injection site can be used to visualize drug dispersion, and the density of images produced can be used to assess the extent of drug diffusion. Quantitative autoradiography can provide an estimate of the actual amount of drug in different regions following microinjection. The visualization of drug dispersion with this method is time consuming because it requires serial sectioning of the brain and because adequate exposure times must be used to insure proper visualization. Furthermore, quantitative autoradiography is difficult to perform making estimates of actual drug amounts very tenuous.

Another method of physically determining the degree of drug spread following intracranial injections combines the micro-punch assay procedure of Palkovits (1973) with liquid scintillation counting. As with the autoradiographic method, the brain is sliced in serial sections. Small brain areas are then removed with a micro-punch and the amount of radioactivity present can be determined using standard liquid scintillation procedures. This method has the advantage of accurately measuring the amount of drug found at various regions around the microinjection site without introducing the complications associated with quantitative autoradiography. An excellent description of the use of this technique can be found in Myers and Hoch (1978) who used this approach to determine the dispersion kinetics of radiolabeled dopamine following intracranial injections. Although this method is relatively simple and affords an accurate assessment of drug spread, it can be very laborious if a large number of brain regions are measured.

Probably the best approach to studying physical drug spread is to perform both autoradiographic visualization and micro-punch liquid scintillation counting. Initial work could be done with autoradiography, and the results of this procedure used to direct the micro-punch assays. This way, the overall dispersion pattern will be determined and accurate quantification of drug concentrations in the target areas can also be provided. It should be noted that only autoradiography performed on a broad range of serial sections is likely to reveal drug diffusion to extremely distal sites. Such drug diffusion may occur if the microinjections encroach on cerebral vascular supplies or the cerebral ventricles. In this case drug may diffuse much further than the area likely to be included in micro-punch assays.

Functional Tests of Drug Diffusion

A different approach to determining the anatomical specificity of a response produced by intracranial injections focuses on functional tests of drug spread. Here, the physical spread of drug is considered less important, and the assessment of spread of behaviorally relevant concentrations considered the primary objective. In tests of physical drug spread, it is erroneous to conclude that the drug is acting at a distal site just because drug is present there. The behaviorally relevant concentration of drug would have to be known to make such a conclusion. Functional tests of drug spread vary the microinjection sites around the brain region found to be effective in producing the behavioral response and determine if proximal microinjections are also effective. Areas where the drug is most likely to reach by diffusion (e.g., cerebral ventricles, up the cannula shaft) are particularly important test sites (see Bozarth & Wise, 1984). If the behavior is not produced with microinjections into adjacent brain sites, then the response is likely to be produced by a drug action in the target area.

This approach has two important advantages over physical tests of drug spread. First, it is very easy to perform and does not require any facilities except those necessary to perform the intracranial self-administration experiments. The use of radiolabeled compounds requires that certain safety precautions be followed, and facilities to measure the radioactivity are required. Second, it determines if behaviorally relevant concentrations of drug are diffusing to a distal site of action. Methods measuring physical drug spread cannot determine if behaviorally relevant concentrations are being reached at distal sites but only reveal that some quantity of drug has spread to other regions.

Anatomical Mapping

One of the most important contributions that intracranial self-administration studies can make to the understanding of drug reward is the identification of brain regions where drug injections are directly reinforcing. The brain can be mapped for sites that support intracranial self-administration of a test compound using a standard protocol. If behavioral and pharmacological specificity of the intracranial self-administration has been established, this should indicate the location of receptors that initiate the rewarding actions of a given compound (see Bozarth, 1983). Tests of drug diffusion are also necessary to determine if the reinforcing effect is due to a local drug action.

The observation that a drug is not intracranially self-administered into a given brain region does not eliminate that region as a potential site for drug reward. A higher drug dosage may support intracranial self-administration, or competing responses may be produced by the central drug injections (e.g., sedation) and inhibit lever pressing. Nonetheless, mapping the brain using a standard protocol that has been shown to be effective in supporting intracranial self-administration into one or more brain regions is a first approximation to delineating the anatomical localization of reward-relevant receptors. Tests of behavioral and pharmacological specificity and tests of drug diffusion to a distal site of action must be conducted for each brain region and compound that supports intracranial self-administration.

METHODOLOGICAL CONSIDERATIONS

There are a number of methodological considerations that are important in studies of intracranial self-administration. These include the method of drug delivery and the parameters selected for studying intracranial self-administration. In this rapidly developing field, these factors have not always been given adequate attention and each laboratory appears to have developed its own standards for conducting intracranial self-administration studies.

Drug Delivery System

The topics of cannula systems and general considerations for drug microinjections have been extensively reviewed (e.g., Myers, 1972, 1974; Routtenberg, 1972) and will not be addressed here. One factor that is unique to intracranial self-administration studies and deserves special mention, however, is the method of intracranial drug delivery. Intracranial self-administration requires that low volume, response-contingent drug be delivered immediately following the lever-press response and that drug not be infused when the animal is not emitting the appropriate response. If drug is not injected immediately following the behavioral response to be reinforced or if drug is delivered at times other than immediately following the appropriate response, it is very unlikely that the subject will learn the response-reinforcement contingency. For example, a delay of reinforcement of only a few seconds is sufficient to disrupt performance in operant paradigms (see Renner, 1964; Tarpy & Sawabini, 1974). The availability of drug delivery systems that can assure the contingency of reinforcement has been perhaps the most serious limitation to the development of intracranial self-administration as a standard laboratory procedure.

Several methods are available for centrally injecting drugs into freely moving animals. The traditional approach is a direct adaptation of intravenous self-administration procedures and involves connecting the subject's injection cannula to a microsyringe via flexible plastic tubing. A fluid commutator positioned between the microsyringe and the injection cannula permits unrestricted movement of the subject during behavioral testing. A motor-driven syringe pump advances the syringe plunger a predetermined amount following each lever press, thus displacing a known volume of drug. The presumption made by most investigators using this technique is that the amount of drug displaced from the microsyringe is centrally injected into the freely moving subject. Unfortunately, this may be an erroneous assumption.

Movement of the subject can compress and expand the plastic tubing connecting the microsyringe to the injection cannula. This can cause the injection of an undetermined quantity of drug as the subject freely moves about the test chamber. Attempts have been made to prevent the twisting and compression of the connecting tubing by using an outer cable to relieve the strain produced by the subject's movement. The flexibility of the connecting line, however, is the reason why plastic tubing is used. Thus, making the connecting tubing sufficiently rigid to prevent stretching and compression is likely to inhibit the animal's movement about the test chamber. Another source of potential problem with this method is the fluid swivel. If the swivel is not absolutely gas tight, leakage can occur and drug can siphon into the subject's brain.

Various approaches have been used to increase the reliability of drug microinjections into freely moving animals. The original studies of J. Olds (e.g., 1962) used a specially developed injection technique to improve the reliability of microinjections. E. Stein and Rodd (1980) have also developed a technique that eliminates the fluid swivel which is one source of variance in drug microinjections. Both of these procedures, however, retain the flexible tubing which is likely to be the major source of variability in small volume drug delivery.

Another approach to the problem of small volume drug delivery in freely moving animals uses a technique that eliminates both the fluid swivel and flexible connecting tubing. This system uses a small gas-tight drug reservoir filled with drug and attached to an injection cannula. The entire unit is mounted directly on the subject's head. Drug injections are accomplished by passing a small direct current between two electrodes contained in the drug reservoir. This causes the production of a specific amount of hydrogen and oxygen gas which displaces drug from the reservoir through the injection cannula. The amount of drug injected is controlled by the current intensity and duration. The animal's injection unit is connected to the current source with light electrical leads. This eliminates the necessity of both the fluid swivel and flexible injection tubing; thus the major sources of injection volume variability are functionally circumvented while maintaining unrestricted movement of the subject during testing. (See Bozarth and Wise, 1980, for details of this procedure.) This technique has been used for studies of morphine self-administration into the ventral tegmental area (e.g., Bozarth & Wise, 1981) and for studies of cocaine self-administration into the frontal cortex (Goeders & Smith, 1983).

Testing Parameters

Intracranial self-administration studies have involved both animals previously trained to lever-press for another reinforcer and animals that were experimentally naive. Animals that are already trained to lever-press can emit high levels of responding for no reinforcer (i.e., extinction). This situation may be advantageous in initial screening for drug reinforcement from new brain sites or new compounds--the high levels of responding insure that the subject emits enough lever presses to deliver drug and may enhance the subject's learning of the lever-press/drug-effect contingency. Also, if the drug delivery method is unreliable, high baseline rates of lever-pressing may facilitate the subject learning to respond on an intermittent reinforcement schedule. However, there is a serious limitation of using lever-trained subjects with studies involving drug effects. Animals frequently emit high levels of responding during extinction and this effect may be prolonged by certain drug treatments. Furthermore, noncontingent drug injections have been shown to reinstate lever pressing in animals only receiving saline injections (see Stewart & de Wit, this volume). Although this is likely to reveal important information regarding the nature of the drug reward, it does not establish behavioral specificity of the intracranial self-administration behavior. To satisfy this criterion, it is necessary to show that response-contingent drug delivery is maintaining the lever-pressing behavior.

Studies of direct acquisition of a lever-pressing response to receive intracranial drug provide the strongest demonstration of drug reinforcement from central injections. Although it may not always be possible to establish intracranial self-administration in experimentally naive animals, this preparation is preferred to approaches using subjects previously trained to lever press for other reinforcers.

Another important factor to consider is the concentration of the test compound injected following each lever press. In addition to the problem of nonspecific physico-chemical drug action that is usually increased with larger drug concentrations, the problem of drug spread is also exacerbated by the use of large injection doses. Drugs diffuse down their concentration gradient, and the rate and quantity of drug diffusion is determined partially by the law of mass action: The larger the concentration at the injection site the larger will be the concentration some distance from that site. Morphine is self-administered into the ventral tegmental area in picomolar unit doses (i.e., dose/microinjection), and this dose level is generally not effective in supporting intracranial morphine self-administration into other brain regions (Bozarth & Wise, 1982). Methionine enkephalin (Goeders & Smith, 1984) and cocaine (Goeders & Smith, 1983) are also self-administered into other brain sites in picomolar doses, and this suggests that this dose range may be applicable for initial tests involving the intracranial self-administration of different compounds. The use of larger injection doses may result in the diffusion of pharmacologically relevant amounts of drug to distal sites of action. For intracranial self-administration studies (as in other studies involving central drug microinjections), it is advantageous to use the lowest effective dose of a test compound. Picomolar unit doses appear to be the effective dose range for these studies. The arbitrary selection of larger injection doses is likely to invalidate any conclusions drawn regarding the anatomical specificity of the effect and may cause appreciable nonspecific effects.

The last factor to be considered here is the selection of the injection volume. In general, it might appear that the smaller the injection volume the better the anatomical resolution of intracranial microinjection studies. In fact, one study has reported a behavioral response from the microiontophoretic application of a substance (Aghajanian & Davis, 1975) suggesting that extremely small drug doses and injection volumes may be capable of producing a behavioral response. There are, however, practical considerations that also need to be taken into account. Intracranial microinjection studies require that the performance of the injection cannula be routinely checked before and after behavioral testing. For this, the volume of drug needs to be sufficient to permit easy visualization so that the injection reliability can be assured. The use of a 100 nl injection volume appears to be a reasonable trade-off between a small volume that maintains good anatomical resolution and a volume that can be visualized to determine if the microinjection system is functioning properly. Although the reliable microinjection of smaller volumes may be feasible, volumes in the low nanoliter range do not permit visual confirmation of individual drug infusions following behavioral testing. Because the single most important consideration for establishing intracranial self-administration is response contingent drug delivery, the reliability of single infusions must be assessed before and after behavioral testing. To accomplish this, it is necessary to visually confirm drug delivery following each lever press and not just the cumulative effect of numerous lever presses.

CONCLUSIONS

Provided that certain conditions are satisfied to insure the validity of intracranial self-administration studies, there are several advantages that can be gained by using this approach to the study of drug reinforcement. It is critical, however, that the limitations of this technique are considered in concert with the potential advantages and that the criteria for assuring the validity of these studies outlined in the previous section are fulfilled.

The first obvious advantage of using this approach is that drugs with limiting pharmacokinetic properties can be adequately tested for their rewarding effects. Compounds that do not readily cross the blood-brain barrier, that are slowly absorbed or distributed in the central nervous system, or that are rapidly metabolized or excreted are difficult to assess with systemic self-administration techniques. The direct application of these drugs into the brain should circumvent the limiting pharmacokinetic factors that preclude adequate assessment with methods such as intravenous self-administration. For example, the enkephalins and some other peptides poorly penetrate the blood-brain barrier and are rapidly inactivated. These compounds can be more effectively screened for reinforcing effects with direct microinjection into the brain.

Second, compounds that are available only in limited quantities can be screened for reinforcing effects with intracranial methods. The use of intracranial microinjection procedures should minimize the quantity of a compound required to assess its reinforcing properties. Because distribution to the critical site of action and minimal loss to irrelevant pharmacokinetic compartments result from direct drug microinjection into the brain, substantially less compound is required to produce a behavioral response. Thus, compounds that are expensive or available in limited quantities can be adequately tested if the central site of drug action is known or if it lies proximal to the cerebral ventricles.

Third, multiple actions of a drug can potentially be minimized with intracranial microinjection procedures. When a drug is injected systemically, the drug is distributed to a number of brain and peripheral sites where it may produce various effects. Many of the actions of a drug may be unrelated to its rewarding action and some of these side-effects may even obscure the important rewarding effects of a drug. For example, when opiates are intravenously self-administered, drug is distributed to a number of brain sites where several different actions are produced. A periventricular gray action of opiates produces analgesia (Sharpe, Garnett, & Cicero, 1974; Yaksh, Yeung, & Rudy, 1976) and if the dose is sufficient, physiological dependence (Bozarth & Wise, 1984) and sedation (Pert, DeWald, Liao, & Sivit, 1979) may occur. Changes in thermoregulation can be produced by a drug action in the preoptic area of the lateral hypothalamus (Lotti, Lomax, & George, 1965; Teasdale, Bozarth, & Stewart, 1981), and effects on prolactin secretion can accompany an opiate action in the raphe nucleus (Johnson, 1982). The rewarding and locomotor stimulating actions of opiates appear to be derived from an action in the ventral tegmental area which does not involve these other opiate effects (see Bozarth, 1983). Thus, the compound opiate effects produced during systemic drug administration are related to the drug's actions on multiple brain sites and most of these effects are not related to the rewarding action of the compound. Central injections of opiates can isolate the rewarding action from analgesia, physiological dependence, and other opiate effects that may be irrelevant to opiate reinforcement (see Bozarth, 1983).

Fourth, the independent contributions of different reinforcement systems simultaneously activated by systemic drug delivery can be assessed with this technique. Opiates, for example, appear to involve a strong positive reinforcing action in the ventral tegmental area (Bozarth & Wise, 1981, 1982; van Ree & De Wied, 1980). This rewarding effect is independent of physiological dependence mechanisms as revealed by the fact that repeated morphine injections into this region fail to produce physiological dependence (Bozarth & Wise, 1984). It is possible, however, that physiological dependence contributes to the net reinforcing impact of systemically delivered opiates in subjects that have become physically dependent. The relief of withdrawal distress may provide negative reinforcement and may be capable of maintaining lever-pressing behavior. By limiting the distribution of morphine to the brain region where positive reinforcement is initiated (i.e., ventral tegmental area) or the area where relief of withdrawal discomfort is likely to be produced (i.e., periventricular gray region), the contribution of positive and negative reinforcement processes from these two brain systems can be independently evaluated. Similarly, if multiple brain systems are involved in the positive reinforcing actions of a compound (e.g., frontal cortex and nucleus accumbens in the case of cocaine), then the relative importance of each system can be evaluated with the intracranial self-administration paradigm. If several brain sites are capable of initiating the reinforcing effect of a drug, then brain lesion challenges of a single site during intravenous self-administration would be unlikely to reveal the importance of that site in drug reward because the unlesioned brain system may be capable of maintaining the rewarding action of the test compound. Intracranial self-administration permits the systematic determination of the ability of various brain regions to initiate the rewarding actions of a compound and can thus identify brain systems involved in drug reinforcement even if multiple systems are capable of maintaining the behavior.

There are several serious limitations of intracranial self-administration procedures. The most obvious is that this technique is methodologically difficult requiring the precise delivery of nanoliter volumes of drug in freely moving animals. Improvements in microinjection technology can eliminate this problem, but caution needs to be observed when studying the effects of repeated drug microinjections because of the potential problem of tissue trauma. The repeated microinjection of substances in the brain can radically alter the cell environment, and changes in the responsiveness to drug can occur because of physiological changes produced by the injection procedure. These problems, however, can be minimized by the selection of an adequate microinjection procedure and by the use of low volume and low infusion rate injections that are not traumatic to neural tissue.

A limitation of intracranial self-administration studies that is more difficult to circumvent involves the nature of brain reinforcement systems. It is possible that reinforcement from a given drug might involve the concurrent activation of several brain sites that cannot be duplicated by drug injection into a single site. Thus, conventional microinjection studies which examine the effect of a drug injection into one brain site at a time would not reveal a reinforcing action for a compound that requires the concurrent activation of several neural systems. Nonetheless, a number of compounds have been shown to be reinforcing when microinjected into discrete brain regions thus suggesting that reinforcement from at least some substances can result from a drug action initiated at a single brain region (see Table 1).

Table 1

Compounds Intracranially Self-Administered

Compound	Brain Site	Investigators
amphetamine	FCX NAS	Phillips et al., 1981 Monaco et al., 1981 Hoebel et al., 1983
calcium chelators	LHA	J. Olds et al., 1964
cholinergic agent(?)	PFR Spt	Morgane, 1962 Myers, 1963
cocaine	FCX	Goeders & Smith, 1983
fentanyl	VTA	van Ree & De Wied, 1980
iproniazid	LHA	J. Olds & M. Olds, 1958
methionine enkephalin d-ala^2-met-enkephalinamide	NAS LHA	Goeders & Smith, 1984 M. Olds & Williams, 1980
morphine	LHA + others LHA NAS VTA	E. Stein & J. Olds, 1977 M. Olds, 1979 M. Olds, 1982 Bozarth & Wise, 1981, 1982

Abbreviations: FCX, frontal cortex; LHA, lateral hypothalamic area; NAS, nucleus accumbens; PFR, perifornical region; Spt, septal region; VTA, ventral tegmental area.

One limitation of the intracranial self-administration paradigm cannot be circumvented and is inherent in the very nature of this approach to studying drug reinforcement. Intracranial self-administration demonstrates that a drug action in a specific brain region is <u>sufficient</u> for reinforcement. That is, activation of that region by the compound can directly reinforce behavior. The fact that a compound is self-administered into a given brain region does not, however, suggest that activation of that brain region is <u>necessary</u> for reinforcement from systemic application of the test compound (see Bozarth, 1983). It could be the case that several brain systems are involved in the reinforcing action of a single compound and that activation of any one of these systems is sufficient to reinforce behavior. Only studies assessing the effects of blocking drug action in a given brain region during tests of the reinforcing effects of systemically administered drug (e.g., intravenous self-administration) can determine if a drug action in a given brain region is necessary for drug reinforcement.

Intracranial self-administration procedures can provide an important advance in the study of drug reinforcement mechanisms. This paradigm is uniquely suited for determining the anatomical localization of brain sites responsible for the initiation of drug reward and can provide important corroboration of findings revealed with other methods. Intracranial self-administration is a relatively new and unexplored technique, although the first studies using this approach were reported thirty years ago. Because the standards for evaluating these experiments have not been clearly established in the literature, it is especially important to be cautious when interpreting the results of these studies. The criteria of behavioral, pharmacological, and anatomical specificity provide minimal requirements for demonstrating the validity of these studies. In addition to the acceptance of uniform standards for conducting these experiments, further improvements in microinjection technology will undoubtedly permit the more widespread application of this important procedure for studying drug reinforcement.

ACKNOWLEDGMENTS

Preparation of this manuscript was supported by grants from the Natural Science and Engineering Research Council of Canada (NSERC) and by the National Institute on Drug Abuse (U.S.A.). The author is a University Research Fellow sponsored by NSERC.

REFERENCES

Aghajanian, G. K., & Davis, M. (1975). A method of direct chemical brain stimulation in behavioral studies using microiontophoresis. <u>Pharmacology Biochemistry & Behavior</u>, 3, 127-131.

Bozarth, M. A. (1983). Opiate reward mechanisms mapped by intracranial self-administration. In J. E. Smith and J. D. Lane (Eds.), <u>Neurobiology of opiate reward processes</u> (pp. 331-359). Amsterdam: Elsevier/North Holland Biomedical Press.

Bozarth, M. A., & Wise, R. A. (1980). Electrolytic microinfusion transducer system: An alternative method of intracranial drug application. <u>Journal of Neuroscience Methods</u>, 2, 273-275.

Bozarth, M. A., & Wise, R. A. (1981). Intracranial self-administration of morphine into the ventral tegmental area in rats. <u>Life Sciences</u>, 28, 551-555.

Bozarth, M. A., & Wise, R. A. (1982). Localization of the reward-relevant opiate receptors. In L. S. Harris (Ed.), Problems of drug dependence, 1981 (National Institute on Drug Abuse Research Monograph 41, pp. 158-164). Washington, DC: U.S. Government Printing Office.

Bozarth, M. A., & Wise, R. A. (1984). Anatomically distinct opiate receptor fields mediate reward and physical dependence. Science, 244, 516-517.

Goeders, N. E., & Smith, J. E. (1983). Cortical dopaminergic involvement in cocaine reinforcement. Science, 221, 773-775.

Goeders, N. E., Lane, J. D., & Smith, J. E. (1984). Self-administration of methionine enkephalin into the nucleus accumbens. Pharmacology Biochemistry & Behavior, 20, 451-455.

Hoebel, B. G., Monaco, A. P., Hernandez, L., Aulisi, E. F., Stanley, B. G., & Lenard, L. (1983). Self-injection of amphetamine directly into the brain. Psychopharmacology, 81, 158-163.

Johnson, J. H. (1982). Release of prolactin in response to microinjection of morphine into mesencephalic dorsal raphe nucleus. Neuroendocrinology, 35, 169-172.

Joyce, E. M., & Iversen, S. D. (1979). The effect of morphine applied locally to mesencephalic dopamine cell bodies on spontaneous motor activity in the rat. Neuroscience Letters, 14, 207-212.

Lotti, V. J., Lomax, P., & George, R. (1965). Temperature responses in the rat following intracerebral microinjections of morphine. Journal of Pharmacology and Experimental Therapeutics, 150, 135-139.

Monaco, A. P., Hernandez, L., & Hoebel, B. G. (1981). Nucleus accumbens: Site of amphetamine self-injection: Comparison with the lateral ventricle. In R. B. Chronister and J. F. DeFrance (Eds.), Neurobiology of the nucleus accumbens (pp. 338-343). Brunswick, ME: Haer Institute.

Morgane, P. J. (1962). Reinforcing effects of self-injected cholinergic agents into hypothalamic 'drinking' areas in rats. Federation Proceedings, 21, 352.

Myers, R. D. (1963). An intracranial chemical stimulation system for chronic or self-infusion. Journal of Applied Physiology, 18, 221-223.

Myers, R. D. (1972). Methods for chemical stimulation of the brain. In R. D. Myers (ed.), Methods in psychobiology (Vol. 1, pp. 247-280). New York: Academic Press.

Myers, R. D. (1974). Handbook of drug and chemical stimulation of the brain. New York: Van Nostrand Reinhold.

Myers, R. D., & Hoch, D. B. (1978). ^{14}C-dopamine microinjected into the brain-stem of the rat: Dispersion kinetics, site content and functional dose. Brain Research Bulletin, 3, 601-609.

Olds, J. (1962). Hypothalamic substrates of reward. Physiological Reviews, 42, 554-604.

Olds, J., & Olds, M. E. (1958). Positive reinforcement produced by stimulating hypothalamus with iproniazid and other compounds. Science, 127, 1175-1176.

Olds, J., Yuwiler, A., Olds, M. E., & Yun, C. (1964). Neurohumors in hypothalamic substrates of reward. American Journal of Physiology, 207, 242-254.

Olds, M. E. (1979). Hypothalamic substrate for the positive reinforcing properties of morphine in the rat. Brain Research, 168, 351-360.

Olds, M. E. (1982). Reinforcing effects of morphine in the nucleus accumbens. Brain Research, 237, 429-440.

Olds, M. E., & Williams, K. N. (1980). Self-administration of d-ala^2-met-enkephalinamide at hypothalamic self-stimulation sites. Brain Research, 194, 155-170.

Palkovits, M. (1973). Isolated removal of hypothalamic or other brain nuclei of the rat. Brain Research, 59, 449-450.

Pert, A., DeWald, L. A., Liao, H., & Sivit, C. (1979). Effects of opiates and opioid peptides on motor behaviors: Sites and mechanisms of action. In E. Usdin, W. Bunney, Jr., and N. S. Kline (Eds.), Endorphins in mental health research (pp. 45-61). London: MacMillan.

Phillips, A. G., Mora, F., & Rolls, E. T. (1981). Intracerebral self-administration of amphetamine by rhesus monkeys. Neuroscience Letters, 24, 81-86.

van Ree, J. M., & De Wied, D. (1980). Involvement of neurohypophyseal peptides in drug-mediated adaptive responses. Pharmacology Biochemistry & Behavior, 13(Suppl. 1), 257-263.

Renner, K. E. (1964). Delay of reinforcement: A historical review. Psychological Bulletin, 61, 341-361.

Routtenberg, A. (1972). Intracranial chemical injection and behavior: A critical review. Behavioral Biology, 7, 601-642.

Sharpe, L. G., Garnett, J. E., & Cicero, T. J. (1974). Analgesia and hyperactivity produced by intracranial microinjections of morphine into the periaqueductal gray matter of the rat. Behavioral Biology, 11, 303-313.

Stein, E. A., & Olds, J. (1977). Direct intracerebral self-administration of opiates in the rat. Society for Neuroscience Abstracts, 3, 302.

Stein, E. A., & Rodd, D. (1980). A new injection technique for intracerebral drug administration in behaving animals. Pharmacology Biochemistry Behavior, 12, 815-817.

Tarpy, R. M., & Sawabini, F. L. (1974). Reinforcement delay: A selective review of the last decade. Psychological Bulletin, 81, 984-997.

Teasdale, J. A. P., Bozarth, M. A., & Stewart, J. (1981). Body temperature responses to microinjections of morphine in brain sites containing opiate receptors. Society for Neuroscience Abstracts, 7, 799.

Yaksh, T. L., Yeung, J. C., & Rudy, T. A. (1976). Systematic examination in the rat of brain sites sensitive to the direct application of morphine: Observation of differential effects within the periaqueductal gray. Brain Research, 114, 83-103.

CHAPTER 10

PREDICTION OF DRUG ABUSE LIABILITY FROM ANIMAL STUDIES

Tomoji Yanagita

Preclinical Research Laboratories
Central Institute for Experimental Animals
1433 Nogawa, Miyamae-ku, Kawasaki, 213 Japan

ABSTRACT

In this chapter, the pharmacological factors involved in predicting the abuse liability of drugs are discussed with major emphasis on their psychological dependence potential. For prediction of drug abuse liability, it is important to find and compare the drug's effects against those of prototypic drugs. The important pharmacological properties include the following: central nervous system (CNS) effects, including operant behavioral effects; tolerance; physical dependence potential; and psychological dependence potential. It is also important to consider such chemical and pharmacokinetic properties as water solubility and speeds of absorption and elimination. In particular, psychological dependence potential is most relevant to abuse liability. To evaluate psychological dependence potential from animal studies, the reinforcing and discriminative stimulus properties of drugs must be assessed in comparison with those of prototypic drugs. When human data are available, it is important to verify the animal results on such points as pharmacokinetics and CNS drug susceptibility which may differ across species.

Special consideration should also be given to the following in evaluating psychological dependence potential from animal studies: differences in reinforcing effects depending on the experimental procedure used, analysis of reinforcement data obtained in intragastric self-administration, daily dose and CNS manifestation in self-administration experiments, and influence of physical dependence. From a practical viewpoint, it is also important to predict the nature and extent of ill effects which arise as a consequence of abuse. For this, such drug properties as the CNS effects, psychological dependence potential, toxicity, tolerance, and physical dependence potential must be considered.

ABUSE LIABILITY AND PHARMACOLOGICAL PROPERTIES OF DRUGS

The abuse liability of a drug refers to its likelihood of being abused by humans. The abuse liability of a drug is not solely determined by the drug's pharmacological properties but also by many other factors such as its availability, popularity, price, ease and "fashionability" of use. A good example of this is found in the organic solvents. Until the 1960s their abuse liability was regarded to be rather low, but it is now known to have become high. The pharmacological properties of a drug are, nevertheless, the essential factors constituting its abuse liability--no past case of abuse has been reported for a drug that is free of such pharmacological properties.

The kind of pharmacological properties of a drug that have bearing in the prediction of its abuse liability are outlined below.

(1) <u>Chemistry</u>: chemical structure, physical state, active ingredients, water solubility, preparations, etc.

(2) <u>General Pharmacology</u>: general pharmacological effects, particularly central nervous system (CNS) effects, for profiling the class of the drug in comparison with those of the prototypic drugs of abuse

(3) <u>Special Pharmacology</u>: tolerance and physical dependence potential, reinforcing and discriminative stimulus properties, and effects on other operant behaviors

(4) <u>Pharmacokinetics</u>: absorption, distribution, metabolism, and excretion, including the half-life in the blood for comparison with the half-lives of the prototypic drugs of abuse

GENERAL METHODS TO EVALUATE PSYCHOLOGICAL DEPENDENCE POTENTIAL OF DRUGS FROM ANIMAL STUDIES

As discussed in the previous section, abuse liability is constituted by many factors and cannot be predicted from the drug properties alone. Therefore, as a step towards making this prediction, what is usually discussed is the psychological dependence potential of a drug--in other words, the capacity of a drug to produce a psychic (nonphysical) state of dependence. Drug dependence in general is defined in a technical report of the World Health Organization (WHO, 1969) as follows:

A state, psychic and sometimes also physical, resulting from taking a drug, characterized by behavioral and other responses that always include a compulsion to take a drug on a continuous or periodic basis in order to experience its psychic effects, and sometimes to avoid the discomfort of its absence. (p. 6)

In this definition two points are particularly important: (a) The essential state in drug dependence is the psychic state (i.e., psychological or psychic and not physical dependence) and (b) the behavioral responses of compulsive drug-seeking and/or drug-taking form the essential constituent of psychological dependence, although this dependence may include such responses as a strong desire for a drug that is unexpressed in the behavior as well as the physical and mental states contingent upon experiencing certain of the central nervous system effects of a drug.

The first step in evaluation of the psychological dependence potential of a drug is to determine the drug's class from its chemical and pharmacodynamic profiles. If a drug is found to bear similarity to one of the prototypic drug classes, the possibility is then suggested of the drug having psychological dependence potential similar to that of the prototypic drug. The reliability of this evaluation depends on the availability of reliable data. More reliable data usually permit better evaluation but, depending on the class, a limited evaluation may be possible from either the chemical structure or just a few critical data on general pharmacological effects.

The most important animal data used in evaluating psychological dependence potential are those concerning the reinforcing and discriminative stimulus properties of a drug and other behavioral effects reviewed in other chapters of this book. The assessment of these data is the next step after evaluating the compound's chemical and pharmacodynamic profiles. The question to be answered here is whether the drug is reinforcing or not, and if so, then to what extent. Again, comparisons with similar prototypic drugs should be made. Quite often there may be disagreement in the data on a drug or no clear answer may be obtainable, thus making prediction difficult. In addition to this, many complexities exist in the methods of testing and in the assessment of the data; some of these problems will be mentioned later. But as a rule, if the reinforcing intensity of a drug is found to be similar to the reinforcing intensity of a prototypic drug, there is a good possibility that the drug in question has similarly strong psychological dependence potential. This is particularly true when the data on the drug's discriminative stimulus properties and other behavioral effects support the similarity. In assessment of the reinforcing properties, however, some caution must be taken; since the term reinforcement by definition refers to the increment of the response rate, it can be said that in the self-administration experiment the intensity or efficacy of the reinforcing effects of a drug will be indicated by the level of increment, but the determinants of the response rate here are not only the reinforcing properties of a drug and the experimental procedure but also the duration of the drug effects at the unit dose used in the experiment. Therefore, the reinforcing intensity or efficacy in a strict sense may not necessarily represent the intensity of the animals' drug-seeking and drug-taking behavior.

When the reinforcing effect of a drug is found to be weak in a certain experiment, the evaluation has two possible directions: For example, although the reinforcing effects of cyclazocine and nicotine were both found to be weakly positive in an intravenous continuous self-administration experiment in rhesus monkeys (discussed in the following section), it is well known that cyclazocine has no meaningful psychological dependence potential in humans while nicotine definitely does.

In contrast, the lack of a reinforcing effect does not necessarily imply the lack of psychological dependence potential. An example of this can be seen in many of the hallucinogenic drugs such as LSD or mescaline. Although the psychological dependence potential of these drugs does not appear to be very high, it is still high enough for them to be occasionally abused by humans. Thus when a drug is found to belong to the hallucinogenic class, such data as the discriminative stimulus properties and other behavioral effects may be of great importance in making the prediction of abuse liability.

When psychological dependence potential is to be evaluated from animal data, the usual approach in the extrapolation should be applied. Namely, the animal data should be verified by the human data in such points as pharmacokinetics and drug susceptibility, particularly susceptibility to the central nervous system effects. For example, differences between the experimental animal species and humans in the plasma half-life or in the bioproduction of active metabolites may considerably change the reinforcing and other behavioral effects. Another possibility to be considered is the difference in receptor susceptibility to a particular drug. Therefore, where human data on bioavailability and drug response are available, verification of the animal data by the human data will be be indispensable for reliable evaluation of the psychological dependence potential based on animal data.

SPECIFIC PROBLEMS IN EVALUATION
OF PSYCHOLOGICAL DEPENDENCE POTENTIAL FROM ANIMAL STUDIES

When the psychological dependence potential of a drug is evaluated from animal studies, it is necessary to be cautious about the analysis of data on animal responses that are characteristic of self-administration experiments. In this regard, the following four major points are discussed.

Influence of Differences in Experimental Procedure on the Reinforcing Effect

In intravenous self-administration experiments in rhesus monkeys, the reinforcing effects of such drugs as cyclazocine and nicotine were not found to be demonstrable under the cross self-administration procedure but were demonstrable under the continuous self-administration procedure using a fixed ratio-1 schedule (FR-1). Tables 1 and 2 show the results of the cross and continuous self-administration experiments on cyclazocine and nicotine. In the cross-administration procedure, the period is limited to 4 hours daily for 3 days each with the reference drug first, saline next, and then a certain unit dose of the test drug; in the continuous self-administration procedure, the

TABLE 1

Procedurally Related Differences in the Reinforcing Effect of
Intravenous (i.v.) Cyclazocine in Rhesus Monkeys
(Yanagita, unpublished data)

A. Cross self-administration experiment (i.v., FR-1)

Self-administration ratio (%)a

Agent	Saline	Cyclazocine (µg/kg/inj.)				
Unit dose	0.25 ml/kg	0.06	0.25	1	4	15
	7.7 ± 3.8	5.8 ± 3.5	10.0 ± 5.8	7.7 ± 5.7	3.8 ± 2.0	2.3 ± 1.2

a) Mean $\pm$ S.D. of percent ratio against lefetamine 0.1 mg/kg/inj. as 100%

B. Continuous self-administration experiment (i.v., FR-1)

		Average daily number of self-administrations			
Unit dose (µg/kg/inj.)		Saline	15	4	WD[a]
Period (weeks)		2	2	2	2 days
Monkey	No. 669[b]	2.1	16.0	26.1	106
	No. 718[b]	0.9	5.8	8.8	8
	No. 839[b]	10.3	51.5	---	72
	No. 658[c]	0.4	1.1	0.7	2
	No. 858[c]	1.9	15.1	15.4	61

a) Withdrawal observation, number of lever presses
b) Experienced monkey
c) Naive monkey

- 192 -

TABLE 2

Procedurally Related Differences in the Reinforcing Effect
of Nicotine in Rhesus Monkeys
(Adapted from Yanagita et al., 1974, 1983)

A. Cross self-administration experiment (i.v., FR-1)

Self-administration ratio (%)[a]

Agent	Saline	Nicotine (µg/kg/inj.)				
Unit dose	0.25 ml/kg	2.5	10	40	160	640
	14.3 ±5.3	3.8 ± 2.0	7.9 ± 1.7	16.3 ± 8.8	18.5 ± 9.0	7.8 ± 2.1

a) Mean ±S.D. of percent ratio against lefetamine 0.1 mg/kg/inj. as 100%

B. Continuous self-administration experiment (i.v., FR-1)

Unit dose (µg/kg/inj.)		Approximate average daily number of self-administrations		
		20	50	200
Monkey	Experienced (N=6)	35-100	20	15
	Naive (N=4)	50-80	--	20

test drug alone is available almost continuously for several weeks. The reason
for such a procedurally related difference in the demonstrability of the
reinforcing effects is not clear, but it seems to occur when (a) the
reinforcing effect of a test drug is relatively weak, (b) a test drug is
relatively long acting, or (c) the class of the reference drug is markedly
different from that of the test drug.

Assessment of Reinforcing Properties by Intragastric Self-Administration Experiments

Generally speaking, the intravenous route is more reinforcing than the
oral route, probably because of the sharper rise and higher peak value of the
blood level as well as the shorter duration of the CNS effects, which may make
it easier for the animal to discriminate the drug effects and lead to more
frequent responding on the lever. In animal experiments the intragastric route
is mostly used when a drug is water-insoluble. Since the absorption rate of
such drugs is usually lower than those in the intravenous route, relatively
large unit doses are used, which results in further prolongation of the
duration of the drug effects. For this reason the daily response rates tend to
be low in intragastric self-administration experiments. This is particularly
true with a class of drugs such as benzodiazepines. For example, the daily
response rates for diazepam in rhesus monkeys under intragastric continuous
self-administration were not high (see Table 3), but this should not be taken

as indicating a lack of reinforcing properties with the drug, because the result obtained in the progressive-ratio experiment in the rhesus monkeys shows definite reinforcing effect. The progressive-ratio procedure presently used in our laboratory first requires monkeys to press a lever 100 times per intravenous injection (FR-100), and 24 hours later the ratio is gradually increased at each intake so that it is doubled every four intakes; when the number of lever presses in any 24-hour period drops to less than half of that achieved for the preceding period or when no intake is observable for 48 hours, the animals are said to have extinguished the self-administration behavior and the number of the lever presses for the last intake attained is regarded as the final ratio (Yanagita, 1976). This procedure is intended to assess the intensity of animals' drug-seeking behavior as a measure of the psychological dependence potential of a drug, and the final ratios obtained with a test drug, reference drug, and saline or those obtained under physically dependent versus nondependent states are regarded to reflect the relative intensity of the drug-seeking behavior. The final ratios obtained in such experiments with diazepam were generally high as shown in Table 4, and the drug was found to have considerably high reinforcing properties depending on the procedure. This example suggests that even though the increment of the response rate in an intragastric experiment is slight, it may not be judged as negligible.

Importance of Observing the Self-Administered Daily Dose and CNS Manifestation

For evaluation of the psychological dependence potential of a drug and prediction of the ill effects resulting from its abuse (to be discussed later), observations of the daily dose self-administered by the animals and of the behavioral manifestation resulting from self-administration of the drug are very important (Deneau, Yanagita, & Seevers, 1969; Yanagita, 1977). For example, if the self-administered dose level of one drug is higher than another in terms of their minimum effective and toxic doses, it indicates the possibility that a larger daily dose of the former drug is likely to be sought and taken by humans under the condition that the drug is relatively freely available, and thus its psychological dependence potential is evaluated to be that much higher. Similarly, where the drug effects that are sought by the animals are stronger with one drug than another, the former's psychological dependence potential would be evaluated to be analogously higher. The continuous self-administration procedure allowing free access to a drug provides information such as the following in addition to a measure of the reinforcing effect: (a) the total ingestible dose during one day or any fixed period, (b) the property of the drug to produce overt signs of the CNS effects in animals at self-administered dose levels, (c) the long-term trends of intake of the drug, and (d) the drug-seeking behavior and withdrawal manifestation during the withdrawal period.

For observation of the overt signs of the CNS effects, the gross behavioral manifestations are usually scored using standardized observational protocols. Recently, intensive attempts have been made by several investigators to quantify behavioral toxicity in the course of testing for drug dependence potential (Brady & Griffiths, 1983).

Influence of Physical Dependence on the Psychological Dependence Potential

Although the importance of the psychological state in drug dependence has been stressed in the previous sections, the capacity of a drug to produce physical dependence is also important if its development enhances the drug-seeking behavior. With several opioids such as morphine or heroin, it is well known that the drug-seeking behavior in humans becomes compulsive when physical

TABLE 3

Continuous Intragastric Self-Administration of Diazepam in Rhesus Monkeys
(Adapted from Yanagita & Kato, 1983)

	0.5% CMC	Diazepam (mg/kg/inj.)				CMC	Diazepam		CMC
Monkey (experienced)	1 wk	0.25 4 wk	1.0 2 wk	0.25 2 wk	1.0 4 wk	3 days	1.0 4 wk	2.0 2 wk	1 wk
No. 433	0.1	4.5 2.1	4.9	5.1	8.7 3.6	3.3	2.3 2.1	-	3.1
No. 828	4.7	4.9 -	3.4	2.1	10.1 6.4	14.3	9.9 5.9	-	12.7
No. 993	4.3	1.4 -	1.2	-	1.8 0.6	1.7	1.0 -	0.1	0.4
No. 1062	3.3	5.9 -	3.1	-	2.1 3.2	1.7	5.4 2.3	2.5	2.1

Average daily number of self-administrations (per 1 or 2 wks)

TABLE 4

Final Ratios in Progressive-Ratio Experiment on Diazepam in Rhesus Monkeys
(Yanagita, unpublished data)

	Diazepam 1 mg/kg/inj., i.v.		Saline
Monkey	Saline- pretreated[a]	Diazepam- pretreated[a]	0.25 ml/kg/inj., i.v.
No. 966	3,200	1,600	240
No. 1025	950	670	<100
No. 1031	280	340	240
No. 1057	1,350	1,350	400
No. 1058	1,130	1,900	-

a) Pretreated by programmed intravenous administration of diazepam (1 mg/kg/injection) or saline (0.25 ml/kg/injection) every 2 hours for 4 weeks

dependence on these drugs has developed. In the definition of drug dependence, this phenomenon is included in the wording "in order to experience its psychic effects, and sometimes to avoid the discomfort of its absence" (WHO, 1969, p. 6). In predicting the psychological dependence potential of a drug, this factor has to be considered in case the drug has physical dependence potential. Enhancement of drug-seeking behavior under the physically dependent state is also observable in animals by the progressive-ratio procedure. An example of such an experiment on codeine and loperamide is shown in Table 5. Both drugs produced definite physical dependence in rhesus monkeys, but in the progressive-ratio experiment under physically dependent and nondependent states the enhancement of the drug-seeking behavior under the former was observed only with codeine (Yanagita, Miyasato, & Sato, 1980). Such enhancement is also observable with morphine but not with cocaine. Among CNS depressants, alcohol showed a slight enhancement (Table 6) and diazepam did not (Table 4).

TABLE 5

Progressive-Ratio Experiment on Codeine and Loperamide
(Adapted from Yanagita et al., 1980)

Monkey	Saline 0.25 ml/kg/inj.	Codeine 1.0mg/kg/inj., i.v.		Loperamide 0.06mg/kg/inj., i.v.		Saline 0.25 ml/kg/inj.
		Codeine-pretreated[a]	Saline-pretreated	Loperamide-pretreated[a]	Saline-pretreated	
No. 325	140	3,200	2,690	140	670	Died
No. 478	120	12,800	6,400	1,350	670	170
No. 769	170	10,760	4,530	0	570	340

a) Pretreated by programmed intravenous administration of the drug at the indicated unit doses every 20 minutes for 7 days

TABLE 6

Final Ratios in Progressive-Ratio Experiment on Alcohol in Rhesus Monkeys
(Adapted from Yanagita, 1976)

Monkey	Alcohol 0.8 g/kg/inj., i.v.	
	Saline-preceded[a]	Alcohol-preceded[a]
No. 171	3,200	3,200
No. 425	6,400	6,400
No. 466	1,600	6,400
No. 485	3,200	6,400

a) Progressive-ratio tests were preceded by programmed administration of saline for 4 weeks or self-administration of alcohol (0.8 g/kg/injection) at FR-100 for 2 weeks. In this period they ingested 6 to 10 doses of alcohol daily

PREDICTION OF ILL EFFECTS

From a practical viewpoint, when the abuse liability of a drug is predicted, it is necessary to consider the nature and extent of any ill effects which may arise as a consequence of its abuse. The reinforcing and discriminative stimulus properties of a drug are also important in this respect. In the context of international control of drugs under the 1971 Convention on Psychotropic Substances (United Nations, 1977), the following criteria are used in the scheduling of substances:

If a substance
1. has the capacity to produce similar abuse and similar ill effects as a substance in Schedule I, II, III, or IV, or
2. a) has the capacity to produce a state of dependence and central nervous system stimulation or depression resulting in hallucinations or disturbances in motor functions or thinking or behavior or perception or mood, and
   b) is being or is likely to be abused so as to constitute a public health and social problem warranting international control, the World Health Organization shall communicate to the [United Nations Narcotic] Commission an assessment of the substance, including the extent or likelihood of abuse, the degree of seriousness of the public health and social problem and the degree of usefulness of the substance in medical therapy, together with recommendations on control measures, if any, that would be appropriate in the light of its assessment. (p. 9)

As was true for abuse liability, the factors involved in producing such ill effects are not limited to the pharmacological and toxicological properties of a drug alone. Examples of ill effects attributable to other factors will include infection and embolism due to inappropriate handling of the preparation for injection as well as social problems such as smuggling and peddling. However, many ill effects are caused by the pharmacological and toxicological properties. These include (a) the CNS effects, particularly those on mental state and behavior, (b) the psychological dependence potential to produce compulsive drug-seeking behavior, (c) acute and chronic organ toxicity, (d) tolerance as a factor in causing acute toxic death, and (e) physical dependence potential resulting in mentally and physically hazardous withdrawal syndrome.

The general predictive methods here are the same as in the case of abuse liability, and comparative assessment on the above points should be made between the drug in question and some prototypic drugs which cause ill effects that are relatively well-known.

In this chapter the pharmacological factors involved in predicting the abuse liability of drugs were introduced and discussed with major emphasis on their psychological dependence potentials. The predictive methods described here deal for the most part with general methodology rather than actual method. Concerning the actual methods, some considerations and attempts are being made to systematize the assessment of the pharmacological factors by score/point systems and to predict the abuse liability and ill effects from these numerical values. However, at the present time, weighing the scores for each factor is in the trial and error stage because the relationships among the factors are not clear enough to validate the weighing. Progress in behavioral pharmacological research in both animals and humans on the problems of drug dependence will reveal those relationships and make it possible to properly weigh the factors and quantify them.

REFERENCES

Brady, J. V., & Griffiths, R. R. (1983). Testing drugs for abuse liability and behavioral toxicity: Progress report from the laboratories at the Johns Hopkins University School of Medicine. In L. S. Harris (Ed.), Problems of drug dependence, 1982 (National Institute on Drug Abuse Research Monograph 43, pp. 99-124). Washington, DC: U.S. Government Printing Office.

Deneau, G., Yanagita, T., & Seevers, M. H. (1969). Self-administration of psychoactive substances by the monkey: A measure of psychological dependence. Psychopharmacologia, 16, 30-48.

United Nations (1977). Convention on psychotropic substances, 1971. New York: United Nations.

WHO Expert Committee on Drug Dependence. (1969). World Health Organization technical report series (No. 407).

Yanagita, T. (1976). Some methodological problems in assessing dependence-producing properties of drugs in animals. Pharmacological Reviews, 27, 503-509.

Yanagita, T. (1977). Brief review on the use of self-administration techniques for predicting drug dependence potential. In T. Thompson & K. R. Unna (Eds.), Predicting dependence liability of stimulant and depressant drugs (pp. 231-242). Baltimore: University Park Press.

Yanagita, T., Ando, K., Kato, S., & Takada, K. (1983). Psychopharmacological studies on nicotine and tobacco smoking in rhesus monkeys. Psychopharmacology Bulletin, 19(3), 409-412.

Yanagita, T., Ando, K., Oinuma, N., & Ishida, K. (1974). Intravenous self-administration of nicotine and an attempt to produce smoking behavior in monkeys. Committee on Problems of Drug Dependence, 567-578.

Yanagita, T., & Kato, S., (1983). Dependence studies on zopiclone. In L. S. Harris (Ed.), Problems of drug dependence, 1982 (National Institute on Drug Abuse Research Monograph 43, pp. 164-170). Washington, DC: U.S. Government Printing Office.

Yanagita, T., Miyasato, K., & Sato, J. (1980). Dependence potential of loperamide studied in rhesus monkeys. In L. S. Harris (Ed.), Problems of drug dependence, 1979 (National Institute on Drug Abuse Research Monograph 27, pp. 106-113). Washington, DC: U.S. Government Printing Office.

CHAPTER 11

CONDITIONED REINFORCEMENT AS A MEASURE OF
THE REWARDING PROPERTIES OF DRUGS

W. Marvin Davis and Stanley G. Smith*

Department of Pharmacology
School of Pharmacy
The University of Mississippi
University, Mississippi 38677

Abstract

A review is presented of the development and application of a conditioned reinforcement measure for evaluating drug-based primary reinforcement. This procedure has employed both contingent and noncontingent association of the initially neutral stimulus with repeated doses of the drug reinforcer. Evidence for primary reinforcement by doses of drug is later demonstrated by the behavior of a subject when the stimulus is presented contingent to lever-pressing responses. This method allowed testing of potential antagonist drugs for an ability to oppose or cancel the reinforcing action of agents such as dexamphetamine, morphine, and ethanol. Inhibitors of critical enzymes in catecholamine biosynthetic pathways (e.g., tyrosine hydroxylase or dopamine β-hydroxylase) were found to oppose the reinforcing action of such classical drugs of abuse. The ability of conditioned reinforcement tests to avoid the factor of performance deficits induced by many potential antagonist drugs constitutes a major advantage over a more direct evaluation of drugs for possible interactions with primary reinforcing actions of abuse agents.

Introduction

At the beginning of the 1970s, we began investigations of the role that central nervous system (CNS) biogenic amines play in the production of drug-based reinforcement. Our initial efforts centered on the development of experimental protocols to ensure the validity and reliability of planned research on opiate- and amphetamine-based reinforcement. We perceived that previous self-administration research had not ruled out completely the possibility that such drugs were only pseudo-reinforcers, functioning as performance facilitators. That is, previous studies had not controlled for the possibility that drug delivery might merely have increased the general baseline of motor behavior, thus mimicking reinforcement. Also, we soon became aware that pharmacological tools that we wished to employ for the study of CNS adrenergic functions could alter a data baseline via inhibition of motor function, independently of their effects in the central processes related to

*Present address: Choctaw Community Mental Health Center, Philadelphia, Mississippi

drug-based reinforcement. Again, this raised the possibility that data generated using such agents might reflect pharmacological side-effects. Therefore, it seemed imperative to find methods that could validly demonstrate drug-based reinforcement without performance artifacts and that would allow the manipulation of the CNS neurotransmitter systems by means of pharmacological tools without unwanted actions such as motor inhibition, motor disinhibition, or the introduction of nonreinforcement factors into the reinforcement measure.

The area of intracranial self-stimulation research seemed both to suffer parallel problems and to provide a means for circumventing such problems in valid measurement of reinforcement associated with nonclassical sources of reward (Liebman, 1983; Valenstein, 1964). Stein (1958) reported that electrical stimulation of the brain in rats had the capacity to impart secondary reinforcing properties to an originally neutral stimulus. This was accomplished by means of four daily pairing sessions with 100 presentations of a 1.0-second tone given concurrently with a 0.5-second train of electrical stimuli delivered to the brain. Three days following the pairings, a 1-hour test session was conducted in which the rats had access to two levers, and only one lever activated the same 1.0-second tone as in the pairings. This lever had been nonpreferred in a baseline session before the pairings. The no-tone lever only measured general motor activity. Test results showed that the lever-pressing on the tone-producing lever had increased significantly in subjects for whom the brain stimulations were subsequently proven (by giving an opportunity to lever-press for the brain stimulation) to have been positively reinforcing. Subjects whose electrodes were found to give a neutral response (i.e., lacking positive reinforcement) showed neither a change in lever preferences nor an increase in rate of lever-pressing subsequent to tone-stimulation pairings.

We saw Stein's experimental design to be applicable to our aims, substituting small intravenous (i.v.) drug doses for electrical brain stimulation. It provided a means of testing for reinforcement, allowing simultaneous recording of data to control for drug-produced changes in motor activity and thus avoiding performance interpretations. It permitted testing for the reinforcer's stimulus control in the acquisition of a newly learned response, further weakening the performance interpretation. It allowed testing for an interaction between the primary reinforcer and a pharmacological tool several days after the pairings. This would permit actions of the drug or tool to be dissipated and CNS functions to be restored to normal. Therefore, we employed these procedures in a conditioned reinforcement approach to studying intravenous doses of morphine and amphetamine for their reinforcing capacities.

Conditioned Reinforcement After Noncontingent Intravenous Doses of Morphine and Amphetamine

At the outset we established conditions under which drug-naive rats would show apparent evidence of primary reinforcement (i.e., would develop self-administration behavior for intravenous doses of either morphine sulfate or dexamphetamine sulfate solutions; Davis & Smith, 1972). Then, using the drug doses found effective in that situation, we demonstrated conditioned reinforcement produced concurrently with acquisition of self-administration behavior for each of these agents by drug-naive rats (Smith & Davis, 1973a; Davis & Smith, 1974a). Subsequently, we tested for the establishment of conditioned reinforcement with a buzzer stimulus when pairing of the buzzer sound was contingent with programmed drug infusion (i.e., drug effects were noncontingent with behavior; Davis et al., 1972; Davis & Smith, 1974a). We will focus our attention herein on this latter paradigm.

An initial experiment aimed at validating the conditioned reinforcement approach was to demonstrate a magnitude of reinforcement or dose response relationship for intravenous doses of morphine employed to establish a conditioned reinforcer (Crowder, Smith, Davis, Noel, & Coussens, 1972). The subjects were allowed a baseline period for determining the operant level of bar-pressing. Here there were no drug contingencies associated with such behavior. However, a 0.2-second neutral buzzer stimulus occurred with each response on the lever, concurrently with an injection of saline solution. At the end of the operant-level period, the lever was removed from the chamber. After one hour a second session began with 100 noncontingent morphine injections given concurrently with buzzer presentations. Morphine doses (as the sulfate) were given to three groups at either 0.0032, 0.032, or 0.32 mg/kg in the same volume and duration as for the prior saline doses. These small morphine doses, shown to generate high responding for self-administration (Weeks & Collins, 1971), were delivered randomly without regard to behavior. The sessions lasted about 200 minutes.

After the pairing sessions the lever had remained out of the chambers until the following day, when it was restored at the same time of day as the initial operant level session. Conditions of that first session were repeated: A lever-response produced the buzzer stimulus plus a saline infusion. This comprised a test for establishment of secondary reinforcing potency for the buzzer stimulus. Immediately after this test a further session began in which lever-pressing led to delivery of the buzzer stimulus plus the same dose of morphine as had been given on the previous day. This period was used to detect any subjects that did not respond for morphine solution as a primary reinforcer. Rats not sensitive to morphine as a primary reinforcer could not be expected to develop conditioned reinforcement. The data for six subjects were eliminated on this basis.

Results of the test for conditioned reinforcement are shown in Figure 1. The baseline operant responses of the groups did not differ, but after the buzzer-morphine pairings their responses were elevated in a dose-related manner (ANOVA, $p < 0.01$); there was a significant linear trend with log dose ($p < 0.01$). These results confirmed that repeated small intravenous doses of morphine sulfate paired with a buzzer stimulus had imparted reinforcing properties to the buzzer stimulus and that the magnitude of this reinforcement increased linearly with the unit dose of morphine injected. Absence of withdrawal signs indicated that the amount of morphine administered was insufficient to induce acute physical dependence (Coussens, Crowder, & Smith, 1973).

Another validating study (Davis & Smith, 1974a) used a two-lever condition like the procedure employed by Stein (1958). This was conducted with dexamphetamine sulfate as the reinforcer at a dose of 0.015 mg/kg; 100 pairing trials were given on Day 2, and the test for conditioned reinforcement was on Day 6 rather than Day 3. Half of the subjects received the buzzer stimulus plus saline infusions for responses on the left lever, and the other half received the same combination for responses on the right lever. Responding on the inactive lever had no scheduled consequence, but it was recorded as a measure of nonspecific activity. A much higher number of responses occurred on the reinforced lever than on the other (mean 147.2 vs. 17.2), attesting to the specificity of this behavior as measuring conditioned reinforcement. This demonstration eliminated conditioned activation or disinhibition of motor performance as explanations of the conditioned effect. More extensive data for dexamphetamine were reported later (Davis, Smith, & Khalsa, 1975) along with similar results for morphine in the two-lever design (see Figure 2).

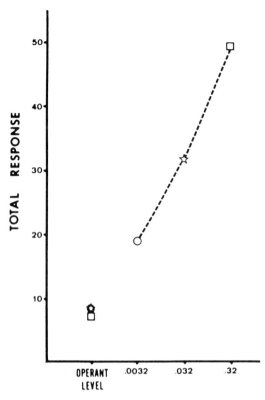

Figure 1: Mean number of lever presses during a 6-hour test for conditioned reinforcement with a buzzer-saline infusion contingency 24 hours after 100 buzzer-morphine infusion pairings. Morphine sulfate in the indicated doses was rapidly injected intravenously in a small volume coincident with a 0.5-second buzzer presentation. The lever was out of the chamber during pairings. (n = 7 or 8/group.) Reprinted with permission from Crowder, Smith, Davis, Noel, and Coussens, 1972. Copyright 1972 by Denison University.

TREATMENTS

Another study confirmed that the level of responding in a test for conditioned reinforcement did not diminish if the test was delayed further-- even to 8 or 16 days after the pairing trials--provided that no extinction procedure intervened (Davis & Smith, 1974a). This finding is in accord with what is known for traditional, nondrug reinforcers used as the basis for secondary reinforcement.

Conditioned Reinforcement Method in Studies
for Antagonism of Morphine or Amphetamine Actions

The successful application of a conditioned reinforcement method to measure a dose-related variation in magnitude of reinforcement from intravenous morphine, and the several other initial validation studies, encouraged our further use of this approach to test whether depletion of CNS catecholamines (CA) might prevent the primary reinforcing action of morphine and dexamphetamine. Despite indications that this might be the case based on our self-administration studies (Davis & Smith, 1972), we felt the need to verify such data by means of the conditioned reinforcement paradigm to preclude motor inhibition or performance factors having possibly contaminated the former data. The general procedure of the initial studies described above was adopted following a 4-step, 7-day format; Day 1 consisted of a 6-hour operant baseline

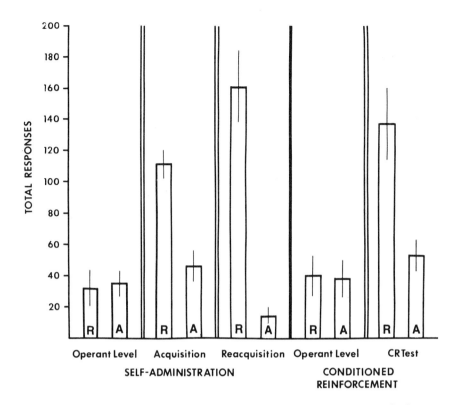

Figure 2: Two-lever validation data for self-administration (SA) and
conditioned reinforcement (CR) paradigms with rats receiving morphine
sulfate in intravenous doses of 0.032 mg/kg during SA or in 100
noncontingent pairings with buzzer 1 day before the CR test. **R**
indicates responses on the reinforced lever for the SA test or the
lever producing the buzzer in the CR test; **A** indicates responses on
the lever having no contingencies associated, providing only an index
of general activity. Adapted with permission from Davis, Smith, and
Khalsa, 1975.

session in which lever presses caused saline infusions. On Day 2 the response
levers were removed from the chambers, and the rats received three
intraperitoneal injections of either alpha-methyl-para-tyrosine (AMT) or saline
solution at 8, 4, and 0 hours before starting an experimental session
consisting of 100 noncontingent pairings of the buzzer stimulus and a rapid
intravenous injection of morphine sulfate solution (0.032 mg/kg) on a variable-
frequency programmed schedule. On Day 6 the rats were again placed in the
chamber for the test of conditioned reinforcement under the buzzer-saline
contingency as on Day 1. The interval between second and third stages (Day 2 to
Day 6) of the experiment permitted recovery from the depression of brain CA
levels produced by AMT (Davis & Smith, 1974b). On Day 7 the rats were given a
test for possible failure to show primary reinforcement with the dose of
morphine used. Only one of 20 rats failed this test and was consequently
excluded.

The results of the Day 6 test showed that the group of rats (n = 9) receiving AMT before the morphine-buzzer pairings did not respond above their initial operant level on the saline-buzzer condition. However, subjects receiving only saline pretreatment prior to morphine-buzzer pairings showed lever-pressing nearly three times their baseline level, a highly significant difference (p < 0.001) both from their own baseline and from the AMT group. These data indicate that AMT blocked the primary reinforcing action of morphine and thus prevented the establishment of conditioned reinforcement associated with the buzzer stimulus, which was clearly present for the saline pretreated rats. As the test for reinforcement was 4 days after the dosing with AMT, it is not reasonable to suppose that the failure to show reinforcement was caused by an impairment of performance. Thus, these data added strong confirmation to the self-administration data, supporting the conclusion that AMT did indeed block the rewarding effects associated with small intravenous doses of morphine (Davis & Smith, 1973a).

Parallel studies performed with dexamphetamine sulfate and AMT (Davis & Smith, 1973b), as with morphine, gave results also parallel to those for morphine. Not only the data for self-administration but also those for the conditioned reinforcement procedure showed a blocking of dexamphetamine-associated primary reinforcement.

Further application of the conditioned reinforcement paradigm was directed to the possible discrimination between noradrenergic and dopaminergic components in the effects of AMT on reward from both morphine and dexamphetamine. Both sodium diethyldithiocarbamate (DDC) and U-14,624 (inhibitors of dopamine β-hydroxylase, which is the enzyme that controls the biosynthetic step between dopamine and norepinephrine) were employed for this purpose (see Figure 3). On the basis of studies with DDC and U-14,624 analogous to those with AMT, it appeared that production of a noradrenergic deficit in this manner could prevent the rewarding action of either morphine or dexamphetamine (Davis et al., 1975).

A particular advantage of the conditioned reinforcement test may be seen in the results of an interaction study of morphine and the dopamine-receptor blocking agent haloperidol (Smith & Davis, 1973b). In this case pretreatment with two large doses (5 and 10 mg/kg) of haloperidol prevented reacquisition of morphine self-administration behavior. However, the same and even higher doses of haloperidol failed to impair the responding in the conditioned reinforcement test of rats that had received haloperidol before the morphine-buzzer pairings. Thus, it was concluded that the former results had reflected a motor inhibitory action of haloperidol rather than a blocking of morphine's rewarding action. This is particularly noteworthy in light of the fact that a lower haloperidol dose (0.5 mg/kg) in both paradigms showed evidence for enhancement of the reward potency of morphine.

In contrast to morphine, dexamphetamine-associated reinforcement was effectively blocked in both experimental designs by haloperidol (Davis & Smith, 1975). Moreover dopamine-receptor antagonism by means of haloperidol also appeared to explain the antagonism of reinforcement associated with two dopaminergic agonists, apomorphine and piribedil (ET-495), both in self-administration and conditioned reinforcement tests (Davis & Smith, 1977). Depletion of brain norepinephrine via U-14,624 treatment, however, was ineffective in altering the rewarding potency of apomorphine (see Figure 4). Similarly, a noradrenergic agent, clonidine, which supported both self-administration and conditioned reinforcement, could be blocked from exerting its primary reinforcing action by the noradrenergic receptor blocker

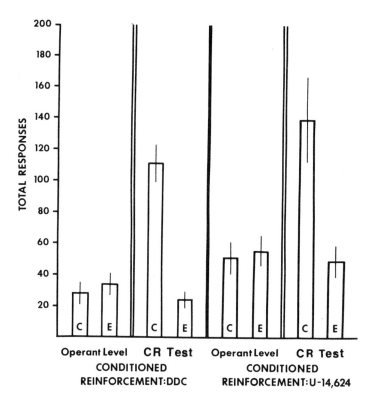

Figure 3: Effects of two dopamine β-hydroxylase inhibitors (DDC and U-14,624) on establishment of a conditioned reinforcer in rats based on intravenous doses (0.032 mg/kg) of morphine sulfate paired 100 times with a neutral buzzer stimulus. Groups C received the drug vehicle treatment, while Groups E received one of the inhibitors before the pairings session. The CR test was 4 days after the pairings. Data are means (±SEM) for groups of 8 subjects. Adapted with permission from Davis, Smith, and Khalsa, 1975.

phenoxybenzamine. A lack of cross-effectiveness both of phenoxybenzamine versus apomorphine and piribedil, and of haloperidol versus clonidine, was demonstrated solely on the basis of the conditioned reinforcement procedure. These results constituted a pharmacological validation for the earlier studies of this paper (Davis & Smith, 1977).

Conditioned Reinforcement Method in Research on Intragastric Ethanol

Ethanol is a considerably weaker reinforcer than is morphine or dexamphetamine even if they are compared by intravenous injection (Smith & Davis, 1974; Smith, Werner, & Davis, 1975a). Moreover, to model its human use/misuse, the oral rather than intravenous route of administration is much to be preferred (see also Amit, Smith, & Sutherland, this volume). In order to

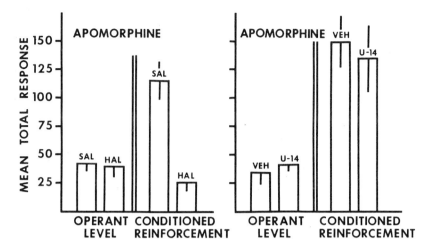

Figure 4: Conditioned reinforcement in rats based on intravenous doses of apomorphine (0.06 mg/kg) paired with a neutral buzzer stimulus in a 100-trial session. Group indicated HAL received 5 mg/kg of haloperidol before beginning the pairings session, while group marked U-14 received U-14,624 before pairings. Reprinted with permission from Davis and Smith, 1977. Copyright 1977 by Pergamon Press Inc.

avoid problems associated with voluntary oral intake of ethanol solutions by rats while maintaining the intragastric mode of absorption, we developed an intragastric (i.g.) cannulation technique that proved applicable to self-administration experiments (Smith, Werner, & Davis, 1975b). The delay imposed by the intragastric route caused a different dose-response relationship for self-administration than resulted if the same doses were made available intravenously (Smith, Werner, & Davis, 1976). Despite these facts the buzzer stimulus that overlaid self-administered 100 mg/kg intragastric doses of ethanol was found to act as a conditioned reinforcer, increasing responding during extinction on saline contingency trials (Smith, Werner, & Davis, 1977; see Figure 5). Furthermore, the response-noncontingent pairing of a buzzer stimulus with experimenter-delivered doses of ethanol (25, 50, or 100 mg/kg, i.g.) 50 times per day for 4 days resulted in a dose-related gradation of responding in a subsequent 10-hour test of conditioned reinforcement on buzzer-saline contingency (see Figure 6).

Experiments regarding the role of brain catecholaminergic systems in the rewarding action of ethanol were conducted in analogous fashion to those described above for morphine and dexamphetamine. The differences were the use of the intragastric route and a longer (10-hour) session for acquisition of self-administration behavior and in testing for conditioned reinforcement. First studied were AMT and U-14,624, which blocked ethanol self-administration (Davis, Smith, & Werner, 1978). This was followed by a similar study of FLA-57, another inhibitor of dopamine β-hydroxylase, which was fully effective against both reacquisition of self-administration behavior and responding in the test for conditioned reinforcement (Davis, Werner, & Smith, 1979).

Figure 5: Demonstration of effects on extinction-responding of a conditioned reinforcer established by intragastric doses of 25 or 100 mg/kg of ethanol given contiguously with a buzzer stimulus during five daily 10-hour self-administration sessions. Data are means (± SEM) of lever responses under extinction on Day 6. Buzzer and saline injection were contingent upon lever pressing in one-half of each dose group, while the other half received saline injection but no buzzer. Reprinted with permission from Smith, Werner, and Davis, 1977. Copyright 1977 by Springer-Verlag.

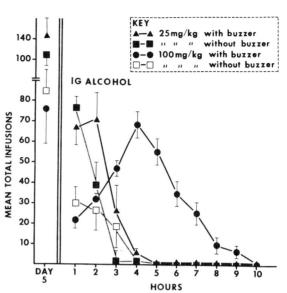

Discussion

Research on conditioned reinforcement and opiates prior to or at the time of our initial studies (Schuster, & Woods, 1968; Stolerman & Kumar, 1972; Wikler, Pescor, Miller, & Norrell, 1972) employed physically dependent organisms that required a lengthy dependence induction phase. Thus, our data first demonstrated conditioned reinforcement in nondependent subjects. Prior researchers also had required an operant-response-contingent relationship between the neutral stimulus (to become the conditioned reinforcer) and the primary reinforcer, morphine. We introduced the classically conditioned relationship. A reinforcement interpretation requires evidence of learning. The conditioned reinforcer must be validly demonstrated to control the dependent variable--in this case the lever-response or drinking rate--as a learned phenomenon. Since the putative conditioned reinforcers in the early studies cited were tested during opiate abstinence, increased responding could have been caused by disinhibitory factors (such as increased motor or drinking activity) related to withdrawal stress or facilitation of locomotor activity or drinking patterns introducing performance artifacts. Therefore, at the time of our studies, no unconfounded data were available which clearly showed that truly learned, secondary reinforcement phenomena were demonstrable in drug-reward research.

Thus, our first efforts were to demonstrate opiate-based primary reinforcement and conditioned reinforcement in nondependent organisms in such ways as to avoid both dependency and performance factors probably contaminating previous data. Next, we undertook to develop valid measures for the study of drug-based conditioned reinforcement, valid being defined as methods uncontaminated by performance variables. This was accomplished by our Pavlovian pairing method which incorporated a new learned instrumental response as its basic measure. Furthermore, we examined the reliability of our results in terms

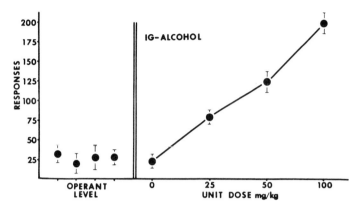

Figure 6: Dose-relationship in a test for conditioned reinforcement with groups that received 0, 25, 50, or 100 mg/kg intragastric doses of ethanol paired with a buzzer stimulus. Pairings were 50 per day for 4 days with the lever removed from the apparatus. The conditioned reinforcement test was a 10-hour session with levers restored and a buzzer-saline contingency like the operant baseline period. Reprinted with permission from Smith, Werner, and Davis, 1977. Copyright 1977 by Springer-Verlag.

of ability to replicate our data. This was accomplished not only by direct replications of our original results but also by means of cross-reliability studies--by showing magnitude of reinforcement effects, by delayed testing for acquisition of conditioned reinforcer, and by systematic replication showing conditioned reinforcers associated with orthogonal primary reinforcers (i.e., other drugs such as amphetamine and apomorphine and later ethanol).

Beyond these methodological considerations there is a considerable significance of drug-based conditioned reinforcement to the clinical bases of drug abuse syndromes. We have described animal experiments directed to the analysis of roles played by conditioned reinforcers in maintenance and/or relapse to drug-seeking behavior (Davis & Smith, 1976). Not only the latter research area but also the utilitarian applications of conditioned reinforcement as a measure of reward from abused drugs merit further attention and exploitation by researchers on drug abuse.

Acknowledgments

This research was supported by research grants MH 13570, MH 11295, and DA 00018 from the National Institute of Mental Health/National Institute on Drug Abuse and by the Research Institute of Pharmaceutical Sciences of the University of Mississippi.

References

Coussens, W. R., Crowder, W. F., & Smith, S. G. (1973). Acute physical dependence upon morphine in rats. Behavioral Biology, **8**, 533-543.

Crowder, W. F., Smith, S. G., Davis, W. M., Noel, J. T., & Coussens, W. R. (1972). Effect of morphine dose size on the conditioned reinforcing potency of stimuli paired with morphine. Psychological Record, **22**, 441-448.

Davis, W. M., & Smith, S. G. (1972). Alpha-methyltyrosine to prevent self-administration of morphine and amphetamine. Current Therapeutic Research, **14**, 814-819.

Davis, W. M., & Smith, S. G. (1973a). Blocking of morphine based reinforcement by alpha-methyltyrosine. Life Sciences, **12**, 185-191.

Davis, W. M., & Smith, S. G. (1973b). Blocking effect of alpha-methyltyrosine on amphetamine based reinforcement. Journal of Pharmacy and Pharmacology, **25**, 174-177.

Davis, W. M., & Smith, S. G. (1974a). Behavioral control exerted by an amphetamine based conditioned reinforcer. In J. M. Singh & H. Lal (Eds.), Drug addiction Volume 3: Neurobiology and influences on behaviors (pp. 209-219). New York: Stratton Intercontinental Medical Book Corp.

Davis, W. M., & Smith, S. G. (1974b). Noradrenergic basis for reinforcement associated with morphine action in nondependent rats. In J. M. Singh & H. Lal (Eds.), Drug addiction Volume 3: Neurobiology and influences on behavior (pp. 155-168). New York: Stratton Intercontinental Medical Book Corp.

Davis, W. M., & Smith, S. G. (1975). Effect of haloperidol on (+)-amphetamine self-administration. Journal of Pharmacy and Pharmacology, **27**, 540-542.

Davis, W. M., & Smith, S. G. (1976). Role of conditioned reinforcers in the initiation, maintenance and extinction of drug-seeking behavior. Pavlovian Journal of Biological Science, **11**, 222-236.

Davis, W. M., & Smith, S. G. (1977). Catecholaminergic mechanisms of reinforcement: Direct assessment by drug self-administration. Life Sciences, **20**, 483-492.

Davis, W. M., Smith, S. G., & Crowder, W. F. (1972). Morphine-based conditioned reinforcement. Abstracts of Volunteer Papers, 5th International Congress on Pharmacology, p. 52.

Davis, W. M., Smith, S. G., & Khalsa, J. H. (1975). Noradrenergic role in the self-administration of morphine or amphetamine. Pharmacology Biochemistry & Behavior, **3**, 477-484.

Davis, W. M., Smith, S. G., & Werner, T. E. (1978). Noradrenergic role in the self-administration of ethanol. Pharmacology Biochemistry & Behavior, **9**, 369-374.

Davis, W. M., Werner, T. E., & Smith, S. G. (1979). Reinforcement with intragastric infusions of ethanol: Blocking effect on FLA 57. Pharmacology Biochemistry & Behavior, **11**, 545-548.

Kumar, R. (1972). Morphine dependence in rats: Secondary reinforcement from environmental stimuli. Psychopharmacologia, **25**, 332-338.

Liebman, J. M. (1983). Discriminating between reward and performance: A critical review of intracranial stimulation methodology. Neuroscience & Biobehavioral Reviews, **7**, 45-72.

Schuster, C. R., & Woods, J. H. (1968). The conditioned reinforcing effects of stimuli associated with morphine reinforcement. International Journal of the Addictions, **3**, 223-230.

Smith, S. G., & Davis, W. M. (1973a). Behavioral control by stimuli associated with acquisition of morphine self-administration. Behavioral Biology, **9**, 777-780.

Smith, S. G., & Davis, W. M. (1973b). Haloperidol effects on morphine self-administration: Testing for pharmacological modification of the primary reinforcement mechanism. Psychological Record, 23, 215-221.

Smith, S. G., & Davis, W. M. (1974). Intravenous alcohol self-administration in the rat. Pharmacological Research Communications, 6, 397-402.

Smith, S. G., Werner, T. E., & Davis, W. M. (1975a). Intravenous drug administration in rats: Substitution of ethyl alcohol for morphine. Psychological Record, 25, 17-20.

Smith, S. G., Werner, T. E., & Davis, W. M. (1975b). Technique for intragastric delivery of solutions: Application for self-administration of morphine and alcohol by rats. Physiological Psychology, 3, 220-224.

Smith, S. G., Werner, T. E., & Davis, W. M. (1976). Comparison between intravenous and intragastric alcohol self-administration. Physiological Psychology, 4, 91-93.

Smith, S. G., Werner, T. E., & Davis, W. M. (1977). Alcohol-associated conditioned reinforcement. Psychopharmacology, 53, 223-226.

Stein, L. (1958). Secondary reinforcement established with subcortical stimulation. Science, 127, 466-467.

Stolerman, I. P., & Kumar, R. (1972). Secondary reinforcement in opioid dependence. In J. M. Singh, L. H. Miller, & H. Lal (Eds.), Drug addiction, Volume 1: Experimental pharmacology (pp. 49-50). New York: Futura.

Valenstein, E. S. (1964). Problems of measurement and interpretation with reinforcing brain stimulation. Psychological Reviews, 71, 415-437.

Weeks, J. R., & Collins, R. J. (1971). Primary addiction to morphine in rats. Federation Proceedings, 30, 277.

Wikler, A., Pescor, F. T., Miller, D., & Norrell, H. (1971). Persistent potency of a secondary (conditioned) reinforcer following withdrawal of morphine from physically dependent rats. Psychopharmacologia, 20, 103-117.

CHAPTER 12

REINSTATEMENT OF DRUG-TAKING BEHAVIOR AS A METHOD OF ASSESSING INCENTIVE MOTIVATIONAL PROPERTIES OF DRUGS

Jane Stewart and Harriet de Wit

Center for Studies in Behavioral Neurobiology
Department of Psychology
Concordia University
Montreal, Quebec, Canada   H3G 1M8
and
Department of Psychiatry
University of Chicago
Chicago, Illinois   60637

ABSTRACT

Noncontingent "priming" presentations of positive reinforcers (or incentive events) can enhance and reinstate previously acquired instrumental responding for these reinforcers. We describe how this phenomenon may be used to study the motivational control of drug-taking behavior and the relapse to drug-taking in drug-free individuals.

INTRODUCTION

Positive reinforcers (or incentive events) produce motivational effects that outlast their presentation. These appetitive motivational consequences are reflected in post-incentive behaviors such as locomotion and exploration of the environment, repeated visits to a place associated with the presentation of the incentive, and activation of learned behaviors in the presence of stimuli previously associated with the incentive event (reinstatement). These post-incentive behaviors are thought to result from the activation, by the incentive event, of central appetitive motivational states involved in the initiation and maintenance of instrumental or voluntary behavior.

Both experimental evidence and casual observation suggest that the simple presentation of a reinforcing or incentive event is followed by a transient period of motivational change. Even the first presentation of an incentive event can alter the organism's responsiveness to its environment. In the animal laboratory it is common practice to give noncontingent priming presentations of a reinforcer at the beginning of a session to "create interest" in the environment and to facilitate responding. The enhancement of responding after noncontingent delivery of a reinforcer has been reported for a wide range of events, including food, electrical brain stimulation (EBS) and self-administered drugs.

In animals that have been trained to self-administer drugs such as heroin or cocaine and that are then exposed to a period of extinction, the presentation of noncontingent priming injections of the self-administered drug leads to reinstatement of responding (de Wit and Stewart, 1981, 1983). In our studies of reinstatement, rats implanted with intravenous catheters are trained to self-administer a drug intravenously and are then given test sessions consisting of a period of self-administration followed by extinction conditions. Following cessation of responding, priming injections of the training drug or of test drugs are delivered intravenously by the experimenter. The temporal pattern and the frequency of responding following these priming drug injections are monitored. A similar methodology is used to specify the neural site of action of drugs responsible for the priming effects (Stewart, 1982, 1984). In rats trained to self-administer heroin or cocaine intravenously, the priming effects of drugs applied via intracerebral cannulae to specific sites within the central nervous system can be assessed. The results of studies using this technique suggest that priming and reinforcing properties of self-administered drugs are mediated by common mechanisms and that it is possible to separate these actions from other central and peripheral effects. We have argued that these priming effects of self-administered drugs reflect their incentive motivational properties.

PRIMING EFFECTS OF REINFORCERS OTHER THAN DRUGS

The stimulating effects of appetizers were discussed by Pavlov (1919) who pointed to the familiar phenomenon that "a person who at first displays indifference to his customary meal, afterwards begins to eat with gusto if his taste has been stimulated by something piquant" (p. 108). Konorski (1967) demonstrated the priming effect by offering a small portion of food to hungry dogs in an environment where they had never previously received food. While the dogs were initially impassive and calm before the presentation of food, they afterwards displayed a strong "hunger reflex" characterized by motor restlessness and increased attention to gustatory and olfactory stimuli. Konorski demonstrated the specificity of this priming effect by training dogs to perform two different movements, one for food and one for water. When the dogs were subsequently tested while both hungry and thirsty, a small quantity of food led to the food movement whereas water delivery led to the water movement. He suggested that there was a similar priming effect in humans, that of the so-called "peanut phenomenon" in which "one nut will arouse a selective appetite for eating another one" (Konorski, 1967, p. 20). Despite the familiarity of this phenomenon as illustrated by such anecdotal examples, surprisingly few experimental studies have been undertaken to study it.

One laboratory example of such an effect is the local rate-enhancing effect of "free" food delivery in rats responding for food as the reinforcer (Deluty, 1976). Rats were trained to respond on a random interval schedule for food pellets, and then additional food pellets were delivered noncontingently at fixed or random times. Immediately after noncontingent delivery of food, there was an increase in response rate of 33% to 75% over baseline rates. One way to interpret these results is in terms of the priming or response-enhancing aftereffects of free food delivery.

Another example of the response-facilitatory effect of free food delivery is the reinitiation of responding that is seen when free food pellets are given during extinction (Eiserer, 1978; Reid, 1958; Skinner, 1938). In Eiserer's (1978) experiment, rats were trained to bar press for food under food deprivation conditions and were then given a period of free-feeding before being tested in the extinction phase of the experiment. The animals were allowed to extinguish their bar pressing in the satiated condition, and when a period of two minutes occurred with no responses, a free food pellet was delivered. Animals reinitiated responding within one minute after the priming food delivery with a probability of 0.44 while the baseline probability of a response was only 0.19. Eiserer also scored the occurrence, following a free food delivery, of subthreshold components of the bar-press response (e.g., rearing and orienting to the bar) in addition to counting successfully executed bar presses. Ninety percent of the priming food deliveries were followed by either a completed bar press or by a subthreshold component of the response, whereas the baseline occurrence of these responses was only 42%. It is noteworthy that the delivery of a food pellet retained its effectiveness in restoring responding even though the animals were tested while in a sated condition.

In another demonstration of the priming effect of "free" reinforcers during extinction, Panksepp and Trowill (1967) used intraorally-delivered chocolate milk as the reinforcer in rats that were either food deprived or not food-deprived. Rats were prepared with fistulas to their mouths and were then trained to bar press for chocolate milk delivered intraorally. They were subsequently put under extinction conditions until their responding had ceased and then tested with noncontingent delivery of the chocolate milk. Both the deprived and the nondeprived rats reinitiated responding following delivery of chocolate milk (83% and 71% respectively of the animals in each group responded).

While in each of these studies free reinforcement delivery resulted in an enhancement of responding, the basis of this priming effect is not clear. In both Eiserer's and Panksepp and Trowill's experiments, the animals had been trained on a continuous reinforcement schedule, in which a delivery of the reinforcer usually immediately precedes the next reinforced response. It has been argued (e.g., Reid, 1958) that under these circumstances each reinforcement delivery constitutes a discriminative stimulus that "sets the occasion" for the next response. However, the phrase "setting the occasion" does not specify how the response is elicited. An implicit assumption in this conception is that presentation of a certain stimulus directly elicits the appropriate motoric response (the one that has been reinforced). Such an explanation is, however, ruled out by the flexibility and variability seen in the topography of responses. The data are more consistent with the idea that a motivational state is elicited by stimuli that signal reinforcers. It has been argued that presentation of any reinforcer or of a stimulus that predicts a reinforcer has motivationally arousing properties (e.g., Bindra, 1969; Bolles, 1972; Killeen, 1975, 1982). The increase in the vigor of responding that is seen after noncontingent food delivery may reflect, therefore, a general phenomenon of motivational arousal that occurs after delivery of a reinforcer or of a stimulus previously associated with a reinforcer (Bindra & Campbell, 1967; Bindra & Palfai, 1967, Sheffield & Campbell, 1954).

One of the most striking and the most thoroughly studied examples of the priming phenomenon occurs with electrical brain stimulation (EBS). Operant responding (e.g., bar pressing and runway running) for EBS is greatly facilitated by priming brain stimulation pulses delivered shortly before the opportunity to respond (Gallistel, 1973). Both magnitude of the response facilitation and the rate of decay of the effect are directly related to the intensity of the priming stimulation. The brain stimulation priming effect is so powerful that some theorists (e.g., Deutsch, 1960) have postulated that the initiation of self-stimulation behavior actually depends on the direct electrophysiological activation of a "drive" pathway by the priming (or immediately preceding) train of stimulation. A considerable amount of research has been undertaken concerning the question of whether the drive-inducing and reinforcing effects of brain stimulation are mediated by one or more neurophysiological systems. Recent data would suggest that these apparently separate phenomena are mediated, at least at some level, by the same set of neurons (see Hawkins, Roll, Puerto, & Yeomans, 1983). Furthermore, the findings that electrical stimulation of brain sites mediating reinforcing effects can enhance the positive incentive properties of species-typical objects of motivation (for a review, see Glickman & Schiff, 1967) suggests that motivational change is a primary property of reinforcer action. From a behavioral point of view, data on the response-enhancing effects of noncontingent trains of brain stimulation are consistent with the data from studies of conventional reinforcers and support the notion that noncontingent reinforcement delivery specifically enhances the tendency to respond to stimuli associated with that reinforcer at least for a short period of time.

In another set of studies, reinstatement by priming presentations of ethologically significant stimuli has been demonstrated. In ducklings (Eiserer & Hoffman, 1973) the brief presentation of an imprinted stimulus (a potent reinforcer) enhanced responding that had been reinforced previously by the presentation of the imprinted stimulus. Responding following the presentation increased as the duration of the presentation was increased. Distress vocalizations which occurred after withdrawal of the stimulus also increased with longer stimulus presentations. These results point to the specific motivational aftereffects that are aroused by both the presentation and the withdrawal of the positive incentive event, the priming stimulus.

Using cockroaches trained to cross an illuminated runway to darkness, Eiserer and Ramsay (1981) found that a brief priming presentation of the reinforcer (darkness) enhanced runway performance. The effect decayed rapidly if a delay was introduced between presentation of the priming stimulus and the opportunity to respond. As in the experiments with ducklings, stimulus presentations of longer duration led to greater responding.

In Betta spendens (Siamese fighting fish) trained to swim in a "runway" to view a conspecific stimulus, pre-exposure to a view of the conspecific (priming) decreased swimming time to the goal; longer exposures to the priming stimulus led to a stronger response (Hogan & Bols, 1980). The specificity of the priming effect was demonstrated in a choice experiment in which fish were given a choice between a food goalbox and an aggressive display goalbox. Priming with the display stimulus increased the animals' choice of the display goalbox (at least when the display stimulus was visible at the choice-point). These results suggest that there is some specificity to the motivational state aroused by the priming stimulus but that the expression of the increased response tendency also depends on the contextual stimuli present in the animals' environment.

Another example of priming was reported by Shettleworth (1978) in hamsters. When presentations of sunflower seed or nest paper were made intermittently to animals that were living in cages already supplied with seeds and paper, the animals began rearing at the dispenser panel, gnawing and digging around the dispenser panel, as if seeking further material. Eiserer and Ramsay (1981) have noted that such priming effects obtained with ethologically significant stimuli have characteristics similar to those obtained with rewarding EBS. They are strong, easy to obtain, and are related to the magnitude of the priming event. They have suggested that these similarities may be due to the fact that these incentive events appear to generate fewer satiety effects than do incentives such as food and water (see, for example, van der Kooy & Hogan, 1980). We suggest that priming effects such as those obtained with self-administered drugs also have some of the same characteristics.

PRIMING EFFECTS WITH SELF-ADMINISTERED DRUGS

Informal procedures used in the drug self-administration laboratory suggest that noncontingent infusions of the self-administered drug, presented at a time when the animal's blood level of drug is relatively low, produce a strong facilitation of responding. Experimenters involved in the training of animals to self-administer drug routinely give "free" priming infusions at the beginning of sessions. Pickens and Harris (1968) reported that a single noncontingent priming infusion was sufficient to terminate a self-imposed period of abstinence in rats trained to self-administer amphetamine. A somewhat similar effect has been documented by Davis and Smith (1976) in rats and by Gerber and Stretch (1975) and Stretch and Gerber (1973) in monkeys. Davis and Smith found that presession injection of morphine restored morphine-reinforced bar pressing in rats after a period of extinction. In the Gerber and Stretch experiments, monkeys were trained to self-administer either cocaine or amphetamine. After self-administration training the monkeys were put on extinction conditions for several sessions until their rate of responding fell to low levels. Then test sessions were given in which the extinction conditions remained in effect, but prior to which the monkeys were given either intramuscular or intravenous injections of either the self-administered drug or another drug of the same or different class. Presession injections of the self-administered drug resulted in a powerful reinstatement of responding, producing patterns of responding within the session that were indistinguishable from the drug-reinforced sessions. There was also a strong facilitation of responding after pretreatment with another drug of the same class (i.e., cocaine pretreatment for monkeys trained to self-administer amphetamine, and amphetamine pretreatment for cocaine-trained animals) but only transient effects after pretreatment with drugs from another class (barbiturate or minor tranquilizer). One interpretation of these findings might be that the facilitatory effect of noncontingent drug injections on responding after extinction is an example of the discriminative stimulus control of responding by the drug. That is, the presession infusion of the self-administered drug re-established the stimulus conditions that were present when responding was reinforced in the self-administration sessions. The other drugs tested produced responding only to the extent that their stimulus properties are known to resemble the self-administered drug (Ando & Yanagita, 1978; Colpaert, Niemeegers, & Janssen, 1979).

The similarity between the stimulus properties of different drugs has been examined in drug discrimination experiments (Overton, 1971; Stewart, 1962; Thompson & Pickens, 1971) in which drugs are used as the discriminative stimulus for responding for a positive reinforcer or avoidance of an aversive stimulus. In these experiments animals are trained to make one response (usually a lever press) after a presession injection of a drug, and another response (on a second lever) after a saline injection. Then on test sessions, other drugs are substituted for the training drug, and the animals' tendency to respond on the drug- or saline-lever is taken to indicate the degree of similarity or dissimilarity of the test drug to the training drug. It is important to note here that while results from such drug discrimination experiments can provide useful information about the similarity and dissimilarity of the stimulus properties of a wide range of substances in experimental animals, these experiments do not tell us which actions of drugs form the basis of the discrimination. Do all or any discriminably similar stimulus properties lead to training-drug-related responding, or are some properties more important than others? It may be, for example, that the activation of common motivational states is the critical factor for the reinstatement of responding by drugs with apparently similar stimulus properties. Whether or not this is the case, what the Davis and Smith and the Gerber and Stretch experiments do show is that the presence of drug in the body enhances drug-related behavior in an animal returned to the environment where drug has in the past been available. It was the potential significance of this finding that led us to investigate the basis of the priming effect in the reinstatement of drug-taking in animals trained to self-administer stimulants and opiates intravenously (de Wit & Stewart, 1981, 1983; Stewart, 1982, 1984).

The idea that the ingestion of a formerly self-administered drug induces a strong motivational state or "craving" for the drug and that it retains the ability to do this over an indefinite period of abstinence from the drug is not new. Former cigarette smokers speak of the potential for relapse following the smoking of a single cigarette, and formerly uncontrolled drinkers of alcohol hold that one drink elicits an urge to have another. There is some experimental evidence from studies with human alcoholics that lends support to this idea (Hodgson, Rankin, & Stockwell, 1979). An interesting example of the priming effect in human opiate use comes from a study by Meyer and Mirin (1979) of patterns of heroin self-administration in hospitalized ex-heroin addicts. Ratings of craving for the drug were taken before and after heroin intake in subjects free to self-administer a fixed dose of heroin when they wanted it. Surprisingly, the subjects reported only a very modest decrease in craving from immediately before to after heroin infusion, and levels of craving during heroin self-administration never fell to levels as low as in drug-free periods. It seems likely that drug circulating in the blood acted as a priming stimulus maintaining interest in the drug and in drug-related stimuli.

REQUIREMENTS OF A METHODOLOGY FOR REINSTATEMENT
OF DRUG SELF-ADMINISTRATION BY PRIMING EVENTS

One requirement of a reinstatement methodology is that the effectiveness of the priming manipulation must be tested in animals experienced in drug-taking but which, at the time of test, are drug-free and are not engaging in drug-taking behavior. In order to be able to evaluate the effect of the priming event, however, the animal must be in a situation where it is free to engage in drug-taking or drug-seeking behavior. In short, the animal must be trained, drug-free and not currently responding but free to do so.

One situation in which these conditions might be obtained is in the test box at the beginning of periodic self-administration sessions. Animals returned to the test chamber from their home cages would be trained, drug-free and free to respond. The problem is that most of them do respond, some immediately, others with varying, unpredictable latencies. The effects of priming drug injections would be, therefore, difficult to estimate under these conditions.

Another circumstance in which the effects of priming injections have been observed is when animals are given 24-hour access to a drug. Under these conditions animals spontaneously cease responding for periods of time and priming injections have been reported to reinstate drug-taking (Pickens & Harris, 1968). While the method is attractive in that it seems to approximate quite realistically some human conditions for drug-taking, it is quite impractical from the standpoint of data collection; abstinence periods are unpredictable and maintaining animals in test chambers for long periods of time is difficult and expensive. Furthermore, though of considerable interest, little is known about the factors leading to these periods of spontaneous abstinence. If, for example, neurotransmitter pools were depleted, making a drug temporarily less effective, reinstatement might not occur.

Because of these considerations, the reinstatement paradigm that we have found most satisfactory for evaluating priming is one modified from those used in studies with food reinforcers (see Eiserer, 1978; Panksepp & Trowill, 1967). Animals are trained to self-administer drug intravenously and are then given periodic sessions in which drug self-administration is followed by extinction conditions. When responding has ceased for some standardized time period, the priming manipulations are tested. The added feature of this design is that extinction conditions are maintained throughout the test. The effectiveness of the priming manipulation is evaluated on a baseline of behavior maintained without additional drug intake. We have found with this method that it is possible to test animals repeatedly on both the reinitiation and maintenance of responding following the priming event. One comment made frequently in connection with this methodology is that perhaps the priming infusions act to reinstate behavior by "predicting the availability of drug." If this were the case, it would be expected that animals would learn quickly that priming infusions given during extinction do not lead to further drug availability and animals would cease to respond to them. The fact that we find persistence of responding after many sessions argues against such an interpretation.

Reinstatement of Intravenous Drug Self-Administration
by Intravenous Priming Injections;
Drug Self-Administration: Preparation and Training

Preliminary Handling

Adult male rats weighing 250 to 350 g at the beginning of the experiments are used in our studies. Prior to surgical implantation of intravenous catheters, animals are routinely trained to bar press for food in test chambers used only for that purpose. Animals are introduced to a 23-hour food deprivation schedule for 3 to 5 days and are then placed in the training box for an hour a day until they press regularly for food pellets on a continuous reinforcement schedule. Following this, the deprivation schedule is terminated immediately. This period of training for food reduces the period of training necessary for intravenous drug self-administration. Animals adapt to handling and to being placed in test chambers and tend after such training to react readily to bar mechanism. Following recovery from the food deprivation schedule, animals are subjected to surgery.

Surgical Procedures

Permanent, indwelling intravenous catheters are implanted into the left jugular vein under pentobarbital anesthesia (60 mg/kg). Animals are given, in addition, a 0.1 mg/kg injection of atropine sulphate to prevent saliva accumulation during surgery. Following surgery, animals are given a dose of 60,000 IU Penicillin G.

The catheters are constructed from a 110 mm piece of silastic tubing (0.064 cm inner diameter, 0.119 cm outer diameter). At approximately 33 mm and 37 mm from the tapered end of the tubing, two rings of silastic glue are formed around the outer surface to cause slight swellings in the diameter of the tube. The jugular vein is exposed and the tapered end inserted in the vein just past the point of the first ring. The vein is tied with thread between the rings; the upper end of the vein is also secured to the catheter between the rings. The catheter is then passed subcutaneously to the top of the head where it exits into a connector made from 22-gauge stainless steel tubing that is then mounted on the skull with dental cement. A stainless-steel screw is also mounted in the dental cement, upside-down, with the threaded end exposed. A cap made from a piece of silastic tubing is placed over the open end of the connector when the animal is not in the test chamber. Catheters are flushed daily with heparinized (5 IU/ml) physiological saline for the first week after catheterization; this protects against the formation of embolisms in the vein. If catheter failure occurs (either leakage or blockage), animals are subjected to surgery and catheters are placed in the right jugular vein. During the week following surgery, animals are checked carefully for infections, for normal food and water intake and for urination.

Apparatus

Standard operant chambers are used for self-administration. The boxes are fitted with two bars only one of which is activated to deliver drug. The bars are mounted 9.0 cm from the floor to prevent accidental activation by the animal. A swivel (Brown, Amit, & Weeks, 1976) and the infusion tubing are suspended from the box. The infusion tubing leading from the rat's head to the swivel is enclosed in a coil of stainless steel wire. One end of this wire is attached by a nut to the screw embedded in the cement on the animal's head; the other end is attached to the swivel causing the swivel to move as the animal turns. Further tubing leads from the swivel to an infusion pump outside the chamber. Each depression of the bar starts a timer that activates the infusion pump for the number of seconds needed to deliver the appropriate amount of drug solution. Using a fixed concentration of drug solution, the duration of the infusion is determined by the animal's weight and varies from approximately 9 to 13 seconds. Bar presses during infusions are counted but do not reset the pump delivery mechanism. All presses on both the activated and the "dummy" bar are recorded in time.

Training

During self-administration training animals are connected to the infusion tubing in the test chamber for 2 to 3 hours daily during which the training drug, either cocaine HCl (1.0 mg/kg/infusion) or diacetylmorphine HCl (heroin, 100 μg/kg/infusion), is available for each press on the activated bar. Solutions are made up in physiological saline with 5 IU/ml heparin added. During training priming injections of the drug are deliberately avoided. Occasionally, on the first day of training, a food pellet is placed on the activated bar to elicit interest in the bar. Most importantly, the number of infusions taken by the animals in the early training sessions is closely monitored to avoid overdosing. Animals so learn to space their responses and develop regular patterns of intake.

In order to reduce infection and illness, the entire infusion system is flushed and cleaned regularly. Before being placed in the chambers, the animal's catheter is checked for blockage or leakage by injecting a small amount of heparinized physiological saline directly into the head-mount opening.

Extinction and Test Sessions

Test sessions are begun when animals reliably initiate responding at the beginning of sessions and respond regularly throughout. Each test session consists of a varying period of 1 to 2 hours of self-administration followed by extinction conditions for the remainder of the session. Extinction conditions are introduced by substituting a syringe containing heparinized physiological saline for the one containing drug. After a standardized period of time has passed without responding, usually 30 minutes, priming injection trials are initiated. Frequently, on the first day that extinction conditions are introduced, response rates are high initially and responding continues for a long period of time; priming tests are started, then, on subsequent sessions.

Intravenous priming infusions are delivered by the experimenter from just above the swivel, with minimal disturbance to the animal. Because, however, the experimenter does enter the area, preliminary saline priming infusions are given prior to drug infusions. Thirty minutes later a test drug infusion is delivered. The drug infusions are followed by a saline solution that flushes the drug solution throughout the infusion system. Behavior is monitored for 3 hours following the infusion.

REINSTATEMENT BY PRIMING INFUSIONS OF THE TRAINING DRUG

The effectiveness of priming by infusions of different doses of the training drug can be tested using the method described above. We have found the latency to respond, the peak period of responding and the duration of responding are all affected by the infusion doses. In general, higher doses lead to longer latencies to responding, longer durations of responding and sometimes to delayed peak rates. Figure 1 shows the results obtained using this method when different doses of the training drug are used as the priming event in cocaine- and heroin-trained animals.

REINSTATEMENT BY PRIMING INFUSIONS OF DRUGS OTHER THAN THE TRAINING DRUG

The effectiveness of priming infusions of drugs other than the training drug in reinstating drug-taking behavior can also be evaluated using this method. One can determine whether drugs with common pharmacological actions or drugs which act on common neurochemical pathways or with common stimulus properties (as determined in drug discrimination paradigms) can reinstate responding for the training drug. This method may indicate the relation between discriminable stimulus properties of drugs and their incentive properties. If priming infusions act primarily by reactivating incentive motivational states, then other drugs that also arouse the motivational state would be effective in reinstating drug-taking or drug-seeking behavior. It is known, however, that stimuli that are repeatedly paired with the positive incentive properties of drugs acquire the ability through conditioning to activate a motivational state similar to that activated by the incentive event. Through such a mechanism, drugs without intrinsic incentive properties, but with discriminably similar stimulus properties to a self-administered drug, could bring about reinstatement of drug-taking behavior. By the same token it is possible that drugs having incentive effects similar to those of the training drug, but having additional actions that result in very different stimulus properties, might not bring about reinstatement of the original drug-taking behavior. Results of studies using this methodology can be found in papers by de Wit and Stewart (1981, 1983).

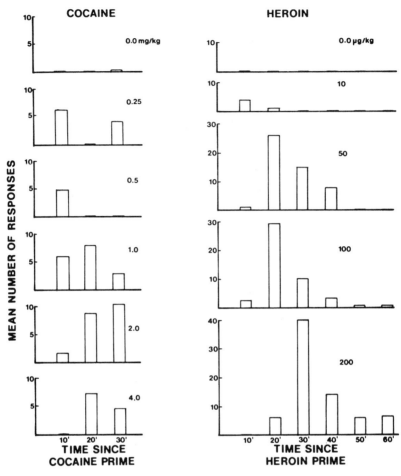

Figure 1: Mean number of responses made under extinction conditions following intravenous priming injections of various doses of cocaine to animals trained to self-administer 1 mg/kg cocaine (left panel) and of heroin to animals trained to self-administer 100 µg heroin (right panel). Adapted with permission from de Wit and Stewart, 1981, 1983.

REINSTATEMENT OF DRUG SELF-ADMINISTRATION BEHAVIOR
BY INTRACEREBRAL APPLICATION OF DRUGS

Two questions arise from the intravenous priming experiments: (1) Can we specify which actions of the drugs are responsible for the priming effects, and (2) can we delineate the specific neural systems of the brain involved? The idea that priming injections reinstate behavior by activating appetitive motivational states suggests that drugs belonging to different pharmacological classes such as stimulants and opiates might have their priming effects via their actions on the same systems of the brain that mediate their positive reinforcing effects. It has been shown that the positive reinforcing properties of the stimulants, cocaine and amphetamine, depend on the integrity of the neurons of the mesolimbic dopamine system where they act to release dopamine from terminals or to block the mechanisms of transmitter inactivation (Creese & Iversen, 1975; de Wit & Wise, 1977; Lyness, Friedle, & Moore, 1979; Roberts, Koob, Klonoff, & Fibiger, 1980; Yokel & Wise, 1976). Further support for the idea that this system is critically involved comes from a study showing that animals will self-administer amphetamine to the terminal regions of these neurons in the nucleus accumbens (Monaco, Hernandez, & Hoebel, 1981). Recent evidence suggests that the reinforcing effects of opiates derive from their actions on these same dopamine neurons. Rats will self-administer morphine directly into the ventral tegmental area of the brain, the cell body region of these mesolimbic dopamine neurons (Bozarth & Wise, 1981a) and will display an increased preference for a place associated with central injections to the area (Bozarth & Wise, 1981b; Phillips & LePiane, 1980). Thus the appetitive motivational or positive incentive properties of opiates, like those of stimulants, appear to be mediated via the mesolimbic dopamine pathway. Opiates appear to excite one subpopulation of these neurons by acting on opiate receptors in the cell body region (Gysling & Wang, 1982, 1983; Matthews & German, 1982). Bilateral application of morphine to the region elicits forward locomotion and exploration of the environment (Joyce & Iversen, 1979; Vezina & Stewart, 1983), behavior normally elicited by positive incentive stimuli. In light of these observations, we have approached the problem of specifying the neural substrate involved in the priming effect by examining the effects of central application of drugs in animals previously trained to self-administer either heroin or cocaine intravenously.

In these experiments animals are trained to self-administer heroin or cocaine intravenously as described above. At the time of surgery, however, animals are prepared with intracerebral guide cannulae directed at different areas of the brain. Cannulae can be implanted either unilaterally or bilaterally, and animals can be prepared with cannulae placed in two or more sites.

Intracerebral Application of Drug

Guide cannulae, cut to appropriate lengths from 22-gauge stainless steel tubing, are lowered stereotaxically to positions 1.00 mm above the target area. The cannulae are held in place by embedding them in dental cement. Drug is delivered to the brain site in crystalline form via 28-gauge stainless steel inner injector tubes that extend 1.00 mm beyond the tip of the guide cannulae. "Dummy" inner tubes with caps are kept in place between drug applications. Drug is tapped into the 28-gauge applicator by making 10 taps on a thin layer of powdered drug placed on a hard surface. We have found by weighing bits of tubing before and after tapping that the amount of drug inserted remains relatively constant (in the case of morphine, for example, at approximately 18 μg). The applicators are checked under a microscope before and after tapping. Used applicators are cleaned in an ultrasonic cleaner containing 70% ethanol.

Using this method, we have found that drugs appear to be released very slowly from the end of the tubing. After being in the brain for up to 3 hours, some drug remains in the tubing. Furthermore, there appears to be little spread of drug into the surrounding areas. This, of course, will depend on cannula sites. We have found that placements as little as 1.00 mm away from an effective target site can prove to be ineffective. Efforts are made to avoid passing the cannulae through cerebral ventricles by lowering them at an angle when necessary.

One disadvantage of using crystalline application of drug is that drug delivery cannot be controlled remotely. In these experiments, therefore, animals are picked up and handled from time to time while in test chambers. This is done to ensure that any changes in responding that occur following the experimental manipulation are not due to merely disturbing the animal. Control injections of saline, intravenously or intraperitoneally, are given appropriately, and removal and reinsertion of the dummy applicators is also done.

Tests For Reinstatement

Test sessions are conducted as described for intravenous priming injections. Following a period of at least 1 hour without responding under extinction conditions, the animal is picked up and the inner dummy tube of one (or two in the case of bilaterally placed cannulae) of the cannulae is removed and replaced by an empty applicator. Thirty minutes later the empty applicator is removed and replaced by one containing drug. Each brain site is tested one or more times on different test days. Behavior is usually monitored for up to 3 hours following the application of the drug.

Specificity of the drug action can be tested in these experiments by pretreatment with specific antagonists of the test drug or with antagonists of the transmitter suspected of being involved in the drug action. Intracerebral application of inactive optical isomers of effective drugs can also be tested when they are available. Some examples of the effects on responding of intracerebral application of morphine to animals trained to self-administer either heroin or cocaine are shown in Figure 2.

What should be noted about these data is that priming effects of morphine applied centrally were specific to sites in the ventral tegmental area; application of morphine to other regions of the brain known to contain opiate receptors did not reinstate behavior. Also, the priming effect of morphine was blocked by pretreatment with the specific opiate antagonist, naltrexone HCl. And, finally, because morphine applied to the cell body region of the mesolimbic dopamine neurons was effective in reinstating behavior in both heroin- and cocaine-trained animals, it would appear that activation of this pathway involved in the appetitive motivational properties of these drugs is critical for the reinstatement by priming effect (see also Stewart, 1984).

Significance of Reinstatement by Priming Events

The fact that priming injections of self-administered drugs can reinstate drug-taking and drug-seeking behavior has important implications for our understanding of the basis of relapse to and maintenance of drug-taking behaviors. We have seen that the presence of the drug in the body has the capacity to activate learned behaviors in the presence of stimuli previously associated with the drug. Furthermore, it appears from the intracerebral studies that the activation of appetitive motivational systems of the brain is responsible for reinstatement by the priming drugs. The question then becomes: Could neutral stimuli, through their association with a self-administered drug, i.e., through conditioning, come to elicit appetitive motivational states similar to those elicited by the drugs themselves and thereby act as priming events to reinitiate drug-taking.

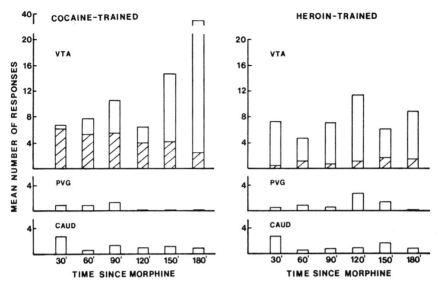

Figure 2: Mean number of responses made under extinction conditions following priming applications of morphine to sites in the ventral tegmental area (VTA), periventricular gray (PVG) and caudate nucleus (CAUD) in cocaine-trained animals (left panel) and heroin-trained animals (right panel). Cross-hatched portions of the bars in the upper part of the figure indicate responses made 30 minutes following pretreatment with naltrexone HCl, 2 mg/kg, intraperitoneally.

Evidence that stimuli associated with self-administered drugs do acquire effects that mimic appetitive actions of drugs comes from studies on conditioned reinforcing effects of drug-paired stimuli in animals (Beach, 1957; Bozarth & Wise, 1981b; Davis & Smith, 1976; Katz & Gormezano, 1978; Phillips & LePiane, 1980; Reicher & Holman, 1977; Rossi & Reid, 1976; Schuster & Woods, 1968; Sherman, Roberts, Roskam, & Holman, 1980; van de Kooy, Mucha, O'Shaughnessy, & Bucenieks, 1982; White, Sklar, & Amit, 1977). Recently we have shown in our laboratory (Vezina & Stewart, 1983, 1984) that the distinctive environmental stimuli paired with morphine applications to the ventral tegmental area elicit increased locomotor activity mimicking the unconditioned action of the drug. Here we see that stimulus events that are associated with the appetitive motivational actions of the drug appear to acquire the ability to activate neural states similar to those activated by the drugs themselves. We would argue that the arousal of these states by conditioned stimuli (as well as by drugs themselves) acts to reinstate and to maintain drug-taking behavior by increasing the salience of other drug-related stimuli (Stewart, de Wit & Eikelboom, 1984).

ACKNOWLEDGMENTS

This paper was prepared with the assistance of a grant to J. S. from the Medical Research Council of Canada (MA 6678).

REFERENCES

Ando, K., & Yanagita, T. (1978). The discriminative stimulus properties of intravenously administered cocaine in rhesus monkeys. In R. C. Colpaert & S. A. Rosecrans (Eds.), Stimulus properties of drugs: Ten years of progress (pp. 125-136). Amsterdam: Elsevier/North Holland.

Beach, H. D. (1975). Morphine addiction in rats. Canadian Journal of Psychology, 11, 104-112.

Bindra, D. (1969). The interrelated mechanisms of reinforcement and motivation and the nature of their influence on response. In W. J. Arnold & D. Levine (Eds.), Nebraska symposium on motivation (pp. 1-33). Lincoln: University of Nebraska Press.

Bindra, D., & Campbell, J. F. (1967). Motivational effects of rewarding intracranial stimulation. Nature, 215, 375-376.

Bindra, D., & Palfai, T. (1967). Nature of positive and negative incentive-motivational effects of general activity. Journal of Comparative and Physiological Psychology, 63, 288-297.

Bolles, R. C. (1972). Reinforcement, expectancy, and learning. Psychological Review, 79, 394-409.

Bozarth, M. A., & Wise, R. A. (1981a). Intracranial self-administration of morphine into the ventral tegmental area in rats. Life Sciences, 28, 551-555.

Bozarth, M. A., & Wise, R. A. (1981b). Localization of the reward-relevant opiate receptors. In L. S. Harris (Ed.), Problems of Drug Dependence 1981 (National Institute on Drug Abuse Research Monograph 41, pp. 158-164). Washington, DC: U.S. Government Printing Office.

Brown, Z. W., Amit, Z., & Weeks, J. R. (1976). Simple flow-thru swivel for infusions into unrestrained animals. Pharmacology Biochemistry & Behavior, 5, 363-365.

Colpaert, F. C., Niemegeers, C. J. E., & Janssen, P. A. J. (1979). Discriminative stimulus properties of cocaine: Neuropharmacological characteristics as derived from stimulus generalization experiments. Pharmacology Biochemistry & Behavior, 10, 535-546.

Creese, I., & Iversen, S. D. (1975). The pharmacological and anatomical substrates of the amphetamine response in the rat. Brain Research, 83, 419-436.

Davis, W. M., & Smith, S. G. (1976). Role of conditioned reinforcers in the initiation maintenance and extinction of drug-seeking behavior. Pavlovian Journal of Biological Sciences, 11, 222-236.

Deluty, M. Z. (1976). Excitatory and inhibitory effects of free reinforcers. Animal Learning and Behavior, 4, 436-440.

Deneau, G., Yanagita, T., & Seevers, M. H. (1969). Self-administration of psychoactive substances by the monkey. Psychopharmacologia, 16, 30-48.

Deutsch, J. A. (1960). The Structural Basis of Behavior. Chicago: University of Chicago Press.

de Wit, H., & Stewart, J. (1981). Reinstatement of cocaine-reinforced responding in the rat. Psychopharmacology, 75, 134-143.

de Wit, H., & Stewart, J. (1983). Drug reinstatement of heroin-reinforced responding in the rat. Psychopharmacology, 79, 29-31.

de Wit, H., & Wise, R. A. (1977). Blockade of cocaine reinforcement in rats with the dopamine receptor blocker pimozide, but not with the noradrenergic blockers phentolamine or phenoxybenzamine. Canadian Journal of Psychology, 31, 195-203.

Eiserer, L. A. (1978). Effects of food primes on the operant behavior of nondeprived rats. Animal Learning and Behavior, 6, 308-312.

Eiserer, L. A., & Hoffman, H. S. (1973). Priming of ducklings' responses by presenting an imprinted stimulus. Journal of Comparative and Physiological Psychology, 82, 345-359.

Eiserer, L. A., & Ramsay, D. S. (1981). Priming of darkness-rewarded runway responses in the American cockroach (periplaneta americana). Journal of General Psychology, 104, 213-221.

Gallistel, C. R. (1973). Self-stimulation: The neurophysiology of reward and motivation. In J. A. Deutsch (Ed.), The physiological basis of memory (pp. 175-267). New York: Academic Press.

Gerber, G. J., & Stretch, R. (1975). Drug-induced reinstatement of extinguished self-administration behavior in monkeys. Pharmacology Biochemistry & Behavior, 175, 1055-1061.

Glickman, S. E., & Schiff, B. B. (1967). A biological theory of reinforcement. Psychological Review, 74, 81-109.

Gysling, K., & Wang, R. (1982). Morphine facilitates the activity of dopaminergic neurons in the rat ventral tegmental area. Society for Neuroscience Abstracts, 8, 777.

Gysling, K., & Wang, R. (1983). Morphine-induces activation of A10 dopamine neurons in the rat. Brain Research, 277, 119-127.

Hawkins, R. D., Roll, P. L., Puerto, A., & Yeomans, J. S. (1983). Refractory periods of neurons mediating stimulation-elicited eating and brain stimulation reward: Interval scale measurement and tests of a model of neural integration. Behavioral Neuroscience, 97, 416-432.

Hodgson, R., Rankin, H., & Stockwell, T. (1979). Alcohol dependence and the priming effect. Behavioral Research and Therapy, 27, 379-387.

Hogan, J. A., & Bols, R. J. (1980). Priming of aggressive motivation in betta splendens. Animal Behaviour, 28, 135-142.

Joyce, E. M., & Iversen, S. D. (1979). The effect of morphine applied locally to mesencephalic dopamine cell bodies on spontaneous motor activity in the rat. Neuroscience Letters, 14, 207-212.

Katz, R. J., & Gormezano, G. (1978). A rapid and inexpensive technique for assessing the reinforcing effects of opiate drugs. Pharmacology Biochemistry & Behavior, 11, 231-233.

Killeen, P. R. (1975). On the temporal control of behavior. Psychological Review, 82, 89-115.

Killeen, P. R. (1982). Incentive theory. In D. J. Bernstein (Ed.), Nebraska symposium on motivation, 1981: Response structure and organization (pp. 169-216). Lincoln: University of Nebraska Press.

Konorski, J. (1967). Integrative activity of the brain. Chicago: University of Chicago Press.

Lyness, W. H., Friedle, N. M., & Moore, K. E. (1979). Destruction of dopaminergic nerve terminals in nucleus accumbens: Effect on d-amphetamine self-administration. Pharmacology Biochemistry & Behavior, 11, 553-556.

Lyness, W. H., Friedle, N. M., & Moore, K. E. (1980). Increased self-administration of d-amphetamine after destruction of 5-hydroxytryptamine neurons. Pharmacology Biochemistry & Behavior, 12, 937-941.

Matthews, R. T., & German, D. C. (1982). Electrophysiological evidence for morphine excitation of ventral tegmental area dopamine neurons. Society for Neuroscience Abstracts, 8, 777.

Meyer, R. E., & Mirin, S. M. (1979). The heroin stimulus. New York: Plenum Press.

Monaco, A. P., Hernandez, L., & Hoebel, B. G. (1981). Nucleus accumbens: Site of amphetamine self-injection; comparison with the lateral ventricle. In R. B. Chronister, & J. F. DeFrance (Eds.), The neurobiology of the nucleus accumbens (pp. 338-342). Brunswick, ME: Haer Institute.

Overton, D. A. (1971). Discriminative control of behavior by drug states. In T. Thompson, & R. Pickens (Eds.), Stimulus properties of drugs (pp. 87-100). New York: Appleton-Century-Crofts.

Panksepp, J., & Trowill, J. A. (1967). Intra-oral self-injection: The simulation of self-stimulation phenomena with conventional reward. Psychonomic Science, 9, 405-408.

Pavlov, I. P. (1957). Lectures on the work of the principal digestive glands. Lecture one (1919). In I. P. Pavlov, Experimental psychology and other essays. New York: Philosophical Library.

Phillips, A. G., & LePiane, F. G. (1980). Reinforcing effects of morphine microinjections into the ventral tegmental area. Pharmacology Biochemistry & Behavior, 12, 965-968.

Pickens, R., & Harris, W. C. (1968). Self-administration of d-amphetamine by rats. Psychopharmacology, 12, 158-163.

Reicher, M. A., & Holman, E. W. (1977). Location preference and flavor aversion reinforced by amphetamine in rats. Animal Learning and Behavior, 5, 343-346.

Reid, R. L. (1958). The role of the reinforcer as stimulus. British Journal of Psychology, 49, 202-209.

Roberts, D. C. S., Koob, G. F., Klonoff, P., & Fibiger, H. C. (1980). Extinction and recovery of cocaine self-administration following 6-hydroxydopamine lesions of the nucleus accumbens. Pharmacology Biochemistry & Behavior, 12, 781-787.

Rossi, N. A., & Reid, L. D. (1976). Affective states associated with morphine injections. Physiological Psychology, 4, 269-274.

Schuster, C. R., & Woods, J. H. (1968). The conditioned reinforcing effects of stimuli associated with morphine reinforcement. The International Journal of the Addictions, 3, 223-230.

Sheffield, F. D., & Campbell, B. A. (1954). The role of experience in the "spontaneous" activity of hungry rats. Journal of Comparative and Physiological Psychology, 47, 97-100.

Sherman, J. E., Pickman, C., Rice, A., Liebeskind, J. C., & Holman, E. W. (1980). Rewarding and aversive effects of morphine: Temporal and pharmacological properties. Pharmacology Biochemistry & Behavior, 13, 501-505.

Shettleworth, S. J. (1978). Reinforcement and the organization of behavior in golden hamsters: Sunflower seed and nest paper reinforcers. Animal Learning and Behavior, 6, 352-362.

Skinner, B. F. (1938). The behavior of organisms. New York: Appleton-Century-Crofts.

Stewart, J. (1962). Differential responses based on the physiological consequences of pharmacological agents. Psychopharmacologia, 3, 132-138.

Stewart, J. (1982). Reinstatement of heroin-reinforced responding in the rat by central implants of morphine in the ventral tegmental area. Society for Neuroscience Abstracts, 8, 589.

Stewart, J. (1984). Reinstatement of heroin and cocaine self-administration behavior in the rat by intracerebral application of morphine in the ventral tegmental area. Pharmacology Biochemistry & Behavior, 20, 917-923.

Stewart, J., de Wit, H., & Eikelboom, R. (1984). The role of unconditioned and conditioned drug effects in the self-administration of opiates and stimulants. Psychological Review, 91, 251-268.

Stretch, R., & Gerber, G. J. (1973). Drug-induced reinstatement of amphetamine self-administration behavior in monkeys. Canadian Journal of Psychology, 27, 168-177.

Thompson, T., & Pickens, R. (Eds.). (1971). Stimulus properties of drugs. New York: Appleton-Century-Crofts.

van der Kooy, D., & Hogan, J. A. (1978). Priming effects with food and water reinforcers in hamsters. Learning and Motivation, 9, 332-346.

van der Kooy, D., Mucha, R. F., O'Shaughnessy, M., & Bucenieks, P. (1982). Reinforcing effects of brain microinjections of morphine revealed by conditioned place preference. Brain Research, 243, 107-117.

Vezina, P., & Stewart, J. (1983). The conditioning of changes in locomotor activity induced by morphine applied to the ventral tegmental area of the rat brain. Society for Neuroscience Abstracts, 9, 275.

Vezina, P., & Stewart, J. (1984). Conditioning and place-specific sensitization of increases in activity induced by morphine in the VTA. Pharmacology Biochemistry & Behavior, 20, 925-934.

White, N., Sklar, L., & Amit, Z. (1977). The reinforcing action of morphine and its paradoxical side effect. Psychopharmacology, 52, 63-66.

Yokel, R. A., & Wise, R. A. (1976). Attenuation of intravenous amphetamine reinforcement by central dopamine blockade in rats. Psychopharmacologia, 48, 311-318.

CHAPTER 13

PLACE CONDITIONING: A SIMPLE AND EFFECTIVE METHOD FOR ASSESSING THE MOTIVATIONAL PROPERTIES OF DRUGS

Derek van der Kooy

Department of Anatomy
University of Toronto
Toronto, Ontario, Canada   M5S 1A8

ABSTRACT

The advantages of the place conditioning paradigm for assessing the reinforcing properties of drugs are presented from historical, procedural, and parametric viewpoints. The importance of employing a "balanced" paradigm is emphasized. The potential of the paradigm to answer basic questions concerning the neural bases of motivation is outlined with examples.

INTRODUCTION

Almost all assessments of the reinforcing properties of stimuli in nonhuman animals depend on learning paradigms. The exceptions involve studying the effects of noncontingent administration of drug reinforcers on ongoing species-typical behaviors such as feeding or locomotion. However, the inferences that the effects of the reinforcing stimuli in these studies are actually due to changes in motivation are very tenuous. In learning paradigms the assessments of the reinforcing properties of stimuli can be classified as either indirect or direct. In the indirect assessment paradigms, animals can be trained to make responses for a reinforcer such as intracranial self-stimulation (see Esposito, Porrino, & Seeger, this volume; Reid, this volume), and then the effects of the reinforcing stimulus of interest (such as a drug) are studied against the baseline responding. Again, the inference is not always obvious that the effects of the drug on baseline responding are due to changes in motivation rather than nonspecific sensory or motor changes.

In the direct assessments paradigms, the essential manipulation is that animals associate a certain stimulus or response with a drug stimulus. This association, in the case of a response learning, produces increased responding for a positive reinforcing drug such as occurs in the self-administration paradigm (see Roberts & Zito, this volume; Yokel, this volume). The association of a positive reinforcing drug with stimuli in the environment produces an increased preference for specific environmental stimuli as opposed to other similar stimuli (this chapter; Phillips & Fibiger, this volume). In both direct assessment paradigms (self-administration and place conditioning), one can formally understand the pairing of the reinforcing drug stimulus as either stimulus-stimulus or stimulus-response depending on one's theoretical view of what is associated during learning. Thus, for example, the lever-pressing self-administration procedure can be seen as animals continually maneuvering themselves as close as possible to stimuli (those proximal to the lever) associated with the drug reinforcer; on the other hand, the place conditioning procedure can be seen as increased locomotor responses to the environment associated with the drug reinforcer. I will argue that place conditioning involves the simplest and quickest association with drug reinforcers and thus minimizes the ambiguity of learning paradigms that inevitably complicate the interpretation of even the direct drug reinforcement assessment procedures. In the following description of the place conditioning method, a number of advantages of the paradigm for assessing the reinforcing properties of drugs will be illustrated. These include the method's rapidity, sensitivity, accurate generation of dose-response curves, avoidance of subject testing under the drug stimulus, possibility of centrally administering drugs, study of both positive reinforcing and aversive properties of drugs, and precise control of the temporal association of drugs with stimuli. Finally, the use of place conditioning to explore two substantive problems in the drug reinforcement field (i.e., the paradoxical reinforcing effects of morphine and the motivational vs. satiety effects of cholecystokinin) will be detailed.

HISTORY OF PLACE CONDITIONING

The history of the place conditioning method is the history of animal conditioning paradigms and can be seen to date from the late 1800s with Thorndike who was the first to establish formal learning paradigms for animals in the laboratory. Thorndike (1911) trained animals to go to a place in a box, to unlock a latch, and to escape. The first use of a place conditioning procedure similar to the one in current use may be that of Garcia, Kimeldorf, and Hunt (1957) who exposed rats to ionizing radiation in a distinctive environment and showed a clear aversion to the cues of this environment. A procedure employing arm choice in a Y-maze, which has some conceptual similarities to the place conditioning method, was first used in 1957 (Beach, 1957) to demonstrate the positive reinforcing properties of morphine. This demonstration predated the classic self-administration study by Weeks (1962) showing operant responding for intravenous morphine injections in rats.

In most place conditioning procedures, animals are treated by explicitly pairing distinctive environmental cues with administration of a drug. The animals are later tested by being presented with an opportunity to spend time in the presence of cues paired with the drug or in the presence of cues not paired with the drug. Animals prefer to spend time in environments paired with a number of drugs that can be classified as positive reinforcers. These include food (Stapleton, Lind, Merriman, Bozarth, & Reid, 1979; Swerdlow, van der Kooy, Koob, & Wenger, 1983), opiates (Bozarth & Wise, 1981; Katz & Gormezano, 1979; Mucha, van der Kooy, O'Shaughnessy, & Bucenieks, 1982; Phillips & Le Paine, 1980; Rossi & Reid, 1976; Sherman, 1980; van der Kooy, Mucha, O'Shaughnessy, & Bucenieks, 1982), amphetamine (Reicher & Holman, 1977; Sherman, Roberts, Roskam, & Holman, 1980b; Spyraki, Fibiger, & Phillips, 1982a), cocaine (Mucha et al., 1982; Spyraki, Fibiger, & Phillips, 1982b), and apomorphine (Spyraki et al., 1982a; van der Kooy, Swerdlow, & Koob, 1983b). On the other hand, animals avoid environments paired with drugs that can be considered aversive. These include lithium chloride (Mucha et al., 1982), naloxone (Mucha et al., 1982), vasopressin (Ettenberg, van der Kooy, Le Moal, Koob, & Bloom, 1983) and cholecystokinin (Swerdlow et al., 1983).

It is important to note that reports exist of both conditioned place preferences and conditioned place aversions with some drugs. Thus, although preferences are usually seen with amphetamine (Reicher & Holman, 1977; Sherman et al., 1980b; Spyraki et al., 1982b), aversions have also been reported

(Martin & Ellinwood, 1974). Similarly, ethanol appears to produce mainly place aversions (Cunningham, 1980; van der Kooy, O'Shaughnessy, Mucha, & Kalant, 1983a), but there is also one report of the conditioning of place preferences (Black, Albiniak, Davis, & Schumpert, 1973). Finally, place preferences are usually seen with apomorphine (Spyraki et al, 1982a; van der Kooy et al., 1983b), but conditioned place aversions also have been seen (Best & Mickley, 1973). In recent work employing intravenous apomorphine administration over a wide dose range, we have primarily seen no motivational effects, neither preferences nor aversions (Mackey & van der Kooy, unpublished observations). One view of these contradictory results is to see the place conditioning paradigm as inherently unreliable. Another viewpoint emphasizes that the three drugs mentioned above (amphetamine, alcohol, and apomorphine) are among the best examples of drugs previously shown (Wise, Yokel, & de Wit, 1976) to have paradoxical reinforcing properties (i.e., positive reinforcing properties as measured in the intravenous self-administration paradigm and yet over the same dose range aversive properties as measured in the conditioned taste aversion paradigm). Thus, perhaps the place preference paradigm can measure both the positive reinforcing and aversive properties of the same drug depending on subtle (and as of yet unknown) procedural differences during conditioning.

For the most part, drugs that are self-administered intravenously by animals also produce place preferences. However, there are some differences between the two methods with certain drugs. For example, dopamine-receptor blockade with neuroleptics attenuates the positive reinforcing effects of cocaine in the self-administration paradigm (de Wit & Wise, 1977) but not the place preference paradigm (Mackey & van der Kooy, 1985; Spyraki et al., 1982b). From one viewpoint this result attests to the exquisite sensitivity of the place preference paradigm; it detects positive reinforcing effects in addition to those blocked by neuroleptics.

PROCEDURAL ISSUES

Place conditioning is really a misnomer for the paradigm under discussion. There is not a stored memory of environmental cues forming a spatial map as in paradigms such as the radial arm maze or Morris water task. In the place conditioning paradigm, as it is routinely used in drug reinforcement studies, rats are tested for their preferences for different environmental cues that are constantly present during testing. In the variation of place conditioning that we use, considerable effort is extended to offer the rat choices between distinctive yet equivalent cues. Thus one side of the box is black with a black Plexiglas floor and a slight smell of vinegar, and the other side is white with a wire mesh floor covered with sawdust. This combination of stimulus choices results in naive rats having no natural or baseline preference for either type of environment. Thus we can counterbalance our drug pairings with half the rats in any experimental condition receiving drug treatments in the black box and vehicle control treatments in the white box, and vice versa for the other half. This counterbalancing is an important point. Other experimenters employ conditioned stimuli that produce a strong "natural" preference for one environment with the result that the drug pairings are almost always with the least preferred side (Ceiling effects usually preclude observing drug conditioned increases in time spent on the preferred side.). Different and sometimes suspicious (see below) results are occasionally seen with "unbalanced" place conditioning paradigms as compared with the "balanced" paradigm we routinely employed.

As noted above, place conditioning is actually conditioning with the differing visual, tactile, and olfactory cues of the two environments. It will be important in the future to determine which modality of sensory stimuli is capturing most of the associative value from the paired drug. For example, rats always show a preference for the visual, tactile, and olfactory cues of the environment paired with morphine (Mucha et al., 1982). Other experimenters report place preferences when morphine is paired with only visual (Rossi & Reid, 1976) or visual and tactile (Bozarth & Wise, 1981; Phillips & Le Paine, 1980) stimuli; however, it is difficult to determine whether these paradigms are as sensitive in revealing the positive reinforcing properties of morphine as paradigms employing visual, tactile, and olfactory conditioned stimuli. On the other hand, when morphine is paired with taste stimuli, as in conditioned taste aversion paradigms, rats avoid the stimulus paired with morphine (Sherman et al., 1980a; van der Kooy & Phillips, 1977). Thus, the motivational properties of morphine seem to depend on the conditioned stimuli used to reveal these properties. A clear understanding of the stimulus modality most important in morphine place conditioning may help in pinpointing the differential associability issue and indeed in solving the problem of the paradoxical reinforcing effects of morphine.

Parametric Data

Place conditioning has been studied most thoroughly by experimenters using morphine as the reinforcing stimulus. Morphine produces place preferences (see Figure 1) over its entire usable dose range (Mucha et al., 1982). A low dose of 0.08 mg/kg (i.v.) produces a preference for the environment in which it was paired (four training trials) although this dose does not produce detectable effects on locomotion or analgesia (measured in the tail flick test) in our hands. More sensitive tests for locomotor or analgesic actions may have revealed effects at this low dose of morphine. High doses (10 and 15 mg/kg, i.v.) also produce strong place preferences, although the animals show marked immobility at these doses which are approaching the lethal range for opiate naive rats. Figure 1 shows that the steep part of the dose-response curve occurs between 0.01 and 0.08 mg/kg (i.v.), although there is a more gentle rise from 0.08 to 10 mg/kg. This can be best appreciated by comparing the differences between the times in the morphine- and saline-paired sides over the dose range. The steep part of the dose response curve for subcutaneously administered morphine occurs between 0.04 and 1.0 mg/kg (Mucha & Iversen, 1985). Thus, place conditioning is a very sensitive measure of the low threshold dose of systemic morphine required for positive reinforcing effects and also shows that there is a gentle increase in the positive reinforcing value of morphine over its entire usable dose range.

Place preferences for morphine can be produced with as little as one pairing of the drug with a distinctive environment (and one pairing of the saline vehicle with the alternate environment; Mucha et al., 1982). In addition, it has recently been shown that after three pairings of morphine with a distinctive environment, the conditioned preferences for that environment were retained for at least one month (Mucha & Iversen, 1985). These properties of one trial learning and long retention suggest that the power and robustness of the place conditioning paradigm for measuring the positive qualities of a drug's reinforcement may be similar to that of the much touted conditioned taste aversion paradigm for measuring the aversive qualities of drugs.

The small numbers of drug pairings necessary in place conditioning is a particular advantage when injections of drugs into the cerebral ventricles (see Figure 2) or brain tissue (see Figure 3) are employed. Damage to the injected brain tissue is a danger especially when large numbers of microinjections are

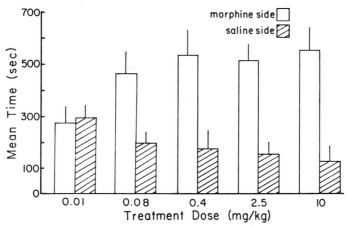

Figure 1: Time spent on the sides of the test box paired with saline and with morphine for rats (n = 8 to 14) treated with different morphine (i.v.) doses. The data were collapsed across the two times in the treatment box. Reprinted with permission from Mucha, Bucenieks, O'Shaughnessy, and van der Kooy, 1982. Copyright 1982 by Elsevier Biomedical Press.

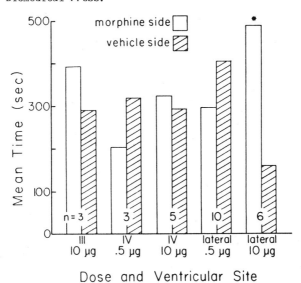

Figure 2: Time spent on the side of the test box paired with saline or morphine for rats given morphine into different cerebroventricular sites and in different doses. The number of animals in each group is indicated near the bottom of each bar. The asterisk indicates that a significant (p < 0.05) place preference was seen. There was also a trend to a significant place preference when 10 μg of morphine was microinjected into the IIIrd ventricle. Reprinted with permission from van der Kooy, Bucenieks, Mucha, and O'Shaughnessy, 1982. Copyright 1982 by Elsevier Biomedical Press.

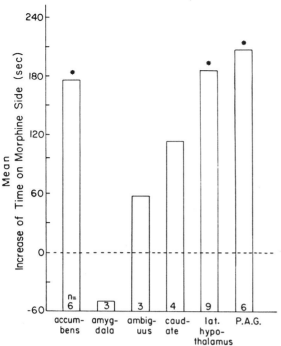

Figure 3: Mean increase of time on the side of the test box paired with morphine (test minus pretest in an unbalanced paradigm) at various cannulae placement sites. The number of animals at each placement site is indicated near the bottom of the corresponding bar. The asterisks indicate that a significant ($p < 0.05$) increase in time spent on the side of the test box paired with morphine was produced by place conditioning. Reprinted with permission from vander Kooy, Bucenieks, Mucha, and O'Shaughnessy, 1982. Copyright 1982 by Elsevier Biomedical Press.

used. A number of investigators have demonstrated place preferences after microinjections of opiates into the ventral tegmental area (Phillips & Le Paine, 1980, 1982), nucleus accumbens (van der Kooy et al., 1982) and periaqueductal gray (van der Kooy et al., 1982). Microinjections of opiates in a number of other areas fail to produce place conditioning (van der Kooy et al., 1982). These studies provide the initial attempt to map specific brain systems where opiates act through their receptors to produce positive reinforcing effects. The place preferences produced by brain microinjections of opiates show stereospecificity, and this provides evidence that a specific opiate receptor is involved (van der Kooy et al., 1982). The possibility of directly probing the neural substrates of motivation with a minimal number of brain microinjections is one of the major advantages of the place preference paradigm.

Unlike some of the indirect methods for assessing the positive reinforcing properties of drugs, place conditioning appears to permit no interpretations of conditioned preferences other than the fact that the drug stimulus has positive reinforcing properties. Testing in place conditioning is done drug-free. This eliminates the problem (in many indirect paradigms) of measuring drug reinforcement while subjects are under the influence of drugs producing various sensory and/or motor changes which can confound and interfere with the reinforcement measurements. The only other conceivable explanation of place preferences might involve the motivational effects of novelty in combination with memory deficits or state-dependent learning. For example, the drug-paired side may not be recalled during testing, because training is under the influence of that drug whereas testing is in its absence. Rats may then spend more time in the presence of the drug-paired cues on the test because these cues are perceived as novel and, for this reason of novelty, possibly positively reinforcing (Berlyne, 1969). These explanations for place preference are untenable for two reasons. First, testing under state-dependent conditions (i.e., under the influence of the drug) produces results no different from those run under normal drug-free testing conditions (Mucha et al., 1982; Mucha & Iversen, 1985). Second, no motivational effects of novelty were seen in the place conditioning paradigm. Rats showed no preferences in place conditioning tests for a novel side over one experienced previously (Mucha & Iversen, 1985; Mucha et al., 1982). Furthermore, when tested in a three-compartment box (the third compartment being novel), rats still preferred the morphine-paired compartment (Mucha & Iversen, 1985).

Different Ways to Run Place Conditioning

There are two ways (i.e., balanced and unbalanced) to do place conditioning. In the balanced paradigm care is taken to choose conditioning stimuli that produce approximately equal preferences for the two sides of the test compartment in naive, untreated rats. This permits counterbalancing of drug pairing with one side of the conditioning box within a group and also obviates the need for pretesting subjects before training begins. In the unbalanced paradigm subjects are pretested and usually show a substantial preference for one side of the test box. Drug pairings are then always on the least preferred side. Because counterbalancing is impossible, a separate control group is often run with vehicle injections to demonstrate that increases in time on the least preferred side are not as large with saline as with morphine (Bozarth & Wise, 1981; Katz & Gormezano, 1980; Phillips & Le Paine, 1980, 1982). Even with morphine, absolute preferences are not often produced in the unbalanced paradigm, just relative increases in time in the least preferred side.

The results of place conditioning studies can vary depending on whether balanced or unbalanced paradigms are used. With the balanced paradigm clear aversions to naloxone (see Figure 4) are observed in both morphine pretreated and morphine naive rats (Mucha et al., 1982). Unbalanced paradigms have generally failed to show conditioned naloxone aversions (Bozarth & Wise, 1981; Phillips & Le Paine, 1980, 1982). Part of the inability to see aversive effects may reflect a baseline problem; naloxone is usually paired with the least preferred side of the test box and an aversion can only be seen by an even greater avoidance of this side.

However, there are more substantial differences between balanced and unbalanced paradigms than can be explained by baseline or ceiling problems. In line with dopamine theories of reward, there have been reports that neuroleptic administration in the unbalanced paradigm blocks the place preferences produced by opiates (Bozarth and Wise, 1981). Employing a balanced paradigm, we have been unable to block with high doses of haloperidol or α-flupenthixol the place preferences produced by various doses of morphine (Mackey & van der Kooy, 1985). At present there is no convincing explanation for these differences. One possible explanation is that the unbalanced paradigm does not really (or at least not only) measure the positive reinforcing properties of morphine. As mentioned above, the normal control group tested in the unbalanced paradigm is one in which saline is paired with the least preferred side, and the increase in time on that side at testing is not as large as when morphine is used. However, this may not be the appropriate control for morphine treatment in the unbalanced paradigm. Because morphine treatment cannot be counterbalanced with both sides of the conditioning box in the unbalanced paradigm, there is no intrinsic control for morphine pairing with the general training environments (test room, handling, common properties of both training compartments). In

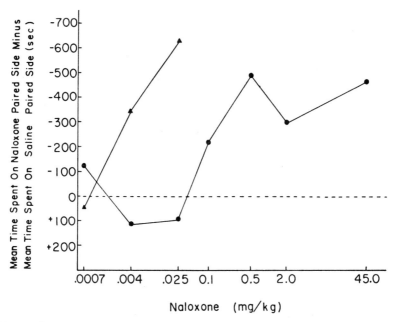

Figure 4: Difference between mean time spent on the side of the test box paired with different doses of naloxone and the mean time spent on the side of the test box paired with saline in morphine naive (circles) and morphine pellet implanted (triangles) rats (n = 5 to 17). Abscissa is a log scale. Reprinted with permission from Mucha, Bucenieks, O'Shaughnessy, and van der Kooy, 1982. Copyright 1982 by Elsevier Biomedical Press.

fact, when an appropriate control is done (pairing of morphine with the least preferred side, preferred side, and general test environment), then increases in time on least preferred side at testing are similar to those seen with rats that received the same number of doses of morphine but only on the least preferred side (Mucha & Iversen, 1985). Presumably, in the unbalanced paradigm morphine is being associated with the entire test environment and the increased time on the least preferred side at testing simply reflects less anxiety about or avoidance of aversive aspects of the conditioned environment. In light of this it is not surprising that experimental differences are seen when the unbalanced paradigm is compared to the balanced paradigm which appears to measure strictly the positive reinforcing properties of the drug stimulus.

USE OF PLACE CONDITIONING TO STUDY PROBLEMS IN DRUG REINFORCEMENT

A major advantage of the place conditioning paradigm over other methods of measuring the reinforcing properties of stimuli is its sensitivity to both the aversive and positive reinforcing properties of drugs. This attribute has allowed the testing of some important questions in the area of motivation. Two examples are described below.

Satiety Versus Aversive Effects of Cholecystokinin

Feeding in food-deprived animals is reduced by injection of cholecystokinin (CCK) in a dose-dependent manner (Gibbs, Young, & Smith, 1973). This evidence has been interpreted either in terms of CCK involvement in satiety (Gibbs et al., 1973) or in terms of a CCK-induced malaise (Deutsch & Hardy, 1977).

These two hypotheses imply opposite predictions concerning the motivational properties of CCK in food-deprived animals. According to the CCK-satiety hypothesis, CCK should reduce the hunger of food-deprived animals. Therefore, hungry rats should learn to prefer an environment associated with CCK over one not associated with CCK. Moreover, sated rats should not learn this preference. On the other hand, according to the CCK-malaise hypothesis, CCK should have only aversive properties in both food-deprived and sated animals. All rats, hungry or not, should therefore learn to avoid environments associated with CCK. We tested these hypotheses using the conditioned place-preference paradigm (Swerdlow, van der Kooy, Koob, & Wenger, 1983). Both food-deprived and sated rats exhibited a dose-dependent conditioned place aversion to CCK (see Figure 5). The malaise interpretation of CCK's effect was therefore

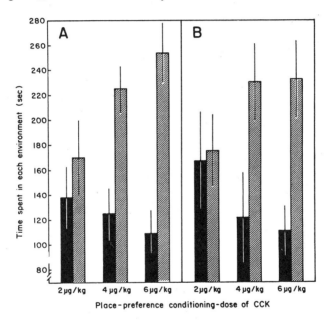

Figure 5: Time spent in environments previously paired with CCK (solid) or saline (stippled) shown as a function of conditioning dose of CCK. All injections were given intraperitoneally in a volume of 3 ml/kg to promote diffusion into the peritoneal cavity. Measurements were made during a 10-minute test period following 8 days of conditioning of (A) sated or (B) food-deprived animals. The value at each dose represents scores from a separate group of six animals. Rats were tested drug-free. Reprinted with permission from Swerdlow, Koob, van der Kooy, and Wenger, 1983. Copyright 1983 by Pergamon Press.

supported (Swerdlow et al., 1983). Thus, the sensitive bidirectional properties of the place conditioning paradigm enabled its use as an independent test of the opposite predictions made by two competing theories concerning CCK's action.

Paradoxical Reinforcing Effects of Opiates

As mentioned above, opiates have been shown to have paradoxical reinforcing qualities--positive reinforcing as measured in the conditioned place preference paradigm and aversive as measured in the conditioned taste aversion paradigm. Recent work showing opiate receptors on primary sensory neurons led us to test the motivational effects of local peripheral administration of opiates. In both the ear scratch and hot plates tests, a local, naloxone-reversible hyperalgesic effect of etorphine was observed (van der Kooy & Nagy, 1985). Thus, we hypothesized that the positive reinforcing properties of opiates are mediated by an action at central opiate receptors (see Figures 2 and 3) whereas the aversive effects of opiates may be mediated by an action at peripherally located opiate receptors. The possibility of measuring both positive reinforcing and aversive effects in the place conditioning paradigm and the availability of naltrexone and its quaternary derivative methyl naltrexone, which does not cross the blood-brain barrier effectively (Valentino, Herling, Woods, Medzihradshy, & Merz, 1981), provided the opportunity to test the hypothesis.

Systemic naloxone has been previously shown to produce place aversions (see Figure 4) in drug naive rats (Mucha et al., 1982). Presumably this aversive effect is due to an antagonism by naloxone of endogenous opioid peptides acting primarily on the dense concentrations of brain opiate receptors. We predicted that systemically administered naltrexone (an opiate antagonist similar to, but longer lasting than, naloxone) would have the same aversive effect. We further predicted that this action on central opiate receptors would overwhelm any action on the much smaller population of peripheral opiate receptors. However, methyl naltrexone, which does not cross the blood-brain barrier effectively, would be expected to primarily block the action of endogenous opiate peptides in peripheral opiate receptors. If the normal action of opiate peptides in the periphery is an aversive or hyperalgesic one, then methyl naltrexone would be predicted to cause conditioned place preferences. Indeed, these predictions were confirmed (Bechara & van der Kooy, 1985). Both subcutaneous and intraperitoneal naltrexone produced dose-dependent conditioned place aversions, whereas both subcutaneous and intraperitoneal methyl naltrexone produced dose-dependent conditioned place preferences. Thus, studies with the place conditioning paradigm provide strong support for the hypothesis that opiates work at central receptors to produce positive reinforcing effects and at peripheral receptors to produce aversive effects.

In conclusion, the place conditioning paradigm provides a rapid, simple, and elegant method of measuring the positive reinforcing or aversive properties of both peripherally and centrally administered drugs. In doing so, the paradigm offers a potent approach to basic questions concerning the neural basis of motivation.

ACKNOWLEDGMENTS

The author acknowledges the wonderful collaboration in the place conditioning studies mentioned of a number of colleagues, including Tony

Bechara, Peter Bucenieks, Aaron Ettenberg, Martha O'Shaughnessy, Harold Kalant, George Koob, Bruce Mackey, Ron Mucha, Neal Swerdlow, and John Wenger. Special thanks to Ron Mucha for innumerable discussions. Thanks also to Dr. H. Merz for his generous gift of methyl naltrexone. This research was supported by grants to the author from the Medical Research Council of Canada and the Natural Sciences and Engineering Research Council of Canada.

REFERENCES

Beach, H. D. (1957). Morphine addiction in rats. Canadian Journal of Psychology, 11, 104-112.

Bechara, A., & van der Kooy, D. (1985). Opposite motivational effects of endogenous opioids in brain and periphery. Nature, 314, 533-534.

Berlyne, D. E. (1969). The reward value of indifferent stimulation. In J. T. Tapp (Ed.), Reinforcement and behavior (pp. 179-214). New York: Academic Press.

Best, P. J., Best, M. R., & Mickley, G. A. (1973). Conditioned aversion to distinct environmental stimuli resulting from gastrointestinal distress. Journal of Comparative and Physiological Psychology, 85, 250-257.

Bozarth, M. A., & Wise, R. A. (1981). Heroin reward is dependent on a dopaminergic substrate. Life Sciences, 29, 1881-1886.

Black, R. W., Albiniak, T., Davis, M., & Schumpert, J. (1973). A preference in rats for cues associated with intoxication. Bulletin of the Psychonomic Society, 2, 423-424.

Cunningham, C. L. (1979). Flavor and location aversions produced by ethanol. Behavioral and Neural Biology, 27, 362-367.

Deutsch, J. A., & Hardy, W. T. (1971). Cholecystokinin produces bait shyness in rats. Nature, 266, 196.

de Wit, H., & Wise, R. A. (1977). Blockade of cocaine reinforcement in rats with the dopamine receptor blocker pimozide, but not with the noradrenergic blockers phentolamine and phenoxybenzamine. Canadian Journal of Psychology, 31, 195-203.

Ettenberg, A., van der Kooy, D., Le Moal, M., Koob, G. F., & Bloom, F. E. (1983). Can aversive properties of (peripherally injected) vasopressin account for its putative role in memory? Behavioral Brain Research, 7, 331-350.

Garcia, J., Kimeldorf, D. J., & Hunt, E. (1957). Spatial avoidance in the rat as a result of exposure to ionizing radiation. British Journal of Radiation, 30, 318-321.

Gibbs, J., Young, R. C., & Smith, G. P. (1973). Cholecystokinin elicits satiety in rats with open gastric fistulas. Nature, 245, 323-325.

Katz, R. J., & Gormezano, G. (1979). A rapid inexpensive technique for assessing the reinforcing effects of opiate drugs. Pharmacology Biochemistry & Behavior, 11, 231-233.

Mackey, W. B., & van der Kooy, D. (1983). Neuroleptics block the reinforcing effects of amphetamine but not of morphine as measured by place conditioning. Pharmacology Biochemistry & Behavior, 22, 101-105.

Martin, J. C., & Ellinwood, E. H. (1974). Conditioned aversion in spatial paradigms following methamphetamine injection. Psychopharmacologia, 36, 323-335.

Mucha, R. F., Bucenieks, P., O'Shaughnessy, M., & van der Kooy, D. (1982). Drug reinforcement studied by the use of place conditioning in rat. Brain Research, 243, 91-105.

Mucha, R. F., & Iversen, S. D. (1985). Reinforcing properties of morphine and naloxone revealed by conditioned place preferences: A procedural examination. Psychopharmacology, 82, 241-247.

Phillips, A. G., & Le Paine, F. G. (1980). Reinforcing effects of morphine microinjection into the ventral tegmental area. Pharmacology Biochemistry & Behavior, 12, 965-968.

Phillips, A. G., & Le Paine, F. G. (1982). Reward produced by microinjection of (D-Ala[2]), Met[5]-enkephalinamide into the ventral tegmental area. Behavioral Brain Research, 5, 225-229.

Reicher, M. A., & Holman, E. W. (1977). Location preference and flavor aversion reinforced by amphetamine in rats. Animal Learning and Behavior, 5, 343-346.

Rossi, N. A., & Reid, L. D. (1976). Affective states associated with morphine injections. Physiological Psychology, 4, 269-274.

Sherman, J. E., Pickman, C., Rice, A., Liebeskind, J. C., & Holman, E. W. (1980a). Rewarding and aversive effects of morphine: Temporal and pharmacological properties. Pharmacology Biochemistry & Behavior, 13, 501-505.

Sherman, J. E., Roberts, T., Roskam, S. E., & Holman, E. W. (1980b). Temporal properties of the rewarding and aversive effects of amphetamine in rats. Pharmacology Biochemistry & Behavior, 13, 597-599.

Spyraki, C., Fibiger, H. C., & Phillips, A. G. (1982a). Dopaminergic substrates of amphetamine-induced place preference conditioning. Brain Research, 253, 185-193.

Spyraki, C., Fibiger, H. C., & Phillips, A. G. (1982b). Cocaine-induced place preference conditioning: Lack of effects of neuroleptics and 6-hydroxydopamine lesions. Brain Research, 253, 195-203.

Stapleton, J. M., Lind, M. D., Merriman, V. J., Bozarth, M. A., & Reid, L. A. (1979). Affective consequences and subsequent effects in morphine self-administration of D-Ala[2]-methionine enkephalin. Physiological Psychology, 7, 146-152.

Swerdlow, N. R., Koob, G., van der Kooy, D., & Wenger, J. R. (1983). Cholecystokinin produces conditioned place-aversions, not place-preferences, in food-deprived rats: Evidence against involvement in satiety. Life Sciences, 32, 2087-2093.

Thorndike, E. L. (1911). Animal intelligence: Experimental studies. New York: Macmillan.

Valentino, R. J., Herling, S., Medzihradshy, F., Merz, H., & Woods, J. H. (1981). Quarternary naltrexone: Evidence for the central mediation of discriminative stimulus effects of narcotic agonists and antagonists. Journal of Pharmacology and Experimental Therapeutics, 219, 652-659.

van der Kooy, D., Bucenieks, P., Mucha, R. F., & O'Shaughnessy, M. (1982). Reinforcing effects of brain microinjections of morphine revealed by conditioned place preference. Brain Research, 243, 107-117.

van der Kooy, D., Kalant, H., Mucha, R. F., & O'Shaughnessy, M. (1983a). Motivational properties of ethanol in naive rats as studied by place conditioning. Pharmacology Biochemistry & Behavior, 19, 441-445.

van der Kooy, D., Koob, G. F., & Swerdlow, N. R. (1983b). Paradoxical reinforcing properties of apomorphine: Effects of nucleus accumbens and area postrema lesions. Brain Research, 259, 111-118.

van der Kooy, D., & Nagy, J. I. (1985). Hyperalgesia mediated by peripheral opiate receptors in the rat. Behavioural Brain Research, 17, 203-211.

van der Kooy, D., & Phillips, A. G. (1977). Temporal analysis of naloxone attenuation of morphine-induced taste aversion. Pharmacology Biochemistry & Behavior, 6, 637-641.

Weeks, J. R. (1962). Experimental morphine addiction: Method for automatic intravenous injections in unrestrained rats. Science, 138, 143-144.

Wise, R. A., de Wit, H., & Yokel, R. A. (1976). Both positive reinforcement and conditioned aversion from amphetamine and apomorphine in rats. Science, 191, 1273-1275.

CHAPTER 14

CONDITIONED PLACE PREFERENCE: A PARAMETRIC ANALYSIS
USING SYSTEMIC HEROIN INJECTIONS

Michael A. Bozarth

Center for Studies in Behavioral Neurobiology
Department of Psychology
Concordia University
Montreal, Quebec, Canada   H3G 1M8

ABSTRACT

A series of experiments is described that explores some of the parametric aspects of place preference conditioning. Several procedures that affect classical conditioning were used, such as increasing the intensity of the unconditioned stimulus and increasing the number of conditioning trials. These manipulations had little effect on the strength of the conditioned response. Alternative explanations for the shift in place preference were also examined, and none of these factors could adequately account for the data. Although place preference is usually tested in drug-free subjects, the strongest place preference was seen when subjects were tested following injections of the conditioning drug. This suggests that the drug cue may be the most salient stimulus associated with the rewarding action of the drug, and the absence of this stimulus may limit the strength of the conditioning seen in most place preference studies.

INTRODUCTION

Many of the methods for assessing drug reward involve examining the ability of a drug to serve as a reinforcer. Frequently, some response is performed by the subject followed by presentation of the drug reward. This approach evaluates the ability of a drug to directly reinforce behavior and is a simple extension of operant psychology. Presentation of the reinforcing stimulus (i.e., rewarding drug) is contingent upon the performance of some behavioral response such as lever pressing. Thus, the drug's capacity to <u>directly</u> control behavior is assessed. An alternative approach involves studying the associations developed between a rewarding drug effect and some arbitrarily selected stimulus. This conditioning approach does not involve the subject "working" for the drug reward, but rather, it examines the behavior of the subject following presentation of stimuli associated with drug reward.

Perhaps the earliest study demonstrating that stimuli associated with drug presentation can elicit behaviors described as drug seeking is Spragg's (1940) study of "Morphine Addiction in Chimpanzees." In this study chimpanzees were injected daily with morphine and Spragg reported signs of drug-seeking behavior when the subjects were brought into the room associated with the injections. No attempt was made to quantify these behaviors, however, and the effect was attributed solely to morphine's ability to relieve withdrawal distress in physically dependent animals. Nonetheless, this study appears to be the first to document drug-seeking behavior in animals and emphasized the importance of stimuli associated with rewarding drug injections in the control of the animals' behavior.

Another early study assessing the ability of stimuli associated with drug reward to influence behavior was reported by Beach (1957). Animals received injections of morphine and were "run into" and remained in an environment paired with the drug effect. After this procedure was repeated for several days, subjects were tested for their attraction to the environment associated with the drug effect. During the test trials, the animals showed a marked preference for the compartment associated with the drug effect. This study involved an instrumental response (i.e., running in a Y-maze), but it is properly considered a conditioning study because the subjects were never reinforced for their performance in the maze; the drug effect was simply associated with "running into" and with the stimuli contained in a specific compartment of the apparatus.

The Beach (1957) study is one of the first demonstrations of drug-reward conditioning, but it involved forcing the animals to "run into" a specific compartment during training. Kumar (1972) reported a study that did not involve an instrumental response associated with the drug effect. In his study, animals were injected with morphine and directly placed in a compartment associated with the drug effect. Thus, the subjects did not run to the drug-associated environment during training. Kumar (1972), however, used very large doses of morphine (i.e., 120 mg/kg) and his data were interpreted as measuring the ability of stimuli associated with the relief of withdrawal distress to serve as a conditioned reinforcer.

Rossi and Reid (1976) reported that a moderate dose of morphine (i.e., 10 mg/kg) associated with a specific environment produced evidence of conditioning that was related to the drug's rewarding effects. In their study animals were injected with morphine and later placed directly into a specific compartment. This method was used as an independent assessment of morphine reward and was offered as corroborative evidence of morphine reward at times-post-injection that corresponded to morphine's facilitation of brain stimulation reward (see Reid, this volume). They further suggested that the conditioned place preference method was a measure of the drug's "affective consequences" and emphasized the positive hedonic impact of morphine administration. This appears to be the first study to employ place preference conditioning in its contemporary fashion. Two factors distinguish their study from the earlier work: (i) no instrumental response was associated with drug conditioning and (ii) a relatively low dose of morphine was used. Considering the current popularity of the conditioned place preference method, it is interesting to note that Rossi and Reid's application of place preference conditioning was not primarily designed to develop a new method of assessing drug reward, but rather, it was designed to provide independent validation of another method (i.e., brain stimulation reward) of assessing the rewarding effects of morphine.

During the past several years, numerous studies have reported evidence of drug reward using place preference conditioning. Because this procedure appears to be relatively simple, it has generated a considerable amount of excitement in the study of drug reward. Surgical preparation of the subjects is not necessary and minimal equipment is required. Data collection can be easily automated using a microcomputer (Bozarth, 1983), and drug testing can be completed in a few days. These factors allow the rapid screening of large numbers of compounds with very little effort. Despite the widespread appeal of this technique, there is controversy regarding the validity of some place preference procedures. Furthermore, the characteristics of this phenomenon have not been systematically examined and are poorly understood.

PARAMETRIC ANALYSIS

The purpose of this series of experiments was to explore some of the variables likely to influence place preference conditioning. The merit of this procedure has relied primarily on its face validity: place preference is an intuitively satisfying statement about the relationship between a rewarding event and stimuli associated with that reward. To assess the validity of this method, it is necessary to characterize the influence of (i) variables known to affect drug reward and (ii) variables known to govern the strength of conditioning. This paper explores the effects of manipulating some variables that have well established effects on classical conditioning. If conditioned place preference studies truly represent a class of behavior governed by the association of drug reward with environmental stimuli, then manipulation of variables known to affect conditioning should influence the development of conditioned place preference. This is one approach to empirically validating conditioned place preference studies. Without such empirical validation, the interpretation of data generated from this technique is questionable.

General Experimental Procedure

Most of the experiments reported in this chapter use the same general procedure. Subjects were experimentally naive, male, Long-Evans rats usually weighing 300 to 400 grams. They were individually housed in cages with a wire mesh bottom. Food and water were available ad libitum, except during conditioning and behavioral testing. A 12-hour light/dark cycle was used, and testing occurred during the light phase of this cycle. The apparatus consisted of a shuttle box measuring 25 x 35 x 25 cm with a smooth, Plexiglas floor on one end of the chamber and a tubular stainless steel floor on the other end. The amount of time spent on the smooth side of the apparatus was automatically recorded as were the number of crosses between the two sides (Bozarth, 1983).

The standard procedure usually consisted of three phases. The initial place preferences of the subjects were recorded for five 15-minute trials during the first week. The last trial of this series served as a measure of the animals' preconditioning place preferences. Next, a barrier was inserted in the shuttle box dividing it into two compartments. The subjects were subcutaneously injected with drug and immediately placed in one compartment of the apparatus (usually their nonpreferred side) for 30 minutes. After three such conditioning trials, place preference was again measured when the subjects were allowed free access to the entire test apparatus. Each subject's change in place preference was computed by subtracting the place preference recorded during the last preconditioning trial from that of the test trial. These data were then grouped according to treatment conditions and the appropriate statistical analysis performed.

There are several points that should be noted with this procedure. First, most subjects (c. 80%) showed a strong preference (c. 70% test duration) for the tubular side of the shuttle box. The reason for this is unclear, but it may be related to the fact that they were housed in cages with a wire mesh floor. Second, subjects were usually conditioned on their nonpreferred sides of the test apparatus. This was done to maximize the potential shift in place preference following conditioning with appetitive rewards. If the objective of the study were to assess place aversions, conditioning on the preferred side would be required to avoid limiting the potential magnitude of the shift. Third, the shuttle boxes were thoroughly washed before each phase of the procedure--prior to preconditioning, conditioning, and test trials. Although olfactory cues are extremely important to rats, this procedure is necessary when large numbers of subjects are tested in the same boxes. Otherwise, the conditioning of one subject may affect the measurement of preference in another; a rat may be responding to the olfactory cues left by earlier rats rather than making a place preference discrimination based on its own conditioning experience.

Reliability of Three-Trial Conditioning

One of the first considerations in the utility of conditioned place preference studies is the reliability of the conditioned effect. Figure 1 illustrates eight independent studies using the same basic conditioning procedure. All subjects, except those in Group A, were subcutaneously injected

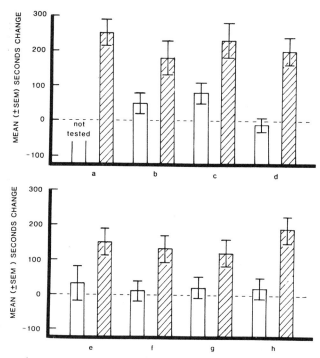

Figure 1: Reliability of the conditioned place preference produced by heroin using a standard conditioning procedure. The various experiments were independently conducted over a 4-year period (n = 11 to 15/group). The figure shows the mean (±SEM) change in place preference following conditioning. Striped bars, heroin conditioned; open bars, saline conditioned.

with 0.3 mg/kg of heroin during three 30-minute conditioning trials. Subjects in Group A were injected with 0.5 mg/kg of heroin during four conditioning trials. Other subjects were injected with physiological saline (1 ml/kg) during their conditioning trials. A single 15-minute test trial measured the place preference following conditioning.

An analysis of variance (ANOVA) performed on the data from Groups B through H showed that conditioning with heroin reliably produced a conditioned place preference [F (1,161) = 54.940, p < 0.001], while saline conditioning resulted in only sporadic shifts in place preference. There was no significant difference across the various replications [F (6,161) = 1.111, p > 0.1], nor was there any Treatment x Replication interaction [F (6,161) = 0.407, p > 0.1].

Statistical Considerations

It is interesting to note that of the several ways that these data could be statistically analyzed, Fisher's (1935) method of specific comparison is perhaps the most appropriate. A series of dependent t-tests can be used to assess shifts in individual groups with the alpha level adjusted to protect against the use of multiple t-tests (i.e., cumulative error rate). By setting $\alpha^* = \alpha/r$ where r = the number of tests, α^* protects against the influence of repeated tests. The use of this method has the advantage of minimizing the effects of unequal numbers of subjects and differences in the homogeneity of variances among treatment conditions. The practical value of this approach can be seen in Table 1 which shows that all of the heroin-conditioned and none of the saline-conditioned groups demonstrated a reliable change in place preference.

For the seven t-tests between groups, $\alpha^* = 0.007$. Two of the seven groups failed to exceed this critical value (i.e., Groups C and E). The within group comparisons consist of 15 individual tests; for this series, $\alpha^* = 0.003$. All drug-treated groups except Group G exceeded this criterion; none of the saline groups even approached this critical value of α^*. Both the t-test for simple main effects (Winer, 1971) and the Tukey's (a) test revealed between group differences for all comparisons.

Although the use of repeated t-tests is very prone to produce Type II errors and some adjustment of the α-level is appropriate, some statisticians (e.g., Lindman, 1974) suggest that the adjusted α-level can be determined on logical grounds and need not rely strictly on statistical approaches. If α is set to 0.005 for each of the 15 specific comparisons across all groups, all of the drug-treated groups show a reliable conditioned place preference while none of the saline-treated groups show significant shifts. This adjustment of α retains much of the power of individual t-tests while minimizing the probability of a Type II error. Furthermore, the results of this approach are very similar to those of both the t-test for simple main effects based on the ANOVA and the more conservative Tukey's (a) test. Thus it would appear that α = 0.005 is a suitable criterion for determining the significance of shifts in place preference, and this approach offers the advantage of minimizing the influence of large, within group variance that sometimes occurs with various treatments. In fact, if an α-level of 0.05 were used to assess changes in place preference, only one saline-conditioned group would have shown a significant shift in place preference (false positive), and even this shift in place preference could have resulted from reward-induced conditioning (see section on Stress-Induced Place Preference).

Table 1

Individual Comparisons of Conditioning Across Various Replications

Group	Condition	t^a	η^2	t^b	Tukey's (a)
A	Drug	p < .001	73%	n/a	n/a
B	Drug	p < .001	82%		
	Saline	p < .25	6%		
	Between	p < .005	22%	p < .005	p < .05
C	Drug	p < .001	81%		
	Saline	p < .01	41%		
	Between	p < .01	26%	p < .025	p < .05
D	Drug	p < .001	65%		
	Saline	p < .35	4%		
	Between	p < .001	41%	p < .001	p < .01
E	Drug	p < .002	58%		
	Saline	p < .35	4%		
	Between	p < .05	14%	p < .025	p < .05
F	Drug	p < .001	62%		
	Saline	p < .45	1%		
	Between	p < .002	32%	p < .005	p < .01
G	Drug	p < .005	57%		
	Saline	p < .35	2%		
	Between	p < .005	25%	p < .025	p < .05
H	Drug	p < .001	63%		
	Saline	p < .25	7%		
	Between	p < .005	25%	p < .001	p < .01

Note: **a,** individual t-tests; **b,** t-tests for simple main effects based on the ANOVA (Winer, 1971); **n/a,** not applicable.

With the ANOVA approach, an extremely high variance in one treatment cell contributes disproportionately to the overall within-cell error variance. Small differences between other cells may be masked, even though their within-cell variances are very small. With the dependent t-test approach, each group is assessed independently for changes in place preference. Extremely high within-cell variance in one group will only affect the statistical outcome of that group and not the others involved in the comparisons. Thus, if the α-level is adjusted to minimize the probability of a Type II error, the use of individual dependent t-tests can greatly enhance the power of the statistical analysis.

Another statistic that is useful in describing the relationship between the experimental manipulation and the observed effect is strength of association measures. For t-tests, η^2 is the appropriate measure (see Linton & Gallo, 1975), and the values of this statistic for each of the comparisons are shown in Table 1. The mean (±SEM) proportion of variance associated with treatment across all groups was 67.6% (±3.5%) for drug treatment, 9.2% (±5.4%)

for saline treatment, and the mean strength of association between groups was 26.4% (±3.2%). The mean strength of association measure based on the between groups t-tests is very close to the strength of association measure based on the ANOVA (ω^2 = 24%; see Linton & Gallo, 1975; Winer, 1971). Although the strength of association measure for the between groups comparisons may not appear to be very large, Linton and Gallo (1975) suggest that most studies fail to account for more than 10% of the variance due to treatment effects. Thus, the overall strength of association for the between groups differences is acceptable.

Stability of Preconditioning Preferences

One factor to consider when assessing the validity of conditioned place preference studies is the stability of the subjects' preconditioning preferences. If these scores were not stable, then shifts in preference might not accurately reflect appetitive conditioning; but, rather, they might result from spontaneous changes in the preconditioning measures. Although the data presented in Figure 1 would suggest that such spontaneous shifts are not significant, an examination of the stability of these scores would help to define the characteristics of place preference testing.

To assess the stability of these preconditioning place preferences, a group of 20 animals was tested for 15 minutes per day for four 5-day blocks of testing. These subjects had free access to the entire shuttle box, and testing was on consecutive 5-day intervals with two days of no testing intervening between each block. Figure 2 reveals that the measure of preconditioning place preference displayed little variation across repeated testing. A similar effect was noted for the measure of locomotor activity (i.e., crosses, data not shown). The mean amount of time spent on the tubular side of the test apparatus was much higher than that spent on the smooth side. An examination of the preconditioning preferences across a large number of groups (i.e., the last trial of the 5-day preconditioning sequence) revealed that this preference is consistent across different groups of experimental subjects tested during the past several years (data not shown).

Dose-Response Analysis

One of the factors that has been shown to influence the strength of a conditioned response is the magnitude of the unconditioned stimulus. In general, increasing the dose of drug tested results in an increase in the behavioral response produced. Following 5 days of preconditioning trials, several groups of rats (n = 19/group) were injected with heroin (0.03 to 1.0 mg/kg) and conditioned for three 30-minute conditioning trials. Various doses of heroin were tested to determine if a graded response might be produced. The data were analyzed by subtracting each subject's preconditioning score from the time spent on the conditioning side during the test trial.

Figure 3 illustrates the influence of drug dosage on the magnitude of the conditioned place preference. The two lowest doses failed to produce a significant place preference as shown by individual t-tests with α^* = 0.01 [t's (18) = 1.113 & 2.229, p's < 0.5 & 0.05, respectively]. The remaining three doses all produced significant shifts in place preference [t's (18) = 4.153 to 5.356, p's < 0.001]. The strength of association measures (computed from the individual dependent t-tests) were: 7%, 21.6%, 48.9%, 59.2%, and 61.4% in ascending dose order. As can be seen in the figure, there is a shallow, but

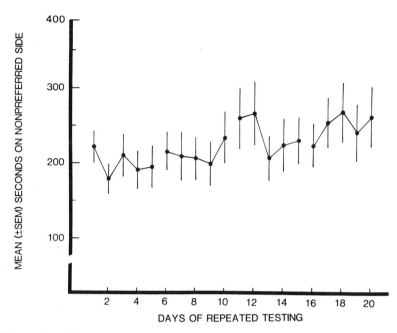

Figure 2: Stability of preconditioning place preference across 20 days of testing. Animals were allowed free access to the test apparatus for 15 minutes per day. The graph shows the mean (±SEM) time spent on the smooth side of the test apparatus.

statistically significant, dose-response effect [$F_{(4,90)} = 4.592$, $p < 0.005$] with little evidence of conditioning produced by 0.03 mg/kg and maximum conditioning produced by 0.3 mg/kg. These data suggest that the conditioning is sensitive to drug dosage, but that there is relatively little difference between the threshold response and maximum response using this conditioning protocol.

Influence of Number of Conditioning Trials

Another variable that has been shown to influence the strength of a conditioned response is the number of stimulus-response pairings. To determine if the number of conditioning trials affected the subsequent conditioned place preference, rats (n = 11 to 12/group) were injected with heroin (0.3 mg/kg) and conditioned for 30 minutes as in the previous experiments. Three groups of subjects were conditioned for one, three, or ten such conditioning trials. Other animals were injected with saline (1 ml/kg) and conditioned for the same number of trials to determine if habituation to the nonpreferred side would affect the measure of place preference.

As with the dose-response analysis, increasing the number of conditioning trials seemed to have little effect on the measure of conditioned place preference [Drug: $F_{(1,66)} = 28.221$, $p < 0.001$; Trials, $F_{(2,66)} = 1.424$, $p > 0.1$]. Despite the failure to find a significant effect for the factor of

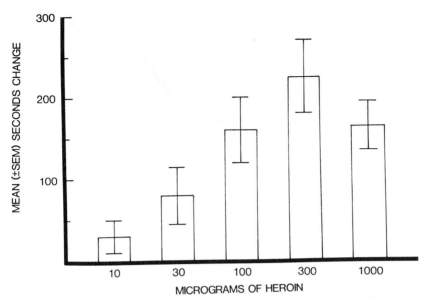

Figure 3: Dose-response analysis of heroin-induced conditioned place preference. The figure shows the mean (±SEM) shifts in place preference after conditioning with various doses of heroin.

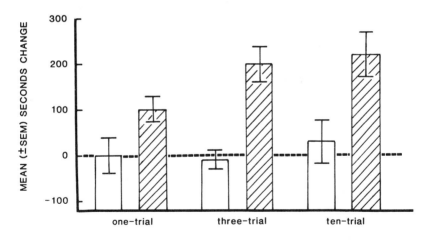

NUMBER OF CONDITIONING TRIALS

Figure 4: Effect of the number of conditioning trials on the strength of the conditioned place preference. The figure shows the mean (±SEM) change in place preference. Striped bars, heroin conditioned; open bars, saline conditioned.

Number of Trials or a significant Drug x Trial interaction [F (2,66) = 0.808, p > 0.1], subjects conditioned for three trials appeared to show a stronger conditioned place preference than subjects receiving only one conditioning trial. This impression is supported by a comparison of the strength of association measures (based on the dependent t-tests) for the one- and three-trial conditioning durations (48% and 65%, respectively). Extending the number of conditioning trials to ten, however, clearly failed to produce a stronger conditioned response (strength of association = 65%).

Influence of Conditioning Trial Duration

The duration of exposure to the unconditioned stimulus is another variable that might influence the magnitude of conditioning seen with this procedure. Longer or shorter conditioning trials might alter the strength of the conditioned place preference. To test this hypothesis, rats (n = 15/group) were injected with heroin (0.3 mg/kg) and conditioned for either 10, 30, or 100 minutes for a total of three conditioning trials. Other groups of rats were conditioned for the same length of time with saline (1 ml/kg) injections. This latter procedure should assess the influence of habituation on any changes in place preference seen with varying the duration of the conditioning trials.

There was an effect for the factor of Drug Treatment [F (1,88) = 6.847, p < 0.05], but neither the factor associated with Trial Duration [F (2,84) = 0.199, p > 0.1] nor the Drug x Duration interaction [F (2,84) = 1.222, p > 0.1] was significant. Subjects conditioned for 10 and 30 minutes showed comparable magnitudes of change in place preference. The rats conditioned for 30 minutes, however, were more uniform in their place preferences as reflected by the variances associated with these two conditioning durations (see Figure 5). Subjects conditioned for 100 minutes appeared to display less preference than subjects conditioned for the two shorter periods of time. This is reflected in the strength of association measures for these three trial durations: 49%, 82%, and 39%, respectively. It is likely that the rewarding drug effect did not last for the entire 100-minute period and that exposure to the conditioning

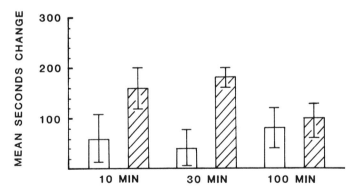

CONDITIONING DURATION

Figure 5: Influence of the duration of individual conditioning trials on the strength of the conditioned response. The figure shows the mean (±SEM) change in place preference. Striped bars, heroin conditioned; open bars, saline conditioned.

environment without this drug action attenuated the conditioned place preference. Alternatively, some aversive effect may accompany the termination of the rewarding drug effect, and this might decrease the net place preference seen with 100-minute conditioning periods. Saline-conditioned rats showed no systematic changes in their place preferences as a function of the duration of the conditioning trials. Thus, habituation to the test apparatus is not likely to be an important factor influencing the animal's place preference.

Effect of Pre-exposure to the Conditioned Stimulus

For a stimulus to serve as an effective conditioned stimulus, it is important that this stimulus be salient during the conditioning trials. Pre-exposure to the test apparatus, which occurs during the preconditioning trials, might decrease the effectiveness of the conditioning environment in serving as a conditioned stimulus. As in the previous studies, rats (n = 7 to 8/group) were injected with heroin (0.3 mg/kg) and conditioned using the standard three-trial conditioning procedure. Other rats were conditioned with saline (1 ml/kg). In this experiment, however, no preconditioning trials were conducted so that the subjects' first exposure to the conditioning environment occurred with the initial presentation of the unconditioned stimulus (i.e., heroin or saline injections).

Figure 6 illustrates the place preferences for rats conditioned with heroin and with saline. Because the preconditioning place preferences were not determined, the data represent the time spent on the conditioning side rather than shifts in place preference. Furthermore, the data are illustrated separately for subjects conditioned on the smooth side of the apparatus (i.e., normally nonpreferred side) and for subjects conditioned on the tubular side of the apparatus (i.e., normally preferred side). For both the heroin- and saline-conditioned subjects, there was a strong preference for the tubular side of the apparatus following conditioning trials [F (1,26) = 169.253, p < 0.001]. A significant change in place preference developed in rats conditioned on what

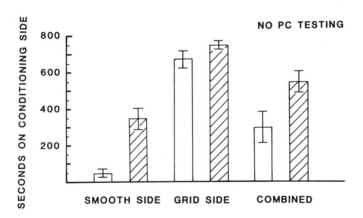

Figure 6: Conditioned place preference seen with no pre-exposure to the test apparatus. Subjects were conditioned using the standard procedure, but no preconditioning trials were conducted. The figure shows the mean (±SEM) time spent on the conditioning side. Striped bars, heroin conditioned; open bars, saline conditioned.

would normally be their nonpreferred side of the test apparatus, while conditioning on the normally preferred side was not effective in altering place preference. The combined results of this experiment suggest that an overall shift in place preference was produced in rats with no prior exposure to the conditioning environment [F (1,26) = 12.863, p < 0.005]. There was a significant Drug x Side interaction [F (1,26) = 13.641, p < 0.005].

The magnitude of the change in preference seen in this experiment appeared somewhat greater than that produced with the usual testing procedure. Figure 1 shows that the standard conditioning procedure produced changes in place preferences ranging from 100 to 200 seconds greater than saline conditioning. Without pre-exposure, heroin-conditioned subjects spent about 250 seconds more on the conditioning side than did saline-conditioned subjects (see Figure 6, combined data). This suggests that a slight increase in the shift in place preference is seen when subjects are not pre-exposed to the conditioning apparatus.

Type of Conditioning

The results of the dose-response analysis and of the experiments concerning the number of conditioning trials, the duration of individual conditioning trials, and conditioning without pre-exposure to the test apparatus were rather disappointing. Although there was some indication of an effect for these manipulations (as would be predicted based on data from classical conditioning experiments), these procedures failed to markedly influence the maximum change in place preference demonstrable with this technique. In fact, ANOVAs failed to reveal significant effects for most of these experimental manipulations, and effects were shown only as changes in strength of association measures. Thus, the data suggest that conditioned place preference studies produce a weak, albeit reliable, index of drug reward.

Animals conditioned with heroin in the previous experiments only had experience with drug in the conditioning side of the apparatus. It might be that contrasting the drug conditioning with experience in the other compartment after saline injections would enhance the preference for the side associated with the drug effect. This discrimination training was investigated in two ways. One group (n = 11) was injected with saline (1 ml/kg), placed on one side of the shuttle box for 30 minutes and then injected with heroin (0.3 mg/kg) and placed on the other side for another 30 minutes. This procedure was repeated once a day for a total of three days. Another group of subjects (n = 12) received heroin (0.3 mg/kg) in the conditioning side of the apparatus for 30 minutes on one day and was injected with saline (1 ml/kg) and placed in the other side for 30 minutes on alternate days. This procedure was repeated three times so that the number of conditioning trials with heroin was equal to that used in the previous experiments. Groups conditioned with saline in both compartments, either within (n = 12) or between (n = 9) sessions, were also tested using this same protocol as were groups under the standard three-trial, drug-only conditioning procedure (n = 14/group). Other groups (n = 15/group) received heroin (0.3 mg/kg) or saline (1 ml/kg) and were allowed free access to both compartments for 30 minutes during each of three conditioning trials.

Significant changes in place preference were seen in both groups receiving heroin and conditioned with discrimination training [Contrast-1, t (11) = 4.493, p < 0.001; Contrast-2, t (10) = 4.939, p < 0.001], while saline injections did not significantly modify place preferences seen with this conditioning procedure [Contrast-1, t (11) = 1.333, p > 0.1; Contrast-2, t (8)

= 1.677, p > 0.05]. Nonassociative conditioning did not produce reliable shifts in either the heroin-treated [t (14) = 1.033, p > 0.1] or the saline-treated [t (14) = 1.181, p > 0.1] groups. The group conditioned with heroin using the standard procedure also showed a significant shift in place preference [t (13) = 4.874, p < 0.001] while the subjects conditioned with saline did not significantly change their place preference [t (13) = 0.973, p > 0.1].

Contrasting the effects of saline with those of heroin did not result in a greater change in preference for either the group receiving saline and heroin conditioning on alternate days or for the group receiving saline and heroin conditioning on the same days. This was surprising because experience with saline in one compartment and heroin in the other would be expected to enhance the contrast, and subsequent preference, for the two compartments. Experiments in classical and operant conditioning have shown that stimulus discrimination can be enhanced by training with similar, but perceptually distinct, stimuli.

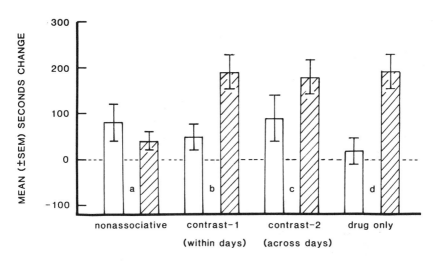

TYPE OF CONDITIONING

Figure 7: Effect of type of conditioning on the magnitude of the conditioned place preference. Nonassociative conditioning represents data from subjects that were not restricted to one compartment in the conditioning apparatus (i.e., were allowed to move freely in both the smooth and tubular sides). Contrast-1 represents subjects that received discrimination training with heroin- and saline-conditioning occurring on the same day. Contrast-2 represents animals that received discrimination training with heroin- and saline-conditioning occurring on alternate days. Drug-only conditioning represents the standard conditioning procedure where subjects did not receive discrimination training. Striped bars, heroin conditioned; open bars, saline conditioned.

Use of an Olfactory Cue

Increasing the salient cues on the conditioning side might be expected to enhance the conditioning seen with this procedure. Because rats are particularly responsive to olfactory cues, a distinctive odor was paired with one side of the apparatus (i.e., the smooth side). Preconditioning place preferences were measured, and rats subsequently conditioned with heroin (0.3 mg/kg, n = 15) or saline (1 ml/kg, n = 14) using the standard conditioning procedure. In addition to the textural cues normally present, three drops of 10% acetic acid were placed on the extreme end of the conditioning side of the apparatus. The odor cue was present throughout all phases of the experiment-- preconditioning, conditioning, and testing.

Reliable shifts in place preference were seen following conditioning with heroin [t (14) = 4.689, p < 0.001] but not following conditioning with saline [t (13) = 0.976, p > 0.1]. The magnitude of the preference change, however, did not appear to be affected by the addition of the olfactory cue. Also, it is interesting to note that the acetic acid cue had little influence on the preconditioning place preferences in these two groups of rats; the subjects spent about 27% of the time on the side associated with the olfactory cue compared with a mean of around 30% of the time for most experiments that did not have an olfactory cue.

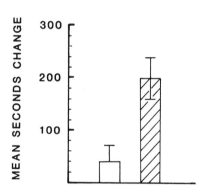

Figure 8: Changes in place preference associated with both textural and olfactory cues. Animals were conditioned using the standard procedure except for the addition of an acetic acid odor on the conditioning side. Striped bars, heroin conditioned; open bars, saline conditioned.

Temporal Analysis of Place Preference

The failure to increase the conditioned change in place preference beyond that produced by the initial conditioning procedure was very surprising. One possible explanation is that the subjects display their maximum change in place preference during the initial minutes of testing and that the remaining test period serves to extinguish the conditioned change in place preferences. That is, the subjects may show a strong conditioned place preference during the first few minutes of testing followed by a return to the preconditioning preferences for the test apparatus. The net place preference would thus include both an initially strong manifestation of conditioning and a later return to the subjects' preconditioning preferences; the average would yield only a modest overall shift for the total test period.

To test this possibility, subjects (n = 20/group) were conditioned with heroin (0.3 mg/kg) or saline (1 ml/kg) for 30 minutes during three conditioning trials. During the test trial, preferences were measured every minute for the duration of the usual 15-minute test period. This temporal analysis of place preference should reveal any decline in preference for the conditioning side as a function of response extinction.

There was a significant effect for Drug Treatment [F (1,570) = 38.221, p < 0.001] with no significant effect associated with Test Period [F (14,570) = 0.72, p > 0.1] or any Treatment x Period interaction [F (14,570) = 0.829, p > 0.1]. The change in place preference produced by heroin-conditioning showed little change over the first ten minutes of testing (see Figure 9). There was no indication that the subjects spent the majority of time on the conditioning side during the first few minutes of testing. The slight decrease in conditioned place preference seen for the last 5 minutes of testing suggests that tests limited to 10 rather than the usual 15-minute period might reveal a somewhat stronger conditioning effect. However, this is unlikely to have a major influence on the strength of the measured shift in place preference.

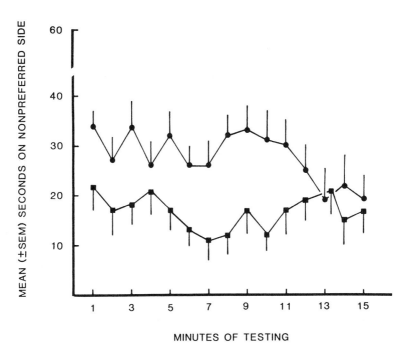

Figure 9: Changes in place preference within a single 15-minute test period. Each data point depicts the mean (±SEM) time spent on the conditioning side for consecutive 60-second intervals. Circles represent heroin-conditioned subjects, and squares represent saline-conditioned subjects.

Alternative Explanations for Shifts in "Place Preference"

The fact that manipulations that influence classical conditioning have little or no effect on the conditioned place preference questions the basis of this phenomenon. Although the dose of drug and number of conditioning trials did affect place preference, these effects were minimal and other variables might account for the apparent shift in place preference following repeated injections of heroin.

Regression Toward the Mean

One factor that might be involved in the increased time spent on the side of putative conditioning is regression toward the mean. Because subjects are usually conditioned on their nonpreferred sides of the test apparatus, spontaneous shifts in the measure of place preference might occur during subsequent testing. An examination of the stability of the preconditioning preferences, however, makes this an unlikely explanation of the shifts in preference. Subjects demonstrated stable preconditioning preferences for 20 days of repeated testing (see Figure 2). Also, animals receiving saline during the conditioning trials failed to show a reliable shift in place preference (see Figure 1) further indicating that spontaneous shifts in preference are not an adequate explanation of this effect.

Habituation or Anxiolytic Drug Action

The strong preference displayed for one side of the test apparatus during the preconditioning trials might also reflect an aversion to the other side. It could be the case that novelty or some other factor inhibits the exploration of the smooth side of the chamber and that forced habituation or the experience of anxiolytic drug effects might decrease the initial aversion to that side. This is consistent with the observation that animals rarely spend over 50% of the time on the smooth side even after heroin conditioning.

The results of the experiment that assessed the influence of the number of conditioning trials is relevant to this alternative explanation of conditioned place preference. Note that in Figure 4, increasing the number of conditioning trials from one to three and to ten did not increase the amount of time saline-conditioned subjects spent on the nonpreferred side. This suggests that forced habituation cannot account for the shift in place preference seen following heroin conditioning. Anxiolytic drug effects would also seem unlikely to account for the observed shifts in place preference because at least a modest decrease in anxiety would be expected following the forced habituation trials. Also, a recent study has shown that diazepam (which has only equivocal rewarding properties, see de Wit & Johanson, this volume; Weeks & Collins, this volume) does not produce a shift in place preference (G. Carr, personal communication, but see Spyraki, Kazandjian, & Varonos, 1985). Because diazepam is a potent anxiolytic agent, this observation appears to directly eliminate anxiolytic effects as a possible explanation of place preference conditioning.

Locomotor Activity

Another potential explanation for the shift in place preference is also related to the strong preconditioning preferences shown by subjects with this procedure. Because the animals spend very little time on the side which will be subsequently used for conditioning and because the change in preference following conditioning seldom results in subjects spending over half of the test trial on the side of putative conditioning, any increase in general activity might be expected to increase the amount of time spent on the nonpreferred side of the apparatus. That is, if the animals increase their locomotor activity, this might result in their spending more time on the nonpreferred side of the shuttle box due to simple exploration.

One way to test this possibility is to increase the subjects' locomotor activity and to measure the amount of time spent on the usual side of conditioning (i.e., nonpreferred side). Subjects (n = 18/group) were given five preconditioning trials, and the last trial served as a measure of the subjects' place preferences. Next, they were injected with either saline (1 ml/kg) or amphetamine (1.0 or 3.0 mg/kg, i.p., 20 minutes prior to testing), and shuttle activity was measured along with the amount of time spent on the smooth side of the test apparatus. The scores derived from this procedure were treated as place preference scores even though the animals never received any conditioning trials and they were tested under the motor-stimulating effect of amphetamine.

The changes in pseudo-place preference are shown in Figure 10. Amphetamine produced a dose-dependent increase in the number of crosses during the 15-minute test trial [$F_{(2,51)}$ = 17.639, $p < 0.001$]; slight, but statistically significant, increases in the amount of time spent on the nonpreferred side of the apparatus were also noted [t's (17) = 2.447 & 2.465, p's < 0.025], although this effect was not dose-dependent [$F_{(2,51)}$ = 1.889, $p > 0.1$]. This suggests that increased activity can influence measures of place preference, but this effect was weak in the present experiment (strength of association = 26%). Nonetheless, the potentially confounding influence of locomotor activity on the measurement of place preference illustrates the importance of assessing changes in locomotor activity during testing.

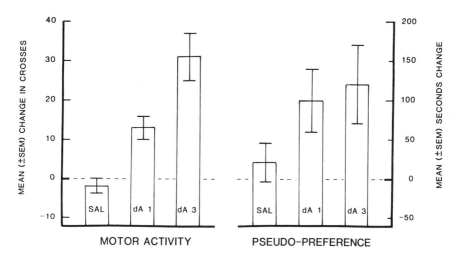

Figure 10: Changes in "pseudo-preference" associated with increases in locomotor activity. The panel on the left shows the changes in locomotor activity produced by amphetamine (dA) injections, while the panel on the right depicts changes in the amount of time spent on the nonpreferred side of the test apparatus during the period of increased locomotor activity.

Large increases in locomotor activity produce marginal shifts in place preference measurement, but the magnitude of this effect is too weak to account for the conditioned place preference seen in most studies. Also, an analysis of locomotor scores obtained from subjects tested in the previous experiments shows only occasional increases in locomotor activity, with the majority of place preferences produced without any concomitant change in motor activity. One group that did show a significant increase in locomotor activity was the group receiving 0.3 mg/kg of heroin in the dose-response analysis (see Figure 3). This group had a mean (±SEM) increase of 7.1 (±1.32) crosses during the 15-minute test period. Although this effect was significant [t (18) = 5.379, p < 0.001], an analysis of the relationship between the increased locomotor activity and the increased time spent on the side of conditioning revealed no significant correlation [r (18) = .105, p > 0.05]. Thus, even in cases where significant changes in locomotor activity do occur, increases in the number of crosses are an unlikely explanation of the increase in time spent on the nonpreferred side of the apparatus.

Cue Reinstatement

The fact that several alternative explanations of place preference described in the preceding section cannot account for this effect supports the notion that this technique can assess the rewarding action of a drug. The failure to find robust effects for factors known to influence classical conditioning, however, questions the conditioning basis of this phenomenon and emphasizes the importance of identifying the factors responsible for limiting the magnitude of conditioning demonstrable with this technique.

Some of the procedures described in the preceding sections were designed to make the conditioned response stronger by increasing the saliency of the environmental stimuli associated with the drug reward. Perhaps the most salient stimulus associated with the rewarding drug-effect is the drug cue itself. That is, the internal stimuli associated with the presence of the drug during conditioning may be the most prominent. These stimuli may be directly related to the rewarding properties of the drug or they may be secondary effects that are simply associated with its presence (e.g., autonomic side-effects, changes in thermoregulation). The purpose of the present study was to determine if testing the subjects under the drug condition would increase the magnitude of the conditioned shift in place preference.

The rats were habituated to the test apparatus for 15 minutes a day for five days. The last day of this series served as a measure of each subject's initial place preference as in the earlier experiments. Next, they received daily injections of heroin (0.3 mg/kg, n = 12) or saline (1 ml/kg, n = 11) and were forced to remain on their nonpreferred side for 30 minutes during three conditioning trials. On the following day, all subjects were injected with saline and tested for changes in place preference during a single 15-minute trial. One day later, each group was injected with the agent used during conditioning (i.e., either heroin or saline) and place preference was measured again.

As shown in the previous studies, heroin injections produced a shift in place preference when the subjects were tested following saline injections [F (1,21) = 19.901, p < 0.001]. When tested following heroin injections, the magnitude of place preference was appreciably greater [F (1,21) = 7.981, p < 0.012]. Figure 11 illustrates the place preference seen across the two measurements. Heroin-conditioned animals spent significantly more time on the drug-associated side than the saline-conditioned subjects [F (1,21) = 12.459, p < 0.001]; the factor of Trials was also significant [F (2,42) = 12.960, p < 0.001] as was the Drug x Trial interaction [F (2,42) = 9.958, p < 0.001]. The changes in place preference were not associated with a reliable change in locomotor activity [F's (1,21) = 0.843 and 1.573, p's > 0.05]. The subjects spent over half of the test time on the side of conditioning when tested under the drug state but not when tested following saline injections (see Figure 12).

When the data were analyzed in terms of the number of subjects showing an absolute preference for the side of conditioning (i.e., spending > 450 seconds on that side), none of the heroin-conditioned subjects during the preconditioning trial and none of the saline-conditioned subjects on any of their three trials spent over half of the total test time on the side of putative conditioning. In the heroin-conditioned group, an absolute preference was demonstrated in 27% of the subjects when tested in the saline state and in 82% of the subjects when the heroin cue was reinstated [χ^2 (2) = 19.56, p < 0.005].

This study shows that a true (i.e., absolute) place preference can be produced in subjects tested under the drug cue. This effect parallels human studies showing that craving is most pronounced when drug is believed to be available (Meyer & Mirin, 1979) and animal studies demonstrating a reinstatement of lever-pressing following priming injections of drug (de Wit & Stewart, 1983; Stewart & de Wit, this volume). Although the exact nature of this effect is not clear, it is possible that overshadowing limits the place preference demonstrable in subjects tested in the drug-free state. If a strong

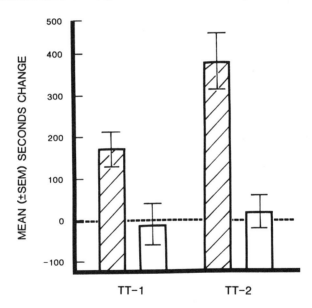

Figure 11: Changes in place preference without (TT-1) and with (TT-2) reinstatement of the drug cue during testing. The data depict mean (±SEM) changes from preconditioning place preferences; the animals were conditioned with the usual conditioning procedure. Striped bars, heroin conditioned; open bars, saline conditioned.

association were developed between the rewarding drug effect and some interoceptive drug cue, this might limit the strength of the response elicited by environmental cues alone. Hence, the absence of the most salient cue (i.e., the interoceptive drug cue) might explain some of the apparent anomalies observed with most procedures used for assessing conditioned place preference.

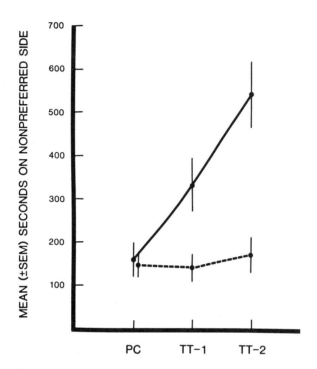

Figure 12: Changes in place preference without (TT-1) and with (TT-2) reinstatement of the drug cue during testing. The data represent the mean (±SEM) time spent on the side of conditioning, with a total test duration of 900 seconds. Solid line, heroin conditioned; dashed line, saline conditioned.

OTHER CONSIDERATIONS

There are a number of other factors that are interesting to examine regarding place preference studies. This section explores some of these factors in an attempt to better understand the basic phenomenon and to help define limitations inherent with this approach to the study of drug reward.

Effect of Home Cage Injections

It has been suggested that the changes in place preference seen with place preference conditioning studies may be unrelated to associative conditioning. That is, shifts in place preference may not depend on a learned association

Figure 13: Effects of home cage injections on place preference. The standard experimental procedure was used, except three daily drug injections were given in the home cage, and the drug effects were never paired with the test apparatus. Abbreviations: Sal, saline; PMZ, pimozide; PMZ & HEROIN, pimozide plus heroin.

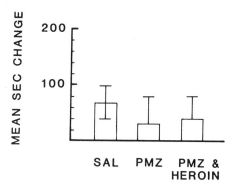

between specific environmental cues and the rewarding action of a drug. One study (Blander, Hunt, Blair, & Amit, 1984) reported a significant shift in place preference following drug injections that were not paired with the environment used to assess place preference. The possibility that place preferences may significantly shift without specific conditioning is potentially a serious problem with place conditioning studies and merits further consideration.

The stability of the preconditioning place preferences illustrated in Figure 2 indicates that large spontaneous shifts in place preference are unlikely to occur with repeated testing. The initial place preference of these rats was stable across 20 days of repeated testing. The experiment summarized in Figure 7 shows that drug injections followed by access to the entire test chamber do not significantly affect place preference. If drug injections caused a shift in place preference independent of explicitly pairing the drug effect with a specific environment, then changes in place preference should have occurred in this study.

Although no attempt has been made to replicate the report of shifts in place preference following rewarding drug injections in an environment other than the one used to measure place preference, a similar condition was tested as part of a control procedure for another study. In this experiment initial place preferences were measured using the standard procedure. Three groups of rats (n = 20/group) then received home cage injections of saline (1 ml/kg), pimozide (0.5 mg/kg), or pimozide (0.5 mg/kg) plus heroin (0.5 mg/kg). After three days of injections, place preferences were remeasured and the data scored in the usual manner even though the drug injections were never paired with the test apparatus. Figure 13 shows the results of this procedure.

There were no significant shifts in place preference for any of the three groups [t's (19) = 0.635 to 1.074, p's > 0.1]. Although this test did not use rewarding drug injections (presuming, of course, that the pimozide injections blocked the heroin reward; see Bozarth & Wise, 1981), drug injections in the home cage failed to modify place preferences. This suggests that neither the handling associated with the injection routine nor a general psychotropic drug action influences the animals' place preferences, and this further corroborates the conclusion from the earlier experiment showing that nonassociative conditioning is insufficient to explain the shifts in place preference.

Stress-Induced Place Preference

Across a large number of studies using essentially the same conditioning procedure, saline-treated animals occasionally showed surprisingly large changes in place preference (see Figures 1, 5, & 7). Although these shifts in place preference can occur without any conditioning trials (as shown in Figures 7 & 13), some groups of saline-treated animals that showed particularly notable shifts appeared to be more difficult to handle than animals not showing such shifts. The possibility exists that handling procedures may vary across different groups of rats (or even within a group of rats) and that differences in handling can influence the place preferences seen after conditioning. Because endogenous opioid peptides can be released by stress and these opioids have also been implicated in motivated behavior (e.g., see Reid, this volume), it is possible that saline-treated animals sometimes experience a rewarding effect from the stress-induced release of these peptides. In this experiment, the ability of a mild stressor to produce a change in place preference was assessed. Pretreatment with a narcotic antagonist (i.e., naloxone) during the conditioning trials was used to determine if any stress-induced effects were dependent on an endogenous opioid peptide.

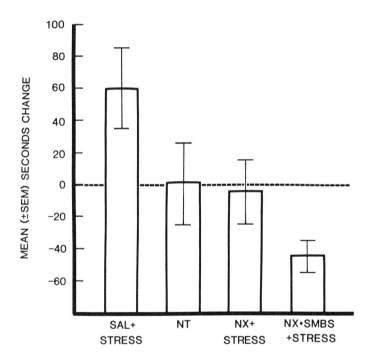

Figure 14: Place preference following a mild stress. Animals were treated with saline (SAL + STRESS), naloxone (NX + STRESS), or naloxone dissolved in an acidic solution (NX*SMBS + STRESS). Other animals were gently placed in the conditioning compartment without any stress or injections (NT).

In this laboratory, animals that are difficult to handle are frequently rocked in a swinging motion just prior to drug injections. This procedure makes the animal docile and facilitates drug injections in active animals. In this experiment preconditioning place preferences were assessed in the usual way for 5 days. Next, three groups of rats (n = 19/group) were rocked in a swinging motion (i.e., gently swinging the arm back and forth) for five repetitions and then injected with saline (1 ml/kg), saline plus naloxone (3 mg/kg), or saline plus naloxone (3 mg/kg) dissolved in sodium metabisulfite (0.1%) which made the solution acidic. A 30-minute conditioning trial immediately followed these injections. Another group of rats (n = 19) were placed in the conditioning compartment without any treatment. After three conditioning trials, place preference was remeasured using a 15-minute trial.

Figure 14 shows the changes in place preference following conditioning. A slight shift in preference was seen after saline injections [t (18) = 2.701, p < 0.02], and this shift was not present in animals injected with naloxone [t (18) = 0.133, p > 0.8]. Injections of naloxone dissolved in an acidic solution produced a strong place aversion [t (18) = 3.101, p < 0.01]. Animals that were simply placed in the conditioning compartment without "rocking" or injections showed no change in place preference [t (18) = 0.145, p > 0.8]. Although the stress-induced change in place preference is very small, it could explain some of the shifts seen in saline-treated animals during the other experiments and illustrates the potential importance of handling procedures in place preference studies. Furthermore, the fact that this shift in preference is blocked by naloxone suggests that endogenous opioid peptides may be important in this effect. The place aversion produced by injections of an acidic naloxone solution shows that drug vehicle and pH can seriously affect place preference and that the drug-vehicle control condition should always be tested concurrently with the experimental groups.

Place Preference with Visual Cues Only

The place preference technique used throughout this chapter employs what has been termed an "unbalanced" procedure (see van der Kooy, this volume). The animals show strong preconditioning place preferences and conditioning is usually done on the nonpreferred side of the test apparatus. The potential side bias inherent with this procedure could produce changes in place preference that are dependent on this initial side preference and not related to the rewarding drug effect. Although the alternative explanations that appear most viable (i.e., habituation, anxiolytic drug action, increased locomotor activity) are insufficient to explain the changes in preference that are seen with this technique (see earlier section), the facts that a "true" place preference is usually not seen following drug conditioning and the possibility that an unbalanced procedure could be measuring an effect other than a rewarding drug action make the test of place preference in a balanced test apparatus important.

The test apparatus was modified so that both sides contained the same type of tubular stainless steel floor. Horizontal black stripes (1 inch wide) were painted on one side of the shuttle box and the other walls remained unpainted. Four groups of rats (n = 10/group) received five 15-minute preconditioning trials and the last trial served as a measure of their preconditioning place preferences. Next, one group received heroin injections (0.3 mg/kg) and were forced to remain on one side of the apparatus for 30 minutes; half of the animals were conditioned on the side with horizontal stripes and half were conditioned on the side without stripes. A second group of rats were treated identically, except saline (1 ml/kg) was injected during the conditioning trials. A third group received discrimination training where saline (1 ml/kg) injections were paired with one side for 30 minutes and followed by heroin (0.3 mg/kg) injections paired with the other side for 30 minutes; half of the rats received saline injections on the side with horizontal stripes and heroin injections on the other side while half of the rats were conditioned with saline injections on the unstriped side and heroin injections on the striped side. A fourth group received conditioning trials with saline on both sides of the apparatus. Two additional groups (n = 10/group) did not receive preconditioning trials and were simply injected with either heroin (0.3 mg/kg) or saline (1 ml/kg) and forced to remain in one compartment for 30 minutes; half of each group was conditioned on the striped side and half on the plain side of the shuttle box.

The use of identical floor textures on both sides of the apparatus produced a procedure with no strong preconditioning preferences (i.e., initial side preferences were balanced). For subjects that received preconditioning trials, the mean (±SEM) time spent on the striped side increased slightly from 411.2 ± 32.8 seconds out of a total test duration of 900 seconds on the first trial to 531.3 ± 38.2 on the last preconditioning trial. Furthermore, because half of the subjects were conditioned on the striped side and half conditioned on the plain side, the side used for drug conditioning was also balanced. Thus this procedure balanced both the initial side preferences and the side used for drug conditioning.

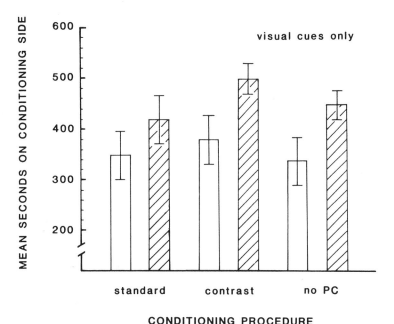

Figure 15: Place preference associated with only visual cues using a "balanced" procedure. Striped bars, heroin conditioned; open bars, saline conditioned.

Subjects conditioned with heroin using the contrast method [i.e., discrimination training; t (18) = 2.148, p < 0.025] or conditioned without preconditioning trials [t (18) = 2.180, p < 0.025] showed reliable shifts in place preferences. Animals conditioned using the standard conditioning procedure, however, failed to show a significant change in place preference [t (18) = 1.119, p > 0.1; see Figure 15]. The only group to show an absolute place preference (i.e., spending over 450 seconds on the drug-associated side) following conditioning was the group conditioned using discrimination training.

When the changes in place preferences seen with the standard conditioning procedure were assessed in reference to which side of the test apparatus the subjects received their conditioning trials, a slight shift in place preference was seen when the subjects were conditioned on the striped side but no change in preference was seen when the subjects were conditioned on the plain side (see Figure 16). It appears that this conditioning procedure was not effective when subjects were conditioned in the absence of the strong visual cue associated with the striped end of the shuttle box. When the data from the contrast conditioning procedure were examined as a function of the conditioning side, a conditioned place preference was seen following conditioning on either the striped or plain side of the apparatus (see Figure 17). In this case the subjects had experience with the striped end whether drug conditioning occurred there or in the other compartment. This probably produces a strong discrimination that is reflected by the place preference either toward or away from the striped cue. A similar effect was seen in animals that did not receive preconditioning trials (data not shown).

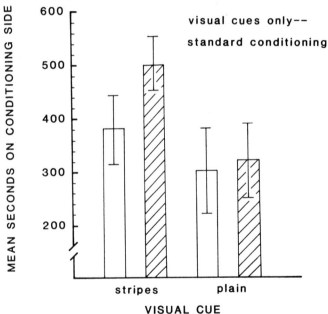

Figure 16: Conditioned place preference associated with only visual cues using the standard (drug only) conditioning procedure. Animals conditioned on the striped side and the plain side are shown separately. Striped bars, heroin conditioned; open bars, saline conditioned.

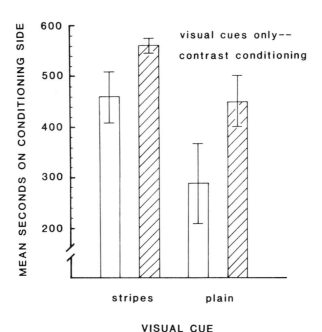

Figure 17: Changes in place preference associated with visual cues only in animals that received discrimination training. Animals conditioned on the striped side or plain side are shown separately. Striped bars, heroin conditioned; open bars, saline conditioned.

GENERAL DISCUSSION

The results of most experiments reported in this chapter were surprising in several ways. First, they failed to reveal strong effects for factors that have been shown to influence classical conditioning. Although there is some indication of a dose-response function, some influence of the number and duration of conditioning trials, and a small effect of pre-exposure to the conditioned stimulus, these manipulations were ineffective in causing a major change in the magnitude of the conditioned place preference. Second, the initial work in this laboratory reported a conditioned place preference from heroin (Bozarth & Wise, 1981) that was based on somewhat arbitrarily selected parameters. The magnitude of this preference remains the same as that produced by more careful selection of testing parameters. Although the strength of association measures reveal that a reasonable proportion of variance is explained by the experimental manipulation, it is disappointing that few of the procedures examined in this chapter produced a significant increase in this measure. Third, similar strengths of conditioning are produced by various laboratories using markedly different procedures as well as by the different conditioning procedures examined in this chapter. Even with different compounds and different routes of administration (e.g., peripheral vs. central injections), most studies report a shift in place preference around 100 to 200 seconds. This is surprising given the variety of methods and drugs that are used in conditioned place preference studies.

Central Topics

There has been considerable discussion regarding "the right way and the wrong way" to conduct conditioned place preference studies. Some investigators suggest that they employ the only method of place preference conditioning that works. Although their logic appears sound and the conclusions they reach sensible, little empirical data are offered to support the strong assertions made by these investigators. The series of experiments reported in this chapter systematically examined variables that seemed likely to influence place preference conditioning. None of these manipulations produced dramatic changes in the observed behavior, except the experiment involving reinstatement of the drug cue. Thus, the present data argue that there is no one method of place preference conditioning that is obviously superior to the other methods used by the various laboratories. Nonetheless, a procedure where the initial side preferences and the side of drug-conditioning are fully balanced may be advantageous (e.g., Mucha, van der Kooy, O'Shaughnessy, & Bucenieks, 1982; van der Kooy, this volume), although the lack of proper "balancing" does not invalidate the conclusions based on other (i.e., unbalanced) conditioned place preference procedures.

Most place preference experiments involve procedures where animals have strong initial preferences for one side of the apparatus. The subjects are usually conditioned on their nonpreferred sides, and a conditioned place preference is reported when a significant increase in the amount of time spent on the drug conditioning side occurs. Even after conditioning, however, the subjects seldom spend over half of the total test time on the conditioning side. Because of this, two controversial issues have emerged. First, it has been argued that the term <u>place preference</u> is a misnomer. Although this observation is correct, the widespread use of the term <u>conditioned place preference</u> to describe increases in the amount of time spent in the compartment associated with drug reward justifies its use <u>de facto</u>. The consistent use of a term to describe an experimental procedure facilitates literature indexing and scientific communication; also, because most investigators are familiar with the lack of an absolute place preference, this term is not generally misleading. Second, some investigators argue that procedures involving strong preconditioning preferences produce a "biased method" of assessing conditioned place preference. Unfortunately, the most common approach to equalizing the amount of time spent by the animals on each side of the apparatus does not really involve removing the "bias" but rather introduces additional biases that result in a more even distribution of time spent in each compartment. For example, other cues (e.g., olfactory, visual, thermal) can be provided that produce a more equal distribution of time spent in each compartment of the apparatus. A potential problem arises if a drug treatment produces a change in reactivity to these cues. This problem could also occur in procedures using a single type of cue, but it is probably more serious in procedures using multiple sensory cues. Another approach to removing strong initial side preferences is to eliminate the stimuli that produce them. The experiment reporting a shift in place preference using only visual cues is one such example (see Figure 15). Perhaps the best solution is to condition some subjects on each side of the apparatus so that half of the subjects are conditioned toward the side of their initial preference while half are conditioned away from the side of their initial preference. This approach may not be successful, however, in procedures with strong initial side preferences

(Schenk, Ellison, Hunt, & Amit, 1985) or in procedures with drug-only conditioning (see Figure 16).

Recommendations

Although conditioned place preference appears to be a reliable measure of the rewarding properties of drugs, caution should be exercised in the use of this technique. Some factors deserve particular attention when conducting place preference experiments: (a) locomotor activity associated with place preference testing should be measured, (b) the effectiveness of a drug treatment known to produce a shift in place preference and the effect of saline should be tested concurrently with the experimental treatments, (c) handling stress should be minimized and equated across all treatment conditions, (d) a priori hypothesis testing and replication of important effects is warranted, and (e) comparisons with other treatment conditions measured at different times should be conservative. As with other measures of drug reward, place preference data are best considered in addition to other lines of evidence supporting a particular hypothesis. Unlike some of the other methods, place preference data are particularly suspect when they are the only supporting evidence for a hypothesis that conflicts with other lines of scientific data. When these and other precautions are observed, conditioned place preference offers an important adjunct to the other methods for assessing drug reward.

Further work is obviously needed to fully understand this method of assessing drug reward. The conditioned place preference technique, however, can offer an additional method of assessing drug reward, and it may provide the opportunity to ask questions that other methods are not well suited to answer. First, place preference studies provide independent corroboration of reward assessed by other measures. This can strengthen the data base that is used to derive important scientific conclusions. Second, large numbers of compounds can be quickly tested using this technique making it an excellent method for the initial screening of drug reward. Drug dosage and other parameters can be estimated from place preference data prior to testing with other more direct methods such as intravenous self-administration. Third, there are applications where a conditioning measure of drug reward is required. For example, the effect of neuroleptic challenge on intravenous opiate self-administration reveals that animals decrease their drug intake, but it has been suggested that this is caused by a sedative drug action and does not reflect an attenuation of opiate reward (Ettenberg, Pettit, Bloom, & Koob, 1982). Place preference conditioning studies permit testing the effect of neuroleptic challenge of drug reward without the potentially confounding influence of sedative effects. These studies have shown that opiate reward is indeed attenuated by neuroleptic treatment (Bozarth & Wise, 1981; Phillips et al., 1982; Schwartz & Marchock, 1974; cf. van der Kooy, this volume) and they help clarify the interpretation of data from intravenous self-administration studies.

CONCLUSION

Despite the failure to fully understand the basis of place preference conditioning, this technique clearly discriminates drug reward from nonreward. The ability of place preference conditioning to reliably distinguish the effect of a rewarding drug (i.e., heroin) from saline treatment was illustrated in Figure 1. Furthermore, Table 2 summarizes some of the studies reporting a conditioned place preference from various compounds, and most of these compounds have rewarding properties that have been confirmed with other

Table 2

Compounds Effective in Producing a Conditioned Place Preference

---

Drug	Reference	Comments
acetaldehyde	Smith et al., 1984	central injections
amphetamine	Asin et al., 1985 Carr & White, 1983 Gilbert & Cooper, 1983 Phillips et al., 1982 Sherman et al., 1980b Spyraki et al., 1982a	central injections
apomorphine	van der Kooy et al., 1983	
beta-phenylethylamine	Gilbert & Cooper, 1983	
clonidine	Asin & Wirtshafter, 1985	
cocaine	Mucha et al., 1982 Spyraki et al., 1982b	
diazepam	Spyraki et al., 1985	
enkephalins	Glimcher et al., 1984a Phillips & LePiane, 1982 Stapleton et al., 1979 Strickrod et al., 1982	enkephalinase inhibitor central injections central injections in utero
ethanol	Bozarth, unpublished observation Reid et al., 1985 Stewart & Grupp, 1981	
etorphine	Mucha et al., 1982	
heroin	Bozarth & Wise, 1981 Bozarth & Wise, 1983 Phillips et al., 1982 Schenk et al., 1985	blocked by pimozide blocked by haloperidol
levorphanol	Mucha et al., 1982	
methylphenidate	Martin-Iverson et al., 1985	
morphine	Advokat, 1985 Bardo et al., 1984 Bozarth & Wise, 1982 Katz & Gormezano, 1979 Kumar, 1972 Mucha et al., 1982 Phillips & LePiane, 1980 Rossi & Reid, 1976 Schwartz & Marchok, 1974 Sherman et al., 1980a Stapleton et al., 1983	central injections central injections blocked by haloperidol central injections

(morphine, continued)	van der Kooy et al., 1982	central injections
neurotensin	Glimcher et al., 1984b	
nicotine	Fudala et al., 1985	
nomifensine	Martin-Iverson et al., 1985	
phencyclidine	Giovino et al., 1983	

procedures. Table 3 shows that not all psychoactive compounds produce a conditioned place preference; most of these compounds have not been reported to be rewarding. Although the shift in place preference is usually not large, the procedure appears to be reliable and yields results consistent with other measures of drug reward.

When used with appropriate precautions, conditioned place preference studies can provide an important addition to the other measures used to assess the rewarding properties of drugs. Because the technique is new and not well understood, most conclusions drawn from this paradigm should be conservative and viewed with regard to the results obtained using other measures of drug reward. Nonetheless, the conditioned place preference method offers an important new tool for studying the rewarding effects of abused drugs.

Table 3

Compounds Ineffective in Producing a Conditioned Place Preference

Drug	Reference	Comments
desipramine	Martin-Iverson et al., 1985	
dextrorphan	Mucha et al., 1982	
ethanol	Asin et al., 1985 Cunningham, 1981 van der Kooy et al., 1983	place aversion
haloperidol	Spyraki et al., 1982b	
hexamethonium	Fudala et al., 1985	
lithium chloride	Kurz & Levitsky, 1983 Mucha et al., 1982	place aversion place aversion
mecamylamine	Fudala et al., 1985	
naloxone	Bozarth & Wise, 1982 Mucha et al., 1985	place aversion
pimozide	Bozarth & Wise, 1981	
saline	most investigators	

ACKNOWLEDGMENTS

Lydia Alessi is thanked for meticulously conducting the experiments described in this chapter. The research was supported by grants from the Natural Sciences and Engineering Research Council of Canada (NSERC) and by the National Institute on Drug Abuse (U.S.A.). The author is a University Research Fellow sponsored by NSERC.

REFERENCES

Advokat, C. (1985). Evidence of place conditioning after chronic intrathecal morphine in rats. Pharmacology Biochemistry & Behavior, 22, 271-277.

Asin, K. E., & Wirtshafter, D. (1985). Clonidine produces a conditioned place preference in rats. Psychopharmacology, 85, 383-385.

Asin, K. E., Wirtshafter, D., & Tabakoff, B. (1985). Failure to establish a conditioned place preference with ethanol in rats. Pharmacology Biochemistry & Behavior, 22, 169-173.

Bardo, M. T., Miller, J. S., & Neisewander, J. L. (1984). Conditioned place preference with morphine: The effect of extinction training on the reinforcing CR. Pharmacology Biochemistry & Behavior, 21, 545-549.

Beach, H. D. (1957). Morphine addiction in rats. Canadian Journal of Psychology, 11, 104-112.

Blander, A., Hunt, T., Blair, R., & Amit, Z. (1984). Conditioned place preference: An evaluation of morphine's positive reinforcing properties. Psychopharmacology, 84, 124-127.

Bozarth, M. A. (1983). A computer approach to measuring shuttle box activity and conditioned place preference. Brain Research Bulletin, 11, 751-753.

Bozarth, M. A., & Wise, R. A. (1981). Heroin reward is dependent on a dopaminergic substrate. Life Sciences, 29, 1881-1886.

Bozarth, M. A., & Wise, R. A. (1982). Localization of the reward-relevant opiate receptors. In L. S. Harris (ed.), Problems of drug dependence, 1981 (National Institute on Drug Abuse Research Monograph 41, pp. 158-164). Washington, DC: U.S. Government Printing Office.

Bozarth, M. A., & Wise, R. A. (1983). Dissociation of the rewarding and physical dependence-producing properties of morphine. In L. S. Harris (Ed.), Problems of drug dependence, 1982 (National Institute on Drug Abuse Research Monograph 43, pp. 171-177). Washington, DC: U.S. Government Printing Office.

Carr, G. D., & White, N. M. (1983). Conditioned place preference from intra-accumbens but not intra-caudate amphetamine injections. Life Sciences, 33, 2551-2557.

Cunningham, C. L. (1981). Spatial aversion conditioning with ethanol. Pharmacology Biochemistry & Behavior, 14, 263-264.

de Wit, H., & Stewart, J. (1983). Drug reinstatement of heroin-reinforced responding in the rat. Psychopharmacology, 79, 29-31.

Ettenberg, A., Pettit, H. O., Bloom, F. E., & Koob, G. F. (1982). Heroin and cocaine intravenous self-administration in rats: Mediation by separate neural systems. Psychopharmacology, 78, 204-209.

Fisher, R. A. (1935). Cited in H. R. Lindman (1974), Analysis of variance in complex experimental designs. San Francisco: W. H. Freeman.

Fudala, P. J., Teoh, K. W., & Iwamoto, E. T. (1985). Pharmacologic characterization of nicotine-induced conditioned place preference. Pharmacology Biochemistry & Behavior, 22, 237-241.

Gilbert, D., & Cooper, S. J. (1983). Beta-phenylethylamine-, d-amphetamine- and l-amphetamine-induced place preference conditioning in rats. European Journal of Pharmacology, 95, 311-314.

Giovino, A. A., Glimcher, P. W., Mattel, C. A., & Hoebel, B. G. (1983). Phencyclidine (PCP) generates conditioned reinforcement in the nucleus accumbens (ACC) but not in the ventral tegmental area (VTA). Society for Neuroscience Abstracts, 9, 120.

Glimcher, P. W., Giovino, A. A., Margolin, D. H., & Hoebel, B. G. (1984a). Endogenous opiate reward induced by an enkephalinase inhibitor, thiorphan, injected into the ventral midbrain. Behavioral Neuroscience, 98, 262-268.

Glimcher, P. W., Margolin, D. H., Giovino, A. A., & Hoebel, B. G. (1984b). Neurotensin: A new 'reward peptide.' Brain Research, 291, 119-124.

Katz, R. J., & Gormezano, G. (1979). A rapid and inexpensive technique for assessing the reinforcing effects of opiate drugs. Pharmacology Biochemistry & Behavior, 11, 231-233.

Kumar, R. (1972). Morphine dependence in rats: Secondary reinforcement from environmental stimuli. Psychopharmacology, 25, 332-338.

Kurz, E. M., & Levitsky, D. A. (1983). Lithium chloride and avoidance of novel places. Behavioral Neuroscience, 97, 445-451.

Lindman, H. R. (1974). Analysis of variance in complex experimental designs. San Francisco: W. H. Freeman.

Linton, M., & Gallo, P. S. (1975). The practical statistician: Simplified handbook of statistics. Monterey, CA: Brooks/Cole Publishing.

Martin-Iverson, M. T., Ortmann, R., & Fibiger, H. C. (1985). Place preference conditioning with methylphenidate and nomifensine. Brain Research, 332, 59-67.

Meyer, R. E., & Mirin, S. M. (Eds.). (1979). The heroin stimulus: Implications for a theory of addiction. New York: Plenum Medical Book Company.

Mucha, R. F., Millan, J. J., & Herz, A. (1985). Aversive properties of naloxone in non-dependent (naive) rats may involve blockade of central beta-endorphin. Psychopharmacology, 86, 281-285.

Mucha, R. F., van der Kooy, D., O'Shaughnessy, M., & Bucenieks, P. (1982). Drug reinforcement studied by the use of place conditioning in rat. Brain Research, 243, 91-105.

Phillips, A. G., & LePiane, F. G. (1980). Reinforcing effects of morphine microinjection into the ventral tegmental area. Pharmacology Biochemistry & Behavior, 12, 965-968.

Phillips, A. G., & LePiane, F. G. (1982). Reward produced by microinjection of (D-ala2), Met5-enkephalinamide into the ventral tegmental area. Behavioural Brain Research, 5, 225-229.

Phillips, A. G., Spyraki, C., & Fibiger, H. C. (1982). Conditioned place preference with amphetamine and opiates as reward stimuli: Attenuation by haloperidol. In B. G. Hoebel & D. Novin (Eds.), The neural basis of feeding and reward. Brunswick, ME: Haer Institute.

Reid, L. D., Hunter, G. A., Beaman, C. M., & Hubbell, C. L. (1985). Toward understanding ethanol's capacity to be reinforcing: A conditioned place preference following injections of ethanol. Pharmacology Biochemistry & Behavior, 22, 483-487.

Rossi, N. A., & Reid, L. D. (1976). Affective states associated with morphine injections. Physiological Psychology, 4, 269-274.

Schenk, S., Ellison, F., Hunt, T., & Amit, Z. (1985). An examination of heroin conditioning in preferred and nonpreferred environments and in differentially housed mature and immature rats. Pharmacology Biochemistry & Behavior, 22, 215-220.

Schwartz, A. S., & Marchok, P. L. (1974). Depression of morphine-seeking behaviour by dopamine inhibition. Nature, 248, 257-258.

Sherman, J. E., Pickman, C., Rice, A., Liebeskind, J. C., & Holman, E. W. (1980a). Rewarding and aversive effects of morphine: Temporal and pharmacological properties. Pharmacology Biochemistry & Behavior, 13, 501-505.

Sherman, J. E., Roberts, T., Roskam, S. E., & Holman, E. W. (1980b). Temporal properties of the rewarding and aversive effects of amphetamine in rats. Pharmacology Biochemistry & Behavior, 13, 597-599.

Smith, B. R., Amit, Z., & Splawinsky, J. (1984). Conditioned place preference induced by intraventricular infusions of acetaldehyde. Alcohol, 1, 193-195.

Spragg, S. D. S. (1940). Morphine addiction in chimpanzees. Comparative Psychology Monographs, 15, 1-132.

Spyraki, C., Fibiger, H. C., & Phillips, A. G. (1982a). Dopaminergic substrates of amphetamine-induced place preference conditioning. Brain Research, 253, 185-193.

Spyraki, C., Fibiger, H. C., & Phillips, A. G. (1982b). Cocaine-induced place preference conditioning: Lack of effects of neuroleptics and 6-hydroxydopamine lesions. Brain Research, 253, 195-203.

Spyraki, C., Kazandjian, A., & Varonos, D. (1985). Diazepam-induced place preference conditioning: Appetitive and antiaversive properties. Psychopharmacology, 87, 225-232.

Stapleton, J. M., Lind, M. D., Merriman, V. J., Bozarth, M. A., & Reid, L. D. (1979). Affective consequences and subsequent effects on morphine self-administration of d-ala^2-methionine enkephalin. Physiological Psychology, 7, 146-152.

Stewart, R. B., & Grupp, L. H. (1981). An investigation of the interaction between the reinforcing properties of food and ethanol using the place preference paradigm. Progress in Neuropsychopharmacology, 5, 609-613.

Strickrod, G., Kimble, D. P., & Smotherman, W. P. (1982). Met-enkephalin effects on associations formed in utero. Peptides, 3, 881-883.

van der Kooy, D., Kalant, H., Mucha, R. F., & O'Shaughnessy, M. (1983). Motivational properties of ethanol in naive rats as studied by place conditioning. Pharmacology Biochemistry & Behavior, 19, 441-445.

van der Kooy, D., Mucha, R. F., O'Shaughnessy, M., & Bucenieks, P. (1982). Reinforcing effects of brain microinjections of morphine revealed by conditioned place preference. Brain Research, 243, 107-117.

Winer, B. (1971). Statistical principles in experimental design. New York: McGraw-Hill.

CHAPTER 15

ANATOMICAL AND NEUROCHEMICAL SUBSTRATES OF DRUG REWARD DETERMINED BY THE CONDITIONED PLACE PREFERENCE TECHNIQUE

Anthony G. Phillips[1] and Hans C. Fibiger[2]

Department of Psychology[1] and
Division of Neurological Sciences
Department of Psychiatry[2]
University of British Columbia
Vancouver, British Columbia, Canada V6T 1W5

ABSTRACT

The conditioned place preference paradigm appears well suited to the analysis of neural pathways involved in drug reward. Current literature on this topic is reviewed with respect to three issues: (1) pharmacological blockade of drug reward, (2) mapping of effective brain loci where microinjection of drugs can be used to condition a place preference, and (3) attenuation of place preference conditioning obtained with systemic or intracerebral administration of drugs and by selective lesions of central dopaminergic pathways. Collectively, these data suggest that a mesotelencephalic dopamine system may serve as one important substrate for the rewarding effects of both psychostimulant and opiate drugs.

INTRODUCTION

Animal models of drug reinforcement and drug dependence have employed both the voluntary and involuntary administration of drugs. For those interested in behavior related to the initial phases of drug acquisition and dependency, the intravenous self-administration procedure developed by Weeks (1962) has been the method of choice. Studies using this technique have demonstrated positive reinforcing effects of a wide variety of drugs including psychostimulants and opiates in many mammalian species (Schuster & Thompson, 1969). Despite the significant advances permitted by this paradigm, it is not without its drawbacks. For example, the implantation of intravenous catheters is laborious and the patency of the catheters can be problematic. In addition, the interpretation of data relating to neural substrates of drug reinforcement can sometimes be difficult as the animals are often required to perform operant responses after pharmacological treatments or brain lesions that may interfere with operant behavior. The rate of operant responding under simple schedules of drug delivery also can be an unreliable measure of the relative efficacy of reinforcement (Johanson & Aigner, 1981). Therefore the development of other procedures for the study of drug-induced reinforcement is desirable.

One alternative procedure, suitable for studying the relation between the rewarding stimulus properties of drugs and environmental stimuli, is the conditioned place preference paradigm (Rossi & Reid, 1976). This procedure is derived from the finding that the association of distinctive environmental stimuli with a primary reward such as food or a drug injection will result in an acquired preference for those specific environmental stimuli in the absence of the primary reward. Some of the advantages of the place preference paradigm include replacement of multiple drug injections by a single systemic or intracerebral injection at the beginning of each daily session. Furthermore, rapid conditioning in one to four trials eliminates the need for extensive behavioral testing. The purpose of the paper is to review recent research utilizing conditioned place preference as a procedure for the identification of anatomical and neurochemical substrates of drug reward.

It is now well established that many of the drugs used to maintain intravenous self-administration also can be used to establish conditioned place preference (Phillips, Spyraki, & Fibiger, 1982). Opiates (Rossi & Reid, 1976) and psychostimulants (Reicher & Holman, 1977) have been studied most frequently, and recent attempts to identify neurochemical correlates of drug reward have used these drugs in conjunction with specific opiate or catecholamine receptor antagonists.

Several laboratories have reported that naloxone disrupts conditioned place preference produced either by systemic administration of morphine (Sherman, Pickman, Rice, Liebeskind, & Holman, 1980) or by heroin (Bozarth & Wise, 1981b), thereby indicating an opiate receptor mediation of the rewarding effects of opiate drugs. This interpretation presumes that naloxone itself does not simply cancel the rewarding effect of opiates by having inherent aversive properties. One body of data indicates that peripheral administration of naloxone (1 to 3 mg/kg) via the intraperitoneal (i.p.) route does not produce a conditioned place aversion (Bozarth & Wise, 1981b; Phillips & LePiane, 1980). However, controversy surrounds this issue as Mucha and colleagues have demonstrated significant conditioned place aversion with both intravenous (0.1 to 4.5 mg/kg) and subcutaneous (0.1 to 0.5 mg/kg) administration of naloxone (Mucha & Iversen, 1984; Mucha, van der Kooy, O'Shaughnessy, & Bucenieks, 1982). In the latter study, a smaller but nevertheless significant place aversion was obtained with intraperitoneal administration of naloxone. The discrepancy between these experiments would appear to reflect both route of drug administration and, to a lesser degree, possible floor effects associated with pairing naloxone injections with confinement to the least preferred compartment of the shuttlebox. On the basis of these studies, it appears that intraperitoneal injections of naloxone can disrupt conditioned place preference produced by opiates by antagonizing the direct action of these drugs on the subclass of opiate receptor that mediates their rewarding effects on behavior. It should also be recognized that the more sensitive procedures employed by Mucha and his coworkers point to the existence of an endogenous opioid peptide system, the modulation of which can result either in reward or in punishment. The identification of such a system has been a high priority in this field of research, and the relevant experiments using intracerebral injections and brain lesions are reviewed below.

In the context of pharmacological antagonism of opiate reward, there have been several independent reports of significant attenuation of opiate-induced place preference by neuroleptic drugs. Morphine place preference has been blocked by pretreatment with the catecholamine synthesis inhibitor alpha-methyl-p-tyrosine or by the dopamine (DA) receptor antagonist haloperidol (0.25 to 1.0 mg/kg) (Schwartz & Marchok, 1974). Similar results have been obtained with heroin induced place preference. In these studies pimozide (Bozarth & Wise, 1981b, 1982) and haloperidol (see Figure 1B) prevented conditioning of a place preference by heroin. Treatment with either neuroleptic alone did not produce a conditioned place aversion. Both pimozide and haloperidol have relatively selective effects on dopamine receptors. Therefore these data

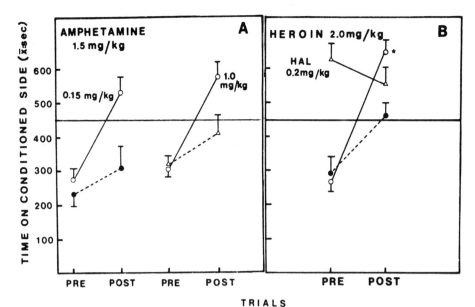

Figure 1: A: Effect of haloperidol (●, 0.15 mg/kg; △, 1.0 mg/kg) or vehicle injections (○) on conditioned place preference with amphetamine (1.5 mg/kg) reward. **B:** Effect of haloperidol (●, 0.15 mg/kg) or vehicle (○) on conditioned place preference with heroin (2 mg/kg) reward. Lack of conditioned aversion to haloperidol (△, 0.2 mg/kg) alone, paired with the initially preferred compartment also is illustrated. Adapted with permission from Spyraki, Fibiger, and Phillips, 1982a, 1983.

clearly implicate a dopaminergic mechanism in opiate reward processes.

As indicated previously, psychostimulant drugs have been used successfully to induce conditioned place preference. Included in this category are d-amphetamine (Sherman, Roberts, Roskam, & Holman, 1980), apomorphine (Spyraki, Fibiger, & Phillips, 1982a), cocaine (Spyraki, Fibiger, & Phillips, 1982b), methylphenidate, and nomifensine (Martin-Iverson, Ortmann, & Fibiger, 1985). Interestingly, d-amphetamine induced place preference is attenuated by dopamine receptor blockade (see Figure 1A) but this treatment fails to block place preference obtained with cocaine (see Figure 2), methylphenidate, or nomifensine (Martin-Iverson et al., 1985). These data are important on two counts. First, they indicate that the neural substrates of the rewarding effect of d-amphetamine are to some extent distinct from those mediating the reinforcing effects of cocaine, methylphenidate, and nomifensine. Furthermore, these data point to possible differences between the intravenous self-administration and conditioned place preference paradigms in their sensitivity to different aspects of drug reward because DA receptor antagonists have similar effects on self-administration maintained by all of these stimulants.

Notwithstanding the useful data provided by the use of selective antagonists, it is clear that more direct and localized manipulation of brain activity is required for the successful identification of the neural

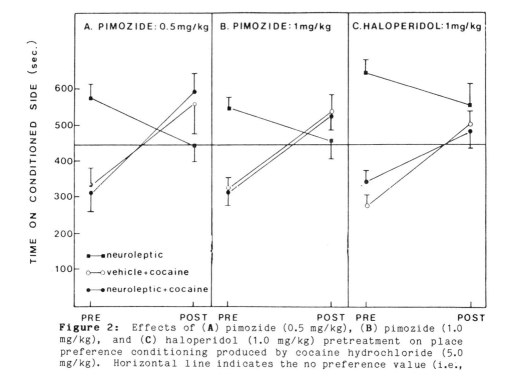

Figure 2: Effects of (**A**) pimozide (0.5 mg/kg), (**B**) pimozide (1.0 mg/kg), and (**C**) haloperidol (1.0 mg/kg) pretreatment on place preference conditioning produced by cocaine hydrochloride (5.0 mg/kg). Horizontal line indicates the no preference value (i.e., half of the 900-second session). Adapted with permission from Spyraki, Fibiger, and Phillips, 1982b.

substrates of drug reward. Some success has been obtained through mapping studies involving intracerebral micro-injection of opiates and psychostimulants. Selective lesions of central catecholamine pathways also have proved useful in this endeavor.

REWARDING EFFECTS OF LOCALIZED INTRACEREBRAL MICROINJECTION OF DRUGS

A major advantage of intracerebral microinjection procedures for identifying neural substrates of drug reward is derived from the ability to place various compounds into specific subcortical loci in a relatively precise manner. When this procedure is coupled with the abundant information on the anatomical location of various receptor types, it becomes feasible to relate receptors for specific synaptic transmitters to reward produced by different drugs. Although intracerebral microinjection can also be used in conjunction with lever pressing to confirm the reinforcing properties of drugs (cf. Bozarth, 1983; Olds, 1979), the conditioned place preference paradigm has several features which recommend its use.

It is now well established that rewarding effects can be demonstrated by the intracerebral technique with as few as one to three individual pairings of drug and environmental stimuli (van der Kooy, Mucha, O'Shaughnessy, & Bucenieks, 1982). Therefore few intracerebral injections need to be made, thus minimizing nonspecific damage to brain tissue at the tip of the injection needle. Perhaps the greatest advantage comes from conducting the tests for conditioned reinforcement when the animals are in a drug free state. This fact along with the minimal response demands of the procedure insures that measures of reward are not confounded by changes in activity or performance.

Opiates and Opioid Peptides

The successful conditioning of a place preference with intraventricular injections of d-ala[2]-methionine enkephalin (D-Ala) (Katz & Gormezano, 1979; Stapleton, Lind, Merriman, Bozarth, & Reid, 1979), a long-acting enkephalin analogue (Pert, Pert, Chang, & Fong, 1976), provided the rationale for similar experiments with more localized microinjection of opiate drugs. Several factors influenced our initial selection of the ventral tegmental area (VTA) as a possible site at which the pharmacological action of opiates could lead to the reinforcement of behavior. A primary consideration was the facilitation of intracranial self-stimulation from electrodes implanted into the lateral hypothalamus by intracerebral injections of morphine at the diencephalic-mesencephalic border (Broekkamp, van den Bogaard, Heynen, Rops, Cools, & van Rossum, 1976). The most effective sites were subsequently localized to the VTA, and D-Ala was shown to mimic the facilitory effects of morphine on electrical self-stimulation (Broekkamp, Phillips, & Cools, 1979a). Locomotor activity, a behavior often linked to activation of dopaminergic neurons in the A_{10} nucleus of the VTA, also was observed after local application of morphine (Joyce & Iversen, 1979) or D-Ala (Broekkamp, Phillips, & Cools, 1979b) to this region of the brain. Other factors included the identification of enkephalinergic nerve terminals in this region of the brain (Johansson, Hokfelt, Elde, Schulzberg, & Terenius, 1978) and the excitation of single unit activity following microinjections of morphine into the region (Finnerty & Chan, 1979).

Successful conditioning of a place preference was established after three daily microinjections of morphine (0.2 to 1.0 µg/0.5 µl) injected bilaterally into the VTA were paired with the less preferred compartment of a shuttlebox (see Figure 3; Phillips & LePiane, 1980). Independent confirmation of this effect was provided by Bozarth and Wise (1982) using unilateral injections of morphine (0.25 µg/0.5 µl). Subsequently, a similar effect was reported with unilateral injections of D-Ala (0.1 to 0.25 µg/0.5 µl) into the VTA (Phillips & LePiane, 1982). Naloxone (2 mg/kg, i.p.) successfully antagonized the rewarding effect of a unilateral injection of 0.1 µg D-Ala. The failure to obtain significant place preference with injection sites located dorsal (Phillips & LePiane, 1980, 1982) or caudal (Bozarth & Wise, 1982) to the VTA suggests that important elements of opiate reward are located in the VTA.

These place preference experiments with intracerebral injections of opiate drugs and enkephalin analogues have been complemented by a study using an enkephalinase inhibitor which protects endogenous opioid peptides from enzymatic degradation (Glimcher, Giovino, Margolin, & Hoebel, 1984). Microinjection of the enkephalinase inhibitor thiorphan (Roques, Fournie-Zaluski, Soroca, Lecomte, Malfroy, Llorens, & Schwartz, 1980) was used to elevate endogenous levels of enkephalin in the VTA by inhibiting dipeptidyl carboxypeptidase, the enkephalinase which normally cleaves enkephalin at the gly[3]-phe[5]-amide bond. Successful conditioning of a place preference following such injections suggested that the release of endogenous enkephalin in the VTA has primary rewarding effects.

It must be emphasized that the localization of a substrate for opiate

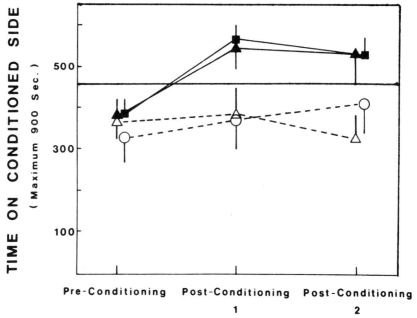

Figure 3: Preference scores expressed as time spent on one side of the test chamber before and after intracerebral microinjection of morphine or saline. The preconditioning scores indicate that the "conditioned" side was the less preferred prior to drug treatment. The amount of time spent on the preferred side may be obtained by subtracting a given group score from the session length of 900 seconds. Postconditioning scores represent the amount of time spent on the same side after association between this environment and microinjection of morphine or saline. Groups: (▲) 0.2 μg morphine, VTA; (■) 1.0 g morphine, VTA; (O) 1.0 μg morphine, dorsal placements; (△) 0.9% saline, VTA. Adapted with permission from Phillips & LePiane, 1980.

reward in the VTA does not preclude other critical sites elsewhere in the brain. In fact, several positive sites have been identified using bilateral injections of morphine (5 μg per side). Significant place preference was conditioned in rats with cannulae placements into the lateral hypothalamus, nucleus accumbens, and periaqueductal gray; no effect was obtained following injections into the central nucleus of the amygdala, caudate-putamen, or nucleus ambiguus (van der Kooy, Mucha, O'Shaughnessy, & Bucenieks, 1982). The most pronounced behavioral effects of morphine observed during these conditioning trials were increased locomotion and excessive rearing and grooming. It is noteworthy that hyperactivity also accompanied morphine injections into the VTA (Joyce & Iversen, 1979). An important control in the study by van der Kooy et al. (1982) was the use of the active (-) and inactive (+) isomers of morphine (Jacquet, Klee, Rice, & Minamikawa, 1977). The establishment of place preference only with (-) morphine provides further evidence for the involvement of specific brain opiate receptors in the rewarding effect of morphine.

To date, the four brain loci noted above have been identified as active sites at which opiates produce primary rewarding effects. Given the limited number of sites tested, it is obviously premature to conclude that these positive loci constitute the neural substrates of opiate reward. As noted by van der Kooy et al. (1982), it is possible that greater diffusion of a drug within a given nucleus or that refinement of the place conditioning procedure may be used to condition significant place preference at loci that so far have failed to yield positive results. It also should be stated that identification of positive sites need not infer an action of morphine in that specific area of the brain. Intraventricular injections of morphine at a dose of 10 µg into the lateral ventricle can be used to obtain conditioned place preference, whereas a dose of 0.5 µg is below threshold (cf. van der Kooy et al., 1982). Consequently, care must be exercised to avoid penetration of the ventricles during stereotaxic implantation into regions such as the nucleus accumbens and lateral hypothalamus. Inadvertent damage to the ventricles in conjunction with relatively high doses of morphine (i.e., 10 µg) would preclude localization of effects to specific brain nuclei. Such factors may account for some of the positive results reported by van der Kooy et al. (1982).

Amphetamine

The conditioned place preference paradigm is now used routinely in conjunction with peripheral routes of drug administration to confirm the rewarding effects of both opiates and psychostimulants. In contrast, to date there has been only one report of conditioned place preference with intracerebral injections of a stimulant drug. A significant preference was produced by d-amphetamine sulphate (10 µg/0.5 µl) for the drug environment after six daily injections of the drug unilaterally into the nucleus accumbens (Carr & White, 1983). These cannulae were implanted on an angle to avoid penetration of the ventricles. Comparable injections into the head of the striatum did not have a significant effect. The results of this study along with the earlier report of conditioned place preference after morphine injections into the nucleus accumbens suggest that a common mechanism in this region of the brain may mediate the rewarding effects of both psychostimulants and opiates. As already alluded to above in reviewing the effects of neuroleptics on conditioned place preference, the common denominator may well involve activation of certain mesotelencephalic dopaminergic neurons.

Neurotensin

One of the most significant findings of all of the mapping studies conducted to date with the conditioned place preference procedure is the consistent overlap between reward placements and the trajectory of the dopaminergic neurons arising from the VTA. Positive results have been obtained with all compounds known to influence the activity of these neurons, be they opiate drugs, opioid peptides, or stimulants. Given this pattern of results, it follows that other endogenous neuropeptides with direct excitatory effects on dopaminergic neurons in the VTA may have rewarding effects on behavior. Neurotensin, a tridecapeptide, has been shown to have excitatory effects on the neurophysiological activity of DA neurons (Andrade & Aghajanian, 1982), and neurotensin-like immunoreactivity has been seen in the VTA (Uhl, Goodman, & Snyder, 1979). These characteristics of neurotensin led to the hypothesis that it may serve as a novel "reward" peptide. This conjecture has received initial support from the demonstration that neurotensin can be used to induce a place preference when injected into the VTA (Glimcher, Margolin, Giovino, & Hoebel, 1984).

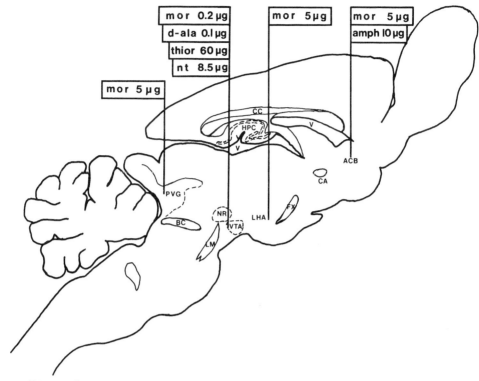

Figure 4: Sagittal section of the rat brain indicating subcortical regions from which intracerebral microinjection of drugs can be used to induce a conditioned place preference. Abbreviations: Amph = d-amphetamine sulphate; D-Ala = D-Alanine ^{2}-Met ^{5}-enkephalinamide; Mor = Morphine sulphate; NT = Neurotensin; Thiorp = Thiorphan, an enkephalinase inhibitor; ACB = Nucleus Accumbens; BC = brachium conjunctivum; CA = anterior commissure; CC = corpus callosum; FX = fornix; HPC = hippocampus; LHA = lateral hypothalamus; LM = medial lemniscus; NR = red nucleus; PVG = periventricular gray; VTA = ventral tegmental area.

BLOCKADE OF CONDITIONED PLACE PREFERENCE WITH SELECTIVE LESIONS

Major advances in identifying neurochemical substrates of drug reward have come from the use of selective lesions to transmitter-specific pathways in the brain. The neurotoxin 6-hydroxydopamine (6-OHDA) has been used routinely to lesion various catecholamine terminal areas and axons. Bilateral injections of 6-OHDA into the dopaminergic terminal field of the nucleus accumbens produced extinction-like responding in animals with a stable history of intravenous self-administration of cocaine (Roberts, Koob, Klonoff, & Fibiger, 1980). In contrast, lesions to ascending noradrenergic pathways did not affect cocaine self-administration (Roberts, Corcoran, & Fibiger, 1977). In a related study, rats in which dopaminergic nerve terminals in the nucleus accumbens had been destroyed by 6-OHDA failed to initiate self-administration of d-amphetamine

- 282 -

despite nearly three weeks of post-lesion testing (Lyness, Friedle, & Moore, 1979). Together these data point to an involvement of central DA neurons in the rewarding properties of amphetamine and cocaine. Similar studies now have been conducted with these drugs as primary reinforcers in the conditioned place preference paradigm, and these results have identified possible differences in the substrates of amphetamine and cocaine reward.

Amphetamine, Cocaine, and Apomorphine

The attenuation of amphetamine-induced place preference by neuroleptic treatment (Spyraki et al., 1982a) and the lack of effect when cocaine is used as the primary reward (Spyraki et al., 1982b) provided the initial indication of a dissociation between the mechanisms by which these two drugs can be used to reinforce behavior. A similar pattern of results again emerged with animals receiving 6-OHDA lesions of the nucleus accumbens. In the experiment with amphetamine-induced place preference, there was a significant correlation ($r = 0.76$) between the absence of conditioned place preference and the magnitude of DA depletion in the nucleus accumbens (Spyraki et al., 1982a). No significant correlation was observed with the DA content in the striatum. Depletion of peripheral catecholamines by systemic injections of 6-OHDA did not affect d-amphetamine-induced place preference conditioning. In contrast to the effects obtained with amphetamine, neither 6-OHDA lesions of DA terminals in the nucleus accumbens nor 6-OHDA-induced destruction of central and/or peripheral noradrenergic systems affected cocaine-induced place preference conditioning (Spyraki et al., 1982b).

Resolution of these anomalous results may have been provided by the demonstration of significant place preference conditioning with the local anesthetic procaine at doses that did not affect locomotor activity (Spyraki et al., 1982b). Cocaine too has significant local anesthetic properties; and for reasons yet to be determined, the local anesthetic or other, non-dopaminergic effects of both procaine and cocaine after intraperitoneal administration may be sufficient to produce place preference conditioning. On the other hand, if it were possible to block selectively the local anesthetic properties of cocaine, then conceivably the drug could still produce place preference conditioning solely on the basis of the facilitation of dopaminergic neurotransmission. That is, cocaine may produce place preference by two independent mechanisms, with only one being dopaminergic.

The place-preference paradigm has been used to confirm the rewarding effects of apomorphine (Spyraki et al., 1982a; van der Kooy, Swerdlow, & Koob, 1983), reported previously with the intravenous self-administration procedure (Baxter, Gluckman, Stein, & Scerni, 1974). A dose of 0.5 mg/kg subcutaneously produced a clear preference (i.e., > 50% of time in compartment paired with the drug) when paired explicitly with a nonpreferred compartment (Spyraki et al., 1982a). Ambiguous results were obtained when apomorphine injections (0.01 to 10.0 mg/kg) were paired randomly with two distinct environments regardless of initial preference. Control rats with or without prior experience of apomorphine did not spend more time in the apomorphine as compared to the vehicle-paired side of the test chamber (van der Kooy et al., 1983). Despite the absence of a clear place preference in sham-operated controls, rats with bilateral 6-OHDA lesions of the nucleus accumbens did show a significant preference for the drug compartment over the environment associated with vehicle injections. This effect could be attributed to the development of DA receptor supersensitivity (Creese & Snyder, 1978) following destruction of the dopaminergic innervation of the nucleus accumbens. The fact that this result paralleled the potentiation of apomorphine-induced locomotion in the same subjects may again point to a common dopaminergic substrate for both the rewarding and locomotor effects of psychostimulant drugs.

Opiates and Opioid Peptides

Given the attenuation of heroin-induced place preference by pretreatment with neuroleptics (Spyraki et al., 1983), an obvious complement was to examine the effect of 6-OHDA lesions of the mesolimbic dopaminergic pathway at the level of the nucleus accumbens. Pairing of heroin (2.0 mg/kg) with the initially "nonpreferred" side of the shuttlebox produced a strong conditioned preference for the environmental cues associated with this drug. The percentage of time in the "drug" compartment switched from a 30% preconditioning score to 72% postconditioning. Bilateral lesions caused a 73% reduction of DA in the nucleus accumbens and olfactory tubercle. These depletions were accompanied by a significant reduction in time spent in the drug-paired compartment to approximately 50% of the test session (Spyraki et al., 1983).

Although the 6-OHDA lesions in the nucleus accumbens caused a partial lesion of the noradrenergic projection to the cortex and hippocampus, damage to these projections could not account for the attenuation of place preference. In a separate experiment neonatal injections of 6-OHDA were used to produce far more severe depletions of noradrenaline in cortex and hippocampus, and yet this treatment had no effect on heroin-induced place preference. These data are consistent with the lack of effect of noradrenergic lesions on cocaine self-administration (Roberts et al., 1977) and add to the growing skepticism about the role of noradrenaline in reward (Fibiger, 1978; Wise, 1978).

Successful conditioning of place preference with unilateral injections of the enkephalin analogue D-Ala (Phillips & LePiane, 1982) sets the stage for a more direct assessment of the role of the mesotelencephalic DA neurons in opioid induced reward (Phillips, LePiane, & Fibiger, 1983b). Two groups of rats, each with unilateral cannulae aimed at the VTA, were prepared with 6-OHDA lesions of the DA pathways either ipsilateral or contralateral to the injection site. Upon completion of the place preference conditioning with unilateral injections of D-Ala, the extent of each lesion was assessed biochemically. Eight of the 15 animals with ipsilateral lesions had greater than 95% depletion of forebrain DA levels. Seven animals had partial lesions (mean = 74.5% of control values). A similar dichotomy was observed with contralateral lesions. The behavioral data for the four groups revealed successful place preference conditioning in both of the contralateral lesion groups and the ipsilateral group with partial lesions. Conditioned place preference was not observed with animals receiving nearly complete lesions of the ipsilateral DA system (see Figure 5).

COMPARISON OF DIFFERENT PROCEDURES FOR IDENTIFYING NEURAL SUBSTRATES OF DRUG REWARD

Three different approaches currently are being used to identify the neural mechanism of drug reward. These include the use of the various mapping and lesion techniques in conjunction with the conditioned place preference paradigm as described in the present chapter, studies of lesion effects on intravenous self-administration (see Roberts & Zito, this volume), and intracranial self-administration procedures (see Bozarth, this volume). Although each procedure has been discussed separately and in detail in this volume, there are a number of important similarities and differences in the conclusions drawn from the use

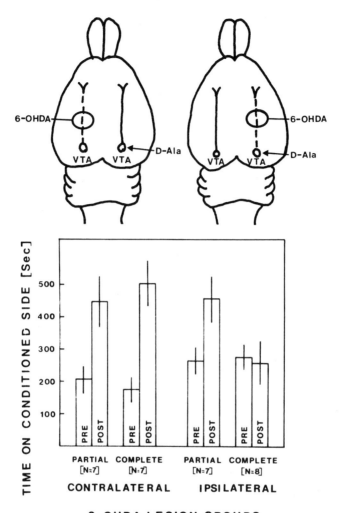

6-OHDA LESION GROUPS

Figure 5: Upper: Schematic representation of unilateral 6-OHDA lesions of forebrain dopamine pathways contralateral or ipsilateral to microinjection sites in the VTA. **Lower:** Effects of partial (< 90%) or complete (> 90%) ipsilateral or contralateral depletion of forebrain dopamine on conditioned place preference induced by unilateral injections of D-Ala (0.2 µg) into the VTA. Adapted with permission from Phillips, LePiane, and Fibiger, 1983b.

of these various procedures. These points will be discussed briefly with respect to an accurate description of the neural substrates of drug reward.

There appears to be a clear consensus from studies using each of the strategies described above that a dopaminergic projection to the nucleus accumbens is important for the rewarding effects of amphetamine. Lesions of these dopaminergic neurons block acquisition of amphetamine self-administration (Lyness et al., 1979); amphetamine is self-administered directly into the nucleus accumbens (Monaco, Hernandez, & Hoebel, 1981); and local injections of amphetamine at this site can be used to induce a place preference (Carr & White, 1983).

Much more uncertainty surrounds the critical involvement of the nucleus accumbens in cocaine reward. On one hand studies with the place preference procedure and neuroleptics or denervation of DA neurons in the nucleus accumbens found no evidence for an exclusive role for DA in mediating the rewarding effects of cocaine (Spyraki et al., 1982b). These data contrast with those showing an attenuation of cocaine self-administration after similar treatments (Roberts et al., 1977, 1980) and may reflect the fact that several mechanisms underlie cocaine reward. One effect may not lend itself to an association with lever pressing in a response contingent manner and as a consequence is not detected by the intravenous self-administration paradigm. The failure to observe intracranial self-administration of cocaine into the nucleus accumbens, despite a clear indication of self-administration into the medial prefrontal cortex (Goeders & Smith, 1983), is also problematic for the nucleus accumbens hypothesis. It is likely that 6-OHDA lesions of the nucleus accumbens would also damage the dopaminergic projection to the prefrontal cortex; this damage may contribute to the blockade of cocaine self-administration following such lesions. Studies with selective lesions of the medial and sulcal prefrontal cortex would resolve this issue. The frontal cortex may contribute to the rewarding effects of both cocaine and amphetamine because rhesus monkeys have been shown to self-administer amphetamine directly into the orbitofrontal cortex (Phillips, Mora, & Rolls, 1981). It still remains to be determined if DA is essential for these effects.

Although a strong case can be presented in support of a dopaminergic substrate for opiate reward processes, this too is still subject to debate. Bilateral 6-OHDA lesions of the dopaminergic axons and terminals in the nucleus accumbens did not attenuate intravenous self-administration of heroin, although similar lesions blocked cocaine self-administration (Pettit, Ettenberg, Bloom, & Koob, 1984). Similarly, pretreatment with high doses of the DA antagonist alpha-flupenthixol blocked responding for cocaine but only produced a slight reduction in heroin self-administration (Ettenberg, Pettit, Bloom, & Koob, 1982). One possible explanation for the discrepancy between these data and the results from place conditioning studies (Phillips et al., 1983b) may be the existence of multiple neural substrates of opiate reward, only one of which is located in the VTA. Systemic administration of opiates would influence many different substrates and would therefore be relatively unaffected by damage to only one subsystem. In contrast, reward produced by direct intracranial activation of a specific substrate would be critically dependent upon the integrity of that single element.

All of the opiate studies with both the conditioned place preference paradigm and intracranial self-administration procedure (cf. Bozarth, 1983) provide strong complementary evidence for a ventral tegmental-nucleus accumbens (i.e., mesolimbic) dopaminergic substrate of opiate reward. An opiate drug presumably gains access to this system through an action at either the nucleus accumbens (Olds, 1982) or the VTA (Bozarth & Wise, 1981a; Phillips & LePiane, 1980). Given the failure to obtain intracranial self-administration of morphine in the lateral hypothalamus (Bozarth & Wise, 1982) despite initial reports of success (Olds, 1979), it seems unlikely that opiate reward is mediated by an action in the hypothalamus. The lack of effect of kainic acid lesions of hypothalamic neurons on heroin self-administration via the intravenous route (Britt & Wise, 1980) is consistent with this conclusion.

In summary, data from many laboratories using a variety of different procedures appear to support a dopaminergic involvement in some of the rewarding effects of both psychostimulants and opiate drugs. Part of the normal physiological function of this system may involve mediation of positive affective states in both humans and animals (Phillips, Broekkamp, & Fibiger, 1983a). If these two premises are correct, the acquisition and maintenance of drug self-administration is best attributed to the artificial induction of euphoria as distinct from the alleviation of withdrawal stress. This conjecture has received strong support from the recent demonstration that anatomically distinct opiate receptor fields mediate reward and physical dependence (Bozarth & Wise, 1984). Withdrawal symptoms appear to involve opiate action in the periventricular gray region independently from reward. In contrast, the rewarding effects of opiate injections into the VTA are not accompanied by any signs of physical dependence. Together these results confirm that dependence is not a prerequisite for opiate reward and that the latter is probably mediated to an important degree by a mesotelencephalic DA system.

ACKNOWLEDGMENTS

The fruitful collaboration of F. G. LePiane, M. Martin-Iverson, R. Ortmann, and C. Spyraki on various phases of our experiments with conditioned place preference is acknowledged with pleasure. This research was funded by a program grant (PG-23) from the Medical Research Council of Canada.

REFERENCES

Andrade, R., & Aghajanian, G. K. (1982). Neurotensin selectively activates dopaminergic neurons of the substantia nigra. Society for Neuroscience Abstracts, 7, 753.

Baxter, B. L., Gluckman, I. I., Stein, L., & Scerni, R. A. (1974). Self-injection of apomorphine in the rat: Positive reinforcement by a dopamine receptor stimulant. Pharmacology Biochemistry & Behavior, 2, 387-391.

Bozarth, M. A. (1983). Opiate reward mechanisms mapped by intracranial self-administration. In J. E. Smith & J. D. Lane (Eds.), The neurobiology of opiate reward processes (pp. 331-359). Amsterdam: Elsevier.

Bozarth, M. A., & Wise, R. A. (1981a). Intracranial self-administration of morphine into the ventral tegmental area in rats. Life Sciences, 28, 551-555.

Bozarth, M. A., & Wise, R. A. (1981b). Heroin reward is dependent on a dopaminergic substrate. Life Sciences, 29, 1881-1886.

Bozarth, M. A., & Wise, R. A. (1982). Localization of the reward-relevant opiate receptors. In L. S. Harris (Ed.), Problems of drug dependence, 1981 (National Institute on Drug Abuse Research Monograph 41, pp. 158-164). Washington, DC: U.S. Government Printing Office.

Bozarth, M. A., & Wise, R. A. (1984). Anatomically distinct opiate receptor fields mediate reward and physical dependence. Science, 224, 516-517.

Britt, M. D., & Wise, R. A. (1980). Effects of hypothalamic kainic acid lesions on self-administration of heroin and cocaine. Society for Neuroscience Abstracts, 6, 105.

Broekkamp, C. L., Phillips, A. G., & Cools, A. R. (1979a). Facilitation of self-stimulation behavior following intracerebral microinjection of opioids into the ventral tegmental area. Pharmacology Biochemistry & Behavior, 11, 289-295.

Broekkamp, C. L., Phillips, A. G., & Cools, A. R. (1979b). Stimulant effects of enkephalin microinjection into the dopaminergic A10 area. Nature, 278, 560-562.

Broekkamp, C. L. E., van den Bogaard, J. H., Heynen, H. J., Rops, R. H., Cools, A. R., & van Rossum, J. M. (1976). Separation of inhibiting and stimulating effects of morphine on self-stimulation behavior by intracerebral microinjections. European Journal of Pharmacology, 36, 443-450.

Carr, G. D., & White, N. M. (1983). Conditioned place preference from intra-accumbens but not intra-caudate amphetamine injections. Life Sciences, 33, 2551-2557.

Creese, I., & Snyder, S. H. (1978). Behavioral and biochemical properties of the dopamine receptor. In M. A. Lipton, A. Di Mascio, and K. F. Killam (Eds.), Psychopharmacology: A generation of progress (pp. 377-388). New York: Raven Press.

Ettenberg, A., Pettit, H. O., Bloom, F. E., & Koob, G. F. (1983). Heroin and cocaine intravenous self-administration in rats: Mediation by separate neural systems. Psychopharmacology, 78, 204-209.

Fibiger, H. C. (1978). Drugs and reinforcement mechanisms: A critical review of the catecholamine theory. Annual Review of Pharmacology and Toxicology, 18, 37-56.

Finnerty, E. P., & Chan, S. H. H. (1979). Morphine suppression of substantia nigra zona reticulata neurons in the rat: Implicated role for a novel striato-nigral feedback mechanism. European Journal of Pharmacology, 59, 307-310.

Glimcher, P. W., Giovino, A. A., Margolin, D. H., & Hoebel, B. G. (1984). Endogenous opiate reward induced by an enkephalin inhibitor, thiorphan, injected into the ventral midbrain. Behavioral Neuroscience, 98, 262-268.

Glimcher, P. W., Margolin, D. H., Giovino, A. A., & Hoebel, B. G. (1984). Neurotensin: A new 'reward peptide.' Brain Research, 291, 119-124.

Goeders, N. E., & Smith, J. E. (1983). Cortical dopaminergic involvement in cocaine reinforcement. Science, 221, 773-775.

Jacquet, Y. F., Klee, W. A., Rice, K. C., & Minamikawa, J. (1977). Stereospecific and nonstereospecific effects of (+) and (-) morphine: Evidence for a new class of receptors? Science, 198, 842-845.

Johanson, C. E., & Aigner, T. (1981). Comparison of reinforcing properties of cocaine and procaine in rhesus monkeys. Pharmacology Biochemistry & Behavior, 15, 49-53.

Johansson, D., Hokfelt, T., Elde, R. P., Schulzberg, M., & Terenius, L. (1978). Histochemical distribution of enkephalin neurons. Advances in Biochemical Psychopharmacology, 18, 51-70.

Joyce, E. M., & Iversen, S. D. (1979). The effect of morphine applied locally to mesencephalic dopamine cell bodies on spontaneous motor activity in the rat. Neuroscience Letters, 14, 207-212.

Katz, R. J., & Gormezano, G. (1979). A rapid and inexpensive technique for assessing the reinforcing effects of opiate drugs. Pharmacology Biochemistry & Behavior, 11, 231-234.

Lyness, W. H., Friedle, N. M., & Moore, K. E. (1979). Destruction of dopaminergic nerve terminals in nucleus accumbens: Effect on d-amphetamine self-administration. Pharmacology Biochemistry & Behavior, 11, 553-556.

Martin-Iverson, M. T., Ortmann, R., & Fibiger, H. C. (1985). Place preference conditioning with methylphenidate and nomifensine. Brain Research, 332, 59-67.

Monaco, A. P., Hernandez, L., & Hoebel, B. G. (1981). Nucleus accumbens: Site of amphetamine self-injection: Comparison with the lateral ventricle. In R. B. Chronister and J. F. De France (Eds.), The neurobiology of the nucleus accumbens (pp. 338-343). Brunswick, ME: Haer Institute.

Mucha, R. F., & Iversen, S. D. (1984). Reinforcing properties of morphine and naloxone revealed by conditioned place preference: A procedural examination. Psychopharmacology, 82, 241-247.

Mucha, R. F., van der Kooy, D., O'Shaughnessy, M., & Bucenieks, P. (1983). Drug reinforcement studied by use of place conditioning in rat. Brain Research, 243, 91-105.

Olds, M. E. (1979). Hypothalamic substrates for the positive reinforcing properties of morphine in the rat. Brain Research, 168, 351-360.

Olds, M. E. (1982). Reinforcing effects of morphine in the nucleus accumbens. Brain Research, 237, 429-440.

Pert, C. B., Pert, A., Chang, J. K., & Fong, B. T. W. (1976). (D-Ala^2) met-enkephalinamide: A potent long-lasting synthetic pentapeptide analgesic. Science, 194, 330-332.

Pettit, H. O., Ettenberg, A., Bloom, F. E., & Koob, G. F. (1984). Destruction of dopamine in the nucleus accumbens selectively attenuates cocaine but not heroin self-administration in rats. Psychopharmacology, 84, 167-173.

Phillips, A. G., Broekkamp, C. L., & Fibiger, H. C. (1983a). Strategies for studying the neurochemical substrates of drug reinforcement in rodents. Progress in Neuro-Psychopharmacology and Biological Psychiatry, 7, 585-590.

Phillips, A. G., & LePiane, F. G. (1980). Reinforcing effects of morphine micro-injection into the ventral tegmental area. Pharmacology Biochemistry & Behavior, 12, 965-968.

Phillips, A. G., & LePiane, F. G. (1982). Reward produced by microinjection of (D-Ala^2) Met^5-enkephalinamide into the ventral tegmental area. Behavioural Brain Research, 5, 225-229.

Phillips, A. G., LePiane, F. G., & Fibiger, H. C. (1983b). Dopaminergic mediation of reward produced by direct injection of enkephalin into the ventral tegmental area of the rat. Life Sciences, 33, 2505-2511.

Phillips, A. G., Mora, F., & Rolls, E. T. (1981). Intracerebral self-administration of amphetamine by rhesus monkeys. Neuroscience Letters, 24, 81-86.

Phillips, A. G., Spyraki, C., & Fibiger, H. C. (1982). Conditioned place preference with amphetamine and opiates as reward stimuli: Attenuation by haloperidol. In B. G. Hoebel and D. Novin (Eds.), The neural basis of feeding and reward (pp. 455-464). Brunswick, ME: Haer Institute.

Reicher, M. A, & Holman, E. W. (1977). Location preference and flavor aversion reinforced by amphetamine in rats. Animal Learning and Behavior, 5, 343-346.

Roberts, D. C. S., Corcoran, M. E., & Fibiger, H. C. (1977). On the role of ascending catecholamine systems in intravenous self-administration of cocaine. Pharmacology Biochemistry & Behavior, 6, 615-620.

Roberts, D. C. S., Koob, F. G., Klonoff, P., & Fibiger, H. C. (1980). Extinction and recovery of cocaine self-administration following 6-hydroxydopamine lesions of the nucleus accumbens. Pharmacology Biochemistry & Behavior, 12, 781-787.

Roques, B., Fournie-Zaluski, M., Soroca, E., Lecomte, J., Malfroy, B., Llorens, C., & Schwartz, J. C. (1980). Thiorphan shows antinociceptive activity in mice. Nature, 288, 286-288.

Rossi, N. A., & Reid, L. D. (1976). Affective states associated with morphine injections. Physiological Psychology, 4, 269-274.

Schuster, C. R., & Thompson, T. (1969). Self-administration of and behavioral dependence on drugs. Annual Review of Pharmacology, 9, 483-502.

Schwartz, A. S., & Marchok, P. L. (1974). Depression of morphine seeking behavior by dopamine inhibition. Nature, 248, 257-258.

Sherman, J. E., Roberts, T., Roskam, S. E., & Holman, E. W. (1980). Temporal properties of rewarding and aversive behaviors of amphetamine in rats. Pharmacology Biochemistry & Behavior, 13, 597-599.

Spyraki, C., Fibiger, H. C., & Phillips, A. G. (1982a). Dopaminergic substrates of amphetamine-induced place preference conditioning. Brain Research, 253, 185-193.

Spyraki, C., Fibiger, H. C., & Phillips, A. G. (1982b). Cocaine-induced place preference conditioning: Lack of effects of neuroleptics and 6-hydroxydopamine lesions. Brain Research, 253, 195-203.

Spyraki, C., Fibiger, H. C., & Phillips, A. G. (1983). Attenuation of heroin reward in rats by disruption of the mesolimbic dopamine system. Psychopharmacology, 79, 278-283.

Stapleton, J. M., Lind, M. D., Merriman, V. J., Bozarth, M. A., & Reid, L. D. (1979). Affective consequences and subsequent effects on morphine self-administration of d-Ala methionine enkephalin. Physiological Psychology, 7, 146-152.

Uhl, G. R., Goodman, R. R., & Snyder, S. H. (1979). Neurotensin containing cell bodies, fibers, and nerve terminals in the brain stem of the rat: Immunohistochemical mapping. Brain Research, 167, 77-92.

van der Kooy, D., Mucha, R. F., O'Shaughnessy, M., & Bucenieks, P. (1982). Reinforcing effects of brain microinjections of morphine revealed by conditioned place preference. Brain Research, 243, 107-117.

van der Kooy, D., Swerdlow, N. R., & Koob, G. F. (1983). Paradoxical reinforcing properties of apomorphine: Effects of nucleus accumbens and area postrema lesions. Brain Research, 259, 111-118.

Weeks, J. R. (1962). Experimental morphine addiction: Method for automatic intravenous injections in unrestrained rats. Science, 138, 143-144.

Wise, R. A. (1978). Catecholamine theories of reward: A critical review. Brain Research, 152, 315-347.

CHAPTER 16

APPLICATIONS AND LIMITATIONS OF THE DRUG DISCRIMINATION METHOD FOR THE STUDY OF DRUG ABUSE

Donald A. Overton

Departments of Psychiatry and Psychology
Temple University
Philadelphia, Pennsylvania 19122

ABSTRACT

This paper describes the advantages and disadvantages of drug discrimination (DD) procedures as methods for obtaining information about the properties of drugs that underlie drug abuse. The paper (1) describes the DD behavioral procedures that are available, (2) enumerates the properties of these procedures that are advantageous for the study of drug effects that cause drug abuse, (3) summarizes properties of DD procedures that are disadvantageous for the study of preclinical psychopharmacology in general and of drug abuse in particular, (4) discusses the face validity of DD procedures, (5) reviews evidence supporting the idea that "sensory" or subjective effects of drugs mediate the formation of DDs, (6) reviews evidence that is not supportive of this explanation for DDs, and (7) describes the types of studies relevant to drug abuse that can be conducted with DD procedures.

HISTORICAL OVERVIEW

In the early nineteenth century, Combe (1830) reported that ethanol could produce state-dependent learning (SDL). Specifically, he reported the case of an Irish deliveryman who had left a parcel at an incorrect address while drunk and could not remember where he had left it until several days later when he was once again intoxicated. No theoretical explanation for this phenomenon was advanced until 1882 when Ribot postulated that "organic sensations" were responsible for drug induced SDL and also for the temporary amnesias observed in cases of multiple personality, somnambulism, and fugue. According to Ribot's theory, sensations reflecting the current physiological and pharmacological state of the body were powerful determinants of which memories could, and could not, be retrieved at any particular moment in time. Specifically, the memories that could be retrieved were those that had been encoded on previous occasions when the body was in the same state as that present at the time of retrieval (Ribot, 1882, p. 115; 1891, p. 34). Ribot's theory was later revised by Semon (1904, 1909) who stated that the retrievability of memories was determined by the "energetic condition of the brain." In Semon's model the influence on memory retrieval of the brain's energetic condition was not assumed to be mediated by sensory events. Apparently, the idea that drugs could influence memory retrieval via an SDL-like process was generally accepted in nineteenth century England (Collins, 1868; Elliotson, 1840, p. 646; Macnish, 1835, p. 30; Siegel, 1982, 1983;

Winslow, 1860, p. 338). No one has reviewed the subsequent literature to determine how widely this idea continued to be accepted during the first third of the twentieth century, although the inclusion of SDL in the plot of Charlie Chaplin's movie City Lights indicates that the idea was not entirely lost (McDonald, Conway, & Ricci, 1965, pp. 191-196).

Girden and Culler (1937) reported the first experimental demonstration of SDL, which they called "dissociated" learning, in dogs virtually paralyzed with raw curare or erythroidine. In their dogs, conditioned leg flexion responses (muscle twitches) learned while the animals were drugged subsequently failed to appear during tests while the animals were undrugged and vice versa (Girden, 1942a, 1942b, 1942c, 1947). Girden did not refer to the earlier literature on SDL and did not interpret his observation as an instance of stimulus control. Instead, he proposed an alternate theory suggesting that drug rendered the cortex nonfunctional. Conditioning carried out in the normal undrugged state established associations only in the cortex which was rendered inoperative during tests when the animal was drugged. Conditioning in the drug state was postulated to establish associative connections in subcortical structures which were inhibited by the cortex during subsequent tests without drug. Theoretical models for SDL such as Girden's, which did not postulate a causal role for drug-induced stimuli, were later labeled "neurological" models by Bliss (1974), and we will adopt that notation throughout this paper.

Conger (1951) first reported that ethanol could acquire discriminative control. He showed that in a telescope-alley task rats could learn to run down the alley when drugged and to withhold that response when undrugged or vice versa. He interpreted these results as showing that ethanol produced sensory stimuli that provided the basis for the rats' discriminated responding. Subsequently, as in the nineteenth century, the notion became moderately widespread that drugs could produce SDL and that because they had "stimulus effects," performance of responses learned in a drug condition might be impaired if the drug context was changed (e.g., Auld, 1951; Barry, Wagner, & Miller, 1962; Grossman & Miller, 1961; Holmgren, 1964; Sachs, Weingarten, & Klein, 1966; Shmavonian, 1956). Several investigators reported data which they interpreted as showing SDL effects of this type (Barry, Miller, & Tidd, 1962; Heistad, 1958; Heistad & Torres, 1959; Miller & Barry, 1960), and Heistad (1957) argued that new behaviors learned while a psychiatric patient was drugged might become unretrievable after drug treatment was discontinued. Of these reports Conger's contained the most convincing data. The nature of the postulated drug-induced stimuli was not identified.

A few years later Overton (1961, 1964, 1966) and Stewart (1962) again trained rats to discriminate presence versus absence of drug and additionally conducted for the first time substitution tests. In these tests, after drug versus no-drug (D versus N) training with one drug (D1), the rats were tested under the influence of other drugs (D2, D3, D4 . . .) to determine under these novel drugs whether the rats would make the response that had been reinforced under the training drug or, alternately, the response that had been reinforced in the no-drug condition. Not surprisingly, the rats selected the response reinforced under the training drug during tests with drugs that were pharmacologically similar to the training drug. Only a few tests were conducted with drugs that differed pharmacologically from the training drug, and under those test conditions the rats selected the response that had been reinforced during no-drug training sessions.

These early reports of successful drug discrimination (DD) training raised two questions that were not immediately answered. First, which drugs would allow animals to easily learn DDs, and which drugs would make DD learning difficult or impossible? Second, what degree of "specificity" would be produced by D versus N training? In other words, after D versus N training, how wide a variety of drugs would produce D choices during test sessions, which drugs would produce a mixture of D and N choices, and which drugs would produce only N choices.

Overton (1971) reported on the relative discriminability of about three dozen centrally acting drugs. Also, on the basis of substitution test results primarily obtained with drugs in four pharmacological classes, he for the first time claimed that rats would make D choices during substitution tests if and only if they were tested under the influence of drugs that pharmacologically resembled the training drug. However, it took several more years before enough data accumulated to fully support this statement as a general property of DD-trained rats.

After 1970, the number of reported DD studies started to increase and by the late 1970s it was firmly established (1) that most centrally acting drugs could be discriminated, and (2) that after D versus N training, rats would usually make D choices during substitution tests with drugs that produced pharmacological actions similar to those of the training drug and not when tested with drugs that produced any of a variety of other pharmacological effects. Reviews of work conducted during this period can be found in several books and articles (Barry, 1974, 1978; Bliss, 1974; Colpaert & Rosecrans, 1978; Colpaert & Slangen, 1982; Erdmann, 1979; Ho, Richards, & Chute, 1978; Lal, 1977; Overton, 1968a, 1974, 1978d, 1984; Schuster & Balster, 1977; Stolerman, Baldy, & Shine, 1982; Thompson & Pickens, 1971; Winter, 1978a). The findings of these studies set the stage for the subsequent application of DD procedures as a method for the investigation of a variety of psychopharmacological and neuropharmacological questions, including studies of the effects of drugs that underlie drug abuse.

TYPICAL DRUG DISCRIMINATION PROCEDURES

This section describes the behavioral procedures that have been developed for use in drug discrimination studies and the types of data that each procedure yields.

Drug Discrimination Training Procedures

Drug discriminations usually involve appetitively or aversively motivated instrumental behaviors. For example, a rat may be trained to turn left in a T-maze to escape shock when drugged (D) and to turn right in the same T-maze during sessions conducted without drug (N). Typically a series of training sessions are conducted in which the drug condition is varied in an alternating sequence (NDNDND . . .). Training sessions are usually conducted daily with drug elimination occurring overnight, thus allowing the D or N condition to be reinstated freshly during the next training session. Usually each daily session lasts 5 to 30 minutes, and responding during the first trial of each session (before any reinforcers are administered) is considered to reflect the degree to which the rat can select the state-appropriate response on the basis of the imposed drug condition.

The DD training procedure is analogous to procedures that are used to establish sensory discriminations (e.g., turn right when the cue light is on and turn left when it is off) except that the differential sensory conditions are replaced by drug conditions which are said to have <u>stimulus effects</u>. When the rat has learned to reliably perform the response appropriate to the current drug state, a drug discrimination is said to have been learned, and the drug is said to be discriminable. The term <u>degree of discriminability</u> is used to refer to the strength, amount, or salience of the drug's stimulus effects, as reflected by the speed at which discriminative control is established or by the stability and accuracy of the resulting discrimination.

Many variations of this procedure are possible. Instead of alternating, the D and N conditions may be imposed in a pseudorandom or double alternation sequence. Rats can be trained to perform a response in one drug condition and to withhold it in a second condition (Ando, 1975; Conger, 1951; Harris & Balster, 1971; Winter, 1973, 1974, 1975, 1977). They can be trained to discriminate among three different drug conditions in a task where three different responses are possible (Overton, 1967; White & Holtzman, 1981, 1983a, 1983b). More generally, any of the following conditions may be discriminated.

D   vs. N
D1 vs. D2
D1 vs. D2 vs. N   (in a three-response task)
D1 vs. D2 vs. D3   (in a three-response task)
D1 vs. (D2 or N)   (in a two-response task)
D1 vs. (D2 or D3 or D4 or N)   (in a two-response task)

The task may involve a series of discrete trials or continuous instrumental behavior as in lever-pressing operant paradigms. Reinforcement contingencies may be the same in each training condition (e.g., reinforce correct responses and extinguish incorrect responses) or may be different (e.g., use an FR-10 schedule of reinforcement of correct responses during D sessions and an FR-20 during N sessions).

Selection from among these procedures is based on empirical data showing the relative advantages of each procedure with respect to various criteria including the following: (1) Discriminations are more rapidly learned with some procedures than with others. (2) Higher asymptotic accuracy of discrimination is obtained with some procedures than with others. (3) Some procedures are more sensitive than others (i.e., rats can discriminate lower doses). (4) Some procedures yield a different degree of specificity than others. At this time the most widely used DD method employs appetitively motivated operant responding in a compartment with two levers mounted side by side on one wall. Every tenth press on the correct lever is reinforced (FR-10 schedule), and presses on the incorrect lever are recorded but have no programmed consequence (Colpaert & Rosecrans, 1978; Lal, 1977; Overton, 1979b).

Performance during DD training sessions yields two major indices of interest: (1) speed of acquisition under each training condition, as reflected by sessions to criterion or number of errors during acquisition and (2) asymptotic accuracy of discrimination.

Substitution Test Procedures

After rats have learned to discriminate a particular training drug and dose versus the no-drug condition, test sessions can be scheduled with various novel drug conditions imposed. During these test sessions responses on either lever are reinforced (or sometimes extinguished) and any of the following drug conditions may be imposed.

        Training Drug (TD) at a novel dose
        TD with various time intervals after injection
        TD plus putative antagonist
        TD plus transmitter manipulator
        TD plus synergistic drug
        Metabolite of TD
        Proposed precursor(s) of TD
        One or more novel drugs

Typically, test sessions are of short duration and allow the rat to make only a few responses. Usually test sessions are interspersed between continuing training sessions in the original training states, which serve to demonstrate and to maintain response control by the training conditions. It is generally assumed that the results of sequentially administered test sessions are independent of one another (i.e., that the conduct of a test session with a particular compound does not alter the probability that the rat will make D choices during subsequent test sessions conducted with the same or different compounds; but see Modrow, Holloway, & Carney, 1981).

The two major types of data obtained from test sessions are (1) percentage of trials under each test condition when the D response is performed and (2) rate (or latency) of responding. The first index typically allows the investigator to subdivide the tested drug conditions into three categories: (1) drugs that mimic the effects of the training drug sufficiently so that D responses regularly occur, (2) drugs with which some intermediate percentage of D choices (25 to 75%) are observed, and (3) drugs which produce no D responses. The second index (rate) is usually considered to indicate the rate-suppressing effects of the test compound, although it is sometimes interpreted as reflecting the degree of novelty of the test condition (Barry, McGuire, & Krimmer, 1982).

ADVANTAGEOUS PROPERTIES OF DRUG DISCRIMINATIONS

As methods for studying the drug effects that underlie drug abuse, drug discriminations have both advantages and disadvantages. This section will review the advantages.

DDs Are Rapidly Learned

A priori one might think that DDs would be learned more slowly than sensory discriminations since specialized receptors, sensory pathways, and brain mechanisms have evolved to mediate the perception of sensory stimuli, whereas corresponding structures designed to mediate the perception of drug effects are not known to exist. Contrary to this prediction, however, the speed of acquisition of drug and of sensory discriminations is similar when comparable training procedures are employed (Duncan, Phillips, Reints, & Schechter, 1979; Kilbey, Harris, & Aigner, 1971, Overton, 1964, 1968b, 1971; Spear, Smith, Bryan, Gordon, Timmons, & Chiszar, 1980).

Most Centrally Acting Drugs Are Discriminable

Most centrally acting drugs are measurably discriminable, and perhaps 75% of centrally acting drugs produce effects sufficiently discriminable so that DD training paradigms can establish stable response control. Table 1 indicates the relative degree of discriminability of various types of centrally acting drugs. Virtually all abused drugs are readily discriminated. The only known

Table 1

Relative Degree of Discriminability of Various Drugs
as Indicated by Speed of Acquisition of Drug Versus No-Drug Discriminations

----

Highly Discriminable

Anesthetics
Antimuscarinics
Benzodiazepines
Dissociative anesthetics
Muscle relaxants
Nicotinics
Tetrahydrocannabinols

Moderately Discriminable

Adrenergics
Adrenergic blockers
Anticonvulsants
Antihistamines
Antitussives
Behavioral stimulants
Convulsants
Hallucinogenics
Histamine blockers
MAO inhibitors
Muscarinics
Narcotic agonists
Narcotic mixed agonist/antagonists
Serotonin blockers
Tricyclic antidepressants

Weakly Discriminable

Antipsychotics
GABA blockers
Some nonnarcotic analgesics

Virtually Undiscriminable

Lithium
Narcotic antagonists
Nicotinic blockers
Salicylates

Note: Highly discriminable drugs frequently produce SDL in 2x2
        experiments. Moderately discriminable drugs are occasionally
        reported to produce SDL. Classification based on data
        published by Overton, 1982a.

exceptions are the occasionally abused salicylates such as aspirin which are
discriminated only with difficulty (Overton, 1982a; Weissman, 1976).

Drugs which act only outside the central nervous system have usually been
found to be much less discriminable than centrally acting drugs (Colpaert,
Kuyps, Niemegeers, & Janssen, 1976; Colpaert, Niemegeers, & Janssen, 1975a;
Downey, 1975; Hazell, Peterson, & Laverty, 1978; Ho, Richards, & Chute, 1978;
Miksic, Shearman, & Lal, 1980; Overton, 1971; Schuster & Balster, 1977;
Valentino, Herling, Woods, Medzihradsky, & Merz, 1981).

A few transmitter blockers such as naltrexone and mecamylamine are
discriminable only at doses considerably higher than those required to produce
the antagonistic actions characteristic of these drugs. Apparently we can
conclude that the antagonistic actions per se of these drugs are not very
discriminable (Carter & Leander, 1982; Overton, 1982a).

Sensitivity Is Relatively High

For several years DDs were a phenomenon most commonly produced by high doses of drugs (e.g., Overton, 1966). Subsequently, the two-lever fixed-ratio operant procedure (Colpaert, Niemegeers, & Janssen, 1975a) allowed the use of more moderate dosages of most drugs, and the dosages now used in DD procedures are comparable to those required by other preclinical behavioral techniques.

Several investigators have tried to determine the lowest dosage of drugs that could be discriminated by using a titration paradigm in which rats discriminated progressively lower dosages until a dosage was reached at which DDs no longer could be maintained (Colpaert, Niemegeers, & Janssen, 1980a; Overton, 1979a; Zenick & Goldsmith, 1981). These experiments showed that DDs could be maintained at dosages as low as one tenth those commonly employed in DD experiments. In other studies several groups of rats have been trained, each with a different dose of the training drug, to determine which doses could acquire control of D versus N DDs (Colpaert, Niemegeers, & Janssen, 1980b; Greenberg, Kuhn, & Appel, 1975; Overton, 1964, 1982a). The amount of training required to establish DDs increases as training dose is reduced, and the asymptotic accuracy of discrimination decreases. Therefore discriminations based on the lowest discriminable doses of a drug do not provide a very practical DD assay procedure.

Quantitative Measurement of Discriminable Effects Is Possible

We have referred several times to the degree of discriminability of drugs without describing how this property might be measured. Three indices of DD performance have been used to indicate degree of discriminability: (1) asymptotic accuracy, (2) speed of acquisition, and (3) ability to substitute for another discriminable drug.

Asymptotic accuracy refers to the relative frequency of correct (state appropriate) response selections after prolonged DD training. Investigators have generally categorized asymptotic accuracy as high (consistent selection of the correct response), medium (occasional lapses of discriminative control), or absent (discrimination never learned). Numerical indices computed from asymptotic accuracy have seldom been used to provide quantitative estimates of degree of discriminability, and such indices appear unlikely to be useful inasmuch as asymptotic accuracy is influenced by several factors other than degree of discriminability, including the schedule of reinforcement that is employed (Colpaert, et al., 1980b; Harris & Balster, 1971; Overton & Hayes, 1984; Schuster & Balster, 1977).

The speed of acquisition of a DD can be expressed in terms of the number of training sessions before some criterion level of accuracy is achieved or in terms of the average accuracy during early DD training sessions (i.e., the area under the learning curve). Figure 1 shows plots of sessions to criterion versus dosage for several drugs and indicates that as dosage is increased speed of acquisition also increases in a monotonic fashion (i.e., sessions to criterion decreases). Comparable data have been obtained with a variety of drugs (Colpaert et al., 1980b; Overton, 1974, 1982a), and a detailed comparison of the effectiveness of various indices of degree of discriminability has recently been reported (Overton, Leonard, & Merkle, 1985).

The substitution test procedure is quicker than either of the previously described techniques but is only applicable in special cases. The center curve in the left half of Figure 2 shows the percentage of drug-lever choices during tests with various doses of phenobarbital in rats previously trained to discriminate phenobarbital (40 mg/kg) versus no drug. As the test dosage decreased, the percentage of drug-lever choices also decreased. There is no

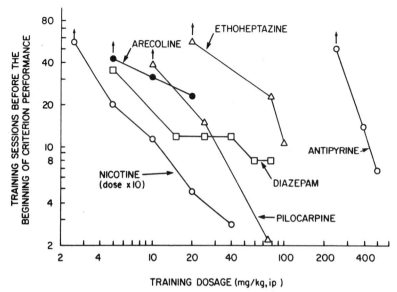

Figure 1: Plots showing the influence of dosage on the speed of acquisition of drug discriminations. In a T-Maze rats were trained to turn right to escape shock when undrugged, and to turn left when drugged. During daily 10-trial sessions, the drug condition alternated (NDNDND . . .) as did the reinforced choice. Criterion was correct choices on the first trial during 8 out of 10 consecutive sessions. Y-axis is the geometric mean number of training sessions before the beginning of criterion performance by three or more rats. Diazepam was suspended and the remaining drugs were dissolved before intraperitoneal injection. With each drug, 11 to 34 rats were trained.

reason to expect a linear relationship between the percentage of presses on the drug lever and the degree of discriminability of the test dosage. However, such substitution test results can indicate the relative ability of various test drugs (or doses) to produce discriminable effects <u>like those of the training drug</u> (Overton, 1974). They are only useful for comparisons between drugs with discriminable effects that are essentially identical to those of the training drug. When this requirement is met, the substitution test technique will provide information about the relative discriminability of various test conditions more rapidly than either the speed of acquisition or the asymptotic accuracy method. For this reason among others, the substitution test method has been frequently employed in DD studies.

DD methods compare favorably with self-administration procedures with regard to their ability to produce quantitative estimates of the strength of subjective drug effects that may underlie drug abuse. Recall that with self-administration procedures it has been difficult to provide more than a yes/no answer to the question of how frequently a drug might be abused. The influence of parameters such as unit dosage and time course of action has made it difficult to provide more quantitative estimates of abuse liability except via certain rather tedious techniques. By comparison, DD procedures can more

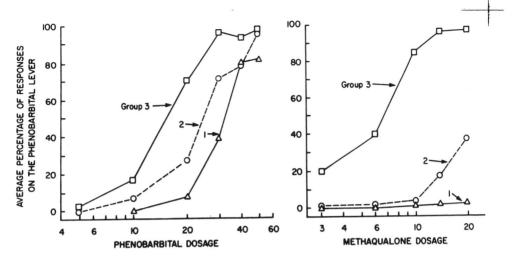

Figure 2: Average percentage of drug-lever presses by three groups
of rats during substitution tests conducted with various doses of two
drugs. The rats were initially trained in a two-lever operant task
with water reinforcement for correct responses (FR-10 schedule) and
extinction of incorrect responses. In Groups 1 to 3, the imposed
drug conditions during bar 1 and bar 2 sessions were as follows:

    Group 1: (Phenobarbital) vs. (Ethanol or Diazepam or Ketamine
             or No Drug)
    Group 2: (Phenobarbital) vs. (No Drug)
    Group 3: (Phenobarbital or Ethanol or Ether or Diazepam) vs.
             (No Drug)

After the required discriminations had been learned, the plotted data
were collected during test sessions in which responses on either
lever were reinforced. Each test session continued until four
reinforcements had been earned. Approximately four test sessions per
drug at each dosage were conducted with each rat. N = 6 rats/group.
Test results with phenobarbital show that the training procedures
produced differing degrees of bias and/or quantitative specificity
such that the dose-response curve was shifted to the right in Group 1
and to the left in Group 3. Test results with methaqualone showed
larger differences in specificity; the Group 3 dose-response curve
shifted further to the left, and substitution failed to occur at any
tested dose in Group 1. Since the dose-response curves obtained with
methaqualone are farther apart than those obtained with
phenobarbital, the results suggest that the groups differed in
qualitative specificity as well as in bias and/or quantitative
specificity.

easily yield data that allows a quantitative comparison of the strength of the
subjective effects of various drugs. Additionally, DD procedures may have the
capability in certain instances to independently measure several different
subjective effects of a drug, including some which promote drug abuse
(euphorigenic) and others that deter drug abuse (nocioceptive).

High Qualitative Specificity Produces Sharp Generalization Gradients

After D versus N DD training with a particular drug and dose, tests may be conducted using drugs that pharmacologically differ from the training drug. Such tests reveal very sharp generalization gradients. Typically the drug choice is not made during tests with any novel drugs except those producing pharmacological effects similar to those of the training drug. The effect is quite striking, and the results are analogous to those which one might expect if animals had been trained using a visual discriminative stimulus and were then tested with the visual stimulus absent and with an auditory stimulus substituted for it. This type of experiment has been repeated many times using a different training drug in each successive group of animals; sharp generalization gradients have been obtained irrespective of the training drug employed (Overton, 1971, 1972, 1978a). The trained animals are said to exhibit high qualitative specificity and can be used as an assay to detect the presence or absence of the actions of the training drug and of its close pharmacological relatives. Indeed, the high qualitative specificity produced by D versus N training is the primary property which has made DD training a useful psychopharmacological assay procedure (Barry, 1974; Colpaert & Slangen, 1982; Lal, 1977). Since a high degree of qualitative specificity has been observed in a variety of DD training paradigms, it appears to reflect some intrinsic property of drug-induced stimuli or of their perception by trained animals rather than a characteristic induced by the particular training paradigm employed (Chance, Murfin, Krynock, & Rosecrans, 1977).

Specificity Can Be Controlled to Some Degree

Until recently, the degree of specificity produced by DD training could not be intentionally varied by the investigator. However methods for controlling specificity are now under development. First, in many drug classes specificity can be decreased (or sometimes increased) by reducing the dose of the training drug that is discriminated. The mechanism by which training dosage influences specificity is not known (Colpaert et al., 1980a, 1980b; Colpaert & Janssen, 1982b; Koek & Slangen, 1982b; Shannon & Holtzman, 1979; Stolerman & D'Mello, 1981; Teal & Holtzman, 1980b; White & Appel, 1982). Second, specificity can be either increased or decreased by training with paradigms that require the rat concurrently to discriminate several drugs (Colpaert & Janssen, 1982c; Overton, 1982c). For example, a rat trained to discriminate chlordiazepoxide (lever 1) versus ethanol, pentobarbital, ketamine or no drug (lever 2) might provide a high specificity assay for new benzodiazepine drugs (see Figure 2). Third, response bias, and perhaps qualitative specificity, can be manipulated by using asymmetrical reinforcement contingencies of various types. With such contingencies the reinforcers applied for correct (or incorrect) presses are different during D than during N training sessions. For example, rats may be punished for incorrect responses in one drug condition and not in the other (Colpaert & Janssen, 1981).

At least two mechanisms can be postulated by which a training procedure might lead to increased specificity. (1) The subjects might discriminate a smaller subset of the discriminable effects of the training drug. (2) The subjects might insist on a closer match between the effects of the training drug and those of a test drug as a condition for making the D response during a test session. At present it is not known which of these mechanisms is operative in the procedures for varying specificity described above. In this context we should mention the breaking point substitution test procedure described by Winter (1981a) in which the subject is subjected to progressively increasing ratios of reinforcement until its exclusive preference for the D lever gives way to mixed responding. Apparently this procedure yields higher specificity than do conventional substitution test paradigms, even though the training paradigm is unaltered. Hence, the second mechanism appears to be operative.

In the past specificity was generally viewed as fixed, and the results of substitution tests were often interpreted as directly reflecting the degree of stimulus overlap between the training drug and a test drug. For example, 100% D choices were often interpreted to mean that the test drug was essentially identical with the training drug, 0% D choices were inferred to mean no overlap in actions, and 50% D choices were interpreted as indicating partial (perhaps 50%) overlap. Unfortunately, no two investigators exactly agreed on the interpretation of test results. The recent discovery that specificity can vary depending on the training paradigm employed should appreciably alter interpretation of test results. We now know that a particular test drug can produce 0, 50, or 100% D choices, depending on the degree of specificity induced by the training procedure (Overton, 1982c). Apparently, the percent D choices observed during a substitution test has no fixed meaning and can only be interpreted with reference to the degree of specificity induced by the training paradigm employed.

Masking Apparently Does Not Occur

During substitution tests after D versus N training, suppose that drug $\underline{X}$ substitutes for the training drug and that substitution does not occur during tests when drugs $\underline{X}$ and $\underline{Y}$ are concurrently administered. One possible interpretation is that $\underline{Y}$ pharmacologically antagonizes or blocks $\underline{X}$ so that the actions of $\underline{X}$ are truly absent during the test. Another possibility, at least in principle, is that the discriminable effects of $\underline{Y}$ somehow mask (occlude, prevent the animal from perceiving) the effects of $\underline{X}$ even though they are present. The term mask is used here to convey the same meaning that it denotes in sensory psychophysics--a situation in which one stimulus prevents the perception of a second concurrently presented stimulus.

After D versus N DD training, rats frequently have been tested while simultaneously drugged with the training drug and with another drug; such tests usually have been performed to identify antagonists of the training drug. In most data thus far reported, the only instances when a second drug prevents the rat from performing the drug response are those in which the second drug pharmacologically antagonizes the effects of the training drug so that its discriminable effects are not present (Altshuler, Applebaum, & Shippenberg, 1981; Browne, 1981; Browne & Ho, 1975a; Browne & Weissman, 1981; Hernandez, Holohean, & Appel, 1978; Hirschhorn & Rosecrans, 1974a, 1974b; Jarbe, 1977; Jarbe & Ohlin, 1977; Romano, Goldstein, & Jewell, 1981; Rosecrans, 1979; Shearman & Lal, 1981; Silverman & Ho, 1980). Thus the results of these experiments suggest that masking seldom if ever occurs. Indeed, in interpreting their data most DD investigators have assumed that masking did not occur, and absence of masking has been an implicitly assumed property of DDs which, surprisingly, has almost never been explicitly discussed or demonstrated (except see Colpaert, 1977a; Witkin, Carter, & Dykstra, 1980).

However, the conclusion that masking does not occur between drug stimuli can hardly be regarded as firmly established. Firstly, experimental designs can be envisaged that should be considerably more sensitive to masking than any of the accidental tests for its occurrence presently in the literature (see below). Secondly, there are a few reported data which suggest that masking may have occurred (e.g., Browne, 1981; Browne & Weissman, 1981; Witkin et al., 1980). Possibly these reports indicate instances of masking; if so, they constitute a first step towards enumerating the conditions under which masking will in fact occur. However, notwithstanding these occasional instances of possible masking, it appears that most drugs do not mask the effects of most other drugs in DD preparations (Overton, 1983, 1984).

DDs Have Some Face Validity for the Study of Drug Abuse

For the study of most psychopharmacological issues, DDs have little or no face validity (see below). However, DDs do appear to provide an animal model which has some face validity for the study of (1) subjective side effects of drugs and (2) subjective or hedonic drug actions which may underlie drug abuse.

With respect to subjective side effects of drugs, it has not been demonstrated that DDs provide accurate preclinical data on such effects. However, it makes sense that if DDs are based on the subjective (perceived) sensory consequences of drug effects in animals, then DDs may be able to provide information about analogous drug effects in humans.

The application of DDs to the investigation of drug abuse has less face validity. Drug abuse is probably based, at least in part, on reinforcing stimulus effects of drugs (e.g., euphorigenic effects), and such reinforcing effects are probably one of the types of subjective effects capable of supporting DDs. Hence, DDs apparently provide a method for measuring and analyzing the sensory effects that underlie drug abuse. However, this application is complicated by the fact that DDs presumably can also be based on noxious subjective effects that would deter drug abuse and on affectively neutral subjective effects that are irrelevant to drug abuse. Also, drug abuse is often ascribed to nonsensory effects of drugs such as reduction of anxiety or selective amnesia for the dysphoric effects of drugs, and the DD preparation has no intrinsic face validity for the investigation of such drug actions. This paper primarily discusses the use of DDs to study the reinforcing stimulus effects of drugs.

Additionally, the DD preparation has been used to investigate the subjective effects of withdrawal in drug-tolerant animals and appears to have face validity for this purpose (Gellert & Holtzman, 1979; Miksic, Sherman, & Lal, 1981; Valentino, Herling, & Woods, 1983; Valentino, Smith, & Woods, 1981).

DISADVANTAGEOUS PROPERTIES OF DRUG DISCRIMINATIONS

This review would be incomplete if it did not describe the most prominent disadvantages and limitations of the DD procedure.

DD Training Procedures Are Cumbersome and Slow

We indicated earlier that DDs are learned as rapidly as sensory discriminations, but even sensory discriminations are learned slowly when animals receive only one training trial per day, as is required in all DD training paradigms to allow drug elimination between sessions. Hence, the process of shaping and training an animal to reliably discriminate a drug typically requires 1 to 3 months. Even longer training is required to establish DDs involving several manipulanda, several drugs, or low doses (Overton & Hayes, 1980; White & Holtzman, 1981). Such training is expensive. Parametric improvements in DD training paradigms have somewhat reduced the duration of training and increased the accuracy of the resulting discriminations, and some further improvement along these lines can be expected (e.g., Overton, 1978c, 1979b; Overton & Hayes, 1984). Nonetheless, the time required to establish DDs will probably continue to be an expensive aspect of the procedure. Apparently, this is only a practical difficulty which does not significantly compromise interpretation of DD results once they are obtained.

Each Substitution Test Yields Only a Bit of Data

With most DD procedures another practical difficulty is posed by the small yield of data produced by each individual substitution test. In the majority of published DD experiments, one substitution test was conducted per day, and each substitution test yielded one binary bit of data per rat as the animal made either a D or an N choice. Hence to measure performance under a particular test condition with 4-bit accuracy, the test procedure had to be repeated four times. Since training sessions must be interspersed between tests and since each test drug is typically evaluated at several doses, more than a month of work is commonly required to generate a dose-response curve showing the ability of a single test compound to substitute for a single training drug. Obviously, such procedures do not always fit conveniently into the life spans of rodents or of investigators.

Fortunately, new substitution test procedures have recently been developed that use repeated tests with cumulatively increasing doses within a single test session. These allow a complete dose-effect curve for a novel compound to be obtained during a single protracted test session. Although these procedures only yield binary data at each individual dose and are not yet fully validated or universally employed, it appears that they will reduce the amount of time required to conduct DD experiments (Herling, Hampton, Bertalmio, Winger, & Woods, 1980; Jarbe, Swedberg, & Mechoulam, 1981; McMillan, 1982; McMillan, Cole-Fullenwider, Hardwick, & Wenger, 1982; Shannon & Holtzman, 1976a, 1976b). A priori, we might expect such procedures to have three disadvantages. First, after a series of injections at various intervals prior to a particular test trial, the blood level of drug is not entirely predictable and is obviously influenced by a variety of factors. Second, the result obtained during a particular test trial within a test session may not be independent of the result obtained during the preceding test trial, and a different percentage of drug choices may be obtained at a given blood level depending on whether the level was higher or lower during the preceding test trial. Finally, the repeated series of test trials that is employed during such cumulative dosing procedures appears more likely to disrupt accurate response control under the training drug conditions than would be the case if only a single test trial was administered. Apparently this effect is most likely to be troublesome in instances where the training conditions are only weakly discriminable, and in such cases it may be necessary to schedule a higher percentage of training sessions than would otherwise be required. In spite of these difficulties, experience with the method thus far suggests that none of its potential problems are terribly serious and that the cumulative dosing procedure does increase the data yield obtained in DD studies.

Other procedures that yield more than one bit of data per substitution test have also been developed. However, these procedures have not been widely adopted, perhaps because they require relatively difficult training and/or test procedures (McMillan et al., 1982; McMillan & Wenger, 1983a; Schechter, 1981a; Shannon & Holtzman, 1976a, 1976b, 1979; Winter, 1981a).

DD Procedure Is Easiest With High Doses

Although DDs can be controlled by relatively low drug doses, DDs based on high doses are more stable and are less likely to be disrupted by substitution tests. Hence, in practice most DD studies use as high a training dose as is possible without disrupting behavioral performance in the DD task. With current DD preparations these doses are usually not outlandish, and they are lower than the doses used in preparations where disruption of ongoing behavior is used to indicate the presence of drug effects. Nonetheless, because high doses make DD experiments easier to conduct, one can recognize in the DD literature a tendency to use relatively high doses, even though this is not absolutely necessary in most cases.

Dose-Response Curves Are Somewhat Unstable

Discriminating a high training dose from no drug is easy because the training dose and the no-drug condition are several JNDs (just noticeable differences) apart (Colpaert & Janssen, 1982a; Overton, 1968b, 1977a). However, it appears that the generalization gradient obtained during tests with intermediate doses is not entirely determined by such D versus N training; hence, the ED50s may vary considerably from rat to rat and within a single rat at different points in time (Colpaert, Niemegeers, & Janssen, 1978a, 1978c; Overton, 1984). Usually these shifts in quantitative specificity are not obvious in the average generalization curves for a group of subjects, as shifts in the ED50s for individual animals tend to cancel one another (Colpaert et al., 1980a). Nonetheless, the preparation would provide more quantitatively reliable results if some method could be found to reduce the variability of the dose response curves both across and within subjects. Colpaert and Janssen (1982a) showed that high dose versus low dose DD training would produce steeper dose response curves and presumably smaller ED50 differences within and between animals, but this technique has not yet been used in enough studies so that its utility can be evaluated.

Specificity Varies in Different Drug Classes

When discussing specificity it is convenient to refer to pharmacological classes of drugs. In this paper the term pharmacological class will be used in its conventional sense to indicate a group of drugs that are generally agreed to produce one or more of the same effects (e.g., depressants, antimuscarinics, tricyclic antidepressants). Obviously, the definitions of these classes change as our knowledge of drug actions improves.

Recent reports suggest that the degree of specificity produced by D versus N training depends on the type of drug used for training (Overton, 1978b). Three cases may be distinguished. (1) With several types of training drugs, specificity approximates the width of the pharmacological class in which the training drug is found. This is the case for antimuscarinics, narcotic agonists, tetrahydrocannabinols, and antihistamines among others (Barry & Kubena, 1972; Colpaert, 1978; Colpaert, Niemegeers, & Janssen, 1975b; Overton, 1977a, 1978a; Woods, Young, & Herling, 1982). (2) In other cases, specificity appears to be higher, and not all drugs in the training drug's pharmacological class will mimic the training drug. This is true for cholinergics, antipsychotics, and narcotic mixed agonist/antagonists among others (Goas & Boston, 1978; Hirschhorn, 1977; Overton & Batta, 1979; Romano et al., 1981; Rosecrans, Spencer, Krynock, & Chance, 1978; Schechter & Rosecrans, 1972a). (3) In still other cases, specificity appears to be lower, as generalization is observed to drugs outside the training drug's pharmacological class. For example, anesthetics, benzodiazepines, muscle relaxants, and some anticonvulsants all tend to generalize to one another, perhaps because they share depressant effects (Barry, 1974; Barry & Krimmer, 1979; Barry & Kubena, 1972; Colpaert, 1977a; Colpaert, Desmedt, & Janssen, 1976; Haug & Gotestam, 1982; Herling, Valentino, & Winger, 1980; Jarbe & McMillan, 1983; Lal & Fielding, 1979; Overton, 1966, 1976, 1977b; Takada, 1982). Other instances of generalization to drugs outside the training drug's class also have been reported (Herling, Coale, Hein, Winger, & Woods, 1981; Herling & Woods, 1981; Holtzman, 1980; Overton, 1974; Shannon, 1981; Teal & Holtzman, 1980a).

In the preceding paragraph we used the breadth of pre-existing drug categories as a standard against which to compare specificity. Alternately, however, it may be the case that a particular D versus N training paradigm produces a fixed degree of specificity in all classes and that some pharmacological classes include a more diverse array of drugs than others, with regard to their discriminable effects, thus allowing cross-generalization between all members in some classes but not in others. At this time we have no way to measure breadth of generalization except by counting the number of drugs to which generalization occurs and by noting their apparent degree of pharmacological similarity to the training drug. Comparison to pharmacological categories established by other psychopharmacological procedures has been very useful in this enterprise and has led to the conclusion that generalization occurs to a greater or smaller portion of the drugs in the training drug's class and sometimes to drugs in other classes depending on the type of drug used for training. Whether this result should be interpreted as showing that some classes are larger than others or as showing that specificity is higher after training in some classes than in others cannot be determined at this time.

The varying degree of specificity produced by D versus N training with different types of drugs is basically a disadvantage of the procedure, since a substantial amount of effort must be devoted to determining the degree of specificity obtained in a drug class before the results of substitution tests can be readily interpreted.

Methods for Controlling Specificity Are Poorly Developed

The methods now available for controlling the degree of specificity produced by DD training have serious limitations and/or have not been tested sufficiently to establish their limitations or capabilities.

Firstly, the method which involves a reduction in training dosage only alters specificity with some types of training drugs·(Shannon & Herling, 1983). Additionally, in some cases a low training dosage may produce qualitatively different discriminable effects than a high dosage, thus changing the basis of the discrimination as well as the degree of specificity achieved (Colpaert, et al., 1976; Emmett-Oglesby, Wurst, & Lal, 1983). Finally, this method usually increases the duration of training and decreases the asymptotic accuracy and stability of DDs, thus making substitution test data more difficult to obtain and to interpret.

Secondly, the method which involves the use of several additional training drugs to manipulate specificity also poses some problems. In order to substantially increase specificity, ancillary training drugs rather similar to the primary training drug must be used. This prolongs training considerably, is only possible in classes where such drugs exist and where the relationship of their discriminable effects to those of the primary training drug is known, reduces the accuracy and stability of asymptotic discrimination, and probably can only be done in drug classes which produce readily discriminable actions (Colpaert & Janssen, 1982c; Overton, 1982c).

Thirdly, the method which uses asymmetrical reinforcement contingencies biases the animals to press either the D or N lever and thereby shifts the ED50 that is obtained during substitution tests with various doses of the training drug as well as with other drugs (Colpaert & Janssen, 1981; Koek & Slangen, 1982a; McMillan & Wenger, 1983b). However in unpublished studies we have found that such procedures do not alter qualitative specificity (the amount of substitution for the training drug obtained with dissimilar drugs) to a degree any greater than the extent to which they modify quantitative specificity (the amount of substitution observed with reduced doses of the training drug). If our results are correct and applicable to all varieties of asymmetrical reinforcement, this will indicate that such procedures are not useful for varying the qualitative specificity of the DD preparation. Further development of methods for controlling specificity will be required before such methods can be employed with confidence.

DD Procedures May Induce Tolerance

In some studies regimens of drug administration have apparently failed to induce tolerance to the discriminable effects of a drug. However, all these studies used a design that was flawed, since DD training continued while tolerance was induced thereby allowing the rats to learn to discriminate the reduced actions produced by drug in the now-tolerant animals (e.g., Bueno & Carlini, 1972; Colpaert, Kuyps, Niemegeers, & Janssen, 1976; Colpaert, Niemegeers, & Janssen, 1978b; Hirschhorn & Rosecrans, 1974c). In other studies which did not suffer from this unfortunate experimental design, tolerance to discriminable drug effects has been observed (Barrett & Leith, 1981; Jarbe & Henriksson, 1973; McKenna & Ho, 1977; Miksic & Lal, 1977; Overton & Batta, 1979; Schechter & Rosecrans, 1972d; Shannon & Holtzman, 1976b; Witkin, Dykstra, & Carter, 1982; York & Winter, 1975). Most of these studies induced tolerance by administration of doses higher than the DD training dosage, and only Miksic & Lal (1977) have shown that the DD training regimen itself induced tolerance.

It is likely that all DD training procedures induce some degree of tolerance to the training drug and that all DD results are thus obtained from "abnormal" rats. Additionally, it appears that whenever the DD training paradigm is interrupted (e.g., over weekends) tolerance may begin to dissipate, thus shifting the pharmacological responsiveness of the subjects. Apparently tolerance may be reduced by the administration of test sessions with reduced doses of the training drug or by tests with drugs that differ from the training drug as well as by more prolonged vacations from training. An additional complexity is posed by the possibility that tolerance to various actions of the training drug may develop (and dissipate) to different degrees and at different rates. Such effects probably do not unduly complicate the interpretation of many DD results. However, Modrow et al. (1981) found different dosage generalization curves during test sessions preceded by D and by N training sessions--an effect possibly produced by short term (24 hour) tolerance induced by the training drug--and other effects of changes in tolerance may go unnoticed in many DD studies. It appears that the role of tolerance is often disregarded in DD experiments, and it would be reassuring if more investigators conducted data analyses designed to identify the effects of shifts in tolerance, if any, in their DD preparations.

Discriminated Effects May Not Be Related to Abuse

As mentioned earlier, not all sensory consequences of drug actions are conducive to drug abuse, and a priori it appears that we can distinguish three categories of subjective drug effects: (1) effects such as euphorigenic actions which promote drug abuse; (2) aversive (nocioceptive) effects which deter drug abuse; and (3) neutral subjective effects which can provide a basis for discriminative control but which neither increase nor decrease a compound's abuse liability.

It would be convenient to speculate that effects in the first category are more frequently produced or are more readily discriminable than those in categories two and three but this apparently is not true. Some time ago this writer performed a rather extensive study designed to determine whether drugs with a high liability for abuse would always be readily discriminated and, conversely, whether drugs with low abuse liability would be relatively nondiscriminable. A high correlation between degree of discriminability and liability for abuse would have suggested that effects in category one were primarily responsible for most drug discriminations. However, the data showed a different result, as only a modest correlation was observed between degree of discriminability and abuse liability (Overton & Batta, 1977). The result clearly suggests that subjective effects in categories two and three form the basis for many, if not most, DDs.

Apparently, the face validity of DDs as a method for studying drug abuse is of a very limited nature. Even though DDs apparently can detect, quantify, and categorize many of the subjective effects that underlie drug abuse, they also detect many other types of subjective effects, and care must be taken to ascertain what type of subjective effect underlies each DD. Thus far, relatively little effort has been directed towards determining which DDs are based on effects related to drug abuse and which are not.

Theoretical Explanations for DDs Are Inadequate

In the next section we will discuss the adequacy of extant theories for DDs. Here, under the topic of disadvantages of the DD method, let us simply note that the primitive nature of DD theories makes it more difficult to interpret certain experimental results and extremely difficult to discover improved DD procedures except via a trial and error approach.

A CRITIQUE OF THEORETICAL FORMULATIONS FOR SDL AND DRUG DISCRIMINATIONS

In spite of about 500 published studies elucidating the empirical properties of SDL and DDs, there is still no generally accepted and adequately detailed theoretical formulation about their causes that satisfactorily predicts all of the observed properties of SDL and DDs. With respect to this issue, it is useful to recall that SDL and DDs are probably based on the same drug effects (Overton, 1964) and that a complete theoretical formulation must predict the properties of both phenomena.

Symmetrical SDL: D Cues Replace N Cues

All early investigators who attributed SDL to drug-induced "stimuli" expected SDL to be symmetrical (i.e., they expected response decrements to be produced by both D-->N and N-->D transitions). This expectation was based on the assumption that "normal" or no-drug interoceptive cues would be replaced by "drug" cues when drug was administered, and that the converse would also be true (Auld, 1951; Barry, Miller, & Tidd, 1962; Barry et al., 1962; Heistad & Torres, 1959; Miller, 1957; Shmavonian, 1956). Model 1 in Table 2 shows this traditional sensory formulation for SDL. In the N-->N and D-->D groups, the same environmental contextual cues (C) and interoceptive cues (N or D cues) are present during training and during the test for retention; hence, test session retrieval and performance are normal. In the N-->D group, learning takes place in the presence of C and N cues; during the retrieval test, N cues are replaced by D cues and hence memory retrieval is impaired. In the D-->N group, training takes place in the presence of C and D cues; during the test, D cues are replaced by N cues and so memory retrieval is impaired here also. The model

Table 2

Effect of the Interactions Between Drug and No-Drug Cues on the Predicted Outcome of 2x2 SDL Experiments

Drug Condition		Salient Cues		Predicted Performance
During Training	During Test	During Training	During Test	During Test Session

Model 1: D cues replace (eliminate) N cues.

N	N	C+N	C+N	1.00
N	D	C+N	C+D	0.50
D	N	C+D	C+N	0.50
D	D	C+D	C+D	1.00

Model 2: D cues superimpose on N cues.

N	N	C+N	C+N	1.00
N	D	C+N	C+N+D	1.00
D	N	C+N+D	C+N	0.66

Model 3: D cues (D1,D2) replace some N cues (N1) and superimpose on others (N2,N3).

N	N	C+N1+N2+N3	C+N1+N2+N3	1.00
N	D	C+N1+N2+N3	C+N2+N3+D1+D2	0.75
D	N	C+N2+N3+D1+D2	C+N1+N2+N3	0.60
D	D	C+N2+N3+D1+D2	C+N2+N3+D1+D2	1.00

Note: The table shows the results predicted by three theoretical models when subjects first learn a response and are subsequently tested for retrieval of that response either in the same drug condition (D or N) that was present during training or in a different drug condition.
C = Exteroceptive contextual cues (apparatus cues)
N = All salient interoceptive cues present in the no drug state
D = All salient drug-induced cues
N1, N2, N3 = Individual salient interoceptive cues present in the no-drug state
D1, D2 = Individual salient drug-induced cues

appears straightforward and has survived for at least twenty-five years--a full century if we count Ribot's initial presentation of the theory. A number of studies have reported data congruent with the theory (e.g., Bustamante, Jordan, Vila, Gonzalez, & Insua, 1970; Cole & Gay, 1976; Overton, 1964).

Asymmetrical SDL

Surprisingly, in many experiments impaired retrieval has been observed only after D-->N state changes and not after N-->D state changes. In other studies retrieval deficits have been observed after both D-->N and N-->D state changes, but they have been larger after D-->N transitions. The term asymmetrical SDL has been used to describe such results in which retrieval deficits were observed primarily in the D-->N group (Overton, 1968a).

Probably because of our theoretical presuppositions, asymmetrical SDL has been a neglected phenomenon. The original stimulus model for SDL predicted symmetrical SDL, and most neurological models for SDL have also been developed to explain symmetrical SDL (Bliss, 1974; Overton, 1973, 1978d). The statistical methods that are most commonly used to test the significance of SDL effects pool results in the D-->N and N-->D groups and do not indicate whether both N-->D and D-->N transitions produce similarly large retrieval deficits (Swanson & Kinsbourne, 1979).

In this context, the frequent reports of data indicating asymmetrical SDL have been problematic, since they appeared to reflect a phenomenon contrary to theoretical expectations. However, the data clearly do suggest that both symmetrical and asymmetrical SDL exist as bona fide phenomena. In the majority of reported SDL studies, some degree of asymmetry is present; in many reports impairment of retrieval is entirely lacking in the N-->D group (Avis & Pert, 1974; Barnhart & Abbott, 1967; Berger & Stein, 1969a, 1969b; Deutsch & Roll, 1973; Eich, Weingartner, Stillman, & Gillin, 1975; Evans & Patton, 1968; File 1974; Goldberg, Hefner, Robichaud, & Dubinsky, 1973; Henriksson & Jarbe, 1971; Holloway, 1972; Overton, 1974; Pappas & Gray, 1971; Peters & McGee, 1982). We will argue here that the sensory model for symmetrical SDL that has been accepted by most investigators since the mid-1950s is inconsistent with contemporary theories regarding the operation of contextual cues and that both symmetrical and asymmetrical SDL are entirely consistent with contemporary theories.

"No-Drug" Cues

First, let us ask what N cues are. Ribot (1882) asserted that they were sensations reflecting the normal functioning of the organs of the body and normal levels of activity in various regions of the brain. Today we might specify that, at a particular instant in time, N cues reflect the current degree of arousal, hunger, thirst, depression, distention of the stomach, vertigo, ringing in the ears (if any), degree of fatigue, et cetera. Next consider a question which is crucial; when a moderate dose of a psychoactive drug is administered, how many N cues are substantially changed? To this writer it appears that the answer is either "some" or "none," depending on the drug and dosage administered. For example, pentobarbital may increase thirst and decrease arousal but may not alter the other interoceptive sensations mentioned. An antihistamine may decrease motion sickness and dry one's mucosa but will probably have no other effects. Most N cues will still be present in the D state. In addition, drugs may create new sensory cues (e.g., hallucinations, euphoria). Such drug-induced cues (a different set of cues for each type of drug) will be superimposed on the still-present N cues and appear to match what contemporary DD investigators apparently have in mind when they refer to drug-induced discriminative stimuli or D cues.

Consequences If D Cues Are Superimposed on N Cues

Model 2 in Table 2 recasts the traditional sensory interpretation of SDL in a more contemporary vein by assuming that drug injection simply adds D cues while leaving N cues unchanged. The N-->N and D-->D groups experience no change in contextual stimuli between training and testing and hence show unimpaired retrieval. So does the N-->D group because, although D cues have been added to its internal environment during the test session, both the C and N cues that were present during training are still present during test sessions and allow efficient retrieval. Only the D-->N group shows a retrieval deficit which occurs because D cues were present during training, became associated with the learned response, and are absent during the test for retrieval. It appears that if drug states simply create D cues without abolishing N cues, then a sensory model for SDL actually predicts asymmetrical SDL--not symmetrical SDL. This idea, incidentally, does not originate with the present writer. It has been repeatedly mentioned in the literature in recent years but has not been generally accepted as yet (Barry, 1978; Boyd & Caul, 1979; File, 1974; Hinderliter, 1978; Hinderliter, Webster, & Riccio, 1975; Mactutus, McCutcheon, & Riccio, 1980; Richardson, Riccio, & Jonke, 1983).

Finally, Model 3 in Table 2 portrays an intermediate case in which some N cues are modified by the drug (N1 becomes D1) and other N cues are unaffected (N2 and N3 remain), and additionally the drug creates some new D cues (D2). The effectiveness of memory retrieval during the test session is considered to be proportional to the number of cues that were present during training and are still present during the test session; all cues are assumed to be equally strong and effects are assumed to be additive. In the N-->N and D-->D groups, no cues change and retrieval is normal. In the N-->D group, the C, N2, and N3 cues are still present during testing, but N1 is missing, yielding somewhat impaired retrieval; the addition of cues D1 and D2 has no effect. In the D-->N group, the C, N2, and N3 cues are present at the time of retrieval, but both D1 and D2 are missing, yielding a larger impairment in retrieval than in the N-->D group. The result is a partially asymmetrical SDL effect. Obviously, we can manipulate the predicted result by varying the assumed relative strength and number of C, N, and D cues and by varying the number of N cues that we assume to be modified by the drug. Depending on the assumptions that we make (the drug and dosage that we use?), the predicted SDL effect may be symmetrical, partially asymmetrical, or entirely asymmetrical.

The theoretical issues raised in the preceding paragraphs have not been empirically addressed in SDL studies. However the vast majority of published SDL results are at least partially asymmetrical and thus inconsistent with the traditional sensory model for SDL (Model 1 in Table 2).

Sensory Theories for DDs

A parallel theoretical problem has existed in the interpretation of the results of DD studies. Early DD investigators often argued that their animals discriminated drug cues versus no-drug cues (Brown, Feldman, & Moore, 1968; Browne & Ho, 1975a; Jones, Grant, & Vospalek, 1976; Schechter, 1973). However, most contemporary investigators apparently believe that animals discriminate presence versus absence of specific drug stimuli; N cues are never mentioned. This formulation is congruent with the common observation that during tests with drugs that are pharmacologically dissimilar from the training drug, the animals usually perform the N response; such results are interpreted as showing that since D cues like those of the training drug are absent, the N response is performed (Colpaert, 1978; Overton, Merkle, & Hayes, 1983).

The change in the nomenclature used to describe DD results has taken place quietly during the past twenty years without any theoretical discussion in the literature and appears to have taken place so that DD investigators' theoretical formulations would not be obviously inconsistent with the data that they obtained. However, a parallel change in theoretical conceptions has not occurred among SDL investigators, most of whom still accept a theory which predicts symmetrical SDL, use statistical tests that can only properly evaluate the occurrence of SDL if it is symmetrical, and regularly obtain results that are asymmetrical. In this paper we are clearly taking the position that SDL theory is in need of revision. However, we might also note that few DD publications have been theoretically oriented and that even DD theory is not very well developed.

One interpretation of DDs likens the occurrence of N choices during tests with a novel drug after D versus N training to results obtained after sensory discrimination training using a discriminative stimulus (Sd) in one modality (e.g., visual Sd) when tests are conducted with the Sd replaced by a stimulus in a different sensory modality (e.g., auditory Sd). This interpretation of DDs implies that each type of drug produces stimuli in a different modality. But what are these modalities, and how can there be so many of them (about 20 have been demonstrated)? By what brain mechanisms do these sensory "modalities" get processed? Why have we been unable to identify sensory events that can mimic the drug stimuli which presumably underlie DDs?

Note that the assumption that each type of drug produces cues in a different modality is counterintuitive (see previous paragraph), as it implies the existence of too many modalities. As an alternative model, we might postulate that all drugs produce stimulus effects in a rather small number of sensory modalities and that each type of drug produces a different pattern of sensory events in these modalities. This alternate hypothesis implies that we should, in time, discover more interactions between the stimulus effects of pharmacologically dissimilar drugs than have thus far been reported. Instances of masking, generalization to pharmacologically dissimilar drugs, and expected generalizations to drug mixtures should all occur, at least occasionally, and patterns of these drug interactions should eventually be discernible.

We face an unpleasant choice between the first model, which claims more distinct modalities of interoceptive experience than appear reasonable, and the second, which fails to predict the high qualitative specificity that D versus N training is usually reported to produce. Neither model appears very satisfactory. It appears that neither DD nor SDL investigators are presently in a very good position to predict or to explain their results on the basis of available theoretical models. Since available theories match available data so loosely, they provide a weak foundation for building a scientific understanding of the subjective drug effects that cause drug abuse, and they do not allow us to precisely interpret the results of many DD experiments or to rationally develop new DD paradigms that have better properties than the ones presently in use. To remedy this problem, we can only hope that future DD research will incorporate substantial efforts directed toward an improved understanding of the effects of behavioral variables in the DD paradigm.

THE PROBLEM OF FACE VALIDITY

The most important disadvantage of the DD procedure is the fact that DDs lack face validity as a method for investigating most psychopharmacological questions. Because this issue is important, we will discuss it at length, beginning with a general discussion of the face validity of DDs as a neuropharmacological research method and then proceeding to special issues involved in the application of DDs to investigate issues related to drug abuse.

Face Validity of DDs as a General Preclinical Assay

DDs have little face validity for the preclinical investigation of many psychopharmacological issues! There is no a priori reason to believe that all antianxiety drugs will produce similar subjective effects in rats that are not fearful or that all phenothiazines will produce shared sensory consequences irrespective of the strength of their extrapyramidal side effects. It is not intuitively obvious that the clinically relevant actions of all of these drugs should be the primary cues used by rats when DDs are learned, nor is it obvious why peripheral side effects should be disregarded by the animals. DDs do, in fact, appear to be based on clinically (or scientifically) important drug actions in many instances. However, this was hardly predictable a priori and is not very well understood even when it occurs.

To clarify this point, Table 3 presents a number of fictitious examples illustrating the varied relationships that may exist between discriminable drug effects and clinically important drug effects. The table assumes that drugs can produce only ten possible actions on the central nervous system, five discriminable and five nondiscriminable; the five discriminable drug effects are assumed to be equally discriminable. The 10 drug effects are classified as clinically relevant (C), referring to important actions that are prototypic of the drug in question, and as side effects (S), referring to actions produced by the drug that are not required in order to achieve its desired clinical actions. Obviously, in some cases the term scientifically important could be substituted for clinically relevant (e.g., competitive blockade of serotonin would be the scientifically important action of cyproheptadine, and this effect might or might not have significant clinical utility).

In general, the table is self-explanatory. Case 2 describes a simple situation in which drugs C and D both produce the same clinically important action (drug action #8) which is discriminable, and where these drugs have no other effects on the brain either discriminable or nondiscriminable. In this instance DDs can be used very effectively to investigate the properties and mechanisms of action of drugs C and D. Case 4 involves two drugs that produce the same clinically relevant effect (drug action #1) which is not discriminable. Additionally, drugs G and H both produce other actions which are discriminable and which differ for the two drugs. In this case DDs will be learned with both G and H but will provide no information relevant to the clinically important actions of these drugs (Rats trained to discriminate G versus N could, however, be used to assist in the development of new drugs that did not produce side effect #6.). Case 6 depicts a situation where DDs will provide some correct and some misleading results. Drugs K and L will be correctly identified as producing effects different than those of drugs M and N, but the differences between the actions of drugs M and N will not be identified by the DD procedure. Finally, in Case 7 drugs O and R will mimic P, but substitution in the reverse direction is not likely as P will produce only one third of the discriminated effects of O or R. Incidentally, this is the only point in this review where we allude to the phenomenon of one-way

Table 3

Hypothetical Examples of Instances in Which Discriminated Drug Effects
Can Provide Useful Information About the Scientifically or Clinically
Important Actions of a Drug and of Instances in Which They Cannot

DRUG	NONDISCRIMINABLE DRUG EFFECTS					DISCRIMINABLE DRUG EFFECTS				
	1	2	3	4	5	6	7	8	9	10

Case 1: DRUGS SHARE NONDISCRIMINABLE CLINICAL EFFECTS.
DDs are not learned with such drugs.

DRUG	1	2	3	4	5	6	7	8	9	10
A			C		C					
B			C		C					

Case 2: DRUGS SHARE CLINICAL ACTIONS THAT ARE DISCRIMINABLE.
DDs correctly indicate drugs C & D to have similar actions.

DRUG	1	2	3	4	5	6	7	8	9	10
C								C		
D								C		

Case 3: CLINICAL EFFECTS ARE DIFFERENT AND NOT DISCRIMINABLE.
SIDE EFFECTS ARE SHARED AND DISCRIMINABLE.
DDs will misleadingly categorize these drugs as similar.

DRUG	1	2	3	4	5	6	7	8	9	10
E	C						S		S	
F			C				S		S	

Case 4: CLINICAL EFFECTS ARE SHARED AND NOT DISCRIMINABLE.
SIDE EFFECTS ARE DIFFERENT AND DISCRIMINABLE.
DDs misleadingly categorize these drugs as dissimilar.

DRUG	1	2	3	4	5	6	7	8	9	10
G	C						S			
H	C							S		

Case 5: CLINICAL EFFECTS ARE SHARED AND DISCRIMINABLE.
SIDE EFFECTS ARE DIFFERENT AND NOT DISCRIMINABLE.
DDs correctly categorize these drugs as similar.

DRUG	1	2	3	4	5	6	7	8	9	10
I	S	S	S				C			C
J	S			S	S		C			C

Case 6: SOME CLINICAL EFFECTS ARE DISCRIMINABLE.
OTHER CLINICAL EFFECTS ARE NOT DISCRIMINABLE.
DD results are determined only by the discriminable effects.

DRUG	1	2	3	4	5	6	7	8	9	10
K		C					C			
L		C					C			
M		C						C		
N			C				C			

Case 7: CLINICAL EFFECTS ARE OVERLAPPING AND DISCRIMINABLE.
NO SIDE EFFECTS ARE PRODUCED.
DDs yield one-way substitution. O and R mimic P.

DRUG	1	2	3	4	5	6	7	8	9	10
O						C	C	C		
P								C		
R								C	C	C

Note: C = Clinically or scientifically important effects of the
drugs
S = Unimportant side effects of the drugs

substitution which is sometimes observed in DD studies (Bueno, Carlini, Finkelfarb, & Suzuki, 1972; Colpaert, Niemegeers, & Janssen, 1976; D'Mello, 1982; Overton, 1966).

The table suggests that the a priori likelihood is low that DDs can provide a useful research paradigm with any particular class of drugs. Hence, it is hardly surprising that widespread adoption of the DD method did not occur until the results of DDs procedures were shown to be useful in several drug classes. Evidence is now available suggesting that DDs are based on clinically or scientifically important drug effects in several pharmacological classes, and from this fact we draw two inferences. First, a relatively high proportion of drug effects on the central nervous system appear to have discriminable consequences. Second, the prototypic or desired effects of drugs in these classes appear to be more discriminable than are the undesired side effects of the same drugs.

Face Validity of DDs for Study of Drug Abuse

DDs may have face validity for investigation of the drug effects that underlie drug abuse if the following three conditions are met.

1. Sensory effects underlie and cause drug abuse.
2. Sensory events underlie DDs.
3. The sensory events underlying DDs are the same as those that underlie drug abuse.

In this paper we will not attempt to deal with the first question--whether and to what degree reinforcing sensory effects are responsible for the abuse of various drugs. Also, we will not attempt a discussion of issue three--an enumeration of the instances where the sensory events underlying DDs are the same as those that cause drug abuse--because a suitable data base for such a discussion is not yet available. We will discuss in detail the second issue--whether DDs are based on the sensory consequences of drug actions--because that issue is of fundamental importance and because a considerable amount of recently reported evidence bears on it.

Are SDL and DDs Based on Sensory Effects of Drugs?

In view of the current popularity of stimulus interpretations of both SDL and DDs, it is probably wise to state explicitly that there are alternative mechanisms that could be responsible for the phenomena; Bliss (1974) referred to these as neurological models. Although the first theoretical explanation for SDL was a sensory theory (Ribot, 1891), the second was a neurological model (Semon, 1904), and Girden (1942a, 1942b, 1942c, 1947) in his pioneering experimental reports on SDL never even mentioned sensory drug effects. The controversy between sensory and neurological models continued throughout the 1970s with most review papers on theories for SDL devoting more space to neurological theories than to sensory theories (Bliss, 1974; Overton, 1978d). Even at this point in time, although a sensory interpretation enjoys wide popularity, the evidence supporting such an interpretation is less than definitive. Hence the decision to devote a substantial portion of this paper to a consideration of this question.

Most of the evidence regarding this issue falls into one of the following three categories: (1) Evidence which is compatible with a sensory interpretation but is equally compatible with some or all of the alternate neurological models. (2) Evidence which is compatible with a sensory interpretation and which is incompatible with many or all of the neurological models. (3) Evidence which is somewhat embarrassing to a sensory interpretation of DDs, although not necessarily strongly supportive of a neurological model. We will devote one section of this paper to each of these categories.

EVIDENCE COMPATIBLE WITH EITHER SENSORY
OR NEUROLOGICAL INTERPRETATIONS OF DRUG DISCRIMINATIONS

This section will enumerate properties of DDs and SDL that are compatible with a sensory interpretation of these phenomena and are equally compatible with most neurological models for SDL and DDs.

Appearance of DD Behavior

The behavior that animals exhibit during the performance of DDs resembles in many respects that seen during the performance of sensory discriminations. In maze tasks vicarious trial and error behavior can be seen. Learning curves showing the acquisition of discriminations are indistinguishable from those obtained when sensory stimuli are discriminated.

Relative Strength of Response Control by Drugs and by Stimuli

The strength of SDL and DD effects is markedly dependent on the drug and dosage employed (Mayse & DeVietti, 1971; Overton, 1982a). Hence an explicit comparison of the degree of response control produced by drug states and by sensory stimuli is difficult. A few SDL and DD studies have attempted this comparison and, depending on the parameters employed, have observed that response control by drug stimuli was either stronger or weaker than response control by sensory stimuli (Balster, 1970; Connelly & Connelly, 1978; Connelly, Connelly, & Epps, 1973; Duncan et al., 1979; Jarbe, Laaksonen, & Svensson, 1983; Kilbey et al., 1971; Overton, 1964, 1968b, 1971; Spear et al., 1980). In general it appears that the strength of drug SDL effects can be considered comparable to the effects of contextual stimuli on memory retrieval.

Broad Generalization Gradients Across Dosage

After D versus N training using a particular drug and dosage, substitution tests can be conducted with various doses of the training drug. Usually the drug response generalizes to doses significantly higher and lower than the training dose with an appreciable percentage of drug responses occurring with doses down to about 30% of the training dose (i.e., rather broad generalization gradients are obtained along the intensity [dosage] continuum; Barry, 1978; Colpaert & Slangen, 1982; Overton, 1966). In a few instances sharp gradients have been obtained, and the particular factors that cause such steep gradients have not yet been determined. To some degree the broad gradients may be artifactual, since levels of drug in the brain vary somewhat during successive training sessions as the result of drug excretion, redistribution in body tissues, and other factors. However, even if this source of variation were controlled, it appears likely that rather broad dosage generalization gradients still would be obtained. Such generalization gradients obtained during test sessions with reduced doses of the training drug are reminiscent of those seen during analogous generalization testing along the quantitative (intensity) dimension of sensory discriminative stimuli.

Peak Shift Is Usually Not Seen

After high-dose versus low-dose DD training, peak shift has been reported during test sessions with various doses of the training drug (Akins, Gouvier, & Lyons, 1980). However, after D versus N training, peak shift is usually not seen (e.g., White & Appel, 1982). This may be an artifact caused by a "ceiling effect" in the vicinity of the training dosage. Additionally, it might be necessary to test with doses as high as twice the training dosage in order to see peak shift, and this is seldom done (but see Emmett-Oglesby et al., 1983). Finally, note that in sensory discrimination paradigms, training to discriminate the presence versus absence of a discriminative stimulus is not the paradigm that most readily allows observation of peak shift. In any case, since some neurological models for DDs predict peak shift, its occurrence versus nonoccurrence is not critical to acceptance of a sensory model.

Overtraining Abolishes SDL

Several studies have shown that a well-learned response will generalize successfully across changes in drug state that would disrupt performance of a response that was not overtrained. In these studies the effect of overtraining on SDL was demonstrated by using several groups of subjects which received different amounts of training before the effects of a change in drug state were evaluated (Bliss, 1973; Eich & Birnbaum, 1982; Iwahara & Noguchi, 1972, 1974; Modrow, Salm, & Bliss, 1982). In most other 2x2 studies where SDL was reported, subjects were in fact only trained to a rather weak criterion. Indeed, in the entire literature reporting SDL effects, all positive findings involve recently mastered responses. Hence, the literature suggests that a change in drug state cannot prevent retrieval and performance of a well-trained, overly practiced response. SDL appears to be demonstrable only with responses that are not overtrained.

SDL Effects Summate With Stimulus Context Effects

Duncan (1979) reported that a simultaneous change in drug state and in stimulus context could impair memory retrieval even though neither change by itself would impair retrieval. Other studies have shown that the addition of sensory retrieval cues or, in human subjects, category cues can prevent SDL effects that would otherwise occur (Connelly et al., 1973; Connelly, Connelly, & Nevitt, 1977; Connelly, Connelly, & Phifer, 1975; Eich, 1977, 1980; Eich et al., 1975; Petersen, 1977). It appears that sensory events and drug state manipulations conjointly determine the efficiency of memory retrieval.

Stimulus Blocking Occurs

Recently, Jarbe showed that initial discriminative training with ethanol would block the subsequent acquisition of discriminative control by the illumination conditions light versus dark. Conversely, discriminative light versus dark training would partially block the subsequent acquisition of control by the conditions pentobarbital versus no drug (Jarbe, Svensson, & Laaksomen, 1983). Although this type of interaction between exteroceptive stimulus control and DDs certainly suggests a sensory interpretation of SDL and DDs, it is compatible with some neurological models for SDL.

Learning Set Phenomena Occur in DD and SDL Experiments

In a T-maze DD task, Overton (1971) demonstrated that light versus dark discriminations could be more rapidly learned if rats had previously mastered an ethanol versus N discrimination in the same task. This suggested that a learning set established by DD training could facilitate subsequent acquisition of sensory discriminations. In a different SDL task Bliss (1974) required monkeys to learn a series of visual discriminations while drugged. Each individual discrimination failed to generalize to the no-drug state, but after several had been learned the resulting learning set did generalize to the no-drug condition. This result appears somewhat counterintuitive since it is usually argued that simple types of learning should generalize more easily across changes in drug state than complex types of learning. However Bliss's data suggest the opposite--the learning set generalized (perhaps because it was overtrained?) even though the individual discriminations failed to generalize. Modrow, Salm, and Bliss (1982) obtained similar results. These learning set phenomena appear to be compatible with both neurological and sensory models for SDL and DDs.

All of the preceding similarities between drug and stimulus control of behavior are compatible with a sensory interpretation of SDL and DDs. However, most of the neurological models for SDL and DDs (reviewed by Bliss, 1974, and by Overton, 1973, 1978d) also predict the same phenomena.

EVIDENCE SUPPORTING A SENSORY INTERPRETATION OF DRUG DISCRIMINATIONS

This section describes several types of evidence that do support the acceptance of a sensory interpretation of SDL and DDs because the data are incompatible with most or all of the proposed neurological models for these phenomena.

No-Drug Responses Are the Default Choice During Substitution Tests

We previously described the fact that during substitution tests conducted after D versus N training, D choices are only observed during tests conducted with drugs that pharmacologically resemble the training drug. In other words, the majority of centrally acting drugs do not produce D choices. We suggested that this result is analogous to what might be expected after training using a discriminative stimulus in one modality (e.g., auditory) if tests were then conducted with the discriminative stimulus replaced by a stimulus from a different sensory modality (e.g., visual). In the present context we should add that most neurological models for SDL and DDs apparently do not predict this outcome but instead predict mixed, random, or confused choice behavior during tests with drugs that pharmacologically differ from the training drug. Hence, the high qualitative specificity produced by D versus N training appears to support a sensory interpretation of DDs. Parenthetically, a few neurological models may predict N responses as the default choice during such substitution tests.

Threshold Dosages for SDL Are Higher Than for DDs

It appears that a determination of the lowest dose that is capable of producing SDL and DDs, respectively, can test whether the mechanism underlying these effects is sensory in nature or involves one of the postulated neurological mechanisms. The argument is as follows.

The literature on contextual control suggests that moderately large sensory changes are required to produce retrieval failures caused by a change in stimulus context. In contrast, after discrimination training it is reasonable to expect that an animal will be able to discriminate much smaller differences between stimuli because prolonged training will allow the animal to gradually learn to attend to the relevant attributes of the discriminated stimuli. Although the literature actually provides little evidence regarding the relative magnitude of the sensory changes that are required to produce (1) retrieval deficits based on changes in sensory context and (2) an adequate basis for discriminative control, some evidence suggests that the threshold for discriminative control is considerably lower than for contextual retrieval effects—perhaps an order of magnitude lower (Riccio, Urda, & Thomas, 1966). Analogously, a sensory interpretation of SDL and DDs appears to predict that the threshold for discriminative control will be considerably lower than the threshold required to produce SDL decrements.

In contrast, all neurological models for SDL predict that the thresholds for DDs and for SDL will be equal. According to these theories, DDs are based on weak (but measurable) SDL effects. During DD training the animal is assumed to learn two responses that have approximately equal habit strengths. During each DD trial both habits are believed to be retrieved from memory. However, the habit that was learned in the currently imposed drug state is retrieved somewhat more efficiently and dominates the overt behavior of the animal (Spear et al., 1980). Clearly, in such a situation where two responses are competing for expression, if the state-appropriate response is consistently performed, then its engram must be appreciably (measurably) more retrievable than that of the other response. Hence, the lowest drug dosage that is capable of controlling discriminative responding should be no lower than the lowest dosage that will produce a measurable SDL effect after D-->N or N-->D state changes.

The differing predictions of the sensory and neurological theories have, to some degree, been experimentally tested. Suppose that one starts with a task, drug, and dosage so selected that both SDL and DDs can be obtained. If SDL and DD experiments are repeated using lower and lower dosages, the SDL effects will disappear first. Then, at lower doses discriminative control will also be lost. Although only a few explicit comparisons of the threshold dose adequate to produce SDL and DDs have been reported (Overton, 1979a, 1982b; Zenick & Goldsmith, 1981), the total literature on these phenomena clearly support the generalization just stated. SDL is only produced by some drugs at the highest doses compatible with sustained behavioral responding (Eich, 1980). In contrast, DDs can be maintained by intermediate doses of the same drugs and by a variety of other drugs which are unable to produce measurable SDL effects at any usable dose. This difference in the threshold dosage for SDL and for DDs is discordant with the predictions of all neurological models for SDL and DDs and supports a sensory interpretation of both phenomena.

EVIDENCE NOT SUPPORTING A SENSORY INTERPRETATION OF DRUG DISCRIMINATIONS

Several types of evidence deter us from an entirely uncritical acceptance of a sensory interpretation for SDL and DDs.

Lack of Direct Supporting Evidence

A substantial embarrassment for sensory theories of SDL and DDs is provided by the fact that no one has been able to identify a sensory stimulus that would mimic or substitute for a drug stimulus or vice versa. If drugs truly achieve contextual and discriminative control via the mechanism of drug-induced stimuli, then it might be possible to duplicate the stimulus conditions produced by drugs via appropriate manipulations of the internal or external milieu, and such a finding would be important for two reasons. First, such results would help identify the specific sensory actions responsible for SDL and DDs produced by the specific drug in question, thus providing a more rational basis than is presently available for evaluating the results of DD experiments conducted with that drug. More importantly, successful identification of the sensory mediators of SDL and DDs, even for a single drug, would more firmly establish the general principle that such effects could be mediated by sensory drug effects--a conclusion presently supported only by indirect evidence.

There are at least three different types of sensory effects which drugs apparently can produce, any or all of which might cause SDL and DDs. (1) Some drugs directly induce changes in peripheral organs, and these changes produce altered sensory input returning to the brain via the classical afferent pathways. For example, antimuscarinics reduce the flow of saliva and produce sensations of "dry mouth." Sedative drugs such as ethanol produce ataxia and the associated altered proprioceptive feedback. (2) Other drugs can modify the processing and perception of interoceptive or exteroceptive stimuli. Blurred or double vision is one example of such a drug-induced modification in sensory processing. Analgesia produced by narcotics provides a second example. (3) Finally, some drugs may directly induce central "sensory" effects by altering the organism's emotions, drive states, arousal level, et cetera.

The first type of mediating mechanism for DDs--drug-produced changes in peripheral organs that cause altered sensory feedback--has been investigated on several occasions with negative results. For example, antimuscarinic drugs produce SDL and DDs and produce altered functioning in a variety of organs innervated by the autonomic nervous system. Tertiary antimuscarinic drugs act at both central and peripheral sites whereas quaternary antimuscarinics cross the blood-brain barrier less easily and thus act only at peripheral sites. After D versus N DD training with scopolamine hydrobromide (which produces both central and peripheral actions), animals fail to generalize the D response to quaternary scopolamine compounds which produce only peripheral actions. Thus it appears that the peripheral actions of scopolamine are not responsible for its discriminable actions (Overton, 1977a). Similarly, after D versus N DD training with pentobarbital, the D response fails to appear during tests with gallamine, a curare-type drug which produces muscular weakness and a lack of coordination vaguely reminiscent of the ataxic actions of pentobarbital (Overton, 1964). Other tests of this type have also been reported, but in no case has a peripheral manipulation been identified that could mimic the discriminable effects of a drug (Downey, 1975; Hazell et al., 1978). Additionally, it has generally been found that drugs which act only on peripheral organs do not produce SDL and are discriminated only with difficulty whereas centrally acting drugs are more likely to produce SDL and are more readily discriminated (Miksic, Shearman, & Lal, 1980; Overton, 1971). This has discouraged further attempts to identify specific peripheral sensory stimuli which might mediate SDL and DDs.

The second possibility--that drug-induced alterations in central sensory processing might mediate SDL and DDs--has also been investigated with negative results. For example, Overton (1968b) hypothesized that blurred vision might mediate the discriminable effects of pentobarbital. To test this possibility, he first blinded rats and then required them to learn a D versus N discrimination in a T-maze. This discrimination was learned as rapidly by blind as by sighted rats, indicating that drug-induced alterations in visual stimuli were not a prerequisite for the establishment of the discrimination. In another experiment sighted rats were required to discriminate pentobarbital versus N; these rats were then blinded, and training was continued. Only a transient disruption in discriminative control was noted at the time of blinding, suggesting that even in sighted rats alterations in visual perception do not mediate discriminative control. In a similar vein Overton hypothesized that pentobarbital versus N discriminations in a shock-escape T-maze task might be mediated by drug-induced analgesia or at least by a drug-induced insensitivity to some of the consequences of electric shock. However, two pieces of evidence contradicted this hypothesis. First, after D versus N training with high shock levels, undrugged rats could not be induced to make D choices by the application of low (less painful) shock intensities (Overton, 1968b). Secondly, after D versus N training with pentobarbital, the D response does not occur during tests with morphine or other narcotic analgesics.

The third type of possible sensory mediator for SDL and DDs--drug induced central sensory effects--implies, as a corollary, that altered states of the central nervous system induced by other manipulations besides drug injections might also produce contextual and discriminative effects analogous to those of drugs. Two questions follow. (1) Which altered CNS states, if any, produce contextual and/or discriminative effects? (2) Do any of the altered CNS states that can be induced by nonpharmacological manipulations produce sensory effects equivalent to those induced by drugs?

Regarding the first question, electroconvulsive shock (ECS) produces SDL, and ECS versus no ECS discriminations are robust (McIntyre & Reichert, 1971; Overton, Ercole, & Dutta, 1976). Alterations in hunger or thirst are discriminable and produce SDL (Bolles, 1958; Nahinsky, 1960; Peck & Ader, 1974). Electrical brain stimulation is discriminable (Colpaert, 1977b; Hirschhorn, Hayes, & Rosecrans, 1975; Stutz & Maroli, 1978). Temporary ablation of certain brain structures can produce SDL (Duncan & Copeland, 1975; Greenwood & Singer, 1974; Langford, Freedman, & Whitman, 1971; Pianka, 1976; Reed & Trowill, 1969; Schneider, 1966, 1967, 1973). REM-sleep deprivation can produce SDL (Joy & Prinz, 1969), and learning that occurs during REM sleep is state dependent (Evans, 1972; Evans, Gustafson, O'Connell, Orne, & Shor, 1966, 1969, 1970). These studies show that a variety of alterations in CNS activity can be discriminated and/or produce SDL.

With regard to the second issue, there are very few studies that we can cite. Huang (1973) trained rats to press one lever after normal sleep and the second lever after REM-deprivation. This discrimination was learned, and subsequent tests showed that amphetamine would cause some REM-deprivation responses in rats that had slept normally and conversely that pentobarbital would cause some responses on the normal-sleep lever in REM-deprived rats. Although the drugs did not completely antagonize (or mimic) the sleep manipulations, the results suggested that the effects of REM deprivation and of normal sleep were to some degree overlapped by the effects of pentobarbital and/or amphetamine. In a related study Schechter (1981b) trained rats to discriminate pentobarbital versus amphetamine and then tested them with saline at various times of day. During midafternoon tests saline caused responding predominantly on the pentobarbital lever, but during saline tests at 2:00 a.m., the rats showed only 50% responses on that lever. Both studies suggest that the drug injections and the time of day (or REM deprivation) manipulations may have moved the animals along some shared "sensory" dimension (arousal level?) which provided at least part of the basis for discriminative control. Finally, Gardner, Glick, and Jarvik (1972) reported some similarities between the SDL effects of ECS, physostigmine, and scopolamine. However, Overton, Ercole, and Dutta (1976) were unable to obtain evidence for analogous effects using a DD paradigm.

In summary, attempts to identify sensory or physiological manipulations that would mimic the postulated sensory effects of drugs have failed, almost without exception, to find such manipulations. This is not entirely surprising because due to the high specificity produced by D versus N training, it might be necessary to rather exactly mimic the sensory effects of a drug in order to observe substitution. Nonetheless, one single explicit demonstration of a DD mediated by identifiable sensory events would make it much easier to accept a sensory interpretation of all DDs.

Masking Has Not Been Reported

We mentioned earlier the less than conclusive evidence suggesting that masking does not occur in the DD preparation. This property is helpful in many DD experiments. However, if DDs are based on sensory events, it appears that masking really should occur. Hence the failure to observe masking can be counted as evidence against a sensory interpretation of DDs.

One should note that attempts to detect masking have not used as yet the drug stimulus conditions that apparently would be most likely to produce masking. For example, it appears that masking will be most likely if a rapidly discriminated drug (with strong sensory effects) is used to mask a training drug with weak, slowly discriminated effects. Additionally, if the sensory literature is a useful guide, it may be the case that drugs producing similar sensory effects (effects in the same modality?) can mask one another more effectively than can drugs that produce markedly dissimilar effects. Even though we know almost nothing about the topography or dimensionality of the sensory modalities in which drugs produce stimuli, it might be feasible to test this possibility by selecting drugs that were sufficiently similar to substitute for one another in a low specificity DD paradigm and by then testing whether these drugs would mask one another in a high specificity paradigm. Tests using such combinations of drugs have not been reported. If future studies detect the occurrence of masking and define the conditions for its occurrence, this will remove an impediment to acceptance of a sensory interpretation of DDs.

Prior Exposure to Drug Does Not Slow the Acquisition of DDs

In several conditioning paradigms prior exposure to a stimulus has been observed to impede the subsequent acquisition of conditioned responses or discriminative control, presumably by habituating the animal to the to-be-conditioned stimulus. However, this effect has not been observed in connection with drug stimuli. In several such studies investigators have repeatedly exposed animals to drugs before commencing D versus N training. Such prior exposure to drug has neither facilitated nor impaired the subsequent acquisition of DDs (Hinderliter, 1978; Jarbe & Henriksson, 1973; Jarbe & Holmgren, 1977; Kilbey et al., 1971; McKim, 1976; Overton, 1972).

Poor Correlation With Human Subjective Reports

One final problem for sensory DD theories is posed by some inconsistencies between data obtained from animal and from human subjects. Recreational, clinical, and experimental drug use in humans have yielded anecdotal and experimental reports on the strength and nature of the subjective effects of drugs including hallucinations, changes in affect, and assorted unpleasant side effects. Somewhat analogous data on the discriminable effects of drugs have been obtained from DD studies in animal subjects (e.g., Overton 1982a). In many instances the two types of data correspond. For example, all morphine-like drugs produce similar subjective effects in humans and similar discriminable effects in rats. However, there are several instances in which data from human and animal subjects are disparate. For example, in rats ethanol is very readily discriminated and chlorpromazine is discriminated only with difficulty whereas in humans both drugs produce more or less equally reportable subjective effects. As another example nicotine and marihuana are both readily discriminated in rats, with nicotine perhaps being more rapidly discriminated. In humans the subjective effects of marihuana appear to be more noticeable than those of nicotine. Instances such as these suggest that subjective drug effects in humans and discriminable drug effects in animals are not entirely isomorphic.

Conclusions Regarding Sensory Mediation of SDL and DDs

Several pages ago we listed the following three prerequisites that had to be met if DDs were to be capable of providing information regarding the causes of drug abuse.

1. Sensory effects must underlie and cause drug abuse.
2. Sensory events must underlie DDs.
3. The same sensory events must underlie both DDs and drug abuse.

Condition one, although not rigorously proven, is widely accepted. At the least, subjective effects of drugs are certainly responsible for many instances of drug abuse. As regards condition two, we have just reviewed the available evidence which, on balance, provides moderate support for the hypothesis that sensory events are responsible for DDs. Most of the evidence supporting this interpretation has been published since 1975, and much of it is indirect in nature. The third condition, for the most part, has to be met by future research efforts. This condition requires that we ascertain which DDs are based on abuse-producing stimulus effects and which are not. Only in the narcotic agonist class of drugs at present is there moderately strong evidence supporting the conclusion that the primary drug effects underlying DDs are also the effects which produce the euphorigenic effects of the same drugs. A similarly advanced degree of understanding of the discriminative stimulus effects of other drug classes and of the relationship between discriminated drug stimuli and reinforcing drug stimuli will require many additional experiments. Hopefully such experiments will be performed, and if they are, DDs should be able to substantially augment our understanding of the causes of drug abuse.

METHODS OF APPLICATION OF DRUG DISCRIMINATIONS TO DRUG ABUSE

This section enumerates the most obvious ways in which DDs can be used to improve our understanding of drug abuse.

Definition of Categories of Drugs

DD investigators have made considerable progress toward developing a new categorization system for psychoactive drugs based entirely on their discriminable properties. In many instances the categories match those already established by other techniques, and one can view these studies as a simple replication of previous work in psychopharmacology (e.g., Barry, 1974; Browne, 1981; Cameron & Appel, 1973; Colpaert, 1977a, 1978; Colpaert & Rosecrans, 1978; Goas & Boston, 1978; Goudie, 1977, 1982; Lal, 1977; Overton, 1977a, 1978a). In other instances DD studies have allowed a subdivision of pre-existing drug classes, thereby defining differences between the actions of drugs that were previously considered to be similar. These results are likely to have relevance to drug abuse since drugs with similar clinical actions but differing subjective effects are likely to have differing liabilities for abuse. Finally, some genuinely new "classes" of compounds have been defined by DD procedures. For example, the class of phencyclidine-like compounds now includes not only phencyclidine (PCP) analogs but also certain narcotic mixed antagonists (dextrorphan, cyclazocine, SK10047) which appear to share some of PCP's discriminable effects (Hein, Young, Herling, & Woods, 1981; Herling et al., 1981). This work provides a good example of the application of DD procedures to obtain information about drugs that is likely to have considerable relevance to their liability for abuse.

Identification of Neuropharmacological Mechanisms of Drug Action

DDs have been used in numerous studies designed to identify the neurotransmitters which mediate the effects of drugs. A typical procedure is to establish a D versus N DD based on the drug in question and then to manipulate various transmitter systems using available agonists, antagonists, depleters, and blockers. The utility of the DD method for such studies derives, as usual, from its relatively high specificity, and a number of rather ingenious and productive studies of this type have been reported (Barrett, Blackshear, & Sanders-Bush, 1982; Barrett & Steranka, 1983; Bennett & Lal, 1982; Browne & Ho, 1975a; Chipkin, Stewart, & Channabasavaiah, 1980; Ho & Huang, 1975; McKenna & Ho, 1980; Schechter, 1977, 1980; Schechter & Cook, 1975; Schechter & Rosecrans, 1972b). Among the most sophisticated of these studies have been those investigating the role of various neurotransmitters in mediating the actions of hallucinogenic drugs (Appel, White, & Holohean, 1982; Glennon, Rosecrans, Young, & Gaines, 1979; White & Appel, 1981, 1982; White, Appel, & Kuhn, 1979; Winter, 1978b).

Some investigators have used DDs to identify the neuroanatomical location where drugs act to produce their subjective effects. However, such studies have been difficult in rats because a long time is required to establish DDs and a relatively small number of tests with intracerebral drugs can be conducted per rat (e.g., Krynock & Rosecrans, 1979; Meltzer & Rosecrans, 1981; Rosecrans & Glennon, 1979).

Identification of Antagonists

Drugs which block or antagonize the actions of the training drug can be easily identified with the DD procedure. Although early reports dealt mainly with well-known antagonists and blockers (e.g., Hirschhorn & Rosecrans, 1974b; Overton, 1966, 1969; Romano et al., 1981; Schechter & Rosecrans, 1972c), more recent studies have identified novel antagonists (Bennett, Geyer, Dutta, Brugger, Fielding, & Lal, 1982; Browne, 1981; Colpaert, 1977a; Dantzer & Perio, 1982; Herling & Shannon, 1982; Shearman & Lal, 1979; Winter, 1981b). Excellent examples are the reports provided by Colpaert, Niemegeers, and Janssen (1982) who identified pirenperone as an LSD antagonist and by Browne who identified compounds which reduced the effects of phencyclidine (Browne & Welch, 1982; Browne, Welch, Kozlowski, & Duthu, 1983). In general, the DD method appears well suited to identify new antagonists and competitive blockers.

Identification of Active Metabolites

The DD method can apparently identify the metabolites of a drug which produce actions similar to those of the parent compound (e.g., Barry, Steenberg, Manian, & Buckley, 1974; Beford, Nail, Borne, & Wilson, 1981; Brady & Balster, 1981; Browne, Harris, & Ho, 1974; Browne & Ho, 1975b; Holtzman, 1979).

Establish Structure-Activity Relationships

DDs can obviously be used to test a series of related chemicals to determine which produce discriminable effects like those of a parent compound (Chance, Kallman, Rosecrans, & Spencer, 1978; Huang & Ho, 1974; Katz, Woods, Winger, & Jacobson, 1982; Meltzer, Rosecrans, Aceto, & Harris, 1980; Shannon, McQuinn, Vaupel, & Cone, 1983; Solomon, Herling, Domino, & Woods, 1982). Industrial DD laboratories have tended not to use DDs as a primary assay, due to the expense of the DD procedure, and have instead used DDs to ask specific questions about compounds already known to have CNS activity. However, Glennon and his associates have used the DD preparation as a primary screen to identify compounds producing hallucinogenic subjective effects (Glennon & Rosecrans, 1982; Glennon, Young, & Jacyno, 1983; Glennon, Young, Jacyno, Slusher, & Rosecrans, 1983; see also Glennon & Young, this volume). Like many other assays, the DD procedure used in this way can only identify compounds that produce effects similar to those of pre-existing drugs. With presently available procedures, it is not feasible to use each new compound as a training drug in order to determine whether it produces any discriminable actions (which might differ from those of pre-existing drugs).

Screen for New Compounds Lacking Abuse Liability

One very promising application of DDs which has been proposed (by J. Woods, personal communication) but not yet employed is screening new compounds to identify those which lack effects already shown to produce abuse. For example, Woods proposes that new analgesics could first be identified in a standard test for analgesic efficacy (e.g., tail flick). Compounds shown to have analgesic efficacy could then be tested in rats that had been trained to discriminate morphine versus no drug. Compounds that substituted for morphine would be rejected on the assumption that they shared with morphine its euphorigenic actions. Compounds that produced analgesia but failed to mimic morphine would remain as candidates for further testing. Note that compounds that survived the dual test procedure might still have liability for abuse due to hallucinogenic or other abuse-producing subjective effects. However they would probably not produce the morphine-like subjective effects which are responsible for a great proportion of the abuse of currently available analgesic drugs.

Characterization of the Sensory Effects That Cause Drug Abuse

It seems likely that a variety of different sensory effects of drugs can cause drug abuse. Investigators using the self-administration method have tended to lump these effects together, referring to all as "reinforcing" stimulus effects, and self-administration procedures have been relatively ineffective in differentiating the various types of drug stimulus effects that could underlie drug abuse. In contrast, DD procedures apparently have the capability to differentiate between the various sensory effects that can underlie drug abuse and have already shown that abused drugs produce at least half a dozen clearly distinct discriminable effects. This research effort is continuing. When attempting to analyze the sensory effects that underlie drug abuse, we appear to face a difficult choice. Self-administration procedures have greater face validity but currently lack the ability to make fine discriminations between different types of sensory effects, some or all of which may underlie self-administration. DD procedures yield data not necessarily based on drug effects that underlie drug abuse, but these procedures have a much greater ability to differentiate between dissimilar drug stimuli. At the very least it appears that DD procedures can be a valuable adjunct to self-administration procedures when attempting to analyze the sensory causes of drug abuse. Possibly DD procedures will become the more important analytic technique with self-administration experiments used as a sort of post hoc test to determine which DD results relate to sensory effects that will promote self-administration and which do not. It seems likely that via a not too well defined series of intermeshed DD and self-administration experiments we could identify and differentiate between the various sensory abuse-inducing effects of drugs. This is not an established use of DDs. Rather, it is an optimistic prediction that a judicious mixture of DD and self-administration experiments might provide much more precise information about the sensory causes of drug abuse than could be produced by either method alone.

It should be obvious that several of the research goals outlined above (e.g., categorization of compounds, identification of neurochemical substrates) can also be accomplished by techniques other than the DD procedure. However, in the context of drug abuse, the DD procedure has the advantage of providing experimental results that are based on the sensory consequences of drug action. Hence, insofar as DD results differ from those obtained by more molecular methods, the DD results are more likely to have relevance to abuse liability.

SUMMARY

Drug discrimination procedures have less face validity than self-administration procedures for investigating the sensory drug effects that presumably underlie drug abuse. However, currently available DD procedures can provide more detailed information comparing and contrasting the subjective effects of drugs than can be produced by self-administration procedures thus far developed. Hence, DDs appear to provide a valuable method for improving our understanding of the subjective effects of drugs that presumably underlie drug abuse.

The utility of DD procedures as methods for understanding drug abuse will be impeded by the currently inadequate theoretical formulations regarding the basis of drug discriminations. Present theories predict only part of the properties of DDs, and we have identified several experimental approaches that should improve our theoretical understanding of DDs.

ACKNOWLEDGMENTS

This paper is dedicated to the memory of David K. Bliss, a careful, dedicated, and innovative investigator who contributed substantially to our understanding of state-dependent learning and drug discriminations and who is recently deceased.

Preparation of this manuscript was supported in part by NIMH grant MH-21536 and NIDA grant DA-02403.

REFERENCES

Akins, F. R., Gouvier, W. D., & Lyons, J. E. (1980). Stimulus control along a drug-dose dimension. Bulletin of the Psychonomic Society, 15, 33-34.

Altshuler, H. L., Applebaum, E., & Shippenberg, T. S. (1981). The effects of opiate antagonists on the discriminative stimulus properties of ethanol. Pharmacology Biochemistry & Behavior, 14, 97-100.

Ando, K. (1975). The discriminative control of operant behavior by intravenous administration of drugs in rats. Psychopharmacologia, 45, 47-50.

Appel, J. B., White, F. J., & Holohean, A. M. (1982). Analyzing mechanism(s) of hallucinogenic drug action with drug discrimination procedures. Neuroscience & Behavioral Reviews, 6, 529-536.

Auld, F. (1951). The effects of tetraethylammonium on a habit motivated by fear. Journal of Comparative and Physiological Psychology, 44, 565-574.

Avis, H. H., & Pert, A. (1974). A comparison of the effects of muscarinic and nicotinic anticholinergic drugs on habituation and fear conditioning in rats. Psychopharmacologia, 34, 209-222.

Balster, R. L. (1970). The effectiveness of external and drug produced internal stimuli in the discriminative control of operant behavior. Unpublished doctoral dissertation, University of Houston.

Barnhart, S. S., & Abbott, D. W. (1967). Dissociation of learning and meprobamate. Psychological Reports, 20, 520-522.

Barrett, R. J., Blackshear, M. A., & Sanders-Bush, E. (1982). Discriminative stimulus properties of L-5-hydroxytryptophan: Behavioral evidence for multiple serotonin receptors. Psychopharmacology, 76, 29-35.

Barrett, R. J., & Leith, N. J. (1981). Tolerance to the discriminative stimulus properties of d-amphetamine. Neuropharmacology, 20, 251-255.

Barrett, R. J., & Steranka, L. R. (1983). Drug discrimination in rats: Evidence for amphetamine-like cue state following chronic haloperidol. Pharmacology Biochemistry & Behavior, 18, 611-617.

Barry, H., III. (1974). Classification of drugs according to their discriminable effects in rats. Federation Proceedings, 33, 1814-1824.

Barry, H., III. (1978). Stimulus attributes of drugs. In H. Anisman & G. Bignami (Eds.), Psychopharmacology of aversively motivated behavior (pp. 455-485). New York: Plenum Press.

Barry, H., III, & Krimmer, E. C. (1979). Differential stimulus attributes of chlordiazepoxide and pentobarbital. Neuropharmacology, 18, 991-998.

Barry, H., III & Kubena, R. K. (1972). Discriminative stimulus characteristics of alcohol, marihuana and atropine. In J. M. Singh, L. H. Miller, & H. Lal (Eds.), Drug addiction: Experimental pharmacology (Vol. 1, pp. 3-16). Mount Kisco, NY: Futura Publishing Company.

Barry, H., III, McGuire, M. S., & Krimmer, E. C. (1982). Alcohol and meprobamate resemble pentobarbital rather than chlordiazepoxide. In F. C. Colpaert & J. L. Slangen (Eds.), Drug discrimination applications in CNS pharmacology (pp. 219-232). Amsterdam: Elsevier/North Holland Biomedical Press.

Barry, H., III, Miller, N. E., & Tidd, G. E. (1962). Control for stimulus change while testing effects of amobarbital on conflict. Journal of Comparative and Physiological Psychology, 55, 1071-1074.

Barry, H., III, Steenberg, M. L., Manian, A. A., & Buckley, J. P. (1974). Effects of chlorpromazine and three metabolites on behavioral responses in rats. Psychopharmacologia, 34, 351-360.

Barry, H., III, Wagner, A. R., & Miller, N. E. (1962). Effects of alcohol and amobarbital on performance inhibited by experimental extinction. Journal of Comparative and Physiological Psychology, 55, 464-468.

Beford, J. A., Nail, G. L., Borne, R. F., & Wilson, M. C. (1981). Discriminative stimulus properties of cocaine, norcocaine, and n-allylnorcocaine. Pharmacology Biochemistry & Behavior, 14, 81-83.

Bennett, D. A., Geyer, H., Dutta, P., Brugger, S., Fielding, S., & Lal, H. (1982). Comparison of the actions of trimethadione and chlordiazepoxide in animal models of anxiety and benzodiazepine receptor binding. Neuropharmacology, 21, 1175-1179.

Bennett, D. A., & Lal, H. (1982). Discriminative stimuli produced by clonidine: An investigation of the possible relationship to adrenoceptor stimulation and hypotension. Journal of Pharmacology and Experimental Therapeutics, 223, 642-648.

Berger, B. D., & Stein, L. (1969a). An analysis of learning deficits produced by scopolamine. Psychopharmacologia, 14, 271-283.

Berger, B. D., & Stein, L. (1969b). Asymmetrical dissociation of learning between scopolamine and Wy4036, a new benzodiazepine tranquilizer. Psychopharmacologia, 14, 351-358.

Bliss, D. K. (1973). Dissociated learning and state-dependent retention induced by pentobarbital in rhesus monkeys. Journal of Comparative and Physiological Psychology, 84, 149-161.

Bliss, D. K. (1974). Theoretical explanations of drug-dissociated behaviors. Federation Proceedings, 33, 1787-1796.

Bolles, R. C. (1958). A replication and further analysis of a study on position reversal learning in hungry and thirsty rats. Journal of Comparative and Physiological Psychology, 51, 349.

Boyd, S. C., & Caul, W. F. (1979). Evidence of state dependent learning of brightness discrimination in hypothermic mice. Physiology & Behavior, 23, 147-153.

Brady, K. T., & Balster, R. L. (1981). Discriminative stimulus properties of phencyclidine and five analogues in the squirrel monkey. Pharmacology Biochemistry & Behavior, 14, 213-218.

Brown, A., Feldman, R. S., & Moore, J. W. (1968). Conditional discrimination learning based upon chlordiazepoxide: Dissociation or cue? Journal of Comparative and Physiological Psychology, 66, 211-215.

Browne, R. G. (1981). Anxiolytics antagonize yohimbine's discriminative stimulus properties. Psychopharmacology, 74, 245-249.

Browne, R. G., Harris, R. T., & Ho, B. T. (1974). Stimulus properties of mescaline and n-methylated derivatives: Difference in peripheral and direct central administration. Psychopharmacologia, 39, 43-56.

Browne, R. G., & Ho, B. T. (1975a). Role of serotonin in the discriminative stimulus properties of mescaline. Pharmacology Biochemistry & Behavior, 3, 429-435.

Browne, R. G., & Ho, B. T. (1975b). Discriminative stimulus properties of mescaline: Mescaline or metabolite? Pharmacology Biochemistry & Behavior, 3, 109-114.

Browne, R. G., & Weissman, A. (1981). Discriminative stimulus properties of delta-9-tetrahydrocannabinol: Mechanistic studies. Journal of Clinical Pharmacology, 21, 227S-234S.

Browne, R. G., & Welch, W. M. (1982). Stereoselective antagonism of phencyclidine's discriminative properties by adenosine receptor agonists. Science, 217, 1157-1159.

Browne, R. G., Welch, W. M., Kozlowski, M. R., & Duthu, G. (1983). Antagonism of PCP discrimination by adenosine analogs. In J. M. Kamenka, E. F. Domino, & P. Geneste (Eds.), Phencyclidine and related arylcyclohexylamines: Present and future applications. Ann Arbor, MI: NPP Books.

Bueno, O. F. A., & Carlini, E. A. (1972). Dissociation of learning in marihuana tolerant rats. Psychopharmacologia, 25, 49-56.

Bueno, O. F. A., Carlini, E. A., Finkelfarb, E., & Suzuki, J. S. (1972). Delta-9-tetrahydrocannabinol, ethanol, and amphetamine as discriminative stimuli-generalization tests with other drugs. Psychopharmacologia, 46, 235-243.

Bustamante, J. A., Jordan, A., Vila, M., Gonzalez, A., & Insua, A. (1970). State dependent learning in humans. Physiology & Behavior, 5, 793-796.

Cameron, O. G., & Appel, J. B. (1973). A behavioral and pharmacological analysis of some discriminable properties of d-LSD in rats. Psychopharmacologia, 33, 117-134.

Carter, R. B., & Leander, J. D. (1982). Discriminative stimulus properties of naloxone. Psychopharmacology, 77, 305-308.

Chance, W. T., Kallman, M. D., Rosecrans, J. A., & Spencer, R. M. (1978). A comparison of nicotine and structurally related compounds as discriminative stimuli. British Journal of Pharmacology, 63, 609-616.

Chance, W. T., Murfin, D., Krynock, G. M., & Rosecrans, J. A. (1977). A description of the nicotine stimulus and tests of its generalization to amphetamine. Psychopharmacology, 55, 19-26.

Chipkin, R. E., Stewart, J. M., & Channabasavaiah, K. (1980). The effects of peptides on the stimulus properties of ethanol. Pharmacology Biochemistry & Behavior, 12, 93-98.

Cole, S. O., & Gay, P. E. (1976). Effects of drug-state change on discrimination performance. Psychopharmacology, 47, 43-47.

Collins, W. (1868). The Moonstone (Reprinted, 1981). New York:Penguin Books.

Colpaert, F. C. (1977a). Discriminative stimulus properties of benzodiazepines and barbiturates. In H. Lal (Ed.), Discriminative stimulus properties of drugs (pp. 93-106). New York: Plenum Press.

Colpaert, F. C. (1977b). Sensitization and desensitization to lateral hypothalamic stimulation. Archives Internationales de Pharmacodynamie et de Therapie, 230, 319-320.

Colpaert, F. C. (1978). Discriminative stimulus properties of narcotic analgesic drugs. Pharmacology Biochemistry & Behavior, 9, 863-887.

Colpaert, F. C., Desmedt, L. K. C., & Janssen, P. A. J. (1976). Discriminative stimulus properties of benzodiazepines, barbiturates and pharmacologically related drugs: Relation to some intrinsic and anticonvulsant effects. European Journal of Pharmacology, 37, 113-123.

Colpaert, F. C., & Janssen, P. A. J. (1981). Factors regulating drug cue sensitivity: The effect of frustrative non-reward in fentanyl-saline discrimination. Archives Internationales de Pharmacodynamie et de Therapie, 254, 241-251.

Colpaert, F. C., & Janssen, P. A. J. (1982a). Factors regulating drug cue sensitivity: The effects of dose ratio and absolute dose level in the case of fentanyl dose-dose discrimination. Archives Internationales de Pharmacodynamie et de Therapie, 258, 283-299.

Colpaert, F. C., & Janssen, P. A. J. (1982b). Factors regulating drug cue sensitivity: Limits of discriminability and the role of a progressively decreasing training dose in cocaine-saline discrimination. Neuropharmacology, 21, 1187-1194.

Colpaert, F. C., & Janssen, P. A. J. (1982c). OR Discrimination: A new drug discrimination method. European Journal of Pharmacology, 78, 141-144.

Colpaert, F. C., Kuyps, J. J. M. D., Niemegeers, C. J. E., & Janssen, P. A. J. (1976). Discriminative stimulus properties of a low dl-amphetamine dose. Archives Internationales de Pharmacodynamie et de Therapie, 223, 34-42.

Colpaert, F. C., Kuyps, J. J. M. D., Niemegeers, C. J. E., & Janssen, P. A. J. (1976). Discriminative stimulus properties of fentanyl and morphine: Tolerance and dependence. Pharmacology Biochemistry & Behavior, 5, 401-408.

Colpaert, F. C., Niemegeers, C. J. E, & Janssen, P. A. J. (1975a). Differential response control by isopropamide: A peripherally induced discriminative cue. European Journal of Pharmacology, 34, 381-384.

Colpaert, F. C., Niemegeers, C. J. E., & Janssen, P. A. J. (1975b). The narcotic cue: Evidence for the specificity of the stimulus properties of narcotic drugs. Archives Internationales de Pharmacodynamie et de Therapie, 218, 268-276.

Colpaert, F. C., Niemegeers, C. J. E., & Janssen, P. A. J. (1976). Fentanyl and apomorphine: Asymmetrical generalization of discriminative stimulus properties. Neuropharmacology, 15, 541-545.

Colpaert, F. C., Niemegeers, C. J. E., & Janssen, P. A. J. (1978a). Changes of sensitivity to the cuing properties of narcotic drugs as evidenced by generalization and cross-generalization experiments. Psychopharmacology, 58, 257-262.

Colpaert, F. C., Niemegeers, C. J. E., & Janssen, P. A. J. (1978b). Studies on the regulation of sensitivity to the narcotic cue. Neuropharmacology, 17, 705-713.

Colpaert, F. C., Niemegeers, C. J. E., & Janssen, P. A. J. (1978c). Factors regulating drug cue sensitivity: A long term study on the cocaine cue. In F. C. Colpaert & J. A. Rosecrans (Eds.), Stimulus properties of drugs: Ten years of progress (pp. 281-299). Amsterdam: Elsevier/North Holland Biomedical Press.

Colpaert, F. C., Niemegeers, C. J. E., & Janssen, P. A. J. (1980a). Factors regulating drug cue sensitivity: Limits of discriminability and the role of a progressively decreasing training dose in fentanyl-saline discrimination. Journal of Pharmacology and Experimental Therapeutics, 212, 474-480.

Colpaert, F. C., Niemegeers, C. J. E., & Janssen, P. A. J. (1980b). Factors regulating drug cue sensitivity: The effect of training dose in fentanyl-saline discrimination. Neuropharmacology, 19, 705-713.

Colpaert, F. C., Niemegeers, C. J. E., & Janssen, P. A. J. (1982). A drug discrimination analysis of lysergic acid diethylamide (LSD): In vivo agonist and antagonist effects of purported 5-hydroxytryptamine antagonists and of pirenperone, a LSD antagonist. Journal of Pharmacology and Experimental Therapeutics, 221, 206-214.

Colpaert, F. C., & Rosecrans, J. A. (Eds.) (1978). Stimulus properties of drugs: Ten years of progress. Amsterdam: Elsevier/North Holland Biomedical Press.

Colpaert, F. C., & Slangen, J. L. (Eds.) (1982). Drug discrimination: Applications in CNS pharmacology. Amsterdam: Elsevier/North Holland Biomedical Press.

Combe, G. (1830). A system of phrenology (3rd ed.). Edinburgh: John Anderson.

Conger, J. J. (1951). The effects of alcohol on conflict behavior in the albino rat. Quarterly Journal of Studies on Alcohol, 12, 1-29.

Connelly, J. F., & Connelly, J. M. (1978). Relative strengths of drug-induced interoceptive cues and emotionally-important exteroceptive cues. In F. C. Colpaert & J. A. Rosecrans (Eds.), Stimulus properties of drugs: Ten years of progress (pp. 397-413). Amsterdam: Elsevier/North-Holland Biomedical Press.

Connelly, J. F, Connelly, J. M., & Epps, J. O. (1973). Disruption of dissociated learning in a discrimination paradigm by emotionally-important stimuli. Psychopharmacologia, 30, 275-282.

Connelly, J. F., Connelly, J. M., & Nevitt, J. R. (1977). Effect of foot-shock intensity in amount of memory retrieval in rats by emotionally-important stimuli in a drug-dependent learning escape design. Psychopharmacology, 51, 153-157.

Connelly, J. F, Connelly, J. M., & Phifer, R. (1975). Disruption of state-dependent learning (memory retrieval) by emotionally-important stimuli. Psychopharmacologia, 41, 139-143.

Dantzer, R., & Perio, A. (1982). Behavioural evidence for partial agonist properties of RO 15-1788, a benzodiazepine receptor antagonist. European Journal of Pharmacology, 81, 655-658.

Deutsch, J. A., & Roll, S. K. (1973). Alcohol and asymmetrical state-dependency: A possible explanation. Behavioral Biology, 8, 273-278.

D'Mello, G. D. (1982). Comparison of the discriminative stimulus properties of clonidine and amphetamine in rats. Neuropharmacology, 21, 763-769.

Downey, D. J. (1975). State-dependent learning with centrally and noncentrally active drugs. Bulletin of the Psychonomic Society, 5, 281-284.

Duncan, P. M. ((1979). The effect of external stimulus change on ethanol-produced dissociation. Pharmacology Biochemistry & Behavior, 11, 377-381.

Duncan, P. M., & Copeland, M. (1975). Asymmetrical state dependency from temporary septal area dysfunction in rats. Journal of Comparative and Physiological Psychology, 89, 537-545.

Duncan, P. M., Phillips, J., Reints, J., & Schechter, M. D. (1979). Interaction between discrimination of drug states and external stimuli. Psychopharmacology, 61, 105-106.

Eich, J. E. (1977). State-dependent retrieval of information in human episodic memory. In I. M. Birnbaum & E. S. Parker (Eds.), Alcohol and human memory (pp. 141-157). Hillsdale, NJ: Lawrence Erlbaum Associates.

Eich, J. E. (1980). The cue-dependent nature of state-dependent retrieval. Memory and Cognition, 8, 157-173.

Eich, J. E., & Birnbaum, I. M. (1982). Repetition, cuing, and state-dependent memory. Memory and Cognition, 10, 103-114.

Eich, J. E., Weingartner, H., Stillman, R. C., & Gillin, J. C. (1975). State-dependent accessibility of retrieval cues in the retention of a categorized list. Journal of Verbal Learning and Verbal Behavior, 14, 408-417.

Elliotson, J. (1840). Human physiology (5th ed.). London: Longman, Orme, Brown, Green, & Longmans.

Emmett-Oglesby, M. W., Wurst, M., & Lal, H. (1983). Discriminative stimulus properties of a small dose of cocaine. Neuropharmacology, 22, 97-101.

Erdmann, G. (1979). State-dependent learning with psychopharmacological agents: A critical review of present studies (German). Psychologische Beitrage, 21, 450-473.

Evans, F. J. (1972). Hypnosis and sleep: Techniques for exploring cognitive activity during sleep. In E. Fromm & R. E. Shor (Eds.), Hypnosis: Research developments and perspectives (pp. 43-83). Chicago: Aldine.

Evans, F. J., Gustafson, L. A., O'Connell, D. N., Orne, M. T., & Shor, R. E. (1966). Response during sleep with intervening waking amnesia. Science, 152, 666-667.

Evans, F. J., Gustafson, L. A., O'Connell, D. N., Orne, M. T., & Shor, R. E. (1969). Sleep-induced behavioral response. Journal of Nervous and Mental Disease, 148, 467-476.

Evans, F. J., Gustafson, L. A., O'Connell, D. N., Orne, M. T., & Shor, R. E. (1970). Verbally induced behavioral responses during sleep. Journal of Nervous and Mental Disease, 150, 171-187.

Evans, H. L., & Patton, R. A. (1968). Scopolamine effects on a one-trial test of fear conditioning. Psychonomic Science, 11, 229-230.

File, S. E. (1974). Sodium pentobarbital and habituation-acquisition and transfer between states. Physiological Psychology, 2, 18-22.

Gardner, E. L., Glick, S. D., & Jarvik, M. E. (1972). ECS dissociation of learning and one-way cross-dissociation with physostigmine and scopolamine. Physiology & Behavior, 8, 11-15.

Gellert, V. F., & Holtzman, S. G. (1979). Discriminative stimulus effects of naltrexone in the morphine-dependent rat. Journal of Pharmacology and Experimental Therapeutics, 211, 596-605.

Girden, E. (1942a). Generalized conditioned responses under curare and erythroidine. Journal of Experimental Psychology, 31, 105-119.

Girden, E. (1942b). The dissociation of blood pressure conditioned responses under erythroidine. Journal of Experimental Psychology, 31, 219-231.

Girden, E. (1942c). The dissociation of pupillary conditioned reflexes under erythroidine and curare. Journal of Experimental Psychology, 31, 322-332.

Girden, E. (1947). Conditioned responses in curarized monkeys. American Journal of Psychology, 60, 571-587.

Girden, E., & Culler, E. A. (1937). Conditioned responses in curarized striate muscle in dogs. Journal of Comparative Psychology, 23, 261-274.

Glennon, R. A., & Rosecrans, J. A. (1982). Indolealkylamine and phenalkylamine hallucinogens: A brief overview. Neuroscience & Biobehavioral Reviews, 6, 489-497.

Glennon, R. A., Rosecrans, J. A., Young, R., & Gaines, J. (1979). Hallucinogens as a discriminative stimuli: Generalization of DOM to a 5-methoxy-N,N-dimethyltryptamine stimulus. Life Sciences, 24, 993-998.

Glennon, R. A., Young, R., & Jacyno, J. M. (1983). Indolealkylamine and phenalkylamine hallucinogens: Effect of alpha-methyl and n-methyl substituents on behavioral activity. Biochemical Pharmacology, 32, 1267-1273.

Glennon, R. A., Young, R., Jacyno, J. M., Slusher, M., & Rosecrans, J. A. (1983). DOM-stimulus generalization to LSD and other hallucinogenic indolealkylamines. European Journal of Pharmacology, 86, 453-459.

Goas, J. A., & Boston, J. E., Jr. (1978). Discriminative stimulus properties of clozapine and chlorpromazine. Pharmacology Biochemistry & Behavior, 8, 235-241.

Goldberg, M. E., Hefner, M. A., Robichaud, R. C., & Dubinsky, B. (1973). Effects of delta-9-tetrahydrocannabinol (THC) and chlordiazepoxide (CDP) on state-dependent learning: Evidence for asymmetrical dissociation. Psychopharmacologia, 30, 173-184.

Goudie, A. J. (1977). Discriminative stimulus properties of fenfluramine in an operant task: An analysis of its cue function. Psychopharmacology, 53, 97-102.

Goudie, A. J. (1982). Discriminative stimulus properties in an operant task of beta-phenylethylamine. In F. C. Colpaert and J. L. Slangen (Eds.), Drug discrimination: Applications in CNS pharmacology (pp. 165-180). Amsterdam: Elsevier/North Holland Biomedical Press.

Greenberg, I., Kuhn, D. M., & Appel, J. B. (1975). Behaviorally induced sensitivity to the discriminable properties of LSD. Psychopharmacologia, 43, 229-232.

Greenwood, P. M., & Singer, J. J. (1974). Cortical spreading depression induced state dependency. Behavioral Biology, 10, 345-351.

Grossman, S. P., & Miller, N. E. (1961). Control for stimulus-change in the evaluation of alcohol and chlorpromazine as fear-reducing drugs. Psychopharmacologia, 2, 342-351.

Harris, R. T., & Balster, R. L. (1971). An analysis of the function of drugs in the stimulus control of operant behavior. In T. Thompson & R. Pickens (Eds.), Stimulus properties of drugs (pp. 111-132). New York: Appleton-Century-Croft.

Haug, T., & Gotestam, K. G. (1982). The diazepam stimulus complex: Specificity in a rat model. European Journal of Pharmacology, 80, 225-230.

Hazell, P., Peterson, D. W., & Laverty, R. (1978). Inability of hexamethonium to block the discriminative stimulus property of nicotine. Pharmacology Biochemistry & Behavior, 9, 137-140.

Hein, D. W., Young, A. M., Herling, S., & Woods, J. H. (1981). Pharmacological analysis of the discriminative stimulus characteristics of ethylketazocine in the rhesus monkey. Journal of Pharmacology and Experimental Therapeutics, 218, 7-15.

Heistad, G. T. (1957). Psychological approach to somatic treatments in psychiatry. American Journal of Psychiatry, 114, 540-545.

Heistad, G. T. (1958). Effects chlorpromazine and electroconvulsive shock on a conditioned emotional response. Journal of Comparative and Physiological Psychology, 51, 209-212.

Heistad, G. T., & Torres, A. A. (1959). A mechanism for the effect of a tranquilizing drug on learned emotional responses. University of Minnesota Medical Bulletin, 30, 518-527.

Henriksson, B. G., & Jarbe, T. (1971). Effects of diazepam on conditioned avoidance learning in rats and its transfer to normal state conditions. Psychopharmacologia, 20, 186-190.

Herling, S., Coale, E. H., Jr., Hein, D. W., Winger, G., & Woods, J. H. (1981). Similarity of the discriminative stimulus effects of ketamine, cyclazocine, and dextrorphan in the pigeon. Psychopharmacology, 73, 286-291.

Herling, S., Hampton, R. Y., Bertalmio, A. J., Winger, G., & Woods, J. H. (1980). A procedure for rapidly evaluating the discriminative stimulus properties of drugs. Pharmacology Biochemistry & Behavior, 13, 313.

Herling, S., & Shannon, H. E. (1982). RO 15-1788 antagonizes the discriminative stimulus effects of diazepam in rats but not similar effects of pentobarbital. Life Sciences, 31, 2105-2112.

Herling, S., Valentino, R. J., & Winger, G. D. (1980). Discriminative stimulus effects of pentobarbital in pigeons. Psychopharmacology, 71, 21-28.

Herling, S., & Woods, J. H. (1981). Discriminative stimulus effects of narcotics: Evidence for multiple receptor-mediated actions. Life Sciences, 28, 1571-1584.

Hernandez, L. L., Holohean, A. M., & Appel, J. B. (1978). Effects of opiates on the discriminative stimulus properties of dopamine agonists. Pharmacology Biochemistry & Behavior, 9, 459-463.

Hinderliter, C. F. (1978). Hypothermia: Amnesic agent, punisher, and conditions sufficient to attenuate amnesia. Physiological Psychology, 6, 23-28.

Hinderliter, C. F., Webster, T., & Riccio, D. C. (1975). Amnesia induced by hypothermia as a function of treatment-test interval and recooling in rats. Animal Learning and Behavior, 3, 257-263.

Hirschhorn, I. D. (1977). Pentazocine, cyclazocine, and nalorphine as discriminative stimuli. Psychopharmacology, 54, 289-294.

Hirschhorn, I. D., Hayes, R. L., & Rosecrans, J. A. (1975). Discriminative control of behavior by electrical stimulation of the dorsal raphe nucleus: Generalization to lysergic acid diethylamide (LSD). Brain Research, 86, 134-138.

Hirschhorn, I. D., & Rosecrans, J. A. (1974a). A comparison of the stimulus effects of morphine and lysergic acid diethylamide (LSD). Pharmacology Biochemistry & Behavior, 2, 361-366.

Hirschhorn, I. D., & Rosecrans, J. A. (1974b). Studies on the time course and the effect of cholinergic and adrenergic receptor blockers on the stimulus effect of nicotine. Psychopharmacologia, 40, 109-120.

Hirschhorn, I. D., & Rosecrans, J. A. (1974c). Morphine and delta-9-tetrahydrocannabinol: Tolerance to the stimulus effects. Psychopharmacologia, 36, 243-253.

Ho, B. T., & Huang, J. T. (1975). Role of dopamine in d-amphetamine-induced discriminative responding. Pharmacology Biochemistry & Behavior, 3, 1085-1092.

Ho, B. T., Richards, D. W., III, & Chute, D. L. (Eds.). (1978) Drug discrimination and state dependent learning. New York: Academic Press.

Holloway, F. A. (1972). State-dependent effects of ethanol on active and passive avoidance learning. Psychopharmacologia, 25, 238-251.

Holmgren, B. (1964). Conditional avoidance reflex under pentobarbital. Boletin del Instituto de Estudios Medicos y Biologicos, 22, 21-38.

Holtzman, S. G. (1979). Discriminative stimulus properties of levo-alpha-acetylmethadol and its metabolites. Pharmacology Biochemistry & Behavior, 10, 565-568.

Holtzman, S. G. (1980). Phencyclidine-like discriminative effects of opioids in the rat. Journal of Pharmacology and Experimental Therapeutics, 214, 614-619.

Huang, J. T. (1973). Amphetamine and pentobarbital effects on the discriminative response control by deprivation of rapid eye movement sleep (REMS). Federation Proceedings, 32, 786.

Huang, J. T., & Ho, B. T. (1974). Discriminative stimulus properties of d-amphetamine and related compounds in rats. Pharmacology Biochemistry & Behavior, 2, 669-673.

Iwahara, S., & Noguchi, S. (1972). Drug-state dependency as a function of overtraining in rats. Japanese Psychological Research, 14, 141-144.

Iwahara, S., & Noguchi, S. (1974). Effects of overtraining upon drug-state dependency in discrimination learning in white rats. Japanese Psychological Research, 16, 59-64.

Jarbe, T. U. C. (1977). Alcohol-discrimination in gerbils: Interactions with bemegride, DH-524, amphetamine, and delta-9-THC. Archives Internationales de Pharmacodynamie et de Therapie, 227, 118-129.

Jarbe, T. U. C., & Henriksson, B. G. (1973). Open-field behavior and acquisition of discriminative response control in delta-9-THC tolerant rats. Experientia, 29, 1251-1253.

Jarbe, T. U. C., & Holmgren, B. (1977). Discriminative properties of pentobarbital after repeated noncontingent exposure in gerbils. Psychopharmacology, 53, 39-44.

Jarbe, T. U. C., Laaksonen, T., & Svensson, R. (1983). Influence of exteroceptive contextual conditions upon internal drug stimulus control. Psychopharmacology, 80, 31-34.

Jarbe, T. U. C., & McMillan, D. E. (1983). Interaction of the discriminative stimulus properties of diazepam and ethanol in pigeons. Pharmacology Biochemistry & Behavior, 18, 73-80.

Jarbe, T. U. C., & Ohlin, G. C. (1977). Stimulus effects of delta-9-THC and its interaction with naltrexone and catecholamine blockers in rats. Psychopharmacology, 54, 193-195.

Jarbe, T. U. C., Svensson, R., & Laaksomen, T. (1983). Conditioning of a discriminative drug stimulus: Overshadowing and blocking like procedures. Scandinavian Journal of Psychology, 24, 325-330.

Jarbe, T. U. C., Swedberg, M. D. B., & Mechoulam, R. (1981). A repeated test procedure to assess onset and duration of the cue properties of (-)delta-9-THC, (-)delta-8-THC-DMH, and (+)delta-8-THC. Psychopharmacology, 75, 152-157.

Jones, C. N., Grant, L. D., & Vospalek, D. M. (1976). Temporal parameters of d-amphetamine as a discriminative stimulus in the rat. Psychopharmacologia, 46, 59-64.

Joy, R. M., & Prinz, P. N. (1969). The effect of sleep altering environments upon the acquisition and retention of a conditioned avoidance response in the rat. Physiology & Behavior, 4, 809-814.

Katz, J. L., Woods, J. H., Winger, G. D., & Jacobson, A. E. (1982). Compounds of novel structure having kappa-agonist behavioral effects in rhesus monkeys. Life Sciences, 31, 2375-2378.

Kilbey, M. M., Harris, R. T., & Aigner, T. G. (1971). Establishment of equivalent external and internal stimulus control of an operant behavior and its reversal. Proceedings of the American Psychological Association, **6**, 767-768.

Koek, W., & Slangen, J. L. (1982a). Effects of reinforcement differences between drug and saline sessions on discriminative stimulus properties of fentanyl. In F. C. Colpaert & J. L. Slangen (Eds.), Drug discrimination: Applications in CNS pharmacology (pp. 343-354). Amsterdam: Elsevier/North Holland Biomedical Press.

Koek, W., & Slangen, J. L. (1982b). The role of fentanyl training dose and of the alternative stimulus condition in drug generalization. Psychopharmacology, **76**, 149-156.

Krynock, G. M., & Rosecrans, J. A. (1979). Morphine as a discriminative stimulus: Role of periaqueductal gray neurons. Research Communications in Chemical Pathology and Pharmacology, **23**, 49-60.

Lal, H. (Ed.). (1977). Discriminative stimulus properties of drugs, advances in behavioral biology (Vol. 22). New York: Plenum Press.

Lal, H., & Fielding, S. (1979). Drug discrimination: A new procedure to evaluate anxiolytic drugs. In H. Lal & S. Fielding (Eds.), Anxiolytics (pp. 83-94). New York: Futura Publishing Company.

Langford, A., Freedman, N., & Whitman, D. (1971). Further determinants of interhemispheric transfer under spreading depression. Physiology & Behavior, **7**, 65-71.

Macnish, R. (1835). The anatomy of drunkenness (5th ed.). New York: Appleton.

Mactutus, C. F., McCutcheon, K., & Riccio, D. C. (1980). Body temperature cues as contextual stimuli: Modulation of hypothermia-induced retrograde amnesia. Physiology & Behavior, **25**, 875-883.

Mayse, J. F., & DeVietti, T. L. (1971). A comparison of state-dependent learning induced by electroconvulsive shock and pentobarbital. Physiology & Behavior, **7**, 717-721.

McDonald, G. D., Conway, M., & Ricci, M. (1965). The Films of Charlie Chaplin. New York: Bonanza Books.

McIntyre, D. C., & Reichert, H. (1971). State-dependent learning in rats induced by kindled convulsions. Physiology & Behavior, **7**, 15-20.

McKenna, M. L., & Ho, B. T. (1977). Induced tolerance to the discriminative stimulus properties of cocaine. Pharmacology Biochemistry & Behavior, **7**, 273-276.

McKenna, M., & Ho, B. T. (1980). The role of dopamine in the discriminative stimulus properties of cocaine. Neuropharmacology, **19**, 297-303.

McKim, W. A. (1976). The effects of pre-exposure to scopolamine on subsequent drug state discrimination. Psychopharmacology, **47**, 153-155.

McMillan, D. E. (1982). Generalization of the discriminative stimulus properties of phencyclidine to other drugs in the pigeon using color tracking under second order schedules. Psychopharmacology, **78**, 131-134.

McMillan, D. E., Cole-Fullenwider, D. A., Hardwick, W. C., & Wenger, G. R. (1982). Phencyclidine discrimination in the pigeon using color tracking under second-order schedules. Journal of the Experimental Analysis of Behavior, **37**, 143-147.

McMillan, D. E., & Wenger, G. R. (1983a). Effects of barbiturates and other sedative hypnotics in pigeons trained to discriminate phencyclidine from saline. Journal of the Experimental Analysis of Behavior, **40**, 133-142.

McMillan, D. E., & Wenger, G. R. (1983b). Schedule-induced bias of phencyclidine (PCP) discrimination in the pigeon. Federation Proceedings, **42**, 1167.

Meltzer, L. T., & Rosecrans, J. A. (1981). Investigations on the CNS sites of action of the discriminative stimulus effects of arecoline and nicotine. Pharmacology Biochemistry & Behavior, **15**, 21-26.

Meltzer, L. T., Rosecrans, J. A., Aceto, M. D., & Harris, L. S. (1980). Discriminative stimulus properties of the optical isomers of nicotine. Psychopharmacology, 68, 283-286.

Miksic, S., & Lal, H. (1977). Tolerance to morphine-produced discriminative stimuli and analgesia. Psychopharmacology, 54, 217-221.

Miksic, S., Shearman, G., & Lal, H. (1980). Discrimination of the interoceptive stimuli produced by phenyl-quinone: A measure of the affective component of pain in the rat. In E. L. Way (Ed.), Endogenous exogenous opiate agonists antagonists (pp. 435-438). Elmsford, NY: Pergamon Press.

Miksic, S., Sherman, G., & Lal, H. (1981). Discriminative response control by naloxone in morphine pretreated rats. Psychopharmacology, 72, 179-184.

Miller, N. E. (1957). Objective techniques for studying motivational effects of drugs on animals. In S. Garattini & V. Ghetti (Eds.), Psychotropic drugs (pp. 83-103). Amsterdam: Elsevier/North Holland Biomedical Press.

Miller, N. E., & Barry, H. (1960). Motivational effects of drugs: Methods which illustrate some general problems in psychopharmacology. Psychopharmacologia, 1, 169-199.

Modrow, H. E., Holloway, F. A., & Carney, J. M. (1981). Caffeine discrimination in the rat. Pharmacology Biochemistry & Behavior, 14, 683-688.

Modrow, H. E., Salm, A., & Bliss, D. K. (1982). Transfer of a learning set between drug states in monkeys. Psychopharmacology, 77, 37-42.

Nahinsky, I. D. (1960). The transfer of a drive intensity discrimination between two drives. Journal of Comparative and Physiological Psychology, 53, 598-602.

Overton, D. A. (1961). Discriminative behavior based on the presence or absence of drug effects. American Psychologist, 16, 453-454.

Overton, D. A. (1964). State-dependent or "dissociated" learning produced with pentobarbital. Journal of Comparative and Physiological Psychology, 57, 3-12.

Overton, D. A. (1966). State-dependent learning produced by depressant and atropine-like drugs. Psychopharmacologia, 10, 6-31.

Overton, D. A. (1967). Differential responding in a three choice maze controlled by three drug states. Psychopharmacologia, 11, 376-378.

Overton, D. A. (1968a). Dissociated learning in drug states (state-dependent learning). In D. H. Efron, J. O. Cole, J. Levine, & R. Wittenborn (Eds.), Psychopharmacology, a review of progress, 1957--1967, (U.S. Public Health Service Publication 1836, pp. 918-930). Washington, DC: U.S. Government Printing Office.

Overton, D. A. (1968b). Visual cues and shock sensitivity in the control of T-maze choice by drug conditions. Journal of Comparative and Physiological Psychology, 66, 216-219.

Overton, D. A. (1969) Control of T-maze choice by nicotinic, antinicotinic, and antimuscarinic drugs. Proceedings of the 77th Annual Convention of the American Psychological Association, 4, 869-870.

Overton, D. A. (1971). Discriminative control of behavior by drug states. In T. Thompson & R. Pickens (Eds.), Stimulus properties of drugs (pp. 87-110). New York: Appleton-Century-Crofts.

Overton, D. A. (1972). State-dependent learning produced by alcohol and its relevance to alcoholism. In B. Kissen & H. Begleiter (Eds.), The biology of alcoholism II: Physiology and behavior (pp. 193-217). New York: Plenum Press.

Overton, D. A. (1973). State-dependent learning produced by addicting drugs. In L. S. Fisher & A. M. Freedman (Eds.), Opiate addiction: Origins and treatment (pp. 61-75). Washington, DC: V. H. Winston and Sons.

Overton, D. A. (1974). Experimental methods for the study of state-dependent learning. Federation Proceedings, 33, 1800-1813.

Overton, D. A. (1976). Discriminable effects of benzodiazepines. Psychopharmacology Communications, 2, 339-343.

Overton, D. A. (1977a). Discriminable effects of antimuscarinics: Dose response and substitution test studies. Pharmacology Biochemistry & Behavior, 6, 659-666.

Overton, D. A. (1977b). Comparison of ethanol, pentobarbital, and phenobarbital using drug vs. drug discrimination training. Psychopharmacology, 53, 195-199.

Overton, D. A. (1978a). Discriminable effects of antihistamine drugs. Archives Internationales de Pharmacodynamie et de Therapie, 232, 221-226.

Overton, D. A. (1978b). Status of research on state dependent learning--1978. In F. C. Colpaert & J. A. Rosecrans (Eds.), Stimulus properties of drugs: Ten years of progress (pp. 559-562). Amsterdam: Elsevier/North Holland Biomedical Press.

Overton, D. A. (1978c). Influence of training compartment design on performance in the two-bar drug discrimination task: A methodological report. In F. C. Colpaert & J. A. Rosecrans (Eds.), Stimulus properties of drugs: Ten years of progress (pp.265-278). Amsterdam: Elsevier/North Holland Biomedical Press.

Overton, D. A. (1978d). Major theories of state dependent learning. In B. T. Ho, D. W. Richards, III, & D. L. Chute (Eds.), Drug discrimination and state dependent learning (283-318). New York: Academic Press.

Overton, D. A. (1979a). Drug discrimination training with progressively lowered doses. Science, 205, 720-721.

Overton, D. A. (1979b). Influence of shaping procedures and schedules of reinforcement on performance in the two-bar drug discrimination task: A methodological report. Psychopharmacology, 65, 291-298.

Overton, D. A. (1982a). Comparison of the degree of discriminability of various drugs using the T-maze drug discrimination paradigm. Psychopharmacology, 76, 385-395.

Overton, D. A. (1982b). Memory retrieval failures produced by changes in drug state. In R. L. Isaacson & N. E. Spear (Eds.), The expression of knowledge, neurobehavioral transformations of information into action (pp. 113-139). New York: Plenum Press.

Overton, D. A. (1982c). Multiple drug training as a method for increasing the specificity of the drug discrimination procedure. Journal of Pharmacology and Experimental Therapeutics, 221, 166-172.

Overton, D. A. (1983). Test for a neurochemically specific mechanism mediating drug discriminations, and for stimulus masking. Psychopharmacology, 81, 340-344.

Overton, D. A. (1984). State dependent learning and drug discriminations. In Iversen, L. L., Iversen, S. D., & Snyder, S. H. (Eds.), Handbook of Psychopharmacology (Vol. 18, pp. 59-127). New York: Plenum Press.

Overton, D. A., & Batta, S. K. (1977). Relationship between abuse liability of drugs and their degree of discriminability in the rat. In T. Thompson & K. R. Unna (Eds.), Predicting dependence liability of stimulant and depressant drugs (pp. 125-135). Baltimore, MD: University Park Press.

Overton, D. A., & Batta, S. K. (1979). Investigation of narcotics and antitussives using drug discrimination techniques. Journal of Pharmacology and Experimental Therapeutics, 211, 401-408.

Overton, D. A., Ercole, M. A., & Dutta, P. (1976). Discriminability of the postictal state produced by electroconvulsive shock. Physiological Psychology, 4, 207-212.

Overton, D. A., & Hayes, M. (1980). Acquisition of four-drug discriminations in the two-bar drug discrimination task. Pharmacology Biochemistry & Behavior, 13, 314.

Overton, D. A., & Hayes, M. W. (1984). Optimal training parameters in the two-bar fixed-ratio drug discrimination task. Pharmacology Biochemistry & Behavior, 21, 19-25.

Overton, D. A., Leonard, W. R., & Merkle, D. A. (1985). Methods for quantifying the discriminable effects of drugs. Neuroscience & Biobehavioral Reviews, (submitted).

Overton, D. A., Merkle, D. A., & Hayes, M. (1983). Are "no drug" cues discriminated during drug discrimination training? Animal Learning and Behavior, 11, 295-301.

Pappas, B. A., & Gray, P. (1971). Cue value of dexamethasone for fear-motivated behavior. Physiology & Behavior, 6, 127-130.

Peck, J. H., & Ader, R. (1974). Illness-induced taste aversion under states of deprivation and satiation. Animal Learning and Behavior, 2, 6-8.

Peters, R., & McGee, R. (1982). Cigarette smoking and state-dependent memory. Psychopharmacology, 76, 232-235.

Petersen, R. C. (1977). Retrieval failures in alcohol state-dependent learning. Psychopharmacology, 55, 141-146.

Pianka, M. J. (1976). Cortical spreading depression: A case of state dependent learning. Physiology & Behavior, 17, 565-570.

Reed, V. G., & Trowill, J. A. (1969). Stimulus control value of spreading depression demonstrated without shifting depressed hemispheres. Journal of Comparative and Physiological Psychology, 69, 40-43.

Ribot, T. (1882). Diseases of memory. London: Kegan, Paul, Trench & Company.

Ribot, T. (1891). The diseases of the personality. Chicago: Open Court Publishing.

Riccio, D. C., Urda, M., & Thomas, D. R. (1966). Stimulus control in pigeons based on proprioceptive stimuli from floor inclination. Science, 153, 434-436.

Richardson, R., Riccio, D. C., & Jonke, T. (1983). Alleviation of infantile amnesia in rats by means of a pharmacological contextual state. Developmental Psychobiology, 16, 511-518.

Romano, C., Goldstein, A., & Jewell, N. P. (1981). Characterization of the receptor mediating the nicotine discriminative stimulus. Psychopharmacology, 74, 310-315.

Rosecrans, J. A. (1979). Nicotine as a discriminative stimulus to behavior: Its characterization and relevance to smoking behavior. In N. A. Krasnegor (Ed.), Cigarette smoking as a dependent process (National Institute on Drug Abuse Research Monograph 23, pp. 58-69). Washington, DC: U.S. Government Printing Office.

Rosecrans, J. A., & Glennon, R. A. (1979). Drug-induced cues in studying mechanisms of drug action. Neuropharmacology, 18, 981-989.

Rosecrans, J. A., Spencer, R. M., Krynock, G. M., & Chance, W. T. (1978). Discriminative stimulus properties of nicotine and nicotine-related compounds. In K. Baettig (Ed.), Behavioral effects of nicotine (pp. 70-82). Basel, Switzerland: Karger.

Sachs, E., Weingarten, M., & Klein, N. W., Jr. (1966). Effects of chlordiazepoxide on the acquisition of avoidance learning and its transfer to the normal state and other drug conditions. Psychopharmacologia, 9, 17-30.

Schechter, M. D. (1973). Ethanol as a discriminative cue: Reduction following depletion of brain serotonin. European Journal of Pharmacology, 24, 278-281.

Schechter, M. D. (1977). Amphetamine discrimination as a test for anti-Parkinsonism drugs. European Journal of Pharmacology, 44, 51-56.

Schechter, M. D. (1980). Effect of neuroleptics and tricyclic antidepressants upon d-amphetamine discrimination. Pharmacology Biochemistry & Behavior, 12, 1-5.

Schechter, M. D. (1981a). Extended schedule transfer of ethanol discrimination. Pharmacology Biochemistry & Behavior, 14, 23-25.

Schechter, M. D. (1981b). Rapid acquisition of a two-drug discrimination: Time of day effect upon saline state. Pharmacology Biochemistry & Behavior, 14, 269-271.

Schechter, M. D., & Cook, P. G. (1975). Dopaminergic mediation of the interoceptive cue produced by d-amphetamine in rats. Psychopharmacologia, 42, 185-193.

Schechter, M. D., & Rosecrans, J. A. (1972a). Nicotine as a discriminative cue in rats: Inability of related drugs to produce a nicotine-like cueing effect. Psychopharmacologia, 27, 379-387.

Schechter, M. D., & Rosecrans, J. A. (1972b). Nicotine as a discriminative stimulus in rats depleted of norepinephrine or 5-hydroxytryptamine. Psychopharmacologia, 24, 417-429.

Schechter, M. D., & Rosecrans, J. A. (1972c). Effect of mecamylamine on discrimination between nicotine- and arecoline-produced cues. European Journal of Pharmacology, 17, 179-182.

Schechter, M. D., & Rosecrans, J. A. (1972d). Behavioral tolerance to an effect of nicotine in the rat. Archives Internationales de Pharmacodynamie et de Therapie, 195, 52-56.

Schneider, A. M. (1966). Retention under spreading depression: A generalization decrement phenomenon. Journal of Comparative and Physiological Psychology, 62, 317-319.

Schneider, A. M. (1967). Control of memory by spreading cortical depression: A case for stimulus control. Psychological Review, 74, 201-215.

Schneider, A. M. (1973). Spreading depression: A behavioral analysis. In J. A. Deutsch (Ed.), The physiological basis of memory (pp.269-303). London: Academic Press.

Schuster, C. R., & Balster, R. L. (1977). Discriminative stimulus properties of drugs. In T. Thompson & P. B. Dews (Eds.), Advances in behavioral pharmacology (Vol. 1, pp. 85-138). New York: Academic Press.

Semon, R. (1904). Die mneme (Reprinted, 1923). London: George Allen & Unwin.

Semon, R. (1909). Mnemic psychology (Reprinted, 1923). London: George Allen & Unwin.

Shannon, H. E. (1981). Evaluation of phencyclidine analogs on the basis of their discriminative stimulus properties in the rat. Journal of Pharmacology and Experimental Therapeutics, 216, 543-551.

Shannon, H. E., & Herling, S. (1983). Discriminative stimulus effects of diazepam in rats: Evidence for a maximal effect. Journal of Pharmacology and Experimental Therapeutics, 227, 160-166.

Shannon, H. E., & Holtzman, S. G. (1976a). Blockade of the discriminative effects of morphine in the rat by naltrexone and naloxone. Psychopharmacology, 50, 119-124.

Shannon, H. E., & Holtzman, S. G. (1976b). Evaluation of the discriminative effects of morphine in the rat. Journal of Pharmacology and Experimental Therapeutics, 198, 54-65.

Shannon, H. E., & Holtzman, S. G. (1979). Morphine training dose: A determinant of stimulus generalization to narcotic antagonists in the rat. Psychopharmacology, 61, 239-244.

Shannon, H. E., McQuinn, R. L., Vaupel, D. B., & Cone, E. J. (1983). Effects of cycloalkyl ring analogs of phencyclidine on behavior in rodents. Journal of Pharmacology and Experimental Therapeutics, 224, 327-333.

Shearman, G. T., & Lal, H. (1979). Discriminative stimulus properties of pentylenetetrazol and bemegride: Some generalization and antagonism tests. Psychopharmacology, 64, 315-319.

Shearman, G. T., & Lal, H. (1981). Discriminative stimulus properties of cocaine related to an anxiogenic action. Progress in Neuro-Psychopharmacology, 5, 57-63.

Shmavonian, B. H. (1956). Effects of serpasil (rauwolfia serpantina) on fear training. Unpublished masters thesis, University of Washington.

Siegel, S. (1982). Drug dissociation in the nineteenth century. In F. C. Colpaert & J. L. Slangen (Eds.), Drug discrimination: Applications in CNS pharmacology (pp. 257-261). Amsterdam: Elsevier/North Holland Biomedical Press.

Siegel, S. (1983). Wilkie Collins: Victorian novelist as psychopharmacologist. Journal of the History of Medicine and Allied Sciences, 38, 161-175.

Silverman, P. B., & Ho, B. T. (1980). The discriminative stimulus properties of 2,5-Dimethoxy-4-Methylamphetamine (DOM): Differentiation from amphetamine. Psychopharmacology, 68, 209-215.

Solomon, R. E., Herling, S., Domino, E. F., & Woods, J. H. (1982). Discriminative stimulus effects of N-substituted analogs of phencyclidine in rhesus monkeys. Neuropharmacology, 21, 1329-1336.

Spear, N. E., Smith, G. J., Bryan, R. G., Gordon, W. C., Timmons, R., & Chiszar, D. A. (1980). Contextual influences on the interaction between conflicting memories in the rat. Animal Learning and Behavior, 8, 273-281.

Stewart, J. (1962). Differential responses based on the physiological consequences of pharmacological agents. Psychopharmacologia, 3, 132-138.

Stolerman, I. P., Baldy, R. E., & Shine, P. J. (1982). Drug-discrimination procedure: A bibliography. In F. C. Colpaert & J. L. Slangen (Eds.), Drug discrimination: Applications in CNS pharmacology. Amsterdam: Elsevier/North Holland Biomedical Press.

Stolerman, I. P., & D'Mello, G. D. (1981). Role of training conditions in discrimination of central nervous system stimulants by rats. Psychopharmacology, 73, 295-303.

Stutz, R. M., & Maroli, A. N. Central mechanisms of reward and the narcotic cue. In F. C. Colpaert & J. A. Rosecrans (Eds.), Stimulus properties of drugs: Ten years of progress (pp. 517-534). Amsterdam: Elsevier/North Holland Biomedical Press.

Swanson, J. M., & Kinsbourne, M. (1979). State-dependent learning and retrieval: Methodological cautions and theoretical considerations. In J. F. Kihlstrom & F. J. Evans (Eds.), Functional disorders of memory (pp. 275-299). Hillsdale, NJ: Lawrence Erlbaum Associates.

Takada, K. (1982). Discriminative stimulus effects of pentobarbital in rats. Japanese Journal of Psychopharmacology, 2, 47-55.

Teal, J. J., & Holtzman, S. G. (1980a). Discriminative stimulus effects of prototype opiate receptor agonists in monkeys. European Journal of Pharmacology, 68, 1-10.

Teal, J. J., & Holtzman, S. G. (1980b). Discriminative stimulus effects of cyclazocine in the rat. Journal of Pharmacology and Experimental Therapeutics, 212, 368-376.

Thompson, T., & Pickens, R. (1971). Stimulus properties of drugs. New York: Appleton-Century-Crofts.

Valentino, R. J., Herling, S., & Woods, J. H. (1983). Discriminative stimulus effects of naltrexone in narcotic-naive and morphine-treated pigeons. Journal of Pharmacology and Experimental Therapeutics, 224, 307-313.

Valentino, R. J., Herling, S., Woods, J. H., Medzihradsky, F., & Merz, H. (1981). Quaternary naltrexone: Evidence for the central mediation of discriminative stimulus effects of narcotic agonists and antagonists. Journal of Pharmacology and Experimental Therapeutics, 217, 652-659.

Valentino, R. J., Smith, C. B., & Woods, J. H. (1981). Physiological and behavioral approaches to the study of the quasi-morphine withdrawal syndrome. Federation Proceedings, 40, 1502-1507.

Weissman, A. (1976). Discriminability of aspirin in arthritic and nonarthritic rats. Pharmacology Biochemistry & Behavior, 5, 583-586.

White, F. J., & Appel, J. B. (1981). A neuropharmacological analysis of the discriminative stimulus properties of fenfluramine. Psychopharmacology, 73, 110-115.

White, F. J., & Appel, J. B. (1982). Training dose as a factor in LSD-saline discrimination. Psychopharmacology, 76, 20-25.

White, F. J., Appel, J. B., & Kuhn, D. M. (1979). Discriminative stimulus properties of quipazine: Direct serotonergic mediation. Neuropharmacology, 18, 143-151.

White, F. J., & Holtzman, S. G. (1981). Three-choice drug discrimination in the rat: Morphine, cyclazocine, and saline. Journal of Pharmacology and Experimental Therapeutics, 217, 254-262.

White, J. M., & Holtzman, S. G. (1983a). Further characterization of the three-choice morphine, cyclazocine and saline discrimination paradigm: Opioids with agonist and antagonist properties. Journal of Pharmacology and Experimental Therapeutics, 224, 95-99.

White, J. M., & Holtzman, S. G. (1983b). Three-choice drug discrimination: Phencyclidine-like stimulus effects of opioids. Psychopharmacology, 80, 1-9.

Winslow, F. (1860). Obscure diseases of the brain and mind. Philadelphia: Blanchard & Lea.

Winter, J. C. (1973). A comparison of the stimulus properties of mescaline and 2,3,4-Trimethoxyphenylethylamine. Journal of Pharmacology and Experimental Therapeutics, 185, 101-107.

Winter, J. C. (1974). Hallucinogens as discriminative stimuli. Federation Proceedings, 33, 1825-1832.

Winter, J. C. (1975). The effects of 2,5-Dimethoxy-4-methylamphetamine (DOM), 2,5-Dimethoxy-4-ethylamphetamine (DOET), d-Amphetamine, and cocaine in rats trained with mescaline as a discriminative stimulus. Psychopharmacologia, 44, 29-32.

Winter, J. C. (1977). Morphine and ethanol as discriminative stimuli: Absence of antagonism by p-Chlorophenylalanine methyl ester, cinanserin, or BC-105. Psychopharmacology, 53, 159-163.

Winter, J. C. (1978a). Drug induced stimulus control. In D. E. Blackman & D. J. Sanger (Eds.), Contemporary research in behavioral pharmacology (pp. 209-237). New York: Plenum Press.

Winter, J. C. (1978b). Stimulus properties of phenethylamine hallucinogens and lysergic acid diethylamide: The role of 5-hydroxytryptamine. Journal of Pharmacology and Experimental Therapeutics, 204, 416-423.

Winter, J. C. (1981a). Drug-induced stimulus control and the concept of breaking point: LSD and quipazine. Psychopharmacology, 72, 217-218.

Winter, J. C. (1981b). The stimulus properties of gamma-hydroxybutyrate. Psychopharmacology, 73, 372-375.

Witkin, J. M., Carter, R. B., & Dykstra, L. A. (1980). Discriminative stimulus properties of d-amphetamine-pentobarbital combinations. Psychopharmacology, 68, 269-276.

Witkin, J. M., Dykstra, L. A., & Carter, R. B. (1982). Acute tolerance to the discriminative stimulus properties of morphine. Pharmacology Biochemistry & Behavior, 17, 223-228.

Woods, J. H., Young, A. M., & Herling, S. (1982). Classification of narcotics on the basis of their reinforcing, discriminative, and antagonist effects in rhesus monkeys. Federation Proceedings, 41, 221-227.

York, J. L., & Winter, J. C. (1975). Assessment of tolerance to barbital by means of drug discrimination procedures. Psychopharmacologia, 42, 283-287.

Zenick, H., & Goldsmith, M. (1981). Drug discrimination learning in lead-exposed rats. Science, 212, 569-571.

CHAPTER 17

DRUG DISCRIMINATION: METHODS OF MANIPULATION, MEASUREMENT, AND ANALYSIS

Francis C. Colpaert

Department of Psychopharmacology
Janssen Pharmaceutica
B-2340 Beerse, Belgium

ABSTRACT

In a typical drug discrimination experiment, laboratory animals are trained to discriminate a given drug from saline; training drug and saline injections serve as pharmacological stimuli which signal which of several operant responses will be reinforced. Drugs are thought to be discriminable on the basis of their sensory-perceptual effects, and tests for stimulus generalization determine whether other pharmacological treatments produce discriminative stimulus effects similar to those of the training drug.

The most commonly used of many possible drug discrimination procedures is one in which food deprived rats press one of two levers for food according to a fixed ratio-10 (FR-10) schedule. The principal dependent variable of the drug discrimination experiment serves to measure discrimination and generalization. It is this author's position, but not the general consensus, that this variable is nominal in nature. The more commonly used dependent variable is quantitative and adheres to Skinnerian tradition in behavioral pharmacology. The two-lever, food-reinforced, FR-10 procedure allows derivation of both these two dependent variables. Both the analysis of drug discrimination and generalization data and the interpretation of these data differ markedly depending on whether the variable being used is nominal or quantitative. The differences in interpretation are particularly apparent with partial generalization and have caused a profound divergence in the pharmacological and molecular interpretations of opiate drug discrimination data (Colpaert, 1984). The phenomenon of partial generalization is very significant (Colpaert & Janssen, 1984), and it is indicated here that its analysis is to be conducted nominally. It is recommended here (i) that the nominal variable be used throughout to measure discrimination and generalization and (ii) that the percentage of responding on the appropriate (in training sessions) or selected lever (in test sessions) be monitored to detect possible drug interferences with the effects of the primary reinforcer.

Finally, it may be pertinent to note that the outcome of generalization tests may vary according to one or several of the independent variables of the experiment. That is, the pharmacological specificity of the paradigm is variable, and the training dose, reinforcement, and discriminandum have been identified

(Colpaert, 1982b) as conditions which co-determine the naloxone-reversibility and the patterns of generalization in opiate drug discriminations. These and, perhaps, additional manipulations open wide but largely unexplored possibilities for the detailed analysis of the discriminative effects of drugs.

INTRODUCTION

It is a distinctive feature of many drugs of abuse that they produce subjective effects in humans. Subjective effects are sensory in nature and differ from many other drug effects in that they are accessible to conscious perception. A familiar example is the feelings of drunkenness and relaxation that can follow the ingestion of ethanol. Also known are the subjective effects of morphine and those of such drugs as cocaine, amphetamines, hallucinogens, cannabinoids, barbiturates, benzodiazepines, and phencyclidine.

It is thought that the ability of opiates (Jasinski, 1977) and many other drugs to produce subjective effects relates intimately to their abuse; in as much as these effects can be euphoric or otherwise reinforcing, they may be involved in the initiation and maintenance of self-administration behavior. The single and, even more so, the repeated exposure to the drug may render the subject drug dependent. That is, the subject's behavioral and physiological homeostasis may come to depend on the intake of the drug in much the same manner as it depends on the intake of gaseous oxygen, fluids, and solid foods. Prominent and particularly powerful among the known drug dependencies is opiate dependence; opiates interfere with respiration (Eckenhoff & Oech, 1960) and with the ingestion of fluids and food (e.g., Holtzman, 1975; Locke, Brown, & Holtzman, 1982; Lowy, Starkey, & Yim, 1981; Ostrowski, Rowland, Foley, Nelson, & Reid, 1981).

Although the production of subjective effects, the occurrence of self-administration behavior, and the development of dependence may thus be relevant to drug abuse, preclinical research on drugs of abuse has been concerned largely with the ability of drugs to produce self-administration and dependence in laboratory animals. Until recently, it has not seemed feasible to study subjective drug effects in any species other than human.

It has been hypothesized (Colpaert, Lal, Niemegeers, & Janssen, 1975a; Colpaert, Niemegeers, Lal, & Janssen, 1975b), however, that the discriminative stimulus properties of opiates in the rat may relate to and can serve as an animal model of opiate-like subjective effects in man. It is not merely incidental that opiates were involved in this original proposal relating discriminative drug properties in animals to subjective drug effects in man. Opiates are a group of drugs of abuse for which formal methods have been developed (Fraser, 1968; Jasinski, 1977) to identify, quantify, and compare their subjective effects. These effects have made it possible that the subjective effects of a number of opiates have been documented and characterized extensively (e.g., Fraser, Van Horn, Martin, Wolbach, & Isbell, 1961; Haertzen, 1970, 1974; Jasinski, 1973; Jasinski & Mansky, 1972; Jasinski, Martin, & Haertzen, 1967; Jasinski, Martin, & Sapira, 1968). More so than with most other drugs of abuse, the clinical evidence on subjective effects of opiates thus offered a data base for comparison to animal data. The initial attempt (Colpaert et al., 1975a, 1975b) to substantiate the hypothesis did in fact consist of a comparison of discriminative effects of morphine, codeine, and diphenoxylate in rat to the results of a clinical study (Fraser & Isbell, 1961) on their subjective effects in man.

The evidence relating the discriminative effects of drugs in laboratory animals to their subjective effects in humans has been the subject of a recent review (Colpaert, 1984). Briefly, two lines of evidence suggest that discriminative drug effects in animals are homologous to subjective drug effects in humans. One similarity is methodological; in both cases the drug acts as a stimulus to behavior, and the formal relationship of the behavioral response to the drug stimulus is similar (Colpaert, 1978a; Schuster, Fischman, & Johanson, 1981). Second, it appears that the pharmacological characteristics of the discriminative effects of drugs in animals may closely match those of their subjective effects in humans. Evidence to this effect is relatively extensive and detailed with opiates (Colpaert, 1977a, 1978a, 1982; Herling & Woods, 1981; Holtzman, 1982a, 1982b) and is also available with such other prominent substances of abuse as CNS stimulants (Ho & Silverman, 1978; Silverman & Ho, 1977), hallucinogens (Appel, White, & Holohean, 1982; Glennon, Rosecrans, & Young, 1982), cannabinoids (Krimmer & Barry, 1977; Weissman, 1978), and ethanol (Barry & Krimmer, 1977).

The aim of the present chapter,[1] then, will be to describe some of the typical as well as the variable features of the drug discrimination experiment. We will also explore how drug discrimination can be used in analyzing the actions of drugs of abuse, and the utility it may have in the preclinical evaluation of drug abuse potential.

DRUG DISCRIMINATION

The Drug Discrimination Experiment

In a typical drug discrimination (DD) experiment, laboratory animals are trained to discriminate injections of a given dose (the training dose) of a particular drug (the training drug) from saline injections. Perhaps the most widely used of many possible procedures is pressing one of two levers according to a fixed ratio-10 schedule which results in food delivery to deprived rats (see Colpaert, Niemegeers, & Janssen, 1976a). That is, rats are trained to press the two levers for food, and the fixed ratio-10 schedule is gradually instituted prior to discrimination training. In any given session only one of the two levers is operative, and the operative lever is alternated between sessions.

Once the two responses--pressing the left and the right of the two levers--are established, discrimination training commences. That is, prior to every daily (5 days/week) 15-minute session, the animal is injected with either the training drug or saline. After the training drug injection only one of the two levers (the drug lever; DL) is operative, and pressing the alternative lever (the saline lever; SL) has no programmed consequences in drug sessions. After injection of saline SL responding is reinforced, and pressing the DL in saline sessions is inconsequential.

The following considerations apply to the sequence in which training drug (D) and saline (S) sessions are administered; (a) D and S sessions occur equally often; (b) simple alternation is avoided; (c) chains of at least two

----
[1]Citations in this chapter are limited in number; useful sources of references are the recent drug discrimination bibliography by Stolerman, Baldy and Shine (1982) and the proceedings of two international symposia (Colpaert & Rosecrans, 1978; Colpaert & Slangen, 1982).

consecutive D and S sessions are thus allowed to appear; this accommodates the nonscheduled occurrence of such chains with later test sessions; finally, (d) the sequence must take into account that rats may learn to use olfactory cues that are left in the operant chamber by preceding animals (Extance & Goudie, 1981). Lever assignments can be: DL, left; SL, right; or DL, right; SL, left. These four conditions are implemented in the following two monthly alternating sequences--(1) D-S-S-D-S, S-D-D-S-S, S-D-S-D-D, D-S-D-S-D and (2) S-D-D-S-S, D-S-D-S-D, D-S-S-D-D, S-D-S-D-S. Rats with even serial numbers are initially run on sequence 1 and the others on sequence 2; the sequence assignments are reversed every 4 weeks (Colpaert, Niemegeers, & Janssen, 1977).

The implementation of these conditions will typically result in a change in behavior that is characteristic of the acquisition of a discrimination; the animals come to reliably press the DL in D sessions and the SL in S sessions. Once a given animal has reached some arbitrarily set criterion, tests of stimulus generalization can be conducted. For the purpose of such tests, the animal is treated with the pharmacological condition that is being studied, and its subsequent operant responding is observed. Stimulus generalization with the training drug is said to occur if the test treatment induces DL responding; generalization is said not to have occurred if the test treatment induces SL responding. Note that the wording "generalization with saline" is not ordinarily used when the test treatment makes the animal respond on the SL.

A built-in precaution against the possible development of state dependency in this procedure is that the two discriminative responses are established prior to the implementation of the pharmacological stimuli. It is also possible to verify whether state dependency occurs by determining if lever selection behavior early in training approaches what is then the chance level (50%) in both D and S sessions (Colpaert, 1977b, 1983).

Typical Features

The DD method consists of a set of experimental conditions whereby one of two or more pharmacological stimuli predicts or signals (Colpaert, 1978b) which of several responses will be associated with reinforcement. Typically, the animals are trained to discriminate a training drug at a given training dose from the drug vehicle. The discrimination involves two responses. These responses are operant--instrumental in the occurrence of reinforcement. The two discriminative responses have a similar morphology (e.g., lever pressing), except for one particular feature such as location (e.g., pressing a left as opposed to a right lever). The responses are mutually exclusive; in the example the FR-10 schedule can be completed for the first time within a session on only one of the two levers.

The reinforcement of the two operant responses is the same; the same schedule of reinforcement is implemented for DL responses in D sessions and SL responses in S sessions. Since the reinforcement of the two responses is the same, it also follows that scheduled reinforcement is symmetrical in D and S sessions.

Another significant typical feature of the DD experiment is that it establishes a nominal (binary, quantal, categorical) relationship between the drug stimulus and the behavioral response (Colpaert, 1982a, 1983); SL responding is reinforced if, and only if, the animal was treated with saline, and DL responding is reinforced if, and only if, the treatment consisted of training drug. Specifically, the pharmacological treatment predicts only which of the two possible, mutually exclusive, locations of responding will yield reinforcement. The treatment is not predictive of any variation in reinforcement that may be consequential to any variation in behavior other than location.

DRUG DISCRIMINATION VARIABLES

Before considering the DD variables, it may be pertinent to note that DD constitutes an extremely simple and straightforward paradigm. Complexities may become apparent with the manipulation of independent variables and with the detailed numerical analysis of dependent variables. But these complexities should not obscure that the utility of the paradigm for pharmacological research owes much to the paradigm's simplicity (Colpaert, 1982a).

Independent Variables

Pharmacological Variables

Pharmacological variables include the training drug, the training dose, and the route and time of drug administration prior to training sessions. Route and time of training drug administration are typically chosen in accordance with what is known about the drug's kinetic properties and are the same for vehicle administration. The training dose is typically chosen to be within a known appropriate or relevant range of doses of the training drug. A wide variety of drugs can be discriminated from saline; suffice it here to indicate that this variety includes many substances of abuse (see Stolerman et al., 1982).

Procedural Variables

A survey of procedural variables is given in Table 1. Though a variety of species, responses, apparatus, reinforcers, and schedules have been used, numerous studies have revealed good agreement across these variables in the data that are obtained in generalization tests. The rat has been the most widely used animal species for obvious reasons. Some effort is involved in the initial DD training, and longevity may be a criterion in the choice of the animal species. The monkey and pigeon may excel the rat at this point, particularly in studies where number of animals is less of a consideration. However, little work has been done on the possible effects of prolonged exposure to the conditions of the DD experiment and of age. Effects of this nature may be significant, especially since the animals are exposed almost continuously either to deprivation schedules or to such stressful manipulations as electric shock. There is yet no evidence of any important change in generalization characteristics in conditions where the discriminandum remains unchanged for protracted periods of time (e.g., Colpaert, Niemegeers, & Janssen, 1976b). But caution must be exerted with the uncontrolled use of the same animals in experiments involving different discriminanda.

Procedures involving an operant chamber, the lever-press response, and food, water, or electric shock have been used more widely than mazes where locomotor responses are reinforced by the escape from or avoidance of electric shock or immersion in water. The operant chamber procedure can perhaps be considered as offering a set of conditions where sizable rates of responding can be maintained while implementing only limited stress. This apparently allows low training doses of drugs to be discriminable (Colpaert & Janssen,

Table 1

Some Procedural Variables of the Drug Discrimination Paradigm

---

animal species	rat, monkey, pigeon
operant response	lever press, locomotor response
apparatus	operant chamber, maze
reinforcer	food, water, electric shock
schedule of reinforcement	fixed ratio, variable interval, differential reinforcement of low rate, continuous reinforcement
deprivation	of food, of water, or none (escape, avoidance)
generalization test	with reinforcement (of selected response, of either response), in extinction (of either response)

Note: The reader is referred to the detailed drug discrimination bibliography recently compiled by Stolerman, Baldy, and Shine, 1982. The listings given here are not exhaustive but indicate conditions that are commonly used.

1982b; Colpaert, Niemegeers, & Janssen, 1980b). Though no truly adequate comparisons have as yet been made, the shock- or water-escape maze procedures typically require much higher training doses for drugs to be discriminable (Overton, 1982). The differences between operant chamber and maze procedures may not be, however, simply quantitative. An (unpublished) experiment in our laboratory revealed that 10 mg/kg of pentobarbital is readily discriminable in both the operant chamber (Colpaert et al., 1976a) and a water-escape maze procedure (Colpaert, Niemegeers, & Janssen, 1978a). Cocaine, in contrast, was readily discriminable (at 2.5 and 10 mg/kg) in the operant chamber procedure but essentially failed to acquire response control in the maze procedure at doses ranging from 0.63 to 40 mg/kg. It would seem possible from these data that severe stress may compromise drug discrimination and that training drugs which alleviate procedure-generated stress may be less vulnerable to this effect than those which do not. The issue deserves analysis but has not as yet been examined.

Fixed ratio (FR), variable interval (VI), differential reinforcement of low rate (DRL), and other schedules of reinforcement have been used in operant chamber procedures; maze procedures have typically utilized continuous reinforcement. Generalization test data have generally been consistent across different schedules. Schedules have often been chosen on the basis of (i) the amount of responding that they generate and (ii) their vulnerability to drug effects on rate. Specifically, schedules yielding modest rates of responding that are abolished by even low doses of drugs are considered undesirable. Overton (1979) has compared FR, VI, and DRL schedules in the two-lever appetitive procedure and concluded that the FR schedule yields relatively rapid acquisition and high asymptotic accuracy. These data add to the attractiveness of the two-lever, food-reinforced FR-10 procedure (Colpaert et al., 1976a); for practical pharmacological purposes, it is desirable to have available a rapid and accurate method which is sensitive to the discriminative effects of low doses and allows exploration of fairly wide ranges of training dose. The availability of this procedure, however, should not act to discourage further methodological research. It would be of interest, for example, to examine and compare stimulus generalization with a given training dose of a given training drug in conditions where its discrimination is rapidly acquired and accurate and in conditions where it is slowly acquired and/or less accurate. In the context of such methodological research, the portrayal of "the ideal" DD procedure (Overton, 1979) obscures the important and interesting fact that the discriminative effects of drugs may vary markedly according to the conditions in which they are being analyzed (Colpaert & Janssen, 1981).

The procedures that have been used in tests of stimulus generalization differ mainly in terms of the delivery of reinforcement. When reinforcement is delivered in test sessions, either the selected response (e.g., Colpaert et al., 1976a) or both responses (e.g., Shannon & Holtzman, 1976) may be reinforced; reinforcing only the response which is alternative to the one selected by the animal is of course uncommon. The other possibility is to institute extinction. One reason for administering reinforcement in generalization tests is that the availability of reinforcement offers the opportunity to analyze the possible effects of test treatments on overall rate of responding (Colpaert et al., 1975a, 1976b; Shannon & Holtzman, 1976). Such data on rate effects are obviously important. The rationale for testing in extinction has been largely intuitive; extinction is often thought to prevent new discrimination learning from taking place in test sessions. There is, however, no a priori reason to assume that less new learning takes place in extinction than with reinforcement; the learning, if any, may simply be opposite in sign. The new learning can be limited by implementing only brief episodes of extinction. But this maneuver does not preclude the possibility that test treatments become a signal for brief sessions of extinction; it may simply discourage responding in later test sessions. At any rate, the overall consistency of results that have been obtained across different test procedures renders it unlikely that much new discrimination learning occurs in test sessions. Consistent with this conclusion are the results of an (unpublished) experiment in which six rats were trained to discriminate 0.04 mg/kg of fentanyl from saline and then tested twice with 1.25 mg/kg of d-amphetamine. In the first test all animals selected the SL but were only reinforced for pressing the DL. The second test was administered one week later and revealed that all animals again selected the SL, despite this previous experience.

Different test procedures may nonetheless yield different results depending on the dependent variable that is being used to measure discrimination and generalization. Figure 1 summarizes earlier (Colpaert, 1977b) and new (unpublished) data on the effects of reinforcement on two different indices of generalization. Nine rats were trained to discriminate 0.04 mg/kg of fentanyl from saline in the two-lever, food-reinforced FR-10 procedure and were tested, eight times in all, with 0.04 mg/kg of fentanyl and saline in four different conditions: (1) Responses on the lever which the animal initially selected were reinforced, a standard practice in this laboratory; (2) responses on both levers were reinforced; (3) only responses on the lever opposite to the selected lever were reinforced; and (4) no reinforcement was delivered (i.e., the test consisted of an extinction episode). The session duration in Conditions 1, 2, and 3 was 15 minutes; the duration in Condition 4 was 60 minutes, but data were recorded after 0.5, 15, and 60 minutes. Two variates were derived from the responding that occurred in test sessions. One is the selected lever (i.e., the lever where the animal totaled 10 responses first); this variate can take one of only two values (i.e., SL and DL) and is nominal. The second variate consisted of the percentage of responding that was appropriate to the training drug (i.e., the

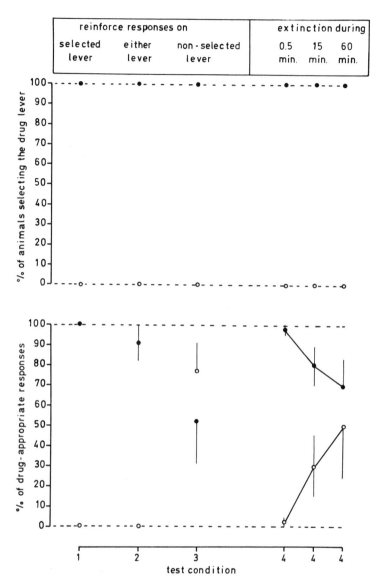

Figure 1: Results of four different stimulus generalization tests with 0.04 mg/kg of fentanyl (●) and saline (O) in nine rats trained to discriminate 0.04 mg/kg of fentanyl from saline. Two dependent variables are presented--the percentage of rats selecting the drug lever (upper panel) and the percentage of drug-appropriate responses (lower panel; mean ±1 SEM). Data points for condition 4 represent data obtained at different intervals of time (i.e., 0 to 0.5 minutes, 0.5 to 15 minutes, and 15 to 60 minutes). See text for details.

percentage of DL responding); this variate is free to vary from 0 to 100% and is quantitative. The results of this experiment indicate that the nominal variate was entirely unresponsive to the manipulations of reinforcement in test sessions (see Figure 1). The reason for this is simple: The variate is based exclusively on responding which occurs **prior** to the time of the first possible delivery of reinforcement. It therefore is entirely independent from reinforcement. The percentage of drug-appropriate responses did vary as a function of the reinforcement procedure used in test sessions. The percentage was entirely treatment-appropriate when reinforcement was instituted on the selected lever. When either lever yielded reinforcement, one fentanyl-treated rat switched from the DL to the SL in the course of the session and continued to press the SL for some time. Behavior became particularly disorganized when pressing the nonselected lever was reinforced (Condition 3). The extinction procedure yielded responding that was almost entirely treatment-appropriate if only the first 30 seconds were considered. This duration corresponds roughly to the length of time it typically takes the animal to complete the first FR-10 schedule; the behavior in extinction at this point, therefore, is essentially identical to the behavior used as the basis for the nominal measure. However, the percentage of drug-appropriate responding rapidly deteriorated as the extinction episode grew longer, and by 60 minutes almost no discrimination was apparent anymore. In summary, the experiment described here utilized the training treatments in tests where the reinforcement procedure was varied. Obviously, adequate test conditions should yield results that are entirely appropriate to the training drug and saline treatments. This occurred at all times with the nominal variate; it also occurred with the quantitative variable when the selected or either lever was reinforced or when only a brief episode of extinction was instituted. The relevance of this data to the use of one or the other dependent variable will be discussed in a subsequent section.

The Discriminandum

The discriminandum specifies what pharmacological treatment is to be discriminated from what alternative treatment(s). This constitutes a third source of independent variability in the DD experiment. Table 2 gives a survey of some of the many possible discriminanda that can be used in drug discrimination (see also Jarbe & Swedberg, 1982) and indicates the additional sources of independent variability that are inherent in each of these discriminanda. The drugs used constitute a further, obvious source of variability but are not listed as such in the table. The DD discriminandum typically involves at least two discriminative responses, but it may also involve three or perhaps even more responses; the discriminanda listed in Table 2 are grouped according to the number of responses involved. Not included in this table is the single response procedure described by Winter (1975). In this procedure an operant response is reinforced for one group of subjects in the presence of drug but extinguished in its absence; reverse conditions apply for a second group. Data obtained with this procedure are, however, confounded by drug effects on rate of responding, and the procedure has been abandoned for this reason.

The drug **vs.** saline discrimination constitutes the single most widely used discriminandum, and its properties have been documented best. Generalization results obtained with this discriminandum are relatively simple to interpret, and the data serve many pharmacological purposes. More than any other single method of behavioral pharmacology, the single drug-saline discrimination offers an exquisitely specific method to characterize the agonist and antagonist activity of a broad range of drugs (Colpaert, 1982a); it is likely that this exceptionally powerful resolving capacity has made the DD paradigm so widely

Table 2

Survey of Some of the Many Possible Discriminanda in Drug Discrimination

----

discriminandum	independent variable(s)

----

discriminanda involving two discriminative responses

drug $\underline{vs}$. saline — training dose

$dose_1$ $\underline{vs}$. $dose_2$ — ratio of $dose_1$ to $dose_2$
absolute magnitude of doses

$drug_A$ $\underline{vs}$. $drug_B$ — training dose of drugs A and B

$drug_A$ AND $drug_B$ $\underline{vs}$. saline — training dose of drugs A and B

$drug_A$ OR $drug_B$ $\underline{vs}$. saline — training dose of drugs A and B

discriminanda involving three discriminative responses

$drug_A$ $\underline{vs}$. $drug_B$ $\underline{vs}$. saline — training dose of drugs A and B

$dose_1$ $\underline{vs}$. $dose_2$ $\underline{vs}$. saline — ratio of $dose_1$ to $dose_2$
absolute magnitude of doses

$drug_A$ $\underline{vs}$. $drug_B$ $\underline{vs}$. $drug_C$ — training doses of drugs A, B, and C

$dose_1$ $\underline{vs}$. $dose_2$ $\underline{vs}$. $dose_3$ — ratio of $dose_1$ to $dose_2$ and $dose_3$
absolute magnitude of doses

----

used in recent years. The drug-saline discrimination is simple also because it has only one independent variable (i.e., training dose). Fragmentary evidence on the effect of training dose originally suggested that it merely sets the sensitivity of the discrimination. Parametric analyses, however, have revealed far more fundamental effects (Colpaert, 1982a). Such analyses have been conducted in detail only on fentanyl (Colpaert, Niemegeers, & Janssen, 1980a; Colpaert et al., 1980b) and cocaine (Colpaert, Niemegeers, & Janssen, 1978c), and parametric data on the effects of training dose with other training drugs remain to be generated.

The $dose_1$ $\underline{vs}$. $dose_2$ discrimination would seem to offer a method for the fine-grained analysis of the differences in discriminative effects of different doses of a given training drug. Two independent variations are inherent in this discriminandum; (i) the dose ratio (i.e., the ratio of the higher to the lower of the two training doses) and (ii) the absolute magnitude of these doses. A parametric analysis of the effects of dose ratio and of dose magnitude in $dose_1$-$dose_2$ discrimination has been carried out with fentanyl (Colpaert & Janssen, 1982a). The study revealed important effects of both factors on parameters of discrimination and generalization. A further study (Colpaert, 1982b) indicated the the $dose_1$-$dose_2$ discrimination may further improve the pharmacological specificity of the DD experiment relative to results obtained in the drug $\underline{vs}$. saline discrimination. The effect is very impressive and challenges the current, intuitive view (Jarbe & Rollenhagen,

1982) that the dose$_1$-dose$_2$ discriminandum represents a discrimination along a simple intensity continuum.

Only limited or no data are available with any of the other discriminanda. The drug$_A$ AND drug$_B$ vs. saline can perhaps demonstrate what can be referred to as residual discriminative effects of an agonist A in the presence of an antagonist B (e.g., Swedberg & Jarbe, 1982) where the combination elicits saline responding in drug vs. saline discrimination. The drug$_A$ OR drug$_B$ vs. saline discriminandum can perhaps be useful as a broadened screen for several types of discriminative effects (Colpaert & Janssen, 1982c). Drug$_A$ vs. drug$_B$ vs. saline may perhaps offer more resolving capacity than a single drug vs. saline discrimination does in otherwise similar conditions (White & Holtzman, 1981).

It will be apparent from this brief survey that the discriminandum presents an exceedingly large source of independent variation in the DD paradigm; discriminative effects of drugs can be examined in any of a great number of discriminanda, and generalization test data may vary accordingly. A potential danger with this large variability is that a given body of generalization data on any particular compound may become difficult to interpret. It has been this author's position, therefore, that it may be appropriate to examine the sources of independent variations in the simplest discriminanda (i.e., drug vs. saline; dose$_1$ vs. dose$_2$) through detailed parametric studies. The insights and concepts derived from such studies are likely to be a condition for comprehending the intricacies produced by the more complex discriminanda. In the meantime the existence of poorly understood generalization data from complex discriminanda may unduly compromise the face validity which DD research has rightfully acquired with the simple drug vs. saline discriminandum.

Subject Variables

A fourth source of independent variation are subject variables. DD research is typically conducted with what are referred to as normal animals, albeit that the subjects are invariably stressed by either deprivation of food or water, by shock, or by some other manipulation. Subjects whose conditions differ from normal may be able to discriminate otherwise nondiscriminable drugs or may show different generalization characteristics. Weissman (1976) has presented data that rats in pain, but not normal animals, may be able to discriminate aspirin. And opiate antagonists may become discriminable in opiate dependent subjects (Gellert & Holtzman, 1979). Subject condition thus has the potential of revealing drug effects that are not accessible otherwise and of establishing unique models of pathology.

Dependent Variables

What is being observed in DD are discrete behavioral responses (e.g., depressions of two or more levers) which occur in the course of an interval of time which is termed a training or test session. What is being inferred from this responding are variates which ascribe some spatial or temporal organization to this responding. The dependent variables of the DD experiment, like those of many other paradigms, must therefore be considered as derived variables; the value which the variable takes is not directly or inherently apparent from what is being observed. Instead, the dependent variables are constructed by the experimenter and are designed to accommodate some (often largely implicit, ill defined) a priori concept or theory. The concepts underlying DD research have differed and so have the dependent variables. Importantly, the difference concerns the dependent variable used to measure discrimination and generalization.

Measures of Discrimination and Generalization

The two most important variables in current use to measure discrimination and generalization are (i) the percentage of drug-appropriate responses and (ii) response selection. These variables will be discussed here as they apply to a drug vs. saline discrimination in the two-lever, food-reinforced FR-10 procedure. The percentage of drug-appropriate responses is most widely used, but an explicit justification of it is not available. Apparently, the use of this variable adheres to a tradition which can be traced to Skinnerian theory (Colpaert, 1983). Skinner (1938) argued that the acquisition of a discrimination represents two reflexes that draw apart in strength and that reflex strength is to be measured by means of response rate. The percentage of drug-appropriate responding occurring in a drug vs. saline discrimination has therefore been taken as a measure of the strength of the drug reflex relative to that of the saline reflex. The measure uses the percentage rather than the absolute number of drug-appropriate responses in an apparent attempt to accommodate possible drug effects on total response output. It is unclear, however, how well this maneuver achieves its goal; the effects of drugs on the rate of operant responding are rate-dependent (e.g., Dews, 1958), and it is conceivable that test drugs have effects on the rates of saline- and drug-appropriate responding which are not simply proportional to the often differing absolute rates.

Response selection, or lever selection as it applies here, has been proposed (Colpaert et al., 1976a) as a more appropriate measure on grounds that the dependent variable of the DD experiment is nominal in nature (for review, see Colpaert, 1983, 1984). Briefly, it is argued (i) that the only programmed variation in behavior which the DD paradigm relates with the pharmacological stimuli is DL as opposed to SL pressing (see above) and (ii) that, therefore, DL as opposed to SL pressing constitutes the only variation in behavior which can be taken to dependably reflect the discriminative effects of pharmacological treatments.

These concepts concerning the observable behavior in the DD experiment have thus given rise to the use of two different measures of discrimination and generalization. A paramount difference between the two measures concerns the level of measurement for scaling behavior: The percentage of drug-appropriate responses scales behavior along a quantitative scale, most often a ratio scale; the response-selection measure scales behavior according to a nominal or classificatory scale. Theory of measurement (Siegel, 1956; Stevens, 1946) specifies what theoretical differences exist between these scales. Some of the differences in data analysis and data interpretation emerging from this distinction will be discussed below.

Other Dependent Variables

In addition to measurements of discrimination and generalization, many DD procedures involve dependent variables that measure other characteristics of animal behavior. Total response output, or overall response rate, can be useful as an indication of possible drug effects on ongoing operant behavior. The training drug itself may have effects on this parameter, and its effects may change in the course of training or at some later point of the experiment. This parameter is often used in the choice of an appropriate dose or dose range of the training drug and of the test drugs. It may also assist in demonstrating the behavioral effectiveness of test drugs in cases where the test drug does not affect the main dependent variable (e.g., does not induce generalization). This parameter can further be used to monitor the subjects' general condition and may at times be instrumental in detecting apparatus failure.

Response latency is another rate measure; it differs from overall response rate by pertaining only to the initial segment of behavior rather than to all behavior occurring during the entire session. In procedures where the main dependent variable is nominal, response latency can be defined as the time which elapses before response choice or response selection occurs and can then perhaps be termed choice rate. Interestingly, it may appear that, relative to saline, a training drug condition decreasing overall rate nonetheless yields a smaller response latency (i.e., a higher choice rate; Colpaert, 1978b). These and other data (Colpaert et al., 1980b) suggest that response latency may perhaps in part reflect the time required for the decision process underlying a nominal response (e.g., Olton & Samuelson, 1974). In addition, however, response latency is also sensitive to what are referred to as nonspecific rate depressant drug effects.

The two-lever, FR-10 procedure and some similar procedures also define two further measures. FRF (first reinforcement responding) represents the total number of responses occurring on either lever prior to the time the animal totals 10 responses on either the appropriate lever (in training sessions) or the selected lever (in test sessions). With an FR-10 schedule median values are typically 10, but individual FRF measures may show variations (Colpaert, 1978b; Colpaert, Niemegeers, & Janssen, 1978b) which suggest that FRF, like choice latency, may at times reflect the varying degrees of certainty for choosing among nominal responses. However, variations of both response latency and FRF often are limited or erratic, and the two measures have as yet found little use in DD research.

Finally, the percentage of responses on the selected lever is a variate which may reflect response control by the reinforcer in test sessions if responding on the selected lever is being reinforced (see Figure 1). Some of the features of this parameter will be demonstrated (see below).

ANALYSIS OF DRUG DISCRIMINATION DATA

The methods used in the analysis of drug discrimination and drug generalization data vary considerably according to whether the main dependent variable is taken to be either quantitative or nominal. Where applicable, the two analytical approaches will be considered below in parallel.

Analysis of Discrimination

The purpose for analyzing a given drug discrimination can be one of at least two different types. One may wish to determine the degree a given discriminandum controls the discriminative responding in one or different sets of experimental conditions, and methods are available to measure response control. Given a particular set of experimental conditions, one may also wish to analyze the discriminability of one or several training drugs, and additional methods are available to measure drug discriminability.

Measurement of Response Control

DD training is typically[2] continued until the animal reaches an arbitrarily chosen criterion of performance in S and D sessions. The conventional method of measuring response control consists of determining the number of sessions required to reach this criterion (sessions-to-criterion: STC; e.g., Overton, 1982). This method may have some practical utility, but it acts to conceal a number of interesting variations in response control. The control of discriminative responding which drugs may exert in the DD paradigm is a somewhat complex, dynamic process which can be divided into two phases-- an acquisition phase and an asymptotic phase.

As indicated above, acquisition can be characterized by the number of (S and D) sessions required to reach some arbitrarily set criterion. When the main dependent variable is taken to be quantitative, the criterion can be the percentage of treatment-appropriate responding (e.g., 70, 80, 90%) or some other value a in 2 or N consecutive S and D sessions. This measurement can be written: $STC_{a; N; S,D}$. Note that DD studies have differed in terms of the values of a and N that were implemented. When a nominal variable is used, the STC can be determined for a criterion requiring that the response was correct (i.e., appropriate to treatment) in n out of N consecutive S and D sessions ($STC_{n/N; S,D}$). Note that measurements of acquisition using this formula may differ according to the length of the criterion run n/N (Colpaert et al., 1980b). STC has also been analyzed for S and D sessions separately (Colpaert, 1978b); such an analysis may be of interest since it may appear that the STC to respond S in S sessions ($STC_{n/N; S}$) is dissimilar to the STC to respond D in D sessions ($STC_{n/N; D}$). Cocaine HCl at 10 mg/kg, for example, is peculiar among many other training drug conditions because rats acquire the D response in cocaine sessions much faster that the S response in saline sessions (Colpaert, 1978b); the asymmetry may vary with training dose and, again, with n/N (Colpaert, 1978b).

Measures of asymptotic performance offer an alternative to measures of acquisition in characterizing response control (Colpaert et al., 1980b). Unlike measures of acquisition, measures of asymptotic performance are independent from the unavoidably arbitrary criterion that must be chosen to define acquisition. This may be important, since speed of acquisition as measured by STC may not strictly covary with asymptotic accuracy; for example, STC is longer with 0.04 mg/kg fentanyl (vs. saline) than with 10 mg/kg of cocaine (vs. saline), but asymptotic accuracy seems to be higher with fentanyl than with cocaine (Colpaert, 1978b). However, it may take a large number of sessions before asymptotic performance is reached (e.g., Colpaert et al., 1980b), and a sizable number of sessions at asymptote is required for measures to be accurate and reliable. The principal measure of asymptotic performance is the percentage of sessions in which the response was treatment appropriate (with the nominal variable) or some measure of central tendency of the percentage of treatment-appropriate responding over sessions (with the quantitative variable). If applied to nominal data, this measure (% $AP_{S,D}$) of asymptotic performance is similar to the measure d' of discriminability in signal detection theory (SDT; Colpaert, 1978b). Further refinement can be achieved by deriving the percentage of errors from saline (% AE_S) and drug sessions (% AE_D) separately. If applied to nominal data, the % AE_D to % AE_S ratio offers a measure of symmetry in performance which is similar to the

----

[2]An alternative possibility to equate acquisition consists of administering a fixed number of training sessions to all subjects (Colpaert & Janssen, 1982a).

measure of response bias in SDT (Colpaert, 1978b). The determination of symmetry in asymptotic performance may be important because generalization data may covary with changes in response bias (Colpaert & Janssen, 1981).

SDT requires[3] the response to be nominal in nature (Green & Swets, 1974), and the DD response may fulfill this requirement (Colpaert, 1978b). This raises the question whether the attractive analytical framework developed for SDT can be applied to DD data. Apart from some practical considerations such as number of observations, a consideration arguing against the application of SDT analyses to DD data is that the threshold dose for generalization varies (Colpaert et al., 1978c; Colpaert, Niemegeers, & Janssen, 1978d). This has led to the argument that the criterion underlying the decision is not stable (Colpaert, Maroli, & Meert, 1982). It is a fundamental assumption of SDT that the criterion be stable (Green & Swets, 1974) and a classical SDT analysis strictly requires that this assumption be satisfied for the analysis to be permissible (Pastore & Scheier, 1974; Treisman, 1976). The discrimination data thus may not be amenable to SDT analysis (Colpaert et al., 1982). It is of interest to note here that the SDT assessment of pain has recently been criticized (Coppola & Gracely, 1983) on similar grounds.

The statistical analysis of the measures of response control discussed above is fairly straightforward. The statistical analysis differs, however, depending on the use of a nominal or quantitative variable, and appropriate nonparametric tests are available (Siegel, 1956) for the comparison of both related and independent samples. Adequate data on the distribution characteristics of the quantitative variable are not available, and it is prudent to use nonparametric statistics as opposed to statistics that make any important assumption about the distribution of the dependent variable.

Measurement of Drug Discriminability

To measure drug discriminability requires (i) that some criterion of response control be defined and (ii) that it be determined to what extent the criterion level of response control is reached at several doses covering the training drug's full dynamic range.

The above has made it apparent that a multitude of criteria of response control can be defined, and the outcome of an analysis of drug discriminability probably varies depending on the criterion implemented. An example of a criterion is that responding be appropriate on 10 out of 10 consecutive sessions and that it be reached within a cut-off number of 100 D and S sessions.

Two general methods are then available to explore the training drug's dynamic range. One consists of using different groups of animals at different training doses and of determining the percentage of animals reaching the criterion of response control (e.g., Overton, 1982). It typically appears that this percentage increases orderly as a function of training dose, and the statistical methods of Litchfield & Wilcoxon (1949) or Finney (1971) are often used to derive ED_{50} values, confidence limits, and slope; these methods can be used further to compare drugs in terms of potency and of slope. A second method consists of initially training a single set of subjects on a relatively high training dose and of determining the percentage of animals reaching

---

[3]This requirement is not being considered in Hayes' (1978) comments on the SDT analysis of DD data.

criterion. The same animals are then retrained on a progressively lowered training dose until a dose is found where none of the animals reach criterion (Colpaert et al., 1980a). The percentage of animals reaching criterion can be used to obtain ED_{50} values, confidence limits, and slope. Fentanyl is the only drug whose discriminability has been examined with both methods, and the two studies (Colpaert et al., 1980a, 1980b) yielded similar ED_{50} values. The method of lowering training dose progressively has the unique feature of establishing the lowest discriminable dose (LDD) in individual animals; it also has revealed characteristics of drug discrimination and generalization which are not accessible by any other method (Colpaert et al., 1980a).

Drug discriminability is often viewed, albeit implicitly, as an immutable drug property (e.g., Overton, 1982), and some caution may be appropriate regarding this view. There is evidence that drug discriminability may vary with the subjects' condition (Weissman, 1976), and it may also depend on other independent variables, including procedural variables (Richards, 1978).

Analysis of Generalization

It is with the analysis and subsequent interpretation of generalization data that the difference in using a quantitative or nominal dependent variable is perhaps most critical; the two variables are for that reason discussed separately here.

Using a Quantitative Measure

The analysis of the percentage of drug-appropriate responding in test sessions is essentially an analysis of group data. In any given test the percentage typically varies anywhere between 0 and 100% among subjects, and some measure of central tendency is taken to represent the group data. The mean (±1 SEM) is used most commonly for this purpose but may be misleading. This is because the distribution of the quantitative variate often is not Gaussian, nor even symmetrical (Colpaert, 1977b; Stolerman & D'Mello, 1981); its typical shape is in fact bimodal, with one peak occurring around 10% (a value similar to what appears in saline sessions) and with a second peak occurring around 90% (a value similar to what is obtained in training drug sessions). Alternative measures of central tendency of the quantitative variate are the median (and 95% confidence limits) and modal values.

The next step in the analysis of quantitative generalization data consists of implementing a (preferably nonparametric) statistical test such as the Wilcoxon test (Siegel, 1956) for related samples to compare the test data with control data; the latter are obtained in saline and training sessions administered prior to or after the test session but in close temporal proximity to it. The test data are thus analyzed by means of two comparisons; the four most common outcomes[4] of the analysis are given in Table 3.

Test data which are similar to saline control and significantly lower than training drug control are simply taken to conclude that generalization did not occur (see Table 3, outcome 1). Test data which are similar to training drug control and higher than saline control are taken to conclude that

----
[4]Cases where the test result is either significantly lower than saline control or significantly higher than training drug control are unusual and will not be considered here.

Table 3

Possible Outcomes of Statistical Comparisons
Between Test and Control Data Using the Quantitative Variable

	vs. saline	vs. training drug	generalization
test data	=	<	no
test data	=	=	?
test data	>	<	?
test data	>	=	yes

generalization did occur (see Table 3, outcome 4). Outcome 2 likely indicates that the number of observations and/or the magnitude of response control were inadequate for any statistical analysis of the data to be conclusive. Outcome 3 may be obtained when the central tendency of drug-appropriate responding is around 50%. Interpretations of this outcome have been that it represents random responding, that it may be due to behavioral drug toxicity, or that it represents some lesser form of stimulus generalization (e.g., Koek & Slangen, 1982). None of these interpretations are entirely satisfactory (Colpaert, 1984), and several authors note that any interpretation of this outcome is troublesome (Holtzman, 1982a; Winter, 1978).

It may be useful to note here that, in addition to the percentage of drug-appropriate responses, some other quantitative measures of discrimination and generalization have also been proposed. One example is the progressive ratio procedure which assesses the breaking point of a ratio schedule (Winter, 1981). Another procedure is termed extended schedule transfer and assesses response perseverance (Schechter, 1981).

Using a Nominal Measure

A test of stimulus generalization using the nominal variable determines whether a given animal selected the training drug-appropriate response following administration of the test treatment; the analysis of generalization with this variable therefore is essentially an analysis of individual data. Generalization testing is, of course, conducted in a number of animals, and the results can be reported concisely by the percentage[5] of animals selecting the drug lever (Colpaert et al., 1975a).

The statistical analysis of nominal generalization data is extremely simple. The analysis often is so straightforward that it is not even reported. Depending on the criterion used for training the animal at the time of acquisition, the actual total (S and D sessions combined) error rate can often be reduced to about 10% to 5%, or even less; as a result, response selection data can be accepted within the 0.10, 0.05, or < 0.05 level of statistical significance. For most practical purposes, therefore, a DL response occurring

---

[5]Note that this procedure turns the nominal variable into a quantitative variate; it serves to simplify data presentation but should not lead to inappropriate interpretation.

in a test session is said to indicate, quite simply, that generalization
occurred in that particular animal; the occurrence of a SL response indicates
that the animal did not generalize the test treatment.

In cases where error rates in S and D sessions differ (Colpaert, 1978b),
it may be useful to refine the analysis. For example, rats discriminating 10
mg/kg of cocaine from saline may show an error rate of 3.7% in saline sessions
and of only 0.6% in training drug sessions (Colpaert et al., 1978c). Thus, in
this study, the conclusion that SL responding in a test session indicates no
generalization could be drawn with 6.2 times more confidence than the
conclusion that DL selection indicates generalization. This refinement is
often felt to be redundant, however, especially when neither the S nor the D
error rate exceeds the universally accepted 5% level. Thus the outcome of a
generalization test using the nominal variable is simply that generalization
occurred in from 0 to 100% of the animals and that no generalization occurred
in the other subjects (see Table 4).

Table 4

Possible Outcomes of Generalization Tests Using the Nominal Variable

---

% of animals responding D	generalization
0%	yes in 0%; no in 100%
10%	yes in 0%; no in 90%
50%	yes in 50%; no in 50%
90%	yes in 90%; no in 10%
100%	yes in 100%; no in 0%

It is clear, then, that although the actual data may be very similar in
appearance the conclusion reached from a generalization test differs markedly
depending on the use of either a quantitative or nominal variable. The
quantitative approach leads to the nominal conclusion that the test treatment
did or did not produce generalization and finds no satisfactory interpretation
for outcomes 2 and 3 in Table 3 [6]. The nominal approach leads to the

---

[6] The problem can, of course, be overcome by manipulations that convert the
quantitative variable into a nominal decision process. For example, 99% drug-
appropriate responding is unlikely ($p < 0.05$) to occur in saline control
sessions, and a 99% test result can therefore be taken to indicate that
generalization did occur in an individual animal. The 50% group result can
thus be re-analyzed to reveal that generalization did occur in some animals
but not in others. But clarity and simplicity then recommend that the
dependent variable be measured nominally in the first place.

conclusion that generalization occurred in a specified percentage or quantity of animals, and that it did not occur in the remaining, complementary quantity of subjects. It will become apparent below that this difference in conclusions presents little problem with unanimous (0 or 100%) data but does become extremely important with all intermediary levels of responding.

Generalization Gradients

When different doses are tested of a treatment that produces stimulus generalization, then the effects of the test drug can be of two general types. The type being considered in this section is that the generalization proceeds orderly from 0 to 100% as a function of test dose (percentage generalization refers to the mean percentage of drug-appropriate responding in the quantitative approach and to percentage of animals selecting the D response in the nominal approach). The percentage-generalization data points are often plotted graphically in log-linear coordinates. The generalization gradient or dose-response curve can then be obtained either by connecting the data points or by fitting them by the function of best fit. The function of best fit may be curvilinear, but it appears that a rectilinear function is often adequate in log-linear coordinates. An important advantage of a rectilinear function is that it allows the description of the data by two simple numericals (i.e., ED_{50} and slope b; the ED_{50} and slope are obtained from the regression equation $y = a + bx$; Colpaert, 1982a).

The methods of Finney (1971) and of Litchfield and Wilcoxon (1946) are usually used in the statistical evaluation of ED_{50} and slope. The use of these methods is not entirely appropriate, however, since both analyses require that the data samples taken at different doses be independent. The problem can, of course, be avoided by obtaining independent samples, but the solution is often impractical since it requires much larger numbers of trained animals. Truly appropriate statistical methods for evaluating ED_{50} doses and slope for related data samples do not seem to be available. The somewhat inappropriate use of these methods, however, is not likely to yield exceedingly misleading results since there is little reason to assume that related generalization data would differ greatly from independent data. It is hoped that alternative statistical methods will be developed to rectify this problem.

The application of the Finney (1971) and Litchfield & Wilcoxon (1946) analyses to quantitative generalization data presents an additional, more important problem. Both analyses have been developed for nominal data, and the analyses' definitions of such terms as ED_{50} values, confidence limits of the ED_{50}, and slope do not apply when data are quantitative.

Partial Generalization

Partial generalization can be said to occur (Colpaert & Janssen, 1984) when test treatments produce levels of discriminative responding which are intermediate between those produced by the treatments which the animals are trained to discriminate. Partial generalization can occur either along a dose-response curve progressing orderly from the 0 to the 100% level of effect, or it may represent the ceiling level of a drug's effect.

A previous section has made it apparent that the analysis of partial generalization is simple with the use of a nominal variate. The use of the nominal variate has revealed (Colpaert, 1984) that (a) the lowest generalized dose (LGD) may differ among rats, (b) the slope of the gradient reflects between-subject variation in terms of LGD, and (c) the occurrence of partial generalization along a curve proceeding from 0 to 100% indicates that the test dose is higher than or equal to LGD in some subjects and lower than LGD in the other subjects (case 1 in Table 5). Where partial generalization represents the ceiling level of a drug's effect, the use of the nominal variate reveals that this can result from one of two sources (Colpaert, 1984; Colpaert, Niemegeers, & Janssen, 1979). First, generalization may occur in only some but not all animals, and generalization can then be specified as partial in terms of subjects (case 2 in Table 5). Secondly, it may occur that all animals generalize the test treatment, but the generalization does not persist at higher doses. In this case the ceiling level of drug effect fails to reach 100% because the doses showing generalization do not coincide among all subjects; this generalization is considered as partial in terms of doses (case 3 in Table 5).

It is difficult, and for many practical purposes impossible, to identify and characterize partial generalization with the quantitative variable. This is because the quantitative variable is responsive both to the discriminative stimulus and to the primary reinforcer (e.g., Figure 1) so that variations in the percentage of drug-appropriate responding cannot simply and directly be attributed to discriminative control alone. The previous section delineates some of the difficulties in data analysis and subsequent interpretation. The examples given below will reveal that converting the quantitative variable into a nominal variate to overcome the problem may be neither adequate nor permissible. It would thus seem that the quantitative variable cannot serve to

Table 5

Schematic Description of Three Instances of Partial Generalization

animal	case 1					case 2					case 3				
	dose					dose					dose				
#	1	2	3	4	5	1	2	3	4	5	1	2	3	4	5
1	−	−	−	+	+	−	−	−	−	−	−	−	−	−	+
2	−	−	−	+	+	−	−	−	−	−	−	−	−	+	−
3	−	−	+	+	+	−	−	+	+	+	−	−	+	+	−
4	−	−	+	+	+	−	−	+	+	+	−	−	+	+	+
5	−	+	+	+	+	−	+	+	+	+	−	+	+	+	+
% generalization	0	20	60	100	100	0	20	60	60	60	0	20	60	80	60

Note: Doses (of test drugs) are represented by the horizontal numerals 1 to 5, where 5 is the highest dose that is being tested. Dose 3 produces partial generalization in all cases 1, 2, and 3, but the apparent mechanism of partial generalization is different in the three cases. Circles indicate the lowest generalized dose in each of three individual animals. The − and + signs indicate S and D response selection, respectively, in animals discriminating a given training drug from saline.

analyze partial generalization because it is co-determined by variables other than the discriminative effects of the treatment being tested.

Other Variables

Overall response rate, response latency, first reinforcement responses, and the percentage of responding on the treatment-appropriate (training sessions) or selected lever (test sessions) are analyzed by conventional methods of statistical analysis. The distributions of these variables may be of a number of different types, and it is prudent to use nonparametric statistics throughout. Latency and first reinforcement responding data have at times been analyzed for subjects individually (Colpaert, 1978b), but it is common practice to only consider group data.

Examples

The foregoing discussions have made it apparent that two dependent variables are currently being used in DD research. The two variables differ greatly in terms of their conceptual origin and in terms of the formal analyses and statistical treatment which they can be given. It has been argued, however, that quantitative and nominal outcomes of generalization tests correlate (Koek & Slangen, 1982; Stolerman & D'Mello, 1981) and that this correlation is reason to suggest that the quantitative and the nominal variable constitute equally adequate measures of discrimination and generalization. The examples given below show that the two variables effectively correlate in some but not in other cases and demonstrate some of the mechanisms for the occurrence of similarities and dissimilarities.

The Fentanyl Gradient

Figure 2 summarizes generalization test data with 0.0025 to 0.04 mg/kg fentanyl obtained (Colpaert et al., 1975a) from 12 rats trained to discriminate 0.04 mg/kg of fentanyl from saline in the two-lever, FR-10, food-reinforced DD procedure. In test sessions responses on the selected lever were reinforced, and the data are expressed both nominally (percentage of animals selecting the DL) and quantitatively (percentage of responses on the DL; mean ±1 SEM). It appears that in this set of data the two variables correlate almost perfectly (see Figure 2). The mechanism of covariation is evident: Whatever the lever that individual animals selected, all or almost all subsequent responding occurred on the selected lever (for detailed individual data, see Table 5 in Colpaert et al., 1975a). Apparently, the pharmacological stimulus controlled lever selection, while the reinforcement of subsequent responding on the selected lever controlled much of the behavior occurring later in the session (see also Figure 1).

Haloperidol and Fentanyl

The following (unpublished) experiment was conducted in seven rats trained to discriminate 0.04 mg/kg of fentanyl from saline, and it is an extension of an earlier study (Colpaert et al., 1977). Before test sessions, the animals were trained with 0.04 mg/kg of fentanyl (subcutaneously, 30 minutes prior to testing) and pretreated (subcutaneously, 60 minutes prior to testing) with a haloperidol dose ranging from 0.0025 to 0.63 mg/kg. All rats pretreated with any dose of haloperidol selected the DL following the injection of fentanyl. The percentage of drug-appropriate responding, however, decreased to reach a

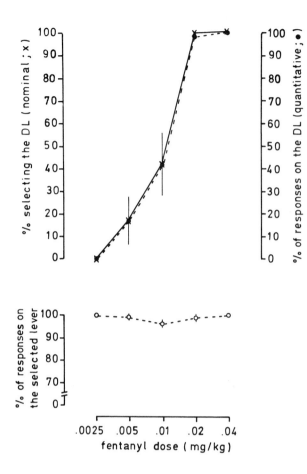

Figure 2: Fentanyl generalization gradient in rats trained to discriminate 0.04 mg/kg of fentanyl from saline. Two dependent variables are presented in the upper graph--the nominal (left ordinate) and the quantitative variable (right ordinate). The lower graph presents the percentage of responding on the lever (i.e., SL or DL) which the animals selected.

level of about 50% at the 0.63 mg/kg dose (see Figure 3). In these data, therefore, there is no correlation between the nominal and the quantitative variable. The lower part of Figure 3 further indicates that the percentage of responses on the selected lever was decreased by haloperidol; this decrease covaried perfectly with the decrease of the quantitative variable and is responsible for it.

The source of this discrepancy is that the quantitative, but not the nominal, variable is responsive to the effects of the primary reinforcer (see Figure 1). In the data in Figure 2, the effects of the primary reinforcer happened to be isodirectional with those of the pharmacological stimulus so that the quantitative variable covaried with the nominal variable. The treatment tested in Figure 3 interfered with the effects of the primary reinforcer and thus caused the quantitative variable to diverge from the nominal variable. These and similar data (Colpaert et al., 1978b) demonstrate the particularly powerful effects that haloperidol and other antipsychotic agents may exert on control of responding by a primary reinforcer.

Figure 3: Effects of haloperidol in rats trained to discriminate 0.04 mg/kg of fentanyl from saline. The symbols S and F are adjacent to data points representing performance on saline and 0.04 mg/kg fentanyl control sessions, respectively. See also legend to Figure 2.

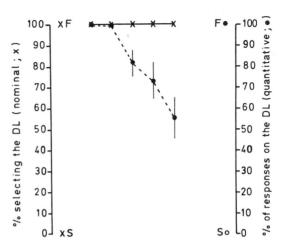

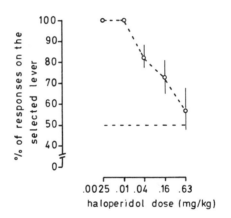

Haloperidol and Cocaine

The data presented in Figure 3 highlight the difficulties which occur with interpreting intermediate quantitative results. The problem originates from the susceptibility of the quantitative variable to the effects of the primary reinforcer. In addition, it is not readily possible to control for the effects of test treatments on the primary reinforcer; in one study (Colpaert et al., 1977) 0.08 mg/kg of haloperidol and 0.04 mg/kg of fentanyl had only limited effects on the percentage of responding on the selected lever, but the percentage dropped very markedly (i.e., to 50%) when the two treatments were combined. To administer haloperidol and fentanyl alone thus would not have served as an appropriate control for the effects of the haloperidol-fentanyl combination on primary reinforcement. The haloperidol-fentanyl combination also reduced overall response rate to about 10% of saline control values (Colpaert et al., 1977). In our experience there is no simple correlation between drug effects on rate and on the percentage of responses on the selected lever. But it often appears that treatments which severely reduce overall response rate also block the effects of the primary reinforcer on responding in at least some animals. The vulnerability of the quantitative variable to such effects renders its use in such conditions particularly adventurous. The nominal variable, of course, is also reinforced; the requirement for the nominal response to occur is that it be reinforced by secondary reinforcement. At sufficiently large doses almost any pharmacological treatment reduces responding altogether and thus blocks the effects of secondary reinforcement; at this point it is no longer possible to measure discrimination and generalization[7].

The interference of the effects of reinforcement with quantitative generalization data has generally been a problem and has been particularly confusing in studies on the effects of neuroleptic agents on discriminative effects of cocaine and other stimulants. Specifically, some authors (Ho & Silverman, 1978) conclude that haloperidol blocks cocaine discrimination, whereas others (Cunningham & Appel, 1982) find any possible haloperidol effect on cocaine discrimination to be of little pharmacological relevance. The confusion is apparent from a set of data (Colpaert et al., 1978b) presented in Figure 4. Haloperidol reduced the value taken by the quantitative variable

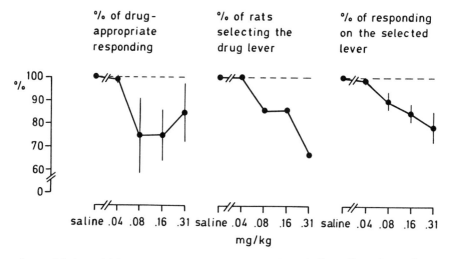

dose of haloperidol pretreatment before injection of 10 mg/kg of cocaine

Figure 4: Effects of pretreatment (60 minutes prior to test) with saline or 0.04 to 0.31 mg/kg of haloperidol on responding in the DD task after injection with 10 mg/kg of cocaine (30 minutes prior to test). The data were obtained from seven rats trained to discriminate 10 mg/kg of cocaine from saline (Colpaert, Niemegeers, & Janssen, 1978).

----

[7] Rate depressant effects thus set a limitation to the DD analysis of drug action. The limitation can be overcome in part, but not entirely, by using schedules of reinforcement that are relatively resistant to rate depressant drug effects.

(see Figure 4) much like it did in the haloperidol-fentanyl experiment (see Figure 3). This time, however, haloperidol also made some animals select the saline lever, indicating that cocaine antagonism occurred. Unlike what appeared in Figure 2, however, the decrease in the quantitative variable in Figure 4 cannot simply be <u>attributed</u> to pharmacological antagonism, because haloperidol also reduced the percentage of responding on the selected lever. The data in Figure 4 thus demonstrate just how confusing and misleading the use of the quantitative variable can be. They also demonstrate, however, the validity of the nominal variable in what are admitted to be difficult experimental conditions. Specifically, that haloperidol does in effect antagonize cocaine could be confirmed in an additional (unpublished) study. Nine rats were trained to discriminate 10 mg/kg of cocaine from saline, and the cocaine gradient (doses 0.63 to 10 mg/kg; administered 30 minutes prior to testing) was determined following pretreatment (60 minutes prior to testing) with saline and 0.04 or 0.16 mg/kg of haloperidol. It appeared that haloperidol made the cocaine dose-response curve shift to the right (see Figure 5). The magnitude of this shift was proportional to haloperidol dose and leaves no doubt that the neuroleptic antagonizes the discriminative effects of cocaine.

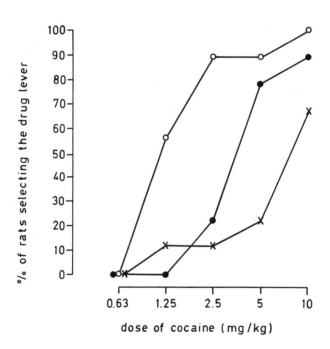

Figure 5: Dose-response curve of cocaine following pretreatment with either saline (O) or 0.04 (●) and 0.16 mg/kg (X) of haloperidol. Data were obtained from nine rats that were trained to discriminate 10 mg/kg of cocaine from saline. See text for details.

DRUG ABUSE POTENTIAL

As indicated in the introduction, many classes of drugs of abuse produce pharmacologically specific discriminative effects in laboratory animals. The preclinical evaluation of drug abuse potential with the DD method essentially consists of determining whether the novel drug produces discriminative effects similar to those of any one or several of the known classes of drugs of abuse. The use of drug discrimination in the preclinical evaluation of drug abuse potential is suggested to proceed along the following phases.

The first phase is determining whether the new drug which is to be evaluated produces stimulus generalization with a training drug (i) that has some significant pharmacological property in common with the new drug and (ii) that belongs to one of the classes of drugs of abuse. For example, a new drug exerting naloxone-reversible inhibition of gastrointestinal motility will be tested for generalization in rats trained to discriminate morphine or another opiate agonist from saline (Colpaert et al., 1975b). The observation that the new drug generalizes with morphine is taken to predict that it may produce opiate-like subjective effects in humans. The alternative outcome is taken to predict that the new drug will not produce such subjective effects but does not guarantee that it is devoid of stimulus properties similar to that of drugs of abuse other than opiates. The latter can be determined in phase two, where the drug is tested for generalization in different sets of rats trained, for example, on cocaine, chlordiazepoxide, Δ^9-THC, LSD, nicotine, and phencyclidine. Phase two testing may require a sizable effort and is required only when there are reasonable grounds to suggest that the new drug shares pertinent pharmacological or structural properties with any of these substances of abuse. In both phase one and phase two, negative outcomes have great face validity, especially if training doses and other conditions have been chosen to yield inclusive generalizations (see Colpaert, 1982a). The significance of positive outcomes can be examined more closely; a new drug producing generalization with a 0.005 mg/kg training dose of fentanyl may produce subjective effects resembling those of cyclazocine (Colpaert et al., 1980b). But the drug is unlikely to produce the more threatening subjective effects of prominent opiates of abuse such as heroin if it fails to generalize with a 0.04-mg/kg training dose of fentanyl (Colpaert, 1984; Colpaert & Janssen, 1984; see also Holtzman, 1982a, 1982b). Much work is currently being undertaken to further develop the drug discrimination methodology such that stimulus properties of drugs can be characterized with extreme refinement in both quantitative and qualitative terms. A third step can be considered if the new drug yields negative outcomes in phases one and two. The third phase is determining whether animals can be trained to discriminate the drug from saline. In as much as it cannot be ascribed to drug impairment of learning at relevant doses, a negative outcome here is strongly suggestive of the drug producing no significant subjective effects. Generalization tests with prototypical agents of all important classes of drugs of abuse are pertinent if training does succeed. Positive outcomes of these tests have a relevance that is similar, but perhaps not identical, to those that may occur in phases one and two. An entirely negative outcome of these tests is essentially inconclusive; it merely indicates the drug to possess discriminative effects that are unlike those of known substances of abuse. Whether these unprecedented stimulus effects are likely to generate an unprecedented drug abuse remains for clinical data to decide.

ACKNOWLEDGMENTS

The preparation of this paper was supported in part by a grant from the I.W.O.N.L.

REFERENCES

Appel, J. B., White, F. J., & Holohean, A. M. (1982). Analyzing mechanism(s) of hallucinogenic drug action with drug discrimination procedures. Neuroscience & Biobehavioral Reviews, 6, 529-536.

Barry, H., III, & Krimmer, E. C. (1977). Discriminable stimuli produced by alcohol and other CNS depressants. In H. Lal (Ed.), Discriminative stimulus properties of drugs (pp. 73-92). New York: Plenum Press.

Colpaert, F. C. (1977a). Narcotic cue and narcotic state. Life Sciences, 20, 1097-1108.

Colpaert, F. C. (1977b). Drug-produced cues and states: Some theoretical and methodological inferences. In H. Lal (Ed.), Discriminative stimulus properties of drugs (pp.5-21). New York: Plenum Press.

Colpaert, F. C. (1978a). Discriminative stimulus properties of narcotic analgesic drugs. Pharmacology Biochemistry & Behavior, 9, 863-887.

Colpaert, F. C. (1978b). Some properties of drugs as physiological signals: The FR procedure and signal detection theory. In F. C. Colpaert & J. L. Slangen (Eds.), Stimulus properties of drugs: Ten years of progress (pp. 217-242). Amsterdam: Elsevier/North Holland Biomedical Press.

Colpaert, F. C. (1982a). The pharmacological specificity of opiate drug discrimination. In F. C. Colpaert & J. L. Slangen (Eds.), Drug discrimination: Applications in CNS pharmacology (pp. 3-16). Amsterdam: Elsevier/North Holland Biomedical Press.

Colpaert, F. C. (1982b). Increased naloxone reversibility in fentanyl dose-dose discrimination. European Journal of Pharmacology, 84, 229-231.

Colpaert, F. C. (1983). Drug discrimination and the behavioral analysis of drug action. In C. F. Lowe, M. Richelle, D. E. Blackman, & C. M. Bradshaw (Eds.), Behaviour analysis and contemporary psychology. Hillsdale, NJ: Lawrence Erlbaum & Associates.

Colpaert, F. C. (1984). Drug discrimination: Behavioral, pharmacological, and molecular mechanisms of discriminative drug effects. In S. R. Goldberg & I. P. Stolerman (Eds.), Behavioral analysis of drug dependence. New York: Academic Press.

Colpaert, F. C., & Janssen, P. A. J. (1981). Factors regulating drug cue sensitivity: The effect of frustrative non-reward in fentanyl-saline discrimination. Archives Internationales de Pharmacodynamie et de Therapie, 254, 241-251.

Colpaert, F. C., & Janssen, P. A. J. (1982a). Factors regulating drug cue sensitivity: The effects of dose ratio and absolute dose level in the case of fentanyl dose-dose discrimination. Archives Internationales de Pharmacodynamie et de Therapie, 258, 283-299.

Colpaert, F. C., & Janssen, P. A. J. (1982b). Factors regulating drug cue sensitivity: Limits of discriminability and the role of a progressively decreasing training dose in cocaine-saline discrimination. Neuropharmacology, 21, 1187-1194.

Colpaert, F. C., & Janssen, P. A. J. (1982c). OR discrimination: A new drug discrimination method. European Journal of Pharmacology, 78, 141-144.

Colpaert, F. C., & Janssen, P. A. J. (1984). Agonist and antagonist effects of prototype opiate drugs in rats discriminating fentanyl from saline: Characteristics of partial generalization. Journal of Pharmacology and Experimental Therapeutics, 230, 193-199.

Colpaert, F. C., Lal, H., Niemegeers, C. J. E., & Janssen, P. A. J. (1975a). Investigations on drug produced and subjectively experienced discriminative stimuli. 1. The fentanyl cue, a tool to investigate subjectively experienced narcotic drug actions. Life Sciences, 16, 705-716.

Colpaert, F. C., Maroli, A. N., & Meert, T. (1982). Parametric effects in the discrimination of intracranial stimulation: Some methodological and analytical issues. Physiology & Behavior, 28, 1047-1058.

Colpaert, F. C., & Rosecrans, J. A. (Eds.). (1978). Stimulus properties of drugs: Ten years of progress. Amsterdam: Elsevier/North Holland Biomedical Press.

Colpaert, F. C., & Slangen, J. L. (Eds.). (1982). Drug discrimination: Applications in CNS pharmacology. Amsterdam: Elsevier/North Holland Biomedical Press.

Colpaert, F. C., Niemegeers, C. J. E., & Janssen, P. A. J. (1976a). Theoretical and methodological considerations on drug discrimination learning. Psychopharmacologia, 46, 169-177.

Colpaert, F. C., Niemegeers, C. J. E., & Janssen, P. A. J. (1976b). Discriminative stimulus properties of fentanyl and morphine: Tolerance and dependence. Pharmacology Biochemistry & Behavior, 5, 401-408.

Colpaert, F. C., Niemegeers, C. J. E., & Janssen, P. A. J. (1977). Differential haloperidol effect on two indices of fentanyl-saline discrimination. Psychopharmacology, 53, 169-173.

Colpaert, F. C., Niemegeers, C. J. E., & Janssen, P. A. J. (1978a). Drug-cue conditioning to external stimulus conditions. European Journal of Pharmacology, 49, 185-188.

Colpaert, F. C., Niemegeers, C. J. E., & Janssen, P. A. J. (1978b). Neuroleptic interference with the cocaine cue: Internal stimulus control of behavior and psychosis. Psychopharmacology, 58, 247-255.

Colpaert, F. C., Niemegeers, C. J. E., & Janssen, P. A. J. (1978c). Factors regulating drug cue sensitivity. A long term study on the cocaine cue. In F. C. Colpaert & J. A. Rosecrans (Eds.), Stimulus properties of drugs: Ten years of progress (pp. 281-299). Amsterdam: Elsevier/North Holland Biomedical Press.

Colpaert, F. C., Niemegeers, C. J. E., & Janssen, P. A. J. (1978d). Changes of sensitivity to the cueing properties of narcotic drugs as evidenced by generalization and cross-generalization experiments. Psychopharmacology, 58, 257-262.

Colpaert, F. C., Niemegeers, C. J. E., & Janssen, P. A. J. (1979). Discriminative stimulus properties of cocaine: Neuropharmacological characteristics as derived from stimulus generalization experiments. Pharmacology Biochemistry & Behavior, 10, 535-546.

Colpaert, F. C., Niemegeers, C. J. E., & Janssen, P. A. J. (1980a). Factors regulating drug cue sensitivity: Limits of discriminability and the role of a progressively decreasing training dose in fentanyl-saline discrimination. Journal of Pharmacology and Experimental Therapeutics, 212, 474-480.

Colpaert, F. C., Niemegeers, C. J. E., & Janssen, P. A. J. (1980b). Factors regulating drug cue sensitivity: The effect of training dose in fentanyl-saline discrimination. Neuropharmacology, 19, 705-713.

Colpaert, F. C., Niemegeers, C. J. E., Lal, H., & Janssen, P. A. J. (1975b). Investigations on drug produced and subjectively experienced discriminative stimuli. 2. Loperamide, an antidiarrheal devoid of narcotic cue producing actions. Life Sciences, **16**, 717-728.

Coppola, R., & Gracely, R. H. (1983). Where is the noise in SDT pain assessment? Pain, **17**, 257-266.

Cunningham, K. A., & Appel, J. B. (1982). Discriminative stimulus properties of cocaine and phencyclidine: Similarities in the mechanism of action. In F. C. Colpaert & J. L. Slangen (Eds.), Drug discrimination: Applications in CNS pharmacology (pp. 181-192). Amsterdam: Elsevier/North Holland Biomedical Press.

Dews, P. B. (1958). Stimulant actions of methamphetamine. Journal of Pharmacology and Experimental Therapeutics, **122**, 137-147.

Eckenhoff, J. E., & Oech, S. R. (1960). The effects of narcotics and antagonists upon respiration and circulation in man. Clinical Pharmacology and Therapeutics, **1**, 483-524.

Extance, K., & Goudie, A. J. (1981). Inter-animal olfactory cues in operant drug discrimination procedures in rats. Psychopharmacology, **73**, 363-371.

Finney, D. J. (1971). Statistical methods in biological assay (2nd ed.). London: Griffin Press.

Fraser, H. F. (1968). Methods for assessing the addiction liability of opioids and opioid antagonists in man. In A. Wikler (Ed.), The addictive states (pp. 176-187). Baltimore: Williams and Wilkins Co.

Fraser, H. F., & Isbell, H. (1961). Human pharmacology and addictiveness of ethyl 1-(3-cyano-3,3-phenylpropyl)-4-phenyl-4-piperidine carboxylate hydrochloride (R-1132, diphenoxylate). Bulletin on Narcotics, **13**, 29-43.

Fraser, H. F., Van Horn, G. D., Martin, W. R., Wolbach, A. B., & Isbell, H. (1961). Methods for evaluating addiction liability. (A) "Attitude" of opiate addicts toward opiate-like drugs, (B) a short-term "direct" addiction test. Journal of Pharmacology and Experimental Therapeutics, **133**, 371-387.

Gellert, V. F., & Holtzman, S. G. (1979). Discriminative stimulus effects of naltrexone in the morphine-dependent rat. Journal of Pharmacology and Experimental Therapeutics, **211**, 596-605.

Glennon, R. A., Rosecrans, J. A., & Young, R. (1982). The use of the drug discrimination paradigm for studying hallucinogenic agents. A review. In F. C. Colpaert & J. L. Slangen (Eds.), Drug discrimination: Applications in CNS pharmacology (pp. 69-98). Amsterdam: Elsevier/North Holland Biomedical Press.

Green, D. M., & Swets, J. A. (1974). Signal detection theory and psychophysics. Huntington: Robert E. Krieger Publishing Co.

Haertzen, C. A. (1970). Subjective effects of the narcotic antagonists cyclazocine and nalorphine in the Addiction Research Center Inventory (ARCI). Psychopharmacologia, **18**, 366-377.

Haertzen, C. A. (1974). Subjective effects of narcotic antagonists. In M. C. Braude, L. S. Harris, E. L. May, J. P. Smith, & J. E. Villarreal (Eds.), Narcotic antagonists (pp. 383-398). New York: Raven Press.

Hayes, R. L. (1978). Experimental design and data analysis in studies of drug discrimination: Some general considerations. In B. T. Ho, D. W. Richards, III, & D. L. Chute (Eds.), Drug discrimination and state dependent learning (pp. 193-201). New York: Academic Press.

Herling, S., & Woods, J. H. (1981). Discriminative stimulus effects of narcotics: Evidence for multiple receptor-mediated actions. Life Sciences, **28**, 1571-1584.

Ho, B. T., & Silverman, P. B. (1978). Stimulants as discriminative stimuli. In F. C. Colpaert & J. A. Rosecrans (Eds.), Stimulus properties of drugs: Ten years of progress (pp. 53-68). Amsterdam: Elsevier/North Holland Biomedical Press.

Holtzman, S. G. (1975). Effects of narcotic antagonists on fluid intake in the rat. Life Sciences, 16, 1465-1470.

Holtzman, S. G. (1982a). Stimulus properties of opioids with mixed agonist and antagonist activity. Federation Proceedings, 41, 2328-2332.

Holtzman, S. G. (1982b). Discriminative stimulus properties of opioids in the rat and squirrel monkey. In F. C. Colpaert & J. L. Slangen (Eds.), Drug discrimination: Applications in CNS pharmacology (pp. 17-36). Amsterdam: Elsevier/North Holland Biomedical Press.

Jarbe, T. U. C., & Swedberg, M. D. B. (1982). A conceptualization of drug discrimination learning. In F. C. Colpaert & J. L. Slangen (Eds.), Drug discrimination: Applications in CNS pharmacology (pp. 327-341). Amsterdam: Elsevier/North Holland Biomedical Press.

Jasinski, D. R. (1973). Effects in man of partial morphine agonists. In H. W. Kosterlitz, H. O. J. Collier, & J. E. Villarreal (Eds.), Agonist and antagonist actions of narcotic analgesic drugs (pp. 94-103). Baltimore: University Park Press.

Jasinski, D. R. (1977). Assessment of the abuse potentiality of morphine-like drugs (methods used in man). In W. R. Martin (Ed.), Drug Addiction I (Handbook of Experimental Pharmacology, Vol. 45, pp. 197-258). Berlin: Springer-Verlag.

Jasinski, D. R., & Mansky, P. A. (1972). Evaluation of nalbuphine for abuse potential. Clinical Pharmacology and Therapeutics, 13, 78-90.

Jasinski, D. R., Martin, W. R., & Haertzen, C. A. (1967). The human pharmacology and abuse potential of n-allylnoroxymorphone (naloxone). Journal of Pharmacology and Experimental Therapeutics, 157, 420-426.

Jasinski, D. R., Martin, W. R., & Sapira, J. D. (1968). Antagonism of the subjective, behavioral, pupillary, and respiratory depressant effects of cyclazocine by naloxone. Clinical Pharmacology and Therapeutics, 9, 215-222.

Koek, W., & Slangen, J. L. (1982). The role of fentanyl training dose and of the alternative stimulus condition in drug generalization. Psychopharmacology, 76, 149-156.

Krimmer, E. C., & Barry, H., III. (1977). Discriminable stimuli produced by marihuana constituents. In H. Lal (Ed.), Discriminative stimulus properties of drugs (pp. 121-136). New York: Plenum Press.

Litchfield, J. T., & Wilcoxon, F. (1949). A simplified method of evaluating dose-effect experiments. Journal of Pharmacology and Experimental Therapeutics, 96, 99-113.

Locke, K. W., Brown, D. R., & Holtzman, S. G. (1982). Effects of opiate antagonists and putative mu- and kappa agonists on milk intake in rat and squirrel monkey. Pharmacology Biochemistry & Behavior, 17, 1275-1279.

Lowy, M., Starkey, C., & Yim, G. (1981). Stereoselective effects of opiate agonists and antagonists on ingestive behavior in rats. Pharmacology Biochemistry & Behavior, 15, 591-596.

Olton, D. S., & Samuelson, R. (1974). Decision making in the rat. Journal of Comparative and Physiological Psychology, 87, 1134-1147.

Ostrowski, N., Rowland, N., Foley, T., Nelson, J., & Reid, L. (1981). Morphine antagonists and consummatory behaviors. Pharmacology Biochemistry & Behavior, 14, 549-559.

Overton, D. A. (1979). Influence of shaping procedures and schedules of reinforcement on performance in the two-bar drug discrimination task: A methodological report. Psychopharmacology, 65, 291-298.

Overton, D. A. (1982). Comparison of the degree of discriminability of various drugs using the T-maze drug discrimination paradigm. Psychopharmacology, 76, 385-395.

Pastore, R. E., & Scheier, C. J. (1974). Signal detection theory: Considerations for general applications. Psychological Bulletin, 81, 945-958.

Richards, D. W., III. (1978). A functional analysis of the discriminative stimulus properties of amphetamine and pentobarbital. In B. T. Ho, D. W. Richards, III, & D. L. Chute (Eds.), Drug discrimination and state dependent learning (pp. 227-247). New York: Academic Press.

Schechter, M. D. (1981). Extended schedule transfer of ethanol discrimination. Pharmacology Biochemistry & Behavior, 14, 23-25.

Schuster, C. R., Fischman, M. W., & Johanson, C. E. (1981). Internal stimulus control and subjective effects of drugs. In T. Thompson & C. E. Johanson (Eds.), Behavioral pharmacology of human drug dependence (National Institute on Drug Abuse Research Monograph 37, pp. 116-129). Washington, DC: U.S. Government Printing Office.

Shannon, H. E., & Holtzman, S. G. (1976). Evaluation of the discriminative effects of morphine in rats. Journal of Pharmacology and Experimental Therapeutics, 198, 54-65.

Siegel, S. (1956). Nonparametric statistics. New York: McGraw-Hill.

Silverman, P. B., & Ho, B. T. (1977). Characterization of discriminative response control by psychomotor stimulants. In H. Lal (Ed.), Discriminative stimulus properties of drugs (pp. 107-119). New York: Plenum Press.

Skinner, B. F. (1938). The behavior of organisms: An experimental analysis. New York: Appleton-Century-Crofts.

Stevens, S. S. (1946). On the theory of scales of measurement. Science, 103, 677-680.

Stolerman, I. P., Baldy, R. E., & Shine, P. J. (1982). Drug discrimination procedure: A bibliography. In F. C. Colpaert & J. L. Slangen (Eds.), Drug discrimination: Applications in CNS pharmacology (pp. 401-441). Amsterdam: Elsevier/North Holland Biomedical Press.

Stolerman, I. P., & D'Mello, G. D. (1981). Role of training conditions in discrimination of central nervous system stimulants by rats. Psychopharmacology, 73, 295-303.

Swedberg, M. D. B., & Jarbe, T. U. C. (1982). Morphine cue saliency: Limits of discriminability and third state perception by pigeons. In F. C. Colpaert & J. C. Slangen (Eds.), Drug discrimination: Applications in CNS pharmacology (pp. 147-164). Amsterdam: Elsevier/North Holland Biomedical Press.

Treisman, M. (1976). On the use and misuse of psychophysical terms. Psychological Review, 83, 246-256.

Weissman, A. (1976). The discriminability of aspirin in arthritic and non-arthritic rats. Pharmacology Biochemistry & Behavior, 5, 583-586.

Weissman, A. (1978). Generalization of the discriminative stimulus properties of ^{9}-tetrahydrocannabinol to cannabinoids with therapeutic potential. In F. C. Colpaert & J. A. Rosecrans (Eds.), Stimulus properties of drugs: Ten years of progress (pp. 99-124). Amsterdam: Elsevier/North Holland Biomedical Press.

White, J. M., & Holtzman, S. G. (1981). Three-choice drug discrimination in the rat: Morphine, cyclazocine and saline. Journal of Pharmacology and Experimental Therapeutics, 217, 254-262.

Winter, J. C. (1975). The stimulus properties of morphine and ethanol. Psychopharmacologia, 44, 209-214.

Winter, J. C. (1978). Drug-induced stimulus control. In D. E. Blackman & D. J. Sanger (Eds.), Contemporary research in behavioral pharmacology (pp. 209-237). New York: Plenum Press.

Winter, J. C. (1981). Drug-induced stimulus control and the concept of breaking point: LSD and quipazine. Psychopharmacology, 72, 217-218.

CHAPTER 18

THE STUDY OF STRUCTURE-ACTIVITY RELATIONSHIPS USING DRUG DISCRIMINATION METHODOLOGY

Richard A. Glennon and Richard Young

Department of Medical Chemistry
School of Pharmacy
Medical College of Virginia
Virginia Commonwealth University
Richmond, Virginia 23298

ABSTRACT

The drug discrimination paradigm, while gaining popularity as a research tool, has been used little for systematic investigations of structure-activity relationships (SAR: the effect of chemical structure on biological activity). This paradigm has been demonstrated to be a highly sensitive and very specific "drug detection" method that provides both quantitative and qualitative results and, as such, is particularly well suited for SAR studies. Using examples from our own work, we attempt to demonstrate our approaches to the study of the SAR of tryptamine, phenylisopropylamine (amphetamine), and benzodiazepine derivatives using drug discrimination methodology.

GENERAL CONCEPTS

Various investigators have employed the drug discrimination paradigm to examine the effects of gross structural modification of drugs on discriminative responding; by and large, however, systematic and detailed investigations of structure-activity relationships (SAR) have not ordinarily been a focal point of these studies. This is rather unfortunate since the drug discrimination paradigm appears to be particularly well suited for such studies. Many techniques generating SAR data are quantitative but not necessarily qualitative; in contrast, drug discrimination is one of the few methods that can afford both quantitative and qualitative results.

Of what value are SAR data? The simplest definition of SAR is the relationship between a given activity and the nature of the molecular entities that produce that activity (i.e., the effect of structural modification on activity). Rarely is such information gathered as an end unto itself; the results of SAR studies can be used, for example, (a) to define which structural features are necessary for activity, (b) to optimize a specific effect (i.e., for the eventual design of new potentially active agents or antagonists), (c) to determine the stereoselectivity or stereospecificity required for an effect, (d) to correlate several types of activity, (e) to determine if members of two or more series of agents act via a similar (i.e., common) receptor interaction, and (f) to study mechanisms of drug action. Conversely, SAR studies can be employed to learn about the sites at which drugs act (e.g., receptor mapping studies). That is, by knowing what features of a molecule are important for activity, insight is gained as to what complementary functionalities might be present at a receptor site in order to effect a productive interaction. The common goal underlying many of these SAR studies is a greater understanding of the physicochemical properties necessary for a molecule to elicit a particular biological effect.

In a specific SAR study, the effects of a series of agents (i.e., structural variants; molecular modifications) on activity are evaluated. Initially, the study might involve members of a class of agents that possess only minor structural differences; ultimately, agents with more dramatic alterations, or even agents of an entirely different chemical class of compounds, might be investigated. SAR data obtained from in vivo studies reflect all of the possible consequences of absorption, distribution, and metabolism (i.e., pharmacokinetics) of a given agent. As a result, caution is advised when comparing SAR derived from whole animal studies with SAR derived from in vitro studies; in the latter the effects of absorption, distribution, and/or metabolism can be minimal, nonexistent, or altered. The results derived from in vitro studies yield incisive and succinct SAR, but they are less likely than in vivo studies to reveal the effects of drug in a "real world" (e.g., clinical) setting. Obviously, there is a need for both types of studies. The SAR generated from drug discrimination represent in vivo SAR and, as such, reflect the involvement of structure and pharmacokinetics as part of the relationship between structure and discriminative stimulus effects.

The drug discrimination paradigm can be used to generate SAR data; however, such data are only valid with respect to a particular dose of a given training drug. Because the sensitivity and duration of effect of a stimulus is related to the training dose of the training drug and because drug stimuli are time dependent, dose-response relationships represent relative, not absolute, relationships between challenge drugs and training drugs. The interested reader is referred to Colpaert and to Overton (this volume and references therein) for a more detailed discussion on the effects of these parameters.

Thus, the SAR for a series of agents is related to the training dose of the training drug and to the conditions present when the data were generated. As a consequence, the results of drug discrimination studies should only be used to formulate SAR for those members of a challenge series where there is evidence for a common effect (i.e., for those agents where stimulus generalization has occurred to a stated training dose of a particular training drug). That is, it is inappropriate to develop an SAR within a series of agents that produced only partial generalization. If a challenge drug produces anything less than stimulus generalization, it is probably safe to assume that the challenge drug is "inactive" with respect to possessing stimulus properties common to the training dose of the training drug under the temporal constraints (e.g., presession injection interval) of the assay. When stimulus generalization has occurred between a training drug and a challenge drug, ED_{50} values can be calculated for comparative purposes. An ED_{50} dose is, normally, the dose of an agent that produces a specific effect in 50% of the animals. Although this is the manner in which ED_{50} values have been used/calculated in some discrimination studies, this is not always the case. In tests of stimulus generalization, it is not uncommon to require, as an endpoint, that all of the animals respond on the drug-appropriate lever. In such studies, then, the ED_{50} dose is defined as that dose (of an agent to which stimulus generalization occurred) at which all of the animals would make 50% of their responses on the drug appropriate lever. The ED_{50} values used in this chapter adhere to the latter definition. Furthermore, when making potency comparisons between two agents that produce similar stimulus effects, it is most appropriate to make these comparisons on a micromole/kg basis, rather than mg/kg basis, when there is a substantial difference in molecular weights of the agents involved.

Ideally, it is desirable to evaluate doses of a challenge drug until either stimulus generalization or disruption of behavior (i.e., no responding) occurs. If, for example, the highest test dose of a challenge drug elicits 50% training-drug-appropriate responding and, for one reason or another, the evaluation of higher doses is precluded, it is incorrect to conclude that the challenge drug is half as active as the training drug (or, for that matter, that it is active at all) when, in fact, there has been no demonstration that the two agents can produce a common effect. In this situation, comparisons can only be made in a qualitative sense. That is, the only valid conclusion that can be reached is that this agent is less effective than the training drug in producing training-drug-like effects (or, correspondingly, that it is less effective than some other challenge drug, which at a dose below the highest test dose produced training-drug-like effects). Likewise, if two challenge drugs produce partial generalization (e.g., 40% and 60% training-drug-appropriate responding) at a given dose, it cannot be stated with certainty that the second challenge drug is more active than the first because the possibility exists that one (or both) agent(s) may not be capable of producing an effect common to that of the training drug.

Another very important consideration is the necessity of a thorough dose-response investigation. It has been our experience in tests of stimulus generalization that certain agents produce saline-like effects at particular doses and disruption of behavior at some higher dose(s). While an initial conclusion to the results of such a study might be that there is a lack of stimulus generalization, we have found in a number of instances that a careful evaluation of additional doses (i.e., doses between the highest dose that resulted in saline-like responding and the lowest dose that produced disruption of behavior) ultimately resulted in stimulus generalization. This has even been observed with agents where the difference in saline-like and disruptive doses has been quite small. Several instances have now been encountered where administration of a challenge drug in a logarithmic progression of doses (e.g., 0.1, 0.3, 1.0, 3.0 mg/kg) resulted in saline-like responding at the lower doses and in disruption of behavior at the highest dose, and examination of the doses between 1.0 and 3.0 mg/kg resulted, ultimately, in stimulus generalization. We believe that these results emphasize the sensitive and specific nature of the drug-induced stimulus.

Finally, it should be recognized that when challenge drugs are being examined the data obtained relate to training-dose-like effects. For example, an investigation of the effects of a series of barbiturates in diazepam-trained animals does not provide SAR of barbiturate activity; rather, the data reflect the SAR of a series of barbiturates to produce diazepam-like results. Thus, this SAR may or may not be the same as the SAR developed for the effects of this same series of barbiturates in, for example, pentobarbital-trained animals.

What follows are fragments of several examples of SAR studies that have been conducted in our laboratory; these involve the SAR of tryptamine derivatives, phenylisopropylamine derivatives (as reflecting DOM-like and amphetamine-like properties), and benzodiazepines. There will be very little discussion as to the interpretation of SAR data (except where a particular point is being emphasized); rather, an attempt is made to describe our approach and to delineate the types of data that might be obtained. Additionally, some of these studies are still in progress and it would be premature to discuss detailed SAR. Nevertheless, each of these studies reveals the value and the limitations of the drug discrimination paradigm in formulating SAR.

SAR STUDIES ON TRYPTAMINE DERIVATIVES

In the course of our studies on the mechanism of action of hallucinogenic agents, it became necessary to determine the in vivo SAR of series of tryptamine derivatives; the drug discrimination paradigm was employed to obtain this information. Using a standard two-lever operant procedure, rats were trained to discriminate 1.0 mg/kg of racemic 1-(2,5-dimethoxy-4-methylphenyl)-2-aminopropane hydrochloride (DOM) from saline under a variable-interval 15-second (VI-15) schedule of reinforcement for food (sweetened condensed milk) reward (Young, Glennon, & Rosecrans, 1981). Generalization studies were then conducted using various doses of a variety of tryptamine derivatives as the challenge series. In this way it was determined which members of the series produced DOM-like effects (i.e., effects similar to that produced by 1.0 mg/kg of racemic DOM when administered 15 minutes prior to a 2.5-minute extinction session). Response rates were monitored and compared with those produced by administration of the training dose of the training drug (i.e., DOM) in order to determine whether or not there was any disruption of behavior. The response rates following DOM were not significantly different from those seen after administration of 1.0 ml/kg of saline.

The study focused on the effects of structural modification in each of three different areas of the tryptamine molecule: the terminal amine group, the aromatic nucleus, and the alkyl side chain (see Figure 1). The first region to be examined was the terminal amine. Administration of tryptamine, up to doses of 25 mg/kg, resulted in saline-like responding, while administration of the N,N-dimethyl derivative of tryptamine (i.e., N,N-dimethyltryptamine: DMT) resulted in DOM-stimulus generalization (ED_{50} = 5.8 mg/kg). Because tryptamine did not result in stimulus generalization at the doses evaluated but because it might have at higher doses, it cannot be concluded that tryptamine is inactive. Nevertheless, DMT is more effective than tryptamine in producing DOM-like effects. This finding is consistent with the results of other pharmacological studies that have concluded that certain primary indolealkylamines, such as tryptamine, penetrate the blood-brain barrier only with difficulty and/or are rapidly metabolized in vivo by oxidative deamination. Dimethylation of tryptamine to produce DMT is known to enhance its ability to penetrate the

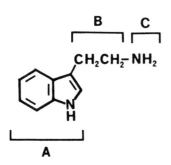

Figure 1: The structure of tryptamine showing the aromatic nucleus (**A**), the alkyl side chain (**B**), and the terminal amine (**C**).

blood-brain barrier and to offer some protection from oxidative deamination; whether the N-methyl groups also contribute to a specific drug-receptor interaction is as yet unknown. (See Glennon, Young, & Jacyno, 1983c, for further discussion of this topic.) Homologation or extension of the terminal amine alkyl groups of DMT to ethyl, propyl, and isopropyl groups (i.e., DET, DPT, and DIPT, respectively; see Table 1) yields derivatives that result in DOM-stimulus generalization when administered to DOM-trained animals. On this basis the relative order of potency is DPT > DET > DIPT > DMT. Thus, the

Table 1

Structures of Tryptamine Derivatives

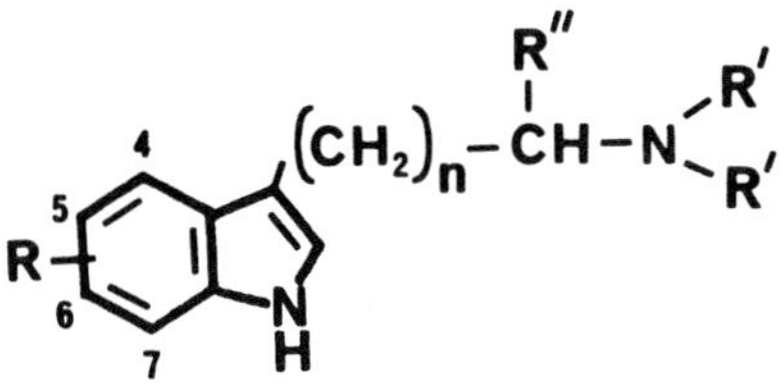

Agent	R'	R"	R$^{\underline{a}}$	n
Tryptamine	H	H	H	1
DMT	CH_3	H	H	1
DET	C_2H_5	H	H	1
DPT	nC_3H_7	H	H	1
DIPT	iC_3H_7	H	H	1
4-OMe DMT	CH_3	H	$4-OCH_3$	1
5-OMe DMT	CH_3	H	$5-OCH_3$	1
6-OMe DMT	CH_3	H	$6-OCH_3$	1
5-OMe DET	C_2H_5	H	$5-OCH_3$	1
5-OMe DIPT	iC_3H_7	H	$5-OCH_3$	1
5-OMe Gramine	CH_3	H	$5-OCH_3$	0
α-MeT	H	CH_3	H	1
5-OMe α-MeT	H	CH_3	$5-OCH_3$	1
α-EtT	H	C_2H_5	H	1

Note: a, Location of substituents is indicated by the position number, except for unsubstituted rings, where R = H.

homologs of DMT are not only active but apparently are more potent than DMT in producing DOM-like effects (Glennon, Young, Jacyno, Slusher, & Rosecrans, 1983d).

Next to be explored was the effect of aromatic substitution (see Figure 1). While a number of different substituents were examined, only the results of methoxy substitution will be discussed here. The 4-methoxylation of DMT (i.e., introduction of a methoxy group at the 4-position of DMT [4-OMe DMT]; see Table 1) somewhat enhanced activity while 5-OMe DMT (ED_{50} = 1.2 mg/kg) was found to be approximately 5 times more potent than DMT in producing DOM-like effects. On the other hand, administration of doses of 6-OMe DMT up to 10 mg/kg resulted in saline-appropriate responding; additional doses were not examined because only limited supplies of this compound were available. Nevertheless, with respect to effectiveness 5-OMe DMT > 4-OMe DMT > DMT > 6-OMe DMT (Glennon et al., 1983d); 5-methoxylation was also found to enhance the potency of DET and DIPT, and 5-OMe DET was more potent than 5-OMe DIPT.

The final tryptamine region to be explored was the alkyl side chain (see Figure 1). All of the tryptamine derivatives discussed to this point possess an unbranched alkyl side chain of two methylene units that separates the aromatic nucleus from the terminal amine; shortening this side chain to one methylene unit results in a series of agents called gramines. For example, 5-OMe DMT might be considered a homolog of its one methylene unit counterpart 5-OMe gramine (see Table 1). Administration of doses of 1.0 to 6.0 mg/kg of 5-OMe gramine to the DOM-trained animals resulted in a saline-like responding; solubility problems preclude administration of higher doses. However, the highest dose evaluated of 5-OMe gramine was 5 times the ED_{50} dose of 5-OMe DMT; thus, it was concluded that 5-OMe gramine was less effective than the latter agent in producing DOM-like effects (Glennon et al., 1983d).

The effect on activity of α-alkylation of the side chain was also investigated. Unlike tryptamine, both the α-methyl and α-ethyl derivatives of tryptamine (i.e., α-methyltryptamine [α-MeT] and α-ethyltryptamine [α-EtT], respectively; see Table 1) produced DOM-like effects with α-MeT (ED_{50} = 3.13 mg/kg) being more potent than α-EtT. Both of these α-alkyltryptamines are primary amines, and yet both produce DOM-like effects at lower doses than those where tryptamine still produces saline-like responding. Further, α-MeT is approximately twice as potent as DMT. These results suggest that the N-methyl groups of DMT do not participate in a specific drug-receptor interaction (and, in fact, that they may actually detract from such an interaction) and that the α-alkyl groups may act either to enhance blood-brain barrier permeability and/or to protect against oxidative deamination of the terminal amine.

This examination can be carried one step further. α-MeT possesses an asymmetric center and, thus, exists as optical isomers (see Figure 2). S(+)-α-MeT was found to be about twice as potent as racemic α-MeT, while R(-)-α-Met produced partial generalization (i.e., 61% DOM-appropriate responding) at 3.25 mg/kg and disruption of behavior at higher doses (Glennon et al., 1983c). Thus, if the role of the α-methyl group was to simply enhance blood-brain barrier permeability, a potency difference between the isomers might not be expected; the observed enantiomeric difference may be explained in one of several ways. It might be speculated that the methyl group of S(+)-α-MeT contributes to an enhanced drug-receptor interaction; alternatively, there may be differences in the metabolism of the two isomers. It is difficult to interpret the results, however, because only one isomer produced DOM-stimulus generalization. Another α-alkyltryptamine examined was 5-OMe α-MeT; as might be expected, 5-methoxylation of α-MeT enhanced its potency (ED_{50} = 0.52 mg/kg).

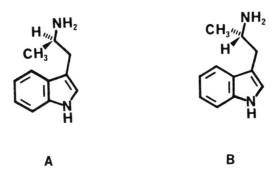

A   **B**

Figure 2: The structure of R(-)-α-methyl-tryptamine (**A**) and S(+)-α-
methyltryptamine (**B**).

However, a strict SAR comparison cannot be made here because, although a 15-
minute presession injection interval was employed for most of the studies, a
90-minute presession injection interval was determined to be optimal for 5-OMe
α-MeT.   Nevertheless, the effect of 5-methoxylation of α-MeT paralleled the
effect observed with 5-methoxylation of DMT (Glennon, Jacyno, & Young, 1983a).
Furthermore, the (+) isomer was found to be approximately twice as potent as
racemic 5-OMe α-MeT; however, in the case of this compound, (-)-5-OMe α-MeT
also produced DOM-like effects although it was several-fold less potent than
its enantiomer.   Although differences in the metabolism of the two isomers
cannot be eliminated at this point, it does appear that the methyl group of
(+)-5-OMe α-MeT contributes in a positive manner to a possible drug-receptor
interaction.

Recently, a series of isotryptamine derivatives was synthesized; these are
analogs of tryptamine where the alkyl side chain and pendant terminal amine are
now attached to the indole nitrogen atom.   Derivatives of the isotryptamines,
such as 5-methoxy-N,N-dimethylisotryptamine (5-OMe isoDMT) and 6-methoxy-N,N-
dimethylisotryptamine (6-OMe isoDMT; see Figure 3), may be viewed either as
tryptamine derivatives where the side chain has been relocated or as
derivatives where the indole nitrogen atom has been moved.   In other words, it
is unclear whether 5-OMe isoDMT would mimic 5-OMe DMT or 6-OMe DMT in
biological situations.

One way to address this problem would be to compare the SAR of the two
series of agents; this was the approach that was taken and the drug
discrimination procedure was used, in part, to obtain some of this information
(Glennon, Jacyno, Young, McKenney, & Nelson, 1984a).   For example,
administration of 5-OMe DMT to DOM-trained animals results in stimulus
generalization, while 6-OMe DMT elicits saline-appropriate responding at doses
up to 10 mg/kg (<u>vide supra</u>).   If the isoDMT derivatives mimic DMT derivatives,
one of the two methoxy derivatives might be anticipated to be more potent than
the other; 5-OMe isoDMT produced saline-like responding at doses to 16 mg/kg,
while the DOM-stimulus generalized to 6-OMe isoDMT (ED_{50} = 7.1 mg/kg.
Furthermore, the time course of effects of 5-OMe DMT and 6-OMe isoDMT was found
to be identical.   Thus, because 6-OMe isoDMT more closely mimics the effects of
5-OMe DMT than does its 5-OMe counterpart, it appears that the isotryptamines

- 379 -

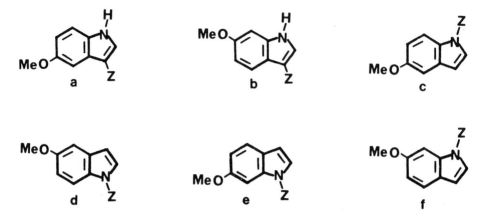

Figure 3: Structural relationships between (**a**) 5-OMe DMT, (**b**) 6-OMe DMT, and, each drawn in two different orientations, (**c,d**) 5-OMe isoDMT and (**e,f**) 6-OMe isoDMT; $Z = CH_2CH_2N(CH_3)_2$.

may be viewed as tryptamine analogs with the indole nitrogen replacing the 3-position carbon atom at the aromatic nucleus. Based on the results of this and other studies, isoDMT derivatives are less potent bioisosteres of DMT derivatives.

SAR STUDIES ON PHENYLISOPROPYLAMINE DERIVATIVES

Phenylisopropylamine or 1-phenyl-2-aminopropane is known as amphetamine; this agent is a CNS stimulant in humans and in animals. Substitution on the aromatic nucleus of amphetamine affords a variety of derivatives that may possess similar or different pharmacological properties. One such derivative is 1-(2,5-dimethoxy-4-methylphenyl)-2-aminopropane or DOM; this agent is known to be hallucinogenic in man. Thus, if given a series of 1-phenyl-2-aminopropane derivatives, it should be possible to develop two independent SARs--an SAR for amphetamine-like activity and an SAR for DOM-like activity. Using the drug discrimination paradigm, it might also be possible to determine if there are any 1-phenyl-2-aminopropane derivatives possessing both amphetamine-like and DOM-like properties.

DOM-Like SAR

Silverman and Ho (1978) were the first to demonstrate that racemic DOM would serve as a discriminative stimulus in rats. Since then, a large number of rats have been trained in our laboratory to discriminate DOM from saline. The training and testing procedures were identical to those discussed for the study of the tryptamine derivatives (for greater detail see Young et al., 1981). Using these DOM-trained animals, we have formulated SAR based on the results of well over one hundred stimulus generalization studies. Silverman and Ho (1978) demonstrated that the DOM-stimulus does not generalize to amphetamine and that an amphetamine-stimulus does not generalize to DOM; results obtained in our laboratory confirm these findings that DOM and amphetamine produce dissimilar discriminative cues.

The general phenylisopropylamine skeletal structure common to DOM and amphetamine can be subdivided into three areas for examination: the terminal amine, the alkyl side-chain, and the aromatic nucleus (see Figure 4). Both monomethylation of DOM (i.e., N-Me DOM) and N,N-demethylation of the α-demethyl derivative of DOM (i.e., DD-DOM) reduce potency. In general, the primary amine derivatives (i.e., derivatives that are unsubstituted on the terminal amine) are more potent than their mono or dimethyl counterparts. Substitution on the aromatic nucleus is also an important factor for DOM-like activity; for example, neither amphetamine nor any of its monomethoxy derivatives (i.e., 2-OMe PIA, 3-OMe PIA, PMA) produce DOM-appropriate responding (see Table 2 for structures).

Within the dimethoxy (DMA) series the DOM-stimulus generalizes only to 2,4-DMA and 2,5-DMA but not to 2,3-DMA, 2,6-DMA, 3,4-TMA or 3,5-DMA. Of the trimethoxyphenylisopropylamines (TMA derivatives), complete DOM-stimulus generalization occurred to all five compounds although 2,4,5-TMA and 2,4,6-TMA were the only derivatives found to be more potent than either 2,4-DMA or 2,5-DMA (Glennon & Young, 1982b; Glennon, Young, Benington, & Morin, 1982b; Glennon et al., 1983c). The 2,4- and 2,5-dimethoxy substitution patterns appear to be important features for DOM-stimulus generalization; as such, additional derivatives of 2,4-DMA and 2,5-DMA were selected for more extensive evaluation.

Without belaboring the detailed SAR of these agents, it might simply be concluded that many derivatives of 2,4-DMA and 2,5-DMA produce DOM-like responding and also constitute some of the more potent agents investigated. For example, substitution of the 4-position of 2,5-DMA by small alkyl groups (e.g., DOET, DOPR) or by halogen (e.g., DOB, DOI) all result in agents that are at least as potent, if not more potent, than DOM itself (Glennon et al., 1982d; Glennon, Young, & Rosecrans, 1982e). However, the 2,5-dimethoxy substitution pattern appears quite sensitive to the presence of substituents at the 3-position. Moving the 4-position methyl or bromo group of DOM or DOB, respectively, to the 3-position (i.e., 3-Me, 2,5-DMA and 3-Br 2,5-DMA) results in agents that produce saline-like responding even at doses of 10 to 20 times the ED_{50} doses of their parent compounds (Glennon et al., 1982d; Glennon, Young, & Rosecrans, 1982f).

Finally, there is the effect of alteration of alkyl side chain (see Figure 4). Removal of the α-methyl groups of those agents that produce DOM-like effects seems to have a common effect--to reduce potency. For example, mescaline is approximately half as potent as its α-methyl analog, 3,4,5-TMA (Glennon & Young, 1982b). Again, it might be speculated that the lack of this methyl function either decreases the ability of a compound to penetrate the blood-brain barrier and/or makes it a better substrate for oxidative

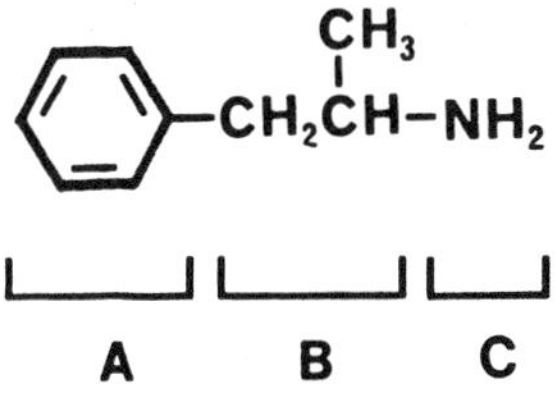

Figure 4: The structure of 1-phenyl-2-aminopropane (phenylisopropylamine) showing the aromatic nucleus (**A**), the alkyl side chain (**B**), and the terminal amine (**C**).

Table 2

Structures of 1-phenyl-2-aminopropane (Phenylisopropylamine) Derivatives

Agent	R'	R_2	R_3	R_4	R_5	R_6
Amphetamine	H	H	H	H	H	H
2-OMe PIA	H	OCH_3	H	H	H	H
3-OMe PIA	H	H	OCH_3	H	H	H
4-OMe PIA (PMA)	H	H	H	OCH_3	H	H
2,3-DMA	H	OCH_3	OCH_3	H	H	H
2,4-DMA	H	OCH_3	H	OCH_3	H	H
2,5-DMA	H	OCH_3	H	H	OCH_3	H
2,6-DMA	H	OCH_3	H	H	H	OCH_3
3,4-DMA	H	H	OCH_3	OCH_3	H	H
3,5-DMA	H	H	OCH_3	H	OCH_3	H
2,3,4-TMA	H	OCH_3	OCH_3	OCH_3	H	H
2,3,5-TMA	H	OCH_3	OCH_3	H	OCH_3	H
2,4,5-TMA	H	OCH_3	H	OCH_3	OCH_3	H
2,4,6-TMA	H	OCH_3	H	OCH_3	H	OCH_3
3,4,5-TMA	H	H	OCH_3	OCH_3	OCH_3	H
DOM	H	OCH_3	H	Me	OCH_3	H
N-Me DOM	Me	OCH_3	H	Me	OCH_3	H
DOET	H	OCH_3	H	Et	OCH_3	H
DOPR	H	OCH_3	H	Pr	OCH_3	H
DOB	H	OCH_3	H	Br	OCH_3	H

DOI	H	OCH_3	H	I	OCH_3	H
3-Me 2,5-DMA	H	OCH_3	Me	H	OCH_3	H
3-Br 2,5-DMA	H	OCH_3	Br	H	OCH_3	H
3,4-MDA	H	H	$-OCH_2O-$		H	H

---

deamination. The presence of an α-methyl group, as in the tryptamine series, appears to be optimal; homologation of the α-methyl to an α-ethyl group reduces potency (Glennon et al., 1983c). The phenylisopropylamines, by virtue of the presence of the α-methyl group, are also optically active. The optical isomers of several of these agents that are capable of producing DOM-like effects have been examined (e.g., DOM, DOB) and in every case the R(-)-isomers have been found to be more potent than either their S(+)-enantiomers and/or racemates (Glennon et al., 1982d).

Thus, in this way it has been possible to determine which phenylisopropylamines produce DOM-like effects and then to develop an SAR based on these results. The interested reader is referred to a review by Glennon, Rosecrans, and Young (1983b) for a more detailed discussion of these SAR.

One of the uses of SAR data is to compare two types of activity. If the SAR for a given series of agents is similar for different measures of activity, this suggests that the two types of activity may be related or may be mediated via a similar mechanism. A comparison of the SAR developed for DOM-like effects reveals similarities with the SAR of these same phenylisopropylamines for human hallucinogenic activity. In fact, there is a significant correlation ($r = 0.96$; $p < 0.001$; $N = 22$) between the ED_{50} values of those phenylisopropylamines with DOM-stimulus generalization and their human hallucinogenic potencies (Glennon, Rosecrans, & Young, 1982a; Glennon et al., 1982d).

Amphetamine-Like SAR

Although our work on the amphetamine-like SAR of these agents is still in progress, sufficient data have been collected to demonstrate that this SAR is quite different from the DOM-like SAR. Various investigators have studied the discriminative stimulus properties of amphetamine and several reviews are available (e.g., Young & Glennon, 1986; Silverman & Ho, 1977).

We have trained rats to discriminate 1.0 mg/kg of (+)-amphetamine sulfate from saline using a VI-15 schedule of reinforcement for food reward. Some of our initial findings are that monomethylation of the terminal amine of amphetamine has little or no effect on amphetamine-appropriate responding and that the S-isomer of amphetamine is more potent than its racemic mixture or corresponding R-enantiomer. These findings are in direct opposition to the DOM-SAR. In general, those agents that elicit DOM-appropriate responding do not elicit amphetamine-appropriate responding and vice versa. For example, agents such as 2-OMe PIA and 3-OMe PIA, that do not result in DOM-stimulus generalization, do produce amphetamine-like effects. Again, this work is currently in progress and detailed SAR must await the results of additional studies. However, there appears to be at least one agent, 3,4-methylenedioxyamphetamine (3,4-MDA) that is capable of producing both DOM-like and amphetamine-like effects. We now take the opportunity to discuss this compound in somewhat greater detail.

MDA-Like SAR

A discriminative stimulus is generally regarded as being quite specific; DOM-stimulus generalization does not occur to amphetamine, for example, nor does amphetamine-stimulus generalization occur to DOM. However, both the amphetamine and DOM stimulus generalize to 3,4-MDA; thus, this compound appears capable of producing both amphetamine-like and DOM-like effects (Glennon, Young, Anderson, & Rosecrans, 1982c; Glennon & Young, 1984c).

Animals were trained to discriminate 1.5 mg/kg of racemic 3,4-MDA hydrochloride from saline employing a VI-15 schedule of reinforcement (Glennon & Young, 1984c). Interestingly, the MDA-stimulus generalized to both amphetamine and DOM. Initial thinking was that 3,4-MDA might represent an agent with a new spectrum of effects and that an SAR might be developed for these MDA-like effects. However, realizing that 3,4-MDA is optically active and drawing upon the above SAR (where those agents producing DOM-like effects have more potent R-isomers than S-enantiomers while the opposite is true for those agents that produce amphetamine-like effects), it was entirely possible that the individual isomers of 3,4-MDA might possess dissimilar properties. In other words, 3,4-MDA might represent a transition agent in a continuum of amphetamine-like to DOM-like agents with the individual isomers being capable of displaying one type of activity or the other.

Using the above mentioned DOM-trained and amphetamine-trained animals, generalization studies were conducted on the individual optical isomers of 3,4-MDA. Substantiation for the presented hypothesis was obtained when it was found that the DOM-stimulus generalized to R(-)-3,4-MDA but not to S(+)-3,4-MDA, while the amphetamine-stimulus generalized to S(+)-3,4-MDA but not to R(-)-3,4-MDA (see Figure 5). Furthermore, in each case the isomer of 3,4-MDA which generalized to the respective training-drug was more potent than racemic 3,4-MDA (Glennon & Young, 1984b). Thus, although an MDA-like SAR was not developed, this series of studies exemplifies the use of previously generated SAR to study a novel agent using drug discrimination methodology.

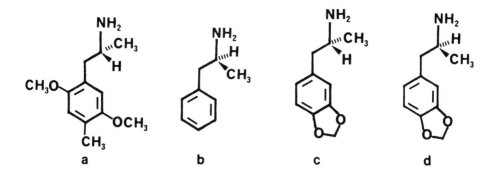

Figure 5: Structures of (**a**) the more isomer of DOM in DOM-trained animals, (**b**) the more active isomer of amphetamine in amphetamine-trained animals, (**c**) the isomer of 3,4-MDA active in DOM-trained animals, and (**d**) the isomer of 3,4-MDA active in amphetamine-trained animals.

SAR STUDIES ON BENZODIAZEPINE DERIVATIVES

The benzodiazepines constitute the most widely prescribed class of compounds in current clinical use; the number of prescriptions for benzodiazepines written annually in the United States alone is thought to exceed 100 million (Tallman, Paul, Skolnick, & Gallager, 1980). The popularity of this class of agents is probably the result of its four major pharmacological actions: anxiolytic, muscle relaxant, sedative, and anticonvulsant. A number of comprehensive reviews have appeared dealing with the behavioral and pharmacological effects of the benzodiazepines (e.g., Haefely, Pieri, Polc, & Schaffner, 1981; Skolnick & Paul, 1982).

Our studies with benzodiazepines were not aimed at delineating structure-activity relationships per se but rather were an attempt to determine if a relationship exists between human potencies and discrimination-derived diazepam-like potencies in animals. A complete SAR study on benzodiazepine derivatives using the drug discrimination paradigm would be an ambitious undertaking. The results of various human and animal studies have already identified several important positions on the benzodiazepine nucleus where the presence of substituents can have a dramatic effect on activity/potency; thus, a comprehensive SAR study might require the investigation of hundreds of compounds. Our studies were limited to a small number of benzodiazepine derivatives (Some are shown in Table 3.) which for the most part are clinically available. As a consequence all of the compounds are active in the drug discrimination paradigm and the overall range of potencies is only two orders of magnitude. Nevertheless, because the SAR for the benzodiazepines is already relatively well established (e.g., Sternbach, 1973), it should be possible to make use of these SARs to determine if the SAR generated from the drug discrimination studies adhere to these same generalities.

Using a two-lever operant choice task, rats were trained to discriminate 3.0 mg/kg of diazepam from saline under a fixed ratio-10 (FR-10) schedule of reinforcement for food (sweetened condensed milk) reward. Once the discrimination was learned, generalization studies were conducted using various doses of a variety of 1,4-benzodiazepine derivatives. Although our goal was to determine which members of the series would produce diazepam-like effects (i.e., effects similar to that produced by 3.0 mg/kg of diazepam administered 10 minutes prior to the test session), one of the by-products of the investigation was an accumulation of data that could be useful for the formulation of limited SAR. As was the case with the phenylisopropylamine derivatives, there was a significant correlation ($r = 0.94$; $p < 0.001$, $N = 15$) between the ED_{50} values of those agents to which the benzodiazepam-stimulus generalized and their previously reported "drug effect" potencies in humans (Zbinden & Randall, 1967).

In describing the SAR of the benzodiazepines, it should be realized that substituents at a number of positions around the benzodiazepine nucleus can influence activity as well as potency. The basic benzodiazepine skeleton is shown in Figure 6 and can be divided into the fused aromatic ring, the 1,4-diazepine ring, and the phenyl ring at the benzodiazepine 5-position; the ring numbering system is also shown. Some of the previously reported SAR generalities will be briefly described; comparisons will then be made between SAR and the results of our discrimination studies in order to determine if similar structure-activity relationships are apparent.

Removal of existing alkyl substituents from the 1-position of the benzodiazepines generally results in a slight decrease in potency (Sternbach,

Table 3

Structure of Benzodiazepine Derivatives

			Substituents at position:		
Agent	1	2	3	7	X
Diazepam	CH_3	O	H	Cl	CH
Oxazepam	H	O	OH	Cl	CH
RO 5-2904	H	O	H	CF_3	CH
Temazepam	CH_3	O	OH	Cl	CH
RO 5-3027	H	O	H	Cl	C-Cl
Desmethyldiazepam	H	O	H	Cl	CH
RO 5-4528	CH_3	O	H	CN	CH
Flunitrazepam	CH_3	O	H	NO_2	C-F
3-Methylflunitrazepam	CH_3	O	CH_3	NO_2	C-F
Lorazepam	H	O	OH	Cl	C-Cl
Medazepam	CH_3	H	H	Cl	CH
RO 5-3590	H	O	H	NO_2	$C-CF_3$
Clonazepam	H	O	H	NO_2	C-Cl
Nitrazepam	H	O	H	NO_2	CH
Bromazepam	H	O	H	Br	N
Flurazepam	a	O	H	Cl	C-F

Note: a, Substituent at 1-position = $CH_2CH_2N(C_2H_5)_2$.

1973); this same effect is evident upon comparing diazepam (ED_{50} = 1.16 mg/kg) with desmethyldiazepam (ED_{50} = 2.33 mg/kg), although the difference in potency between temazepam (ED_{50} = 1.36 mg/kg) and its demethyl counterpart oxazepam

Figure 6: The basic benzodiazepine skeleton showing the fused aromatic ring (**A**), the 1,4-diazepine ring (**B**), and the phenyl ring (**C**) at the 5-position.

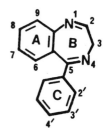

(ED_{50} = 1.35) is minimal. Ordinarily, removal of the 2-position carbonyl group of the benzodiazepines reduces potency somewhat, although the presence of this carbonyl function is not necessary for activity (Sternbach, 1973); a comparison of diazepam with medazepam (ED_{50} = 2.10 mg/kg) reveals a small drop in potency.

Alkyl substitution at the 3-position normally reduces potency while the incorporation of a hydroxyl group at this position has relatively little effect on potency. Flunitrazepam (ED_{50} = 0.05 mg/kg) is clearly 10 times more potent than its alkyl derivative 3-methylflunitrazepam (ED_{50} = 0.65 mg/kg). Comparing diazepam with temazepam, desmethyldiazepam with oxazepam, or RO 5-3027 (ED_{50} = 0.13 mg/kg) with lorazepam (ED_{50} = 0.35 mg/kg) reveals that 3-hydroxylation has relatively little effect (with the greatest effect being a 3-fold increase in potency observed for hydroxylation of RO 5-3027) on potency. The presence of substituents at the 3-position creates a chiral center and hence the possibility of optical stereoisomers (e.g., see Figure 7). Evaluation of the S(+)-isomer of 3-methylflunitrazepam (ED_{50} = 0.34 mg/kg) revealed it to be twice as potent as its racemate; this suggests that it is the S(+)-isomer that is largely responsible for the activity of the racemic mixture.

The benzodiazepines normally possess an aromatic requirement (i.e., a C ring) at the 5-position of the heterocyclic skeleton; ordinarily a phenyl, substituted phenyl, or 3-pyridyl ring is required for optimal activity. Compounds such as diazepam, temazepam, and desmethyldiazepam possess an unsubstituted phenyl ring, while bromazepam (ED_{50} = 0.71 mg/kg) is an example of 2-pyridyl derivative. Substitution on the 5-position phenyl ring at the 3'-

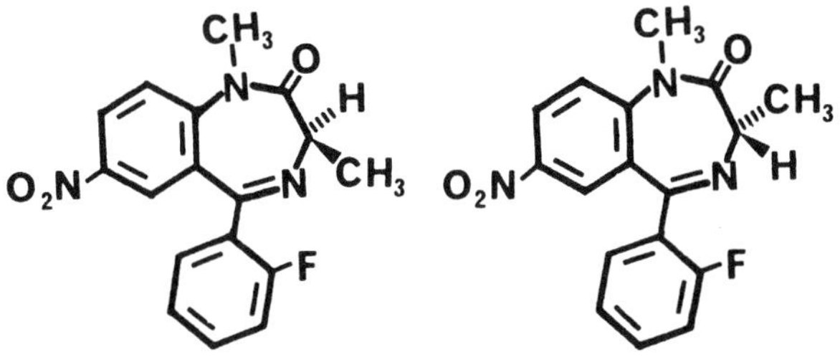

A

B

Figure 7: The structures of the optical isomers of 3-methylflunitrazepam—the R-isomer (**A**) and its S-enantiomer (**B**).

or 4'-position is not well tolerated, whereas a 2'-chloro or 2'-fluoro substituent ordinarily enhances potency. Introduction of a 2'-chloro substituent to oxazepam (i.e., lorazepam), to nitrazepam (ED_{50} = 0.13 mg/kg (i.e., clonazepam, ED_{50} = 0.06 mg/kg), and to desmethyldiazepam (i.e., RO 5-3027), for example, resulted in an increase in potency in each case. Good activity was also shown with 2'-fluoro-substituted derivatives such as flunitrazepam and flurazepam (ED_{50} = 5.1 mg/kg). Substituents at the 2'-position other than chloro or fluoro are reported to cause no significant increase and can even decrease potency (Sternbach, 1973). In agreement with this generality, we found that incorporation of a trifluoromethyl group at the 2'-position of nitrazepam, to yield RO 5-3590 (ED_{50} = 0.22 mg/kg), actually decreased potency somewhat.

Substitutions at positions 6, 8, or 9 of the A ring do not lead to effective compounds; however, the presence of an electron withdrawing group at the 7-position seems essential for optimal activity. We investigated several such derivatives. RO 5-4528 (ED_{50} = 1.18 mg/kg), which possesses a cyano group at the 7-position, appears to be equi-active with diazepam. In the 1-demethyl series a direct comparison can be made between desmethyldiazepam and its trifluoromethyl and nitro derivatives. Both the trifluoromethyl and nitro groups are more electron withdrawing than a chloro group, and, if electron withdrawing effects are important to activity, it might be anticipated that the chloro derivative of desmethyldiazepam would be the least potent of the three. This was found to be the case. Desmethyldiazepam (ED_{50} = 2.33 mg/kg) was less active than either its trifluoromethyl (RO 5-2904, 0.46 mg/kg) or nitro (nitrazepam, 0.13 mg/kg) analogs.

In the formulation of structure-activity relationships, it is desirable to examine as many compounds as possible. Evaluation of large numbers of compounds will provide the most valid SAR and will also serve to identify more readily those agents that may be "exceptions." Although the goal of this present study was not to formulate SAR, the limited SAR that was generated was demonstrated to be consistent with known SAR generalities for the benzodiazepines. This only strengthens the above mentioned correlation between human potencies and discrimination-derived ED_{50} values for benzodiazepine derivatives; if the correlation is valid, structural variation should have similar (barring species differences) effects.

CONCLUSIONS

The drug discrimination paradigm is rapidly gaining popularity as a research tool; however, the use of this paradigm in medicinal chemistry--and in particular its application to investigations of structure-activity relationships--is still in its infancy. Although the potential benefits of this procedure are obvious, additional studies will be required to explore the use of this method as well as to identify its possible shortcomings and limitations for SAR studies. Several factors that can influence the results of such studies have already been described. Perhaps one of the most important factors to be considered is the choice of doses to be examined for a particular challenge compound under investigation; the need for thorough dose-response investigations cannot be over-emphasized. In addition, the formulation of SAR for a series of agents should be reserved only for those members of the series showing generalization to the training-drug stimulus and, even then, only where identical testing conditions (e.g., presession injection interval, route of administration) have been employed. Because the drug discrimination paradigm is an in vivo procedure, SAR data obtained with this method will reflect the pharmacokinetics of the challenge drugs; variation in testing conditions from one challenge drug to another might serve to over-emphasize pharmacokinetic differences. In this respect drug discrimination is no different than any other in vivo method. On the other hand, the sensitive and specific nature of this procedure should make it an excellent tool for studying structure-activity relationships.

ACKNOWLEDGMENTS

Much of the work from our laboratory was supported by Public Health Service grant DA-01642.

REFERENCES

Glennon, R. A., Jacyno, J. M., & Young, R. (1983a). A comparison of the behavioral properties of (±)-, (-)-, and (+)-5-methoxy-α-methyltryptamine. Journal of Biological Psychiatry, 18, 493-498.

Glennon, R. A., Jacyno, J. M., Young, R., & Nelson, D. (1984). Synthesis and evaluation of a novel series of N,N-dimethylisotryptamines. Journal of Medicinal Chemistry, 27, 41-45.

Glennon, R. A., Rosecrans, J. A., & Young, R. (1982a). The use of the drug discrimination paradigm for studying hallucinogenic agents. A review. In F. C. Colpaert & J. L. Slangen (Eds.), Drug discrimination: Applications in CNS pharmacology (pp. 69-96). Amsterdam: Elsevier/North Holland Biomedical Press.

Glennon, R. A., Rosecrans, J. A., & Young, R. (1983b). Drug-induced discrimination: A description of the paradigm and a review of its specific application to the study of hallucinogenic agents. Medicinal Research Reviews, 3, 289-340.

Glennon, R. A., & Young, R. (1982). A comparison of behavioral properties of di- and tri-methoxyphenylisopropylamines. Pharmacology Biochemistry & Behavior, 17, 603-607.

Glennon, R. A., & Young, R. (1984a). Further investigation of the discriminative stimulus properties of MDA. Pharmacology Biochemistry & Behavior, 20, 501-505.

Glennon, R. A., & Young, R. (1984b). MDA: A psychoactive agent with dual stimulus effects. Life Sciences, 34, 379-383.

Glennon, R. A., Young, R., Anderson, G. M., & Rosecrans, J. A. (1982b). Discriminative stimulus properties of MDA analogs. Journal of Biological Psychiatry, 17, 807-814.

Glennon, R. A., Young, R., Benington, F., & Morin, R. D. (1982c). Behavioral and serotonin receptor properties of 4-substituted derivatives of the hallucinogenic 1-(2,5-dimethyloxyphenyl)-2-aminopropane. Journal of Medical Chemistry, 25, 1163-1168.

Glennon, R. A., Young, R., & Jacyno, J. M. (1983c). Indolealkylamine and phenalkylamine hallucinogens: Effect of -methyl and N-methyl substituents on behavioral activity. Biochemical Pharmacology, 32, 1267-1273.

Glennon, R. A., Young, R., Jacyno, J. M., Slusher, M., & Rosecrans, J. A. (1983d). DOM-stimulus generalization to LSD and other hallucinogenic indolealkylamines. European Journal of Pharmacology, 86, 453-459.

Glennon, R. A., Young, R., & Rosecrans, J. A. (1982d). A comparison of the behavioral effects of DOM homologs. Pharmacology Biochemistry & Behavior, 16, 557-559.

Glennon, R. A., Young, R., & Rosecrans, J. A. (1982e). Discriminative stimulus properties of DOM and several molecular modifications. Pharmacology Biochemistry & Behavior, 16, 553-556.

Haefely, W., Pieri, L., Polc, P., & Schaffner, R. (1981). General pharmacology and neuropharmacology of benzodiazepine derivatives. In F. Hoffmeister & G. Stille (Eds.), Psychotropic agents (Part II, pp. 13-262). New York: Springer-Verlag.

Silverman, P. B., & Ho, B. T. (1977). Characterization of discriminative response control by psychomotor stimulants. In H. Lal (Ed.), Discriminative properties of drugs (pp. 107-119). New York: Plenum Press.

Silverman, P. B., & Ho, B. T. (1978). Stimulus properties of DOM: Commonality with other hallucinogens. In F. C. Colpaert & J. A. Rosecrans (Eds.), Stimulus properties of drugs: Ten years of progress (pp. 189-198). Amsterdam: Elsevier/North Holland Biomedical Press.

Skolnick, P., & Paul, S. M. (1982). Benzodiazepine receptors in the central nervous system. International Review of Neurobiology, 23, 103-140.

Sternbach, L. H. (1973). Chemistry of 1,4-benzodiazepines and some aspects of the structure-activity relationships. In S. Garattini, E. Mussini, & L. O. Randall (Eds.), The benzodiazepines (pp. 1-26). New York: Raven Press.

Tallman, J. F., Paul, S. M., Skolnick, P., & Gallager, D. W. (1980). Receptors for the age of anxiety: Pharmacology of the benzodiazepines. Science, 207, 274-281.

Young, R., & Glennon, R. A. (1986) Discriminative stimulus properties of amphetamine and structurally related phenalkylamines. Medicinal Research Reviews, 6, 99-130.

Young, R., Glennon, R. A., & Rosecrans, J. A. (1981). Discriminative stimulus properties of the hallucinogenic agent DOM. Communication in Psychopharmacology, 4, 501-506.

Zbinden, G., & Randall, L. O. (1967). Pharmacology of benzodiazepines: Laboratory and clinical correlations. In S. Garattini & P. A. Shore (Eds.), Advances in pharmacology (Vol. 5, pp. 213-291). New York: Academic Press.

CHAPTER 19

TESTS INVOLVING PRESSING FOR INTRACRANIAL STIMULATION
AS AN EARLY PROCEDURE FOR SCREENING LIKELIHOOD OF ADDICTION[1]
OF OPIOIDS AND OTHER DRUGS

Larry D. Reid

Department of Psychology
Rensselaer Polytechnic Institute
Troy, New York   12181

ABSTRACT

On the basis that the medial forebrain bundle system of the
anterior brainstem is a major component of the system whose activity
is positive affect, it is submitted that any drug that would increase
activity in that system has a high risk of becoming the focus of an
addiction. When an increase in activity of that system is a
contingency of an act (such as imbibing, inhaling, snorting, or
injecting), then that act will occur more and more frequently (i.e.,
positive reinforcement occurs) and this is a basis for an addiction.
The potential for a drug to increase activity in the system is often
manifested by measuring the lever pressing of rats for a fixed
intensity of electrical stimulation of the system. Drugs, therefore,
can be screened for their addiction likelihood by observing their
effects on pressing for brain stimulation.

INTRODUCTION

Thirty years ago the first complete report (Olds & Milner, 1954) of
positive reinforcement from direct electrical stimulation of the brain was
published. We are still a little stunned by that revelation. We were and are
imbued with the idea that the brain is marvelously complicated. We are also
faced with mounting evidence that it is even more complicated then we imagined
(Snyder, 1980, for example, predicted over 200 neurotransmitters will be
discovered). Our own experience tells us that pleasure and reinforcement
processes are varied and subtle. Yet, a gross manipulation by way of

---

[1]The term "abuse liability" is extraordinarily confusing, particularly in the
context of this chapter. Discussing all of the problems with the term is
beyond the scope of this chapter. It will be sufficient to say here, first,
we are concerned with addiction liability. Second, the word liability has two
meanings: likelihood and debt. In this context, and perhaps the entire book,
it seems that we are attempting to assess addiction likelihood rather than
addiction debt or abuse (albeit a likely consequence of addiction).
Consequently, my topic is the use of procedures involving ICS in establishing
likelihood of addiction. In accordance with modern theory of addiction,
particularly opioid addiction (Smith & Lane, 1983), an addiction likelihood,
in turn, is strongly related to the potential for a drug to be positively
reinforcing.

stimulation with a macroelectrode can produce positive affect, and when there is a contingency, this can be reward or positive reinforcement. All that is necessary is to step down the house current to a level that does not destroy neural tissue and to direct it, in brief spurts, to any number of sites in the brain and positive affect is initiated. Furthermore, it seems that in all vertebrates (from samples as diverse as goldfish to human beings) an effect can be elicited by brain stimulation that maintains behavior for that stimulation (Heath, 1964; Olds, 1962).

When the possibility of positive intracranial reinforcement (ICR) was first announced, it was met, not surprisingly, with inordinate skepticism. That skepticism was extant even though the pioneering work of Hess had shown that intracranial stimulation (ICS) elicited a number of motivational and emotional sequences in freely moving animals. Since Olds used in his initial studies small experimental spaces with large manipulanda, it was suggested, for example, that the rats were not voluntarily pressing to get ICS but that they were merely being thrown on the manipulanda by ICS-elicited forced movements. Rats eventually ran mazes, crossed electrified grids, worked a variety of devices, and solved complex discrimination problems for ICS. So, it is no mere automatism that leads rats to work for ICS (Olds, 1962).

To observe ICR, subjects (usually rats) are fixed with chronically indwelling electrodes. The surgical procedures have become standard and electrodes and holders for electrodes are commercially available. In brief, all preparations involve putting wires into the brain so that electric current can stimulate a small amount of neural tissue making that tissue supra-active with respect to the rest of the brain in the freely moving subject.

The standard experimental space is a box similar to the one popularized by Skinner and colleagues. The rat is placed into a box that has a bar or lever extending through one wall. With depression of the lever, events can be programmed, such as delivery of food, water or ICS. Using such an experimental procedure, an extensive body of knowledge has been developed as variables, (e.g., degree of food deprivation and rate of food-delivery relative to lever-pressing) were manipulated. The effects of making ICS a contingency of lever-pressing, therefore, can be understood in the context of this extensive information.

At a site of ICS, intense or prolonged current flowing in one direction destroys neural tissue. The typical ICS, then, is low intensity current with alternating polarity. Even if, however, the current is set so as to not damage tissue, ICS is unambiguously positive only when it is of brief duration. So, the standard experimental arrangement is to put a rat in a box and program it so that a lever-press yields a train of pulsate current with alternating polarity of low intensity lasting 0.5 seconds or less (i.e., train duration = 0.5 seconds).

With ICS set at safe values and brief train durations, sites of ICS were varied while observing the subjects' responsiveness. With some sites rats do not learn to press for ICS. Using other experimental arrangements, it is possible to show that rats will work to avoid getting some ICS that was not positive. ICS, in a standard form, is either positive, neutral, or aversive in affective tone.

Sites of positive ICR differ. Once pressing has been established, the differences are made obvious by changing intensity or duration of ICS. Also, for some sites rats more readily accept experimenter-imposed, frequently

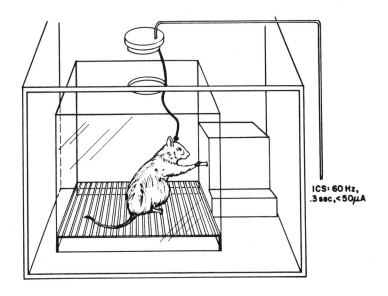

ICS: 60 Hz,
.3 sec,<50μA

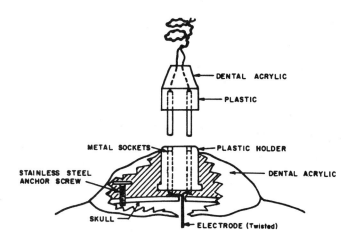

DENTAL ACRYLIC

PLASTIC

METAL SOCKETS — PLASTIC HOLDER

STAINLESS STEEL
ANCHOR SCREW — DENTAL ACRYLIC

SKULL — ELECTRODE (Twisted)

Figure 1: The typical arrangement for observing intracranial reinforcement.

occurring trains of ICS whereas at other sites they will respond to terminate the imposed ICS. Sites are classed a "pure positive" when the rat works to initiate ICS and does little to escape it when imposed and "ambiguous" when it both initiates and escapes the ICS (Olds, 1962). This classification is highly dependent on the ICS used in testing. The ICS at all sites can be made too intense, too frequent, or too prolonged for optimal acceptance by the subject.

We infer that the medial forebrain bundle (MFB) as it extends from the ventral midbrain through the lateral hypothalamus and lateral preoptic areas is particularly relevant to reinforcement processes because MFB ICS is often unambiguously positive. Rats emit many presses for hours each day for MFB ICS. With MFB sites the minimum intensity for eliciting pressing is low. Rats press for MFB ICS across an extensive range of features of the ICS itself (intensity, train duration, frequency of pulses, et cetera). And, rats do not escape imposition of MFB ICS across many variations of its imposition.

One general feature of the behavior emitted for ICS is that the rats work more for greater intensity (more accurately, microcoulombs) of ICS (Keesey, 1964; McIntire & Wright, 1965). For many MFB sites the relationship between rate of pressing and intensity of current is linear up to the point of neural damage. For other sites the function reaches an asymptote so that further increases in intensity produce no further increases in pressing or may even produce a decrease. Observations make it apparent why some rates of pressing may decrease at higher intensities; the higher intensity may elicit seizures or forced movements interfering with pressing.

It appears to be necessary to activate a rather large group of neurons and fibers to elicit ICR. The threshold for perception of ICS (i.e., intensity sufficient for a rat to use it as a conditional stimulus) is less than the intensity that will sustain a minimal rate of pressing. After the threshold for ICR is achieved, it seems that the recruitment of more and more activity in relevant tissue yields more and more intense positive affect which is manifested in greater rates of pressing. When eventually an intensity is reached that elicits activity leading to seizures or other side effects, the affective quality is diluted or the ability to press is hindered.

With the initial studies there were a number of observations indicating that ICR had some peculiar features. In contrast to the behavior of rats working for small bits of food, for example, it was concluded that when a delay was programmed between trains of ICS, operant behavior deteriorated. These peculiarities of ICR, compared to behavior following conventional reinforcement, became known as the anomalies of ICR and were provided in lists to support various theories (Deutsch & Howarth, 1963; Kimble, 1961).

Research on ICR involved an inspection of reputed anomalies (e.g., Reid, 1967). This research was a test, despite some limitations, of the general idea that certain ICS was indeed initiating activity ordinarily initiated by conventional reinforcers. Although it is impossible to prove an identity, the more the two kinds of reinforcers control behavior in the same way, the more confidence one has that they have considerable neural features in common. There is, of course, the obvious difference that one process follows ICS and one follows events such as eating or drinking. Also, with eating and drinking there is the eventual consequence of a full stomach that has no obvious match with ICR. Keeping these differences in mind, it seemed that if ICS was initiating the processes of reinforcement, then ICS should control behavior in nearly the same way as conventional reinforcers.

The first finding of the systematic inspection of the anomalies was that some were not apparent when ICR was from MFB stimulation. For example, on the basis of observations of cats, it was concluded that cats did not show good signs of ICR and, therefore, ICS was not activating a universal reinforcement system present in different species. We (Schnitzer, Reid, & Porter, 1965) merely placed electrodes so that the MFB was stimulated and found that cats worked very hard for ICS.

Also, direct comparisons were made between behavior maintained by food and water and that maintained by ICR. Prior to these experiments, the comparisons were made indirectly by comparing the behavior of rats working for ICR to the generalizations derived from studying rats working for conventional rewards. When rats press for food, the lever press activates a dispenser that delivers food in a dish usually slightly to the side of the lever. When rats pressed for ICS, the ICR was delivered with the depression of the lever. We (Reid & Porter, 1965) then arranged test conditions so that the lever press merely made it possible to get ICS at the dish that usually received food (i.e., the rat broke a photobeam across the dish to receive ICS). Under these comparable conditions of ways of delivering the two kinds of reinforcers and when the ICS was of the MFB, the behaviors maintained by ICS and by conventional reinforcers were indistinguishable in topography (e.g., Gibson, Reid, Sakai, & Porter, 1965).

Rats have been shown to work on periodic schedules of delivery of ICS, to show no peculiarities of extinction (Gibson et al., 1965), and to press without decrement even when intervals between opportunities to press are great (Hunsicker & Reid, 1974; Wasden, Reid, & Porter, 1965). The anomalies of ICR are related to two features: the site of ICS and the comparisons of performance after unequal tasks (Reid, 1967). The site of ICS is a major consideration. There are no gross anomalies of ICR with certain sites of ICS, namely those of the MFB.

Rats do show anomalies when tissue related to positive affect is activated concurrently with other tissue. This can be due to a slightly misplaced electrode or to features of the ICS such as high intensity, prolonged durations, or very brief surges in current that accompany generation of ICS by some stimulators. They perform like rats getting bitter food or food accompanied by low level foot shock. They show vacillation, performance decrements, rapid extinction, et cetera.

By observing when anomalies were and were not present, the features of the system became more defined. When ICS was exclusive to the MFB, anomalies were less apparent or were absent. Arrangements for the clearest cases of ICR supported the idea that activity of the MFB system was, indeed, an important element of the behavior of positive reinforcement.

More recent anatomical study of ICR has both expanded the borders of the MFB system and made more precise the cells and fibers of the system. It has become clear that among the critical tissues are dopaminergic neurons and processes (Wise, 1983). The MFB and adjacent tissue are places where dopaminergic fibers are reasonably densely packed (Jacobowitz & Palkovits, 1974), and ICR is achieved when ICS activates these dopaminergic elements (Wise, 1983).

There are other lines of converging evidence to support a conclusion that the MFB system with its components of dopaminergic cells and fibers is critical to positive affective processes. For example, reward and positive reinforcement procedures fail when the MFB system is debilitated (Wise, 1982a). Experiments showing that the rewards of prototypic addictive drugs have localized, critical effects within the MFB system are, of course, particularly germane (Bozarth, 1983; Wise, 1983). These lines of research have received extensive review and discussion (e.g., Wise, 1980; 1982b; 1983) and this is not the place to repeat them. What is controversial is whether or not the MFB system of dopaminergic elements is part of the brain's only system for expression of positive affect and the consequent events of positive reinforcement.

As the basic information of ICR accumulated, other events happened to produce an interest in the effects of psychotropic drugs on ICR. Most importantly, there was further confirmation of the idea that many, if not all, addictive drugs were taken for their positively reinforcing aspects (Deneau, Yanagita, & Seevers, 1969; Schuster & Thompson, 1969; Thompson & Schuster, 1964; Weeks, 1962).

If drugs of addiction are taken for their positively reinforcing effects and if the MFB system is the only system of positive affect, as retina, optic nerves and geniculate are exclusive to vision, then drugs of addiction must act, either directly or indirectly, on the MFB system. The problem of measuring addiction likelihood then becomes one of measuring drug-induced increases in that functional activity. The MFB system need not be, however, the only system of positive affect for measures of drug effects on the MFB system to be useful. The MFB system need only be a major part of the brain's apparatus for positive affect. A test drug that would increase MFB's functional activity would have high addiction likelihood. Along the same lines the ability of a drug to elicit positive affect need not be the only reason for a drug to be taken recreationally. All that is necessary is that the ability to elicit positive affect be a major component of the addiction syndrome.

I doubt if anyone will challenge the conclusion that the MFB system is a major component of the brain's apparatus for positive affect. (They may challenge the use of the term positive affect; however, they may substitute their favorite synonym without taking away from the conclusion.) I doubt if anyone will challenge in the 1980s that a drug's ability to be positively reinforcing is a major component of a drug's ability to become the focus of an addiction. Given this consensus, it follows that a drug increasing the functional activity of the MFB system is also a drug having high addiction likelihood. If the MFB system is not the only system of positive affect or if other factors besides the ability to elicit positive affect contribute to addiction likelihood, tests of functional activity of the MFB system may fail to index a drug's addiction likelihood. Although there is a consensus concerning the primary conclusions, such a consensus does not translate directly into tests of addiction likelihood. Many problematic theoretical and practical issues remain, some of which, but surely not all, are discussed here. The result is the recommendation of a test, involving drug-induced changes in pressing for ICS by rats, as an initial screening procedure for likelihood of addiction.

No one is satisfied with our current knowledge of the brain's apparatus of positive reinforcement. Little is known, for example, about the afferent patterns of activity that, in ordinary circumstances, set activity in the MFB system. Our lack of knowledge of the brain's apparatus for reinforcement limits all approaches to assessing addiction likelihood. This obvious point is stated because it seems to be a covert criticism of methods using ICS. Perhaps the limitations to our knowledge are merely more focused when considering ICR. This is an advantage rather than a disadvantage.

Although one may develop techniques for measuring the MFB's functional activity in preparations other than those involving behaving subjects (e.g., electrical recording; Nelsen & Kornetsky, 1972), measuring the behavior of subjects is likely to provide a more complete assessment of the relevant functional activity. This also follows from the realization that the MFB system itself is defined behaviorally as well as anatomically.

Two features of responsiveness for MFB ICS seem to index changes in functional activity: measures of threshold for elicitation of ICR and measures of work expended for a fixed intensity of ICS. For either of these indices of MFB activity to be a valid assessment of addiction likelihood, known addictive drugs must have common, systematic effects.

Initial results with the effects of addictive agents on pressing for ICS were confusing. Morphine decreased pressing but amphetamine, cocaine, and barbiturates increased it (Crow, 1970; Olds & Travis, 1960; Reid, Gibson, Gledhill, & Porter, 1964; Stein, 1962). Then, Adams, Lorens, and Mitchell (1972) reported that morphine was capable of increasing pressing. With reports verifying and extending that observation (Bush, Bush, Miller, & Reid, 1976; Holtzman, 1976; Koob, Spector, & Meyerhoff, 1975; Lorens & Mitchell, 1973; Marcus & Kornetsky, 1974; Pert, 1975), the idea was supported that drugs taken frequently for their recreational features by people share two properties. At some doses, these agents are self-administered by laboratory subjects and they facilitated responsiveness for rewarding ICS (Bozarth, 1978; Esposito & Kornetsky, 1978; Reid & Bozarth, 1978).

There were a number of questions concerning morphine's (the prototypic addictive agent) ability to increase pressing for ICS: (a) Was the increase a rebound from initial suppression of pressing? (b) Did the increase reflect morphine's ability to suppress aversive concomitants that could easily accompany ICS? (c) Did the facilitated pressing reflect some increment in positive affect or merely some increased propensity to be active? Each of these questions was addressed experimentally.

With large daily doses of morphine (e.g., 10 or 15 mg/kg/day), the period of facilitation moves forward and the initial depression of press rates wanes. Figure 2 depicts the effects of smaller doses of morphine on pressing for ICS. It is apparent that the effects of morphine, compared to baseline, are characterized by a triple interaction of dose by time after dosing by days of daily dosing (see Figure 3). A further factor is the rate of pressing at baseline. When press rates at baseline are low, the relative increment in pressing can be great. When press rates at baseline are high, there are ceiling effects.

The facilitated pressing is paralleled by a decrease in the lower threshold for ICR, a topic reviewed extensively by Esposito and Kornetsky (1978; Esposito, Porrino, & Seeger, this volume). Morphine shifts the rate of pressing to intensity of ICS function to the left (Esposito & Kornetsky, 1977). Such findings provide an important confirmation for the idea that morphine is increasing the effectiveness of the ICS.

The issue of tolerance to the facilitation effect has received considerable attention (Esposito & Kornetsky, 1978). It is clear that the facilitation in responsiveness to ICS shows nothing approaching complete tolerance (Esposito & Kornetsky, 1977). As daily dosing continues, there is clearly tolerance to the initial suppression (Adams et al., 1972; Bush et al., 1976).

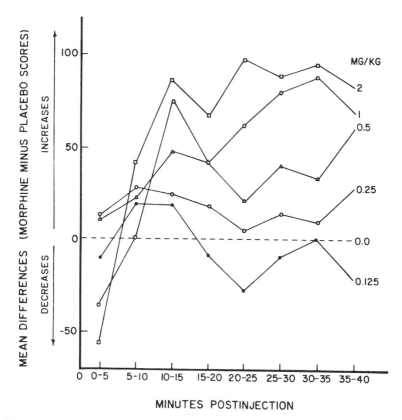

Figure 2: The effects of small doses of morphine on pressing for hypothalamic ICS.

There are a few remaining issues concerning tolerance of the facilitation effect. Quantifying the maximum extent of the facilitation is extraordinarily difficult, because the period of peak facilitation may differ with each dose. We do have enough comparisons to conclude that, in general, facilitation does not diminish much, if any, with repeated doses. In fact, peak effect may become larger with repeated doses.

Along the same lines we do not have enough data to judge whether the period of enhanced positive affect due to morphine actually becomes briefer with repeated doses. There are reasons to suppose it does. With repeated injections the period of facilitated pressing moves forward closer and closer to the time of injections. Withdrawal symptoms do emerge and the events of withdrawal do diminish pressing (Bush et al., 1976). So, with the advent of withdrawal and the movement of the period of facilitation forward, the net result may be that the period of positive affect is shorter.

The data with respect to tolerance provide the first good indication that morphine's ability to induce analgesia and positive affect are separable.

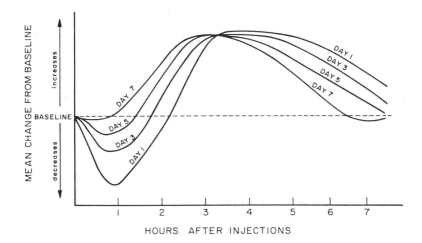

Figure 3: An attempt to depict the triple interaction of the effects of morphine, a standard large dose, on pressing for ICS. Reprinted with permission from Bozarth, 1978.

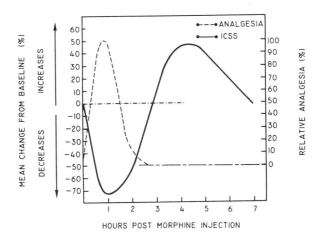

Figure 4: Comparison of time-effect relationship for analgesia and pressing for ICS induced by a single administration of morphine (10 mg/kg). The analgesia data are adapted from Hipps, Eveland, Meyer, Sherman, and Cicero, 1976, and Kayan, Woods, and Mitchell, 1971. The ICR data are extrapolated from Adams, Lorens, and Mitchell, 1972, and Bush, Bush, Miller, and Reid, 1976. Reprinted with permission from Bozarth, 1978.

Also, the time course of analgesia and positive affect (as indexed by pressing for ICS) are not the same (see Figure 4). There are also other kinds of evidence (to be summarized later) to indicate separation of morphine's potential for analgesia and positive affect. So, morphine probably does not facilitate responding for ICS because it reduces some aversive concomitant of ICS that may accompany it.

A direct test (Farber & Reid, 1976) of morphine's ability to affect positive affect independent of its analgesic properties was done by assessing morphine's ability to modify responding for positive ICS that was accompanied by a clearly aversive stimulus. Rats were fixed with two electrodes, one for stimulation of MFB and one for ICS that rats would escape. During one phase of testing, rats had only positive ICS as a contingency. During another phase rats had positive ICS followed immediately by aversive ICS as a single contingency of a lever press. Without drugs the programming of the aversive ICS reduced pressing compared to when only positive ICS was a contingency.

For 20 days rats pressed for positive ICS alone and for combinations of positive and aversive ICS following an injection of morphine. Morphine increased pressing for positive ICS as expected. After a few doses of morphine, morphine did not facilitate pressing for the combination of positive and aversive ICS. If morphine acted by way of diminishing aversiveness, just the opposite would be predicted.

From dose-response data and from data measuring pressing after self-administrated doses or after equivalent small doses (Collaer, Magnuson, & Reid, 1977; Gerber, Bozarth, & Wise, 1981; also, see Bermudez-Rattoni, Cruz-Morales, & Reid, 1983), it is concluded that the facilitated pressing is not a rebound from any initial suppression that may accompany larger doses. This conclusion is compatible with the idea that morphine-induced facilitation of pressing is due to morphine's ability to enhance activity in the MFB system. To confirm this notion an independent test of morphine's capability to produce positive affect was developed.

It was reasoned that if morphine was producing positive affect at the time it facilitated pressing for ICS, then that increment in positive affect should be manifested in some feature of the rat's behavior. If the rat experienced that positive affect in a distinctive place, there is a good possibility that the stimuli of that place would be associated (classically conditioned) to the positive affect and would come to have a positive valence. When given a choice between the place of the drug experience and another place, the subject would choose the place where it had experienced the drug.

Following this reasoning, rats were placed into one side of an alley while under the influence of morphine and, subsequently, were given the choice of being in that side or the other side (Rossi & Reid, 1976). The rats were confined to one side of the alley for conditioning at different times after injection of a large dose of morphine. Among the times chosen was the time that morphine readily facilitated pressing for ICS and times before and after morphine-facilitated pressing. The subjects receiving putative conditioning during the time when morphine facilitated pressing for ICS clearly spent more time on the side of the drug experience compared to rats given saline and treated the same way. Rats receiving putative conditioning at times when morphine did not produce clear signs of facilitated pressing did not show a conditioned preference for a side of the alley.

The test of morphine's ability to establish a preference for the place of a drug experience has come to be called the conditional place preference test (CPP test; Bozarth, this volume; van der Kooy, this volume). The test gave an independent verification that rats were experiencing something (positive affect) that established a preference for a place under the same dosing that facilitated pressing for ICS. Under dosing conditions that facilitate pressing for ICS, a CPP is established, the threshold for initiation of ICR is reduced, and the facilitation is difficult to explain by resorting to explanations other than those involving changing affective-reinforcing properties of ICS. Further, doses comparable to those that are self-administered produce facilitated pressing without an apparent interval of suppressed pressing. So, the conclusion is that morphine's ability to be positively reinforcing is manifested in a number of indices of the rat's behavior, including facilitating pressing for ICS.

TESTS OF ADDICTION LIKELIHOOD

It is one thing to come to the conclusion that a measure of responsiveness to ICS could be an index of addiction likelihood and another thing to devise a reliable, valid, practical test that, indeed, measures or reflects a functional change in reactivity of the MFB system. There are a large number of variables that can be manipulated within the context of assessing a drug's effect on responsiveness to ICS. There are the features of the ICS itself (such as waveform, intensity, train duration, pulse duration, frequency of pulses). There are the variables associated with the subject's performance, for example, difficulty of the task or high versus low rate-dependency tasks. There are, of course, subject variables such as species, gender, age, and drug and testing history. These and other procedural variables (e.g., drug doses) can be combined into a totally overwhelming set of combinations. It is safe to say that no drug will ever be assessed (even in one kind of rat) across all of the potential combinations of procedural variables. The task, then, is to select procedural variables rationally rather than arbitrarily. The rational choice from among this multitude of variables will be discussed in terms of each of the broad categories mentioned starting with the choice of subject.

One definite consideration is the ease and productivity of testing (Liebman, 1983). Any devised system has to be justified on the basis of its ability to screen a large number of drugs, because the medicinal chemists can and are devising more drugs (and, perhaps, food additives) than can be assessed behaviorally even with our most productive procedures. As we shall see, it is on the grounds of practicality that measures of responsiveness to ICR recommend themselves.

Subject Variables

The best predictor of a drug's addiction likelihood for an individual is knowledge concerning how the drug has been responded to by others. If a drug is taken repeatedly for its apparent recreational qualities by a large number of people, then the prediction is made, with some surety, that the drug is likely to be addicting for others. The whole purpose of procedures described in this book, however, is to avoid making the prediction in that way. At this stage, I do not believe anyone has serious objections to concluding that rats show enough of the features of the addiction syndrome seen with human beings to be adequate subjects for screening drugs for their addiction likelihood (e.g., see Collins, Weeks, Cooper, Good, & Russell, 1984; and the drug discrimination data summarized in Woolverton & Schuster, 1983).

Since addictions occur with both genders and across all ages, the choice of rats' gender and age will evidently be of little consequence. The typical, healthy, young adult, male rat has a number of practical features, such as those of price, ease of handling, and ready availability, that recommend its use. Given these considerations, the problem generates into how to use rats to predict addiction likelihood.

ICS Variables

In this context the interest is in testing drug effects rather than ICS effects. So, the problem is to select optimal features of ICS. The choices among ICS variables and among the tasks chosen to index responsiveness to ICS are discussed thoroughly by Liebman (1983). Since Liebman's goal was a discussion of techniques for doing research on the basis of ICR and mine is the more restrictive goal of screening drugs for addiction likelihood, this chapter may be considered an addendum to Liebman's excellent review.

Site of ICS

On the grounds that the MFB system is a major component of the brain's apparatus for positive affect and may even be the only critical part (All other sites of reinforcing ICS may lead to activity that feeds through the MFB or that is part of the field of MFB activity.), the sites of choice are those referred to as the MFB. Aiming an electrode tip to stimulate the anatomically defined MFB of the lateral, posterior hypothalamus has the advantage of aiming the tip toward a relatively large area. If the electrode tip should deviate from MFB itself and be in adjacent areas of the zona incerta or Forel's fields, it is of little consequence. These sites also sustain pressing for ICS without inordinate side effects and have been shown to be appropriately responsive to prototypic addictive agents. These sites also involve the fibers from the ventral tegmental-substantia nigra areas (the meso-limbic dopaminergic system) judged to be particularly relevant to the positive features of conventional rewards and abused drugs (Wise, 1983). This large area, fortunately, allows a high ratio of rats that press for ICS to those fixed with electrodes, a nice practical feature.

Although the size of the electrode's stimulating tip (the uninsulated portion of the indwelling wire) has not been systematically evaluated, it is known that a relatively large area of tissue needs to be stimulated to achieve ICR. An area of ICS which is too large, however, increases the possibility of stimulating tissue that is outside of the MFB system for reinforcement thereby producing side effects. Along the same lines bipolar electrodes provide a more discreet focus of stimulation than unipolar electrodes (Valenstein & Beer, 1961). The recommendation, then, is to use the smallest, commercially available, bipolar macroelectrode.

Waveform

The waveform must have the feature of alternating polarity to prevent neural damage. This has been achieved by using 60 Hz sine waves or by using biphasic square waves. Stimulators made by controlling house current are usually adequate and inexpensive. When devising a stimulator, care must be taken to avoid ground loops (such as those involving oscilloscopes) that can provide very brief but high intensity surges in current.

Duration of Train of ICS

Rats will press one lever to start a train of ICS and then press another to terminate it (Bower & Miller, 1958). There has been considerable research directed toward answering the question why do rats terminate initially positive ICS (see Liebman, 1983, for a review). Among the things to consider is that prolonged durations of ICS, even at low intensities, will destroy neural tissue (Becker & Reid, 1977). The evidence indicates that some feature of prolonged ICS yields aversiveness (Liebman, 1983). All places of positive ICS have extensive connections. Prolonged ICS must, therefore, eventually produce considerable "irrelevant" activity away from the site of ICS. That this other activity and its effects are not positive is, of course, very likely.

A drug-induced increase in the accepted duration of ICS is likely to reflect modification of the side effects. Wauquier, Gilbert, Clincke, and Franson (1983) concluded "There is no reason to sustain that keeping on the stimulation for long times, suggests that the rewarding effect becomes larger, but rather that rats are able to sustain prolonged stimulation which they normally escape because of the building up of aversiveness" (p. 161). It follows that if one wants to measure changes in positivity, only short durations of ICS should be used.

Rats work very well for low intensity ICS of 0.25 seconds, although self-selected durations are usually greater than 0.25 seconds. Since longer durations are apt to also produce aversive side effects, there is no reason to complicate measures of drug-induced changes in responsiveness for ICS by using longer trains of ICS.

Rats escape from places where frequent trains of ICS are delivered as they do prolonged trains. Although task variables are discussed subsequently, it is apparent that any task involving rats working for long durations of ICS or measuring their acceptance of frequently occurring ICS can measure both the positivity of the ICS and the aversiveness of side effects. Since the desire is to measure only changes in positivity, these tasks are inappropriate. If high intensities are used, then brief durations are even more critical. So, the recommendation is the use of low intensity ICS of 0.25 seconds (60 Hz sine waves).

Intensity of ICS

Using ICS of 60 Hz sine waves of 0.25 seconds, pressing for MFB ICS can be easily trained with intensities less than 50 microamperes. With MFB ICS lower thresholds for ICR are less than 15 microamperes. It is only after the introduction of higher intensities or longer durations (seconds rather than fractions of second) that lower thresholds climb beyond that limit. Press rates can be maintained after small lesions at the electrode tip with the use of higher intensities, but this increases the possibility of side effects. When one observes inverted U-shaped pressing-intensity functions, it is a reasonable assumption that the down turn in rates at the high intensities is due to the elicitation of unwanted side effects; hence, these intensities are to be avoided. Some investigators never seem to see low threshold levels, probably because the first intensity used produces a lesion. So, routine testing for a drug's effect on responding for ICS should use low intensity ICS.

Task Variables

The goal is to use some feature of rats' responsiveness to brief MFB ICS to index drug-induced changes in the functional activity of the MFB. A number of ways have been used. One way is to measure the lower threshold for the elicitation of ICR (see Esposito, Porrino, & Seeger, this volume). Another way is to measure the work a rat will engage to get a fixed ICS (i.e., all features of ICS remain the same across testing).

If a drug induces more work for a fixed ICS, the conclusion is that the drug has increased some feature of the activity initiated by the ICS making the ICS more potent. A standard way of indexing work among rats is lever pressing. The question comes down to whether drug-induced changes in lever pressing for a fixed ICS is, indeed, a reliable and practical method for assessing germane functional activity, and, if not, are there viable alternatives.

The issue is not with the reliability of the index of modification in press rates. The arrangement of rats pressing for ICS is relatively easy; consequently, many rats can be tested and the reliability of any resulting drug-induced modification in pressing is assessed by asking, in conventional ways and by using conventional standards, is the change in pressing statistically significant.

The potential confound between reward and performance is the major issue associated with the validity of conclusions made following drug-induced changes in lever pressing. When lever-pressing rates are decreased, it could be because the ICS is less effective or because the rat is debilitated. The procedures one has to engage to prove that decreases in behavioral output are due to decreased reward rather than alternative factors are too laborious for a standard screen of likelihood of addiction. There are, of course, research issues that demand such attention. Wise (1982a), for example, reviews the elaborate series of studies he and his colleagues have engaged to show that pharmacological blockage of dopaminergic systems reduces potential for reward as well as, or rather than, inducing motoric limitations. This work was necessary for development of a theory of the neurochemistry of affect but cannot be done as a routine screen for addiction likelihood.

When a test drug decreases pressing for ICS, no conclusion about its addiction likelihood can be reached. Morphine at some doses and chlorpromazine at many doses both decrease pressing and are different in addiction likelihood. Of course, morphine at other doses and times after dosing increases pressing. So, when a decrease in pressing is seen with a test drug, such a decrease calls for more tests with more doses. If the test involves rats working in sessions of an hour or more, a reasonable sample of behavior following drug administration can be taken. When a wide range of doses are used, particularly within the range of doses that do not produce obvious debility and are reputed to have therapeutic value, then there is a good opportunity to see any increases in pressing that may occur.

When a test drug produces no period of increased pressing across a wide range of doses, the conclusion of low potential for addiction is supported. Such a result, however, is not sufficient by itself to conclude with confidence that the test drug has low addiction likelihood, and it calls for other kinds of tests that are not so dependent on performance. The CPP test is recommended (Hunter & Reid, 1983).

The question might be raised that if one must test a drug eventually with the CPP test, then why not just use that test in the first place. The CPP test involves the arbitrary selection of length of the conditioning period and of the time after dosing of the conditioning period. On the grounds of the principle of delay of reinforcement gradient, it is clear that among the times to be tested is the time shortly after drug administration. This, however, provides only some guidance in selecting periods for conditioning and leaves an inordinate array of choices. A drug, for example, eliciting brief positive affect followed by aversiveness is one that will be difficult to assess in the CPP test. The conditioning period will have to be chosen, before the facts, to exclude the period of negative affect.

When a drug produces an increment in pressing for fixed (but selected) ICS, the conclusion is drawn that the drug has a likelihood of becoming the focus of an addiction. A drug could, however, increase pressing for reasons other than enhancing the potency of ICS. The probable reasons for an increment in pressing, besides the one associated with increased positive affect, fall into two categories: (a) increased arousal and (b) diminished side effects. There has also been critical commentary concerning press rates, themselves, as a measure. Each of these is discussed, in turn, beginning with the last criticism.

The criticism of the measure of rate of lever pressing is based evidently (on the basis of citations given) on the possibility that a rat may choose ICS of one site over that of another and that the chosen site, on occasion, will be pressed for less than the other site (Valenstein, 1964). That $\underline{A}$ is preferred to $\underline{B}$ by one assessment technique, however, says very little about whether or not $\underline{B}$ plus one is greater than $\underline{B}$. Since morphine, for example, will likely increase pressing for $\underline{A}$-ICS as well as $\underline{B}$-ICS, it is irrelevant that $\underline{A}$-ICS is preferred, under some circumstances, to $\underline{B}$-ICS. There are some potential difficulties in interpreting drug-induced increments in pressing, but these difficulties have little to do with the results of some preference testing.

That rates of pressing do not predict everything is surely a truism. Individuals work very hard, on occasion, for a less preferred reward. There are surely circumstances when a measure of work and a measure of choice lead to concordant conclusions. With careful experimental control these two measures can often be made concordant. The fact that they may not be perfectly concordant across tests involving different procedures, however, does not detract from the reliability or the validity of either measure.

To avoid the complications associated with the conclusion that a drug may decrease side effects rather than increase reward potential, the features of the test should be arranged to minimize side effects. As mentioned above, this is done by using low intensity, brief ICS. One should also eliminate rats for which ICS clearly elicits side effects.

As a further procedural variable, it may be desirable to use a variable interval schedule of ICS delivery. If the mean interval is only a few seconds, it is easy to train rats and obtain a steady rate of pressing that is maintained for long testing sessions. This choice of task also has the advantage that the maximum number of ICS, for a session, can be fixed. This eliminates the possibility of side effects occurring with too frequent ICS. The recommendation, then, is to use a lever-pressing task with brief, low intensity ICS delivered on a brief variable interval schedule.

Anticonvulsant drugs produce an increase in pressing for ICS (Reid, Gibson, Gledhill, & Porter, 1964). Evidently, an anticonvulsant drug can act to reduce some side effects of ICS by reducing the spread of activity leaving a more focused effect. In general, we expect drugs eliciting positivity to produce their greatest effect at low intensity. When they do not, alternative explanations seem more reasonable. Once again, the recommendation is to use ICS that is unlikely to elicit side effects such as seizures--low intensity, brief ICS of the MFB (Bogacz, Laurent, & Olds, 1965). If there are still questions concerning whether an increment in pressing is due to anticonvulsant activity, the drug can be tested with the CPP test. After tests with pressing for ICS, the doses and times after dosing are specified.

With the task of pressing for a fixed intensity of ICS, it has been suggested that there is an interpretational problem concerning whether the drug may be merely increasing nonspecific arousal (called incentive by Liebman, 1983) or whether the increases are due to increased reward potential. The screening of drugs for addiction likelihood is not such an issue, provided some care is taken in choosing the task. When there is a small lever in a relatively large box, as in standard experimental spaces, drugs such as morphine and amphetamine (at doses that would increase other measures of activity) do not increase lever pressing when the lever depression yields no ICS.

There is, of course, the possibility of arousal interacting with ICS-elicited processes to produce an increase in pressing. It makes little difference, however, whether a drug-induced increase is due to the interaction or due to only increasing reward potential. A drug doing either has a risk of addiction likelihood. An advantage of the task of pressing for ICS is that it allows for the interaction to be made manifest. A drug, for example, that would increase the basal activity of the MFB system associated with the natural rewards of eating and sexuality is apt to be taken often. Also, in many cases, it may be impossible to separate arousal from reward; rewards by their nature are arousing and have other incentive qualities (Iversen, 1983).

There has been considerable discussion (Liebman, 1983) of using simplified operants (such as nose poking) rather than lever pressing as the task. The reasoning is that simplified tasks are less likely to be disrupted by side effects of ICS or drugs. When a drug reduces any operant, more testing is demanded. There seems to be no inordinate advantage to using simplified operants (Liebman, 1983). Some of the suggested tasks are so novel that considerable research would have to be done to provide an adequate basis for interpreting results (Liebman, 1983).

One can use pressing for ICS to measure thresholds by varying the intensity of ICS and by determining the lowest intensity maintaining pressing. The intensity that produces half of maximum press rates can also be determined. Such testing, however, involves using shortened sessions or an inordinate number of sessions or rats. An advantage of using pressing for a single intensity is that it can easily sample a drug effect across time. Prolonged testing with a range of doses is apt to index any facilitation that may occur. If an increment in pressing is observed, then further testing for threshold will add meaningful data.

There are threshold tracking procedures that allow a continuous sampling of threshold across an extended period. In one situation, two levers are available. Each press of one lever provides ICS and sets the intensity for the next ICS at a lower value. Depression of the other lever resets the intensity to the highest level on the first lever. Rats do press the ICS lever until some low value is reached, then press the reset lever, and again press the ICS lever (Stein & Ray, 1960). The intensity of reset is then monitored with and without drug. The procedure is valuable and was used effectively to show heroin's ability to lower threshold (Bozarth, Gerber, & Wise, 1980). Judgments from this test should be concordant, in most instances, with tests involving pressing for a fixed ICS. Since pressing for a fixed ICS is simpler and since there are unknown complications with threshold tracking (such as the effects of test drug on tendency to perseverate in unrewarding tasks), it seems that there is no marked superiority of this threshold-tracking procedure to those measuring pressing for fixed ICS.

An inspection of some of the myriad variables that may affect the decision of whether or not a drug increases activity in the MFB system leads to the recommendation of using a test involving (a) rats, (b) brief, low intensity MFB ICS, and (c) a lever-pressing task with a short variable interval schedule of delivery of ICS. A drug-induced increment in pressing, under such circumstances, leads to the judgment of risk of addiction. A decrease or no change in pressing leads to the judgment of little or no risk, but that judgment has to be qualified and tested further.

The following procedures are recommended as an economical way of screening novel drugs for addiction likelihood. Among the first tests should be the drug's effects on pressing for ICS. Such tests should follow the procedural guides given and should involve lengthy testing sessions beginning just after drug administration. A wide range of doses should be tested including, of course, a range of reputed therapeutic doses. Because of the test's economics, this is manageable. If a drug increases pressing for a fixed MFB ICS, the judgment is made that it has a risk of becoming the focus of an addiction. To verify that likelihood, other tests can be performed such as a self-administration test or CPP test. The data from the tests with ICS, however, provide guides, which are difficult to derive in other ways, for selection of doses and other procedural variables to use in these other tests.

A drug producing no increment in pressing for ICS has an unknown addiction likelihood. With doses that interfere with ability to bar press, the next test of choice is probably the CPP test, a test that is not dependent upon an animal's ability to move with coordination. Any dose and time after dosing that may appear to be eliciting increments in pressing for ICS, but do not produce large effects, should be assessed in the CPP test.

I submit that measures of responsiveness to ICS are highly sensitive. The CPP test is limited by the necessity to choose before the facts the period of drug-elicited positive affect. The self-administration test is limited by a number of features including its lack of productivity and the necessity to choose doses before the fact. If productivity of self-administration tests is enhanced by using animals already trained to self-administer drugs, mixed agonist-antagonists may produce withdrawal sickness that masks the potential for positive affect (Hunter & Reid, 1983). Measures of responsiveness to ICS, because of their relative ease, can use drug-naive (or nearly drug-naive) subjects with many doses and with measures extending considerably beyond the time after injection. This feature allows the test to index potential for positive affect across a considerable range of variables of drug. With pressing for a low intensity, brief ICS, a very small increment in current can produce marked increases in pressing. Because the test can be sensitive to small increments in elicitation of positive affect and can index such small increments with a variety of doses and times after dosing, the screen is very sensitive. Tests with ICS, for example, would have predicted the likelihood of addictions to commonly used benzodiazepines (Kamei, Yoshinobu, & Schimizu,

1974; Lorens & Sainati, 1978; M. Olds, 1966; 1970).

A highly sensitive test may not be desirable from the view of a manufacturer of drugs. A drug with therapeutic potential for widely occurring disorders such as minor pain, hypertension, obesity, or anxiety and having a low but reliable ability to elicit positive affect with few deleterious side effects (including few withdrawal signs merely because it is not metabolized rapidly) will, if marketed, produce high sales and profits. The use of a highly sensitive test, or group of tests, for likelihood of addiction can surely lead to limiting sales. This is not the place to discuss the issues of management of risk, only the measurement of risk. If the most sensitive tests are not used, however, measurement of risk is bypassed and management of risk is impossible.

PLEASURE AND SPECIFICITY OF EFFECTS OF ICS AND DRUGS

I started with the premise that the MFB system is a major component of the brain's apparatus for pleasure in order to discuss the procedural variables of a test for addiction likelihood. Considerations of those procedural variables, in turn, bring to focus a number of issues concerning the specificity of both ICS and drugs with respect to their ability to induce positive affect or pleasure.

As stated, the MFB system is defined behaviorally as well as anatomically. The MFB system is the system involving elements of or near the MFB, the stimulation of which yields the most unambiguous instances of positive reinforcement. It does not follow from this working definition, however, that the MFB system is homogenous with respect to neurochemical coding or with respect to kinds of pleasure. Smith, Co, and Lane (1984), for example, postulate two reinforcement systems in brain with a variety of relevant neurotransmitters. Interestingly, ICS of the lateral hypothalamic MFB could easily set up relevant activity in both postulated systems (Yardin, Guarini, & Gallistel, 1983). Nevertheless, the advances to be made involve further specification of the relevant tissue and chemical coding. Recent studies lead to the possibility of remarkable specificity of certain opioids for inducing pleasurable affect.

Because all parts of the brain are connected, supra-activity in one part must eventually lead to activity in other parts. This basic feature puts a definite upper limit on the pleasure that can be derived by activating the central circuits, including pharmacological activation. Eventually, specific activity, if intense, has to "spill over" into circuits mediating other events, including negative affect, thereby diluting any elicited pleasure. There also could be activity elicited in the cardiovascular system, gut, muscle, or glands whose activity, in turn, could produce negative feedback (Sakai, Reid, & Porter, 1965). It is for this basic reason that brief duration, moderate intensity ICS is recommended above.

By definition, pleasure is not ambiguous and there can never be too much pleasure (Young, 1967). Experiences involving pleasure can be ambiguous and there surely can be too much of the circumstances initially eliciting pleasure. There are limitations to the achievement of pleasure. The very system (the reward system or pleasure systems) is self-limiting, because it is part of the larger system (brain). Since a number of sites of ICS sustain inordinately high rates of pressing for prolonged times and since the rate-of-pressing to intensity-of-ICS function is linear up to the point of damaging the tissue at the electrode's tip, it seems that the pleasure system's capacity is great.

It is equally clear, however, that driving the system with prolonged trains of ICS, or driving the system with frequent trains, leads to events that rats avoid. Although stimuli that ordinarily are aversive will apparently dampen the positive affect of a fixed ICS (Buckwalter, Gibson, Reid, & Porter, 1967) and although there is probably a gross reciprocal relationship between the systems of pleasure and pain (Miller, Reid, & Porter, 1967), there is no reason to believe that every positive ICS elicits a negative event or dampens the possibility for pleasure of the next ICS, as suggested by Solomon and Corbit (1974). The situation seems much simpler. The limitations to pleasure are related to the system's capacity to be active without engendering supra-normal activity in other systems (manifested by seizures, by forced movements, by high autonomic efferent activity, by preference for brief trains of ICS, et cetera in self-stimulating rats). The limitations to pleasure are due to "spill over."

Since toxic and other side effects are more probable with increasing doses of drugs and since a dose is eventually reached that will produce sickness, coma, or death, large doses of any putative euphorigen will elicit ambiguous effects. It is not surprising, therefore, that large doses of many drugs having some claim to being euphorigens can be used as an unconditioned stimulus for a conditioned aversion to tastes serving as a conditional stimulus (Riley & Baril, 1976). It is also easy to predict that it will be possible to establish conditioned place aversions with drugs having euphorigenic capabilities using the procedures of the CPP test.

The limitation to the development of "pure" euphorigenic drugs (drugs that, until large doses are given, produce unambiguous states) is the specificity of the brain's chemical coding for pleasure. If drug X interacts with chemical system M and if chemical system M has as its only function the transmission of information that is positive affect, then drug X is apt to be a pure euphorigen. If, however, chemical M is part of the information processing of a number of systems, then a drug mimicking the actions of M will produce increments in positive affect and other effects. Since we are finding, for example, that the endogenous opioid systems are extensive and subserve many functions, a drug mimicking the activity of all endogenous opioids has little chance of being a pure euphorigen. Stated another way, if there is an exclusive chemical code in brain for pleasure (or a type of pleasure), then there is a possibility for the development of a pure euphorigen. If a number of pleasures are mediated by a single neurochemical system and if this neurochemical code is exclusive to pleasure systems, then there is a possibility of devising not only a pure euphorigen but also one of extraordinary potency. As related later, there is a possibility for considerable specificity with respect to the brain's opioid systems.

There is an implication to this line of thinking that is at variance with conventional wisdom. In as much as side effects are a major limitation to addiction likelihood and in as much as withdrawal symptoms are side effects, it follows that presence of withdrawal (and of tolerance) is a major limitation to addiction likelihood. From this view heroin is used despite the eventuality of withdrawal, not because of the eventuality of withdrawal. Heroin's long-term, dire consequences, in terms of withdrawal, function as only a weak controller of behavior, as remote consequences do for almost any act (Casper & Reid, 1975; Miller, Reid, & Porter, 1967). A compound that will be self-administered by animals and that is free from the side effects of withdrawal could have, I submit, a greater addiction likelihood than a similar compound readily producing discernible withdrawal symptoms. Along these lines cocaine is apparently more popular than heroin.

It also follows from this line of thinking that a high propensity for withdrawal is as likely to predict limitations on recreational drug use as it is to predict sustained drug use. Also, calling tests of withdrawal potential "a test for dependence" is flawed on the same grounds. Nothing is gained by renaming tests for withdrawal symptoms "tests for physical dependence liability." Actually, considerable precision is lost.

We now know that three genes produce large peptides whose cleavage can yield up to 18 smaller peptides whose actions are similar to one or more actions of morphine and whose effects are antagonized by naloxone. The location of some of the cells producing these endogenous opioid peptides (EOPs) is concentrated in subcortical forebrain and there are widespread connections throughout brain. EOPs interact with specialized receptors in neuronal membranes. There is probably more than one kind of opioid receptor (opioceptor).

The knowledge that the brain has extensive EOP systems provides the basis for a more complete understanding of the actions of morphine, heroin, and related opioids, including their ability to engender signs of positive affect. Morphine has many actions, only some of which are related to its addictive potential. Relatedly, only some parts of the extensive EOP systems are related to positive affect. Only a few of the EOPs have been screened in tests similar to those recommended for assessing addiction likelihood. We can anticipate that future research will delineate the parts of the EOP system that provide information processing relevant to modulation of positive affect, including specification of the EOPs and opioceptors that are involved. All of the methodological issues discussed in this chapter (and, indeed, in this book) are relevant.

As mentioned, there is a possibility for considerable specification of opioids' effects, and this is more likely given that there are many EOPs and opioceptors. There is, however, another topic to be discussed before considering the specificity of opioids--the topic of naloxone's effects on responding for ICS. Naloxone is the prototypic antagonist at the opioceptor. Since naloxone is reputed to have, at doses most often used, no agonist action at opioceptors and no actions at other receptors, the effects of naloxone would, therefore, reveal the functions of the EOPs (Goldstein, 1978). Belluzzi and Stein (1977) reported that administration of naloxone led to substantial reductions in pressing for ICS in rats having had no other drugs. They inferred from their observations that EOPs were major transmitters of reward processes.

Our attempts to replicate Belluzzi and Stein (1977), as well as other attempts (e.g., Lorens & Sainati, 1978; van der Kooy, LePiane, & Phillips, 1977) did not succeed. In some of our tests (Bozarth & Reid, 1977), naloxone, by itself, appeared to have no reliable effects. We then explored with Drs. Stein and Belluzzi the reasons for the apparently conflicting results. We were then using rats pressing at high rates for optimal intensities and short, periodic testing sessions (3 to 5 minutes), while they had rats pressing at low to moderate rates for intensities just above threshold and for longer (30 to 45 minutes) testing sessions. We then started using longer testing sessions and saw slight, but statistically significant, decreases in pressing (Stapleton, Merriman, Coogle, Gelbard, & Reid, 1979).

As mentioned, drug-induced reductions in pressing are difficult to interpret. Before more facts are gathered, however, there is no reason to suppose that naloxone would change a rat's capacity to press. Naloxone may modify rats' responsiveness in other testing situations (e.g., Amir, Solomon, & Amit, 1979); presumably, however, that is due to naloxone modifying motivational and emotional variables (Reid & Siviy, 1982) and not due to naloxone interfering with rats' ability to move with full vigor and coordination. The decreases in pressing for ICS are in situations where the likelihood of seizures and of other interfering side effects is low (i.e., the decreases are seen with low intensity, brief ICS). Also, naloxone does not appear to induce convulsions until extremely high doses are given (Breuker, Dingledine, & Iversen, 1976; Pearl, Aceto, & Harris, 1968). Nevertheless, interpretational problems remain and testing with other procedures is, as we shall see, helpful.

Reliable reductions in pressing rates for ICS under naloxone have been reported for sites within the periaqueductal gray area, area of the lateral hypothalamus (MFB, zona incerta, Forel's fields), accumbens nucleus, substantia nigra-ventral tegmental area, locus coeruleus area, nucleus paratenialis of the thalamus, amygdala, and prefrontal cortex (Belluzzi & Stein, 1977; Bermudez-Rattoni, Cruz-Morales, & Reid, 1983; Cruz-Morales & Reid, 1980; Franklin & Robertson, 1982; Stapleton, 1979; Stein, 1978). There is variability in the extent of reductions across rats with similar placements. Some rats (sites) show very small reductions (about 5% reductions) after large doses, whereas others show much more substantial reductions (upwards to 60%) with a modal reduction of about 20% (Stapleton, 1979). Differences in baseline rates of pressing can probably account for some of this variance. There has not been adequate study of the exact density of opioceptors and the extent of naloxone's effects. There have been few sites tested that have few or no EOP processes. There is no apparent correlation between sites producing analgesia and the extent of the naloxone effect on pressing for ICS (Franklin & Robertson, 1982; Stapleton, 1979).

There is the interesting report of Glick, Weaver, and Meibach (1982) that does specify a relationship between site of ICS and the extent of a naloxone effect. They reported that naloxone's effects are lateralized (i.e., naloxone reduces pressing on the side of the hypothalamus with lower threshold for reward and increases pressing on the side with higher threshold). Thresholds, in this case, were determined by pressing rates in 4-minute sessions with varying intensities of ICS. Given that a 4-minute session is not optimal for seeing a naloxone effect, any potential reductions to be seen with the side of higher threshold may have been missed. Nevertheless, the conclusion is still valid that one side of the hypothalamus may be more sensitive than the other.

Although a full range of doses of naloxone have not been tested with every site, there have been rather extensive testing with lateral hypothalamic sites. Naloxone reliably reduces pressing in doses of 1.25 mg/kg or greater. Within the range of 1 to 60 mg/kg, there are greater reductions with greater doses (references given above). We have recently collected more dose-response data with naloxone and pressing for lateral hypothalamic ICS. We find that doses of 0.1 mg/kg produce about a 30% reduction in pressing, doses of 1.0 mg/kg produce very small or no reduction in pressing, doses greater than 1.25 mg/kg produce about 30% reductions. It seems from the extant results that the dose-response curve is not uniform. This observation has implications for assessing the role of the various EOPs in mediating positive affect.

The naloxone effect on pressing for hypothalamic ICS is not apparent when the testing session is 3 minutes or shorter, is apparent when the session is 5 minutes, and presumably is even more apparent in sessions approaching an hour (Belluzzi & Stein, 1977; Stapleton, 1979). The situation is similar to naloxone's effects on reducing intake of water and food. In water-deprived rats presented water, naloxone does not reduce latency to begin drinking (Cooper & Holtzman, 1983; Siviy, Calcagnetti, & Reid, 1982). It is as if naloxone blocked an action involved in maintaining drinking as it approached the point of satiety. Naloxone has similar effects on eating.

Pressing for ICS is notable because it seemingly does not show quick satiation. In rats with constant access to ICS, however, the median burst of responding is 2.9 minutes with 20 to 60 of these episodes occurring nightly (Katz, 1980). If naloxone reduced each episode a small amount, then the result would be no apparent reduction with short sessions and an effect with longer sessions.

Naloxone does not lead to abolition of responding; it reduces responding rather uniformly across a session (Stapleton, 1979). The resulting pattern is not one of extinction but is more similar to the effect of reducing intensity of ICS a small increment. The conclusion is that the circuitry of EOPs is not critical to elicitation of ICS-produced reward but functions synergistically with other more critical neurotransmitters (Stapleton et al., 1979).

Using a discrete trial procedure, Perry, Esposito, and Kornetsky (1981) did not observe that naloxone lowered the threshold for ICR. Such testing just does not allow for a sample of behavior for which naloxone is likely to have an effect. It is similar to circumstances of drinking (Siviy et al., 1982). If one only observes drinking prior to the approach of satiation under naloxone, then no naloxone effect is apparent.

The reductions following naloxone can be interpreted as a decrease with respect to performance (Franklin & Robertson, 1982) or as a decrease in reward potential (Belluzzi & Stein, 1977; Stapleton et al., 1979). The resolution is to do further testing. Mucha and Iversen (1985) have tested for naloxone's effects in the CPP test. They found that naloxone produced no signs of a preference and actually led rats to spend less time in the place of the drug experience. These results need to be interpreted in the light of Pilcher, Jones, and Browne's (1982) finding that naloxone's ability to condition a taste aversion varied with the circadian cycle. Nevertheless, naloxone's effects are likely due to reduction in affective tone rather than ability to press.

The results with naloxone present an interesting case study demonstrating the limitations of any one procedure and the value of multiple kinds of tests. The reductions in pressing needed to be assessed further to segregate performance from reward. The pressing for ICS in more lengthy test sessions, however, did reveal an interesting drug effect: Naloxone effects were apparent only after the rats had pressed for a number of ICS. The temporal locus of the naloxone effect provides the basis for understanding why the discrete trial testing procedures for threshold yielded a conclusion of no effect of naloxone. The effects of large doses of naloxone on responding for ICS, water, and food do support the idea that one or more of the EOPs are involved with reward processes.

Many addictive agents may increase activity with respect to EOPs; they could mimic one or more EOPs at the receptor or could lead to a release of EOPs. Since naloxone by itself reduces pressing for ICS and establishes an aversion in the CPP test, naloxone cannot be used to assess the involvement of

EOP systems in the reward potential of other drugs. If a test drug produces an increment in pressing for ICS and then if naloxone is given thereby reducing pressing, the reduction may be due only to naloxone's effects (or an interaction involving naloxone's effects). Other ways must be devised to assess the involvement of opioceptors and EOPs in the reward potential of drugs such as diazepam and ethanol. Along these lines it has been shown that morphine produces an increment in pressing for ICS by way of its interaction with a specific opioceptor. Weibel and Wolf (1979) have shown that only one enantiomer of the basic morphine molecule will increase pressing for ICS.

The effects of naloxone are relatively nonspecific with respect to kinds of opioreceptor; in fact, naloxone's ability to antagonize an action of an agent is the defining characteristic for the action and the agent to be classed as opioid. So, naloxone is not the drug of choice for delineating the specificity in the actions of opioids. Other antagonists and mixed agonists-antagonists, however, do seem to show marked specificity.

Naltrexone is very similar to naloxone in structure and in action but is more resistant to degradation. An unpublished study (Merriman & Reid) revealed, however, that naltrexone's effects were more variable than naloxone's. Under naltrexone some rats' press rates were not reliably modified, some were depressed, and some even increased. This finding is similar to that recently reported by Katz (1981).

WIN 44,441 antagonizes the analgesia of some opioids and acts as an antagonist in various bioassays (Ward, Pierson, & Michne, 1983). WIN 44,441 antagonized the depressive actions of large doses of morphine in rats pressing for ICS. WIN 44,441, by itself, leads to reliable increases in pressing (Bermudez-Rattoni et al., 1983).

Diprenorphine is a remarkably potent antagonist for many of morphine and other opioid's effects. We confirmed that doses and times after dosing to be used, subsequently, completely antagonize the analgesia produced by fentanyl (a short acting but powerful opioid analgesic). Using doses that antagonize analgesia (and many other effects of morphine), it was found that diprenorphine facilitated pressing for MFB ICS with doses in the range of 1 to 5 µg/kg (Hunter & Reid, 1983; Pollerberg, Costa, Sherman, Herz, & Reid, 1983).

In summary, naloxone at doses above 1.25 mg/kg decreases pressing. Naltrexone's effects are variable. WIN 44,441 stereoselectively and dose-relatedly increases pressing. Diprenorphine increases pressing and is capable of producing a CPP (Beaman, Hunter, & Reid, 1984). Nalorphine, a compound that has antagonist actions with respect to precipitating withdrawal but also produces analgesia, increases pressing. Other mixed agonist-antagonists and agonists can facilitate pressing for ICS, but their analgesic potency does not correlate well with ability to facilitate pressing for ICS (Bozarth, 1978; Sandberg & Segal, 1978). The ability to facilitate pressing for ICS is unrelated to ability to induce analgesia. In fact, two compounds that clearly antagonize opioid analgesia (WIN 44,441 and diprenorphine) produce strong facilitation in pressing.

The case for the separation of opioid analgesia and opioids' ability to elicit signs of positive affect is very strong. There is tolerance with respect to analgesia but not with respect to facilitation in responsiveness to ICS (Bush et al., 1976; Esposito & Kornetsky, 1978). The time course of analgesia and increments in pressing following morphine differ (see Figure 4). Morphine increases pressing for positive ICS alone but not (after a few doses)

- 413 -

positive and negative ICS given as single contingency for pressing (Farber & Reid, 1976). Morphine is not self-administered intracranially at some sites clearly related to analgesia but is at other sites (Bozarth, 1983). Antagonists of analgesia facilitate pressing for ICS (Bermudez-Rattoni et al., 1983; Pollerberg et al., 1983). These observations are all compatible with the idea that opioid analgesia and an opioid's ability to elicit positive affect are not two facets of the same process.

Some of the more recently developed measures of drug-induced positive affect in the laboratory (i.e., responsiveness to ICS, the CPP test, and intracranial self-administration) have led to the conclusion that opioid analgesia, tolerance, withdrawal symptoms, and catatonia are separable, both anatomically and functionally, from opioids' capability of inducing positive affect. As long as most tests for opioids' specific actions were in preparations that obviated measures of positive affect (e.g., bioassays involving muscle strips, spinal dogs, binding properties of opioids in brain homogenates), there was no reason to devise systems having a specific category for positive affect.

Now that we have measures of opioids' ability to elicit positive affect, classificatory systems of opioid's specific actions can be modified to take into account that facet of the collective actions of nonspecific opioids such as morphine. Any new classificatory system should be built taking into account what is now known about the EOP systems and the idea of multiple kinds of opioceptors. It has been suggested that a particular opioreceptor type might be exclusive to the system of opioid-induced positive affect (Pollerberg et al., 1983). Such a receptor may be particularly responsive to the agonist properties of diprenorphine. Such a possibility leads to the idea that agents can be devised having remarkable specificity with respect to eliciting positive affect.

We have barely begun to assess the implications of the possibility of specificity of chemical coding for pleasure and the inherent possibility of developing euphorigens having few other effects. Measures of addiction likelihood can be used to devise new, subtle, potent euphorigens. One question is whether measures of addiction likelihood will be widely used to manufacture and to market new addictive agents or used to prevent such potentially profitable marketing.

ACKNOWLEDGMENTS

Some of the early work reviewed here was supported by grants from the National Institute on Drug Abuse and subsequent work by a grant from the Health Research Council of the State of New York. I thank the students currently working with me for their work and general encouragement--Carol Beaman, Laura Dunn, Chris Hubbell, and, particularly, George A. Hunter. Jean Bestle and Betty Osganian provided clerical support and helped in many ways, and I appreciate their efforts.

This is the year of retirement of my major professor, Prof. Paul B. Porter. I sincerely wish that I had something more eloquent than this chapter to honor the occasion of his retirement. I have learned, by having students of my own, that professors have only limited effects on the eventual work of their students. So, Paul cannot be held accountable for any foolishness contained here. With that caveat, I dedicate this chapter to the occasion of Prof. Porter's retirement.

REFERENCES

Adams, W. J., Lorens, S. A., & Mitchell, C. L. (1972). Morphine enhances lateral hypothalamic self-stimulation in the rat. Proceedings of the Society of Experimental Biology and Medicine, 140, 770-771.

Amir, S., Solomon, R., & Amit, Z. (1979). The effect of acute and chronic naloxone administration on motor activation in the rat. Neuropharmacology, 18, 171-173.

Beaman, C., Hunter, G. A., & Reid, L. D. (1984). Diprenorphine, an antagonist of opioid-analgesia elicits a positive affective state in rats. Bulletin of the Psychonomic Society, 22, 354-355.

Becker, B. M., & Reid, L. D. (1977). Changes in pressing for intracranial stimulation (ICS) after prolonged ICS. Physiological Psychology, 5, 58-62.

Belluzzi, J. D., & Stein, L. (1977). Enkephalin may mediate euphoria and drive-reduction reward. Nature, 266, 556-558.

Bermudez-Rattoni, F., Cruz-Morales, S., & Reid, L. D. (1983). Addictive agents and intracranial stimulation (ICS): Novel antagonist and agonists of morphine and pressing for ICS. Pharmacology Biochemistry & Behavior, 18, 777-784.

Bogacz, J., Laurent, J., & Olds, J. (1965). Dissociation of self-stimulation and epileptiform activity. Electroencephalography & Clinical Neuro-Physiology, 19, 75-87.

Bower, G. H., & Miller, N. E. (1958). Rewarding and punishing effects from stimulating the same place in the rat's brain. Journal of Comparative and Physiological Psychology, 51, 669-674.

Bozarth, M. A. (1978). Intracranial self-stimulation as an index of opioid addiction liability: An evaluation. Unpublished master's thesis, Rensselaer Polytechnic Institute, Troy, NY.

Bozarth, M. A. (1983). Opiate reward mechanisms mapped by intracranial self-administration. In J. E. Smith & J. D. Lane (Eds.), Neurobiology of opiate reward mechanisms (pp. 331-359). Amsterdam: Elsevier/North Holland Biomedical Press.

Bozarth, M. A., Gerber, G. J., & Wise, R. A. (1980). Intracranial self-stimulation as a technique to study the rewarding properties of drugs of abuse. Pharmacology Biochemistry & Behavior, 13(Suppl. 1), 245-247.

Bozarth, M. A., & Reid, L. D. (1977). Addictive agents and intracranial stimulation (ICS): Naloxone blocks morphine's acceleration of pressing for ICS. Bulletin of the Psychonomic Society, 10, 478-480.

Breuker E., Dingledine R., & Iversen, L. L. (1976). Evidence for naloxone and opiates as GABA antagonists. British Journal of Pharmacology, 120, 458.

Brown, D. R., & Holtzman, S. E. (1981). Suppression of drinking by naloxone in the rat: A further characterization. European Journal of Pharmacology, 69, 331-340.

Buckwalter, M. M., Gibson, W. E., Reid, L. D., & Porter, P. B. (1967). Combining positive and negative intracranial reinforcement. Journal of Comparative and Physiological Psychology, 65, 329-331.

Bush, E. D., Bush, M. F., Miller, M. A., & Reid, L. D. (1976). Addictive agents and intracranial stimulation: Daily morphine and lateral hypothalamic self-stimulation. Physiological Psychology, 4, 79-85.

Casper, N. J., & Reid, L. (1975). Complex contingencies. Physiological Psychology, 3, 9-13.

Collaer, M. L., Magnuson, D. J., & Reid, L. D. (1977). Addictive agents and intracranial stimulation (ICS): Pressing for ICS before and after self-administration of sweetened morphine solutions. Physiological Psychology, 5, 425-428.

Collins, R. J., Weeks, J. R., Cooper, M. M., Good, P. I., & Russell, R. R. (1984). Prediction of abuse liability of drugs using IV self-stimulation by rats. Psychopharmacology, 82, 6-13.

Cooper, S. J., & Holtzman, S. E. (1983). Patterns of drinking in the rat following administration of opiate antagonists. Pharmacology Biochemistry & Behavior, 19, 505-511.

Cox, B. M. (1983). Endogenous opioid peptides: A guide to structures and terminology. Life Sciences, 31, 1645-1658.

Crow, T. J. (1970). Enhancement by cocaine of intracranial self-stimulation in the rat. Life Science, 9, 375-381.

Cruz-Morales, S., & Reid, L. D. (1980). Addictive agents and intracranial stimulation (ICS): Morphine, naloxone, and pressing for amygdaloid ICS. Bulletin of the Psychonomic Society, 16, 199-200.

Deneau, G. A., Yanagita, T., & Seevers, M. H. (1969). Self-administration of psychoactive substances by the monkey: A measure of psychological dependence. Psychopharmacologia, 16, 30-48.

Deutsch, J. A., & Howarth, C. I. (1963). Some tests of a theory of intracranial self-stimulation. Psychological Review, 70, 446-460.

Esposito, R., & Kornetsky, C. (1977). Morphine lowering of self-stimulation thresholds: Lack of tolerance with long-term administration. Science, 195, 189-191.

Esposito, R., & Kornetsky, C. (1978). Opioids and rewarding brain stimulation. Neuroscience & Biobehavioral Reviews, 2, 115-122.

Farber, P. D., & Reid, L. D. (1976). Addictive agents and intracranial stimulation (ICS): Daily morphine and pressing for combinations of positive and negative ICS. Physiological Psychology, 4, 262-268.

Franklin, K. B. J., & Robertson, A. (1982). Effects and interactions of naloxone and amphetamine on self-stimulation of the prefrontal cortex and dorsal tegmentum. Pharmacology Biochemistry & Behavior, 16, 433-436.

Gerber, G. J., Bozarth, M. A., & Wise, R. A. (1981). Small-dose intravenous heroin facilitates hypothalamic self-stimulation without response suppression in rats. Life Science, 28, 557-562.

Gibson, W. E., Reid, L. D., Sakai, M., & Porter, P. B. (1965). Intracranial reinforcement compared with sugar-water reinforcement. Science, 148, 1357-1358.

Glick, S. D., Weaver, L. M., & Meibach, R. C. (1982). Asymmetrical effects of morphine and naloxone on reward mechanisms. Psychopharmacology, 78, 219-224.

Goldstein, A. (1978). Opiate receptors and opioid peptides: A ten year overview. In M. A. Lipton, A. DiMascio, K. F. Killam (Eds.), Psychopharmacology: A generation of progress (pp. 1157-1563). New York: Raven Press.

Heath, R. G. (1964). Pleasure response of human beings to direct stimulation of the brain: Physiologic and psychodynamic consideration. In R. G. Heath (Ed.), The role of pleasure in behavior (pp. 219-243). New York: Hoeber.

Hipps, P. P., Eveland, M. R., Meyer, E. R., Sherman, W. R., & Cicero, T. J. (1976). Moss fragmentography of morphine: Relationship between brain levels and analgesic activity. Journal of Pharmacology and Experimental Therapeutics, 196, 642-648.

Holtzman, S. G. (1976). Comparison of the effect of morphine, pentazocine, cyclazocine and amphetamine on intra-cranial self-stimulation in the rat. Psychopharmacologia, 46, 223-227.

Hunsicker, J. P., & Reid, L. D. (1974). The "priming effect" in conventionally reinforced rats. Journal of Comparative and Physiological Psychology, 87, 618-621.

Hunter, G. A., Jr., & Reid, L. D. (1983). Assaying addiction liability of opioids. Life Sciences, 33(Suppl. 1), 393-396.

Iversen, S. D. (1983). Brain endorphins and reward function: Some thoughts and speculation. In J. E. Smith & J. D. Lane (Eds.), Neurobiology of opiate reward mechanisms (pp. 439-468). Amsterdam: Elsevier/North Holland Biomedical Press.

Jacobowitz, D. M., & Palkovits, M. (1974). Topographic atlas of catecholamine acetylcholinesterase-containing neurons in the rat brain. I. Forebrain (telencephalon, diencephalon). Journal of Comparative Neurology, 157, 13-28.

Kamei, G., Yoshinobu, M., & Schimizu, M. (1974). Effects of psychotropic drugs on hypothalamic self-stimulation behavior in rats. Japanese Journal of Pharmacology, 24, 613-619.

Katz, R. J. (1980). The temporal structure of motivation. Behavioral and Neural Biology, 30, 148-159.

Katz, R. J. (1981). Identification of a novel class of central reward sites showing a delayed and cumulative response to opiate blockade. Pharmacology Biochemistry & Behavior, 15, 131-134.

Kayan, S., Woods, L. A., & Mitchell, C. L. (1971) Morphine-induced hyperalgesia in rats tested on the hot plate. Journal of Pharmacology and Experimental Therapeutics, 177, 509-513.

Keesey, (1964). Duration of stimulation and reward properties of hypothalamic stimulation. Journal of Comparative and Physiological Psychology, 58, 201-207.

Kimble, G. A. (1961). Hilgard and Marquis' conditioning and learning. New York: Appleton-Century-Crofts.

Koob, G. F., Spector, N. H., & Meyerhoff, J. L. (1975). Effects of heroin on lever pressing for intracranial self-stimulation, food, and water in the rat. Psychopharmacologia, 42, 231-234.

Liebman, J. M. (1983). Discriminating between reward and performances: A critical review of intracranial self-stimulation methodology. Neuroscience & Behavioral Reviews, 7, 45-72.

Lorens, S. A., & Mitchell, C. L. (1973). Influence of morphine on lateral hypothalamic self-stimulation in the rat. Psychopharmacologia, 32, 271-277.

Lorens, S. A., & Sainati, S. M. (1978). Naloxone blocks the excitatory effect of ethanol and chlordiazepoxide on lateral hypothalamic self-stimulation behavior. Life Sciences, 23, 1359-1364.

Marcus, R., & Kornetsky, C. (1974). Negative and positive intracranial reinforcement thresholds: Effects of morphine. Psychopharmacologia, 38, 1-13.

McIntire, R. W., & Wright, J. E. (1965). Parameters related to response rate for septal and medial forebrain bundle stimulation. Journal of Comparative and Physiological Psychology, 59, 131-134.

Miller, D. E., Reid, L. D., & Porter, P. B. (1967). Delayed punishment of positively reinforced bar presses. Psychological Reports, 22, 1073-1077.

Mucha, R. F., & Iversen, S. D. (1985). Reinforcing properties of morphine and naloxone revealed by conditioned place preference: A procedural examination. Psychopharmacology, 82, 241-247.

Nelsen, J. M., & Kornetsky, C. (1972). Morphine induced EEG changes in central motivational systems: Evidence for single dose tolerance. Fifth International Congress of Pharmacology, 166.

Olds, J. (1962). Hypothalamic substrates of reward. Physiological Reviews, 42, 554-604.

Olds, J., & Milner, P. (1954). Positive reinforcement produced by electrical stimulation of septal area and other regions of rat brain. Journal of Comparative and Physiological Psychology, 47, 419-427.

Olds, J., & Travis, R. P. (1960). Effects of chlorpromazine, meprobamate, pentobarbital and morphine on self-stimulation. Journal of Pharmacology and Experimental Therapeutics, 128, 397-404.

Olds, M. E. (1966). Facilitory action of diazepam and chlordiazepoxide on hypothalamic reward behavior. Journal of Comparative Physiology and Psychology, 62, 136-140.

Olds, M. E. (1970). Comparative effects of amphetamine, scopolamine, chlordiazepoxide and diphenylhydantoin on operant and extinction behaviour with brain stimulation and food reward. Neuropharmacology, 9, 519-532.

Pearl, J., Aceto, M. D., & Harris, L. D. (1968). Prevention of writhing and other effects of narcotics and narcotic antagonists in mice. Journal of Pharmacology and Experimental Therapeutics, 160, 217-230.

Perry, W., Esposito, R. U., & Kornetsky, C. (1981). Effects of chronic naloxone treatment on brain-stimulation reward. Pharmacology Biochemistry & Behavior, 14, 247-250.

Pert, A. (1975). Effects of opiates on rewarding and aversive brain stimulation in the rat. Problems of Drug Dependence, 963-973.

Pilcher, C. W. T., Jones, S. M., & Browne, J. (1982). Rhythmic nature of naloxone-induced aversions and nociception in rats. Life Sciences, 31, 1249-1252.

Pollerberg, G. E., Costa, T., Sherman, G. T., Herz, A., & Reid, L. D. (1983). Opioid antinociception and positive reinforcement are mediated by different types of opioid receptors. Life Sciences, 33, 1549-1559.

Reid, L. D. (1967). Reinforcement from direct stimulation of the brain. Unpublished doctoral dissertation, University of Utah, Salt Lake City.

Reid, L. D., & Bozarth, M. A. (1978). Addictive agents and pressing for intracranial stimulation (ICS): The effects of various opioids on pressing for ICS. Problems of Drug Dependence, 729-741.

Reid, L. D., Gibson, W. E., Gledhill, S. M., & Porter, P. B. (1964). Anticonvulsant drugs and self-stimulation behavior. Journal of Comparative and Physiological Psychology, 58, 353-356.

Reid, L. D., & Porter, P. B. (1965). Reinforcement from direct electrical stimulation of the brain. Rocky Mountain Psychologist, 1, 3-22.

Reid, L. D., & Siviy, S. M. (1982). Administration of antagonists of morphine and endorphin reveal endorphinergic involvement in reinforcement processes. In J. E. Smith & J. D. Lane (Eds.), Neurobiology of opiate reward mechanisms (pp. 257-279). Amsterdam: Elsevier/North Holland Biomedical Press.

Riley, A. L., & Baril, L. L. (1976). Conditioned taste aversion: A bibliography. Animal Learning & Behavior, 4(Suppl.), 15-35.

Rossi, N. A., & Reid, L. D. (1976). Affective states associated with morphine injections. Physiological Psychology, 4, 269-274.

Sakai, M., Reid, L. D., & Porter, P. B. (1965). Why is reinforcing brain stimulation turned off? In Proceedings of the 73rd Annual Convention of the American Psychological Society (pp. 155-156).

Sandberg, D. E., & Segal, M. (1978). Pharmacological analysis of analgesia and self-stimulation elicited by electrical stimulation of catecholamine nuclei in the rat brain. Brain Research, 152, 529-542.

Schnitzer, S. B., Reid, L. D., & Porter, P. B. (1965). Electrical intracranial stimulation as a primary reinforcer for cats. Psychological Reports, 16, 335-338.

Schuster, C. R., & Thompson, T. (1969). Self-administration of and behavioral dependence on drugs. Annual Review of Pharmacology, 9, 483-502.

Simon, E. J. (1982). History. In J. B. Malick & R. M. S. Bell (Eds.), Endorphins: Chemistry, physiology, pharmacology, and clinical relevance (pp. 1-8). New York: Marcel Decker.

Siviy, S. M., Calcagnetti, D. J., & Reid, L. D. (1982). A temporal analysis of naloxone's suppressant effect on drinking. Pharmacology Biochemistry & Behavior, 16, 173-175.

Smith, J. E., Co, C., & Lane, J. D. (1984). Limbic acetylcholine turnover rates correlated with rat morphine-seeking behaviors. Pharmacology Biochemistry & Behavior, 20, 429-442.

Smith, J. E., & Lane, J. D. (Eds.) (1983). Neurobiology of opiate reward mechanisms. Amsterdam: Elsevier/North Holland Biomedical Press.

Snyder, S. H. (1980). Brain peptides as neurotransmitters. Science, 209, 976-983.

Solomon, R. L., & Corbit, J. D. (1974). An opponent process theory of motivation: Temporal dynamics of affect. Psychological Review, 81, 119-145.

Stapleton, J. M. (1979). Naloxone suppression of intracranial self-stimulation: Evidence for the involvement of endogenous opioids in the modulation of intracranial reward. Unpublished master's thesis, Rensselaer Polytechnic Institute, Troy, NY.

Stapleton, J. M., Merriman, V. J., Coogle, C. L., Gelbard, S. D., & Reid, L. D. (1979). Naloxone reduces pressing for intracranial stimulation of sites in the periaqueductal gray area, accumbens nucleus, substantia nigra, and lateral hypothalamus. Physiological Psychology, 7, 427-436.

Stein, L. (1962). Effects and interactions of imipramine, chlorpromazine, reserpine, and amphetamine on self-stimulation: Possible neurophysiological basis of depression. In J. Wortis (Ed.), Recent advances in biological psychiatry (pp. 288-308). New York: Plenum Press.

Stein, L. (1978). Reward transmitters: Catecholamines and opioid peptides. In M. A. Lipton, A. DiMascio, & K. F. Killam (Eds.), Psychopharmacology: A generation of progress (pp. 569-581). New York: Raven Press.

Stein, L., & Ray, O. S. (1960). Brain stimulation reward "thresholds" self-determined in rat. Psychopharmacologia, 1, 251-256.

Thompson, T., & Schuster, C. R., (1964). Morphine self-administration, food reinforcement and avoidance behavior in rhesus monkeys. Psychopharmacologia, 5, 57-94.

Valenstein, E. S. (1964). Problems of measurement and interpretation with reinforcing brain stimulation. Psychological Review, 71, 415-437.

Valenstein, E. S., & Beer, B. (1961). Unipolar and bipolar electrodes in self-stimulation experiments. American Journal of Physiology, 201, 1181-1186.

van der Kooy, D., LePiane, F. E., & Phillips, A. E. (1977). Apparent independence of opiate reinforcement and electrical self-stimulation systems in rat brain. Life Sciences, 29, 981-986.

Ward, S. J., Pierson, A. K., & Michne, W. F. (1983). Multiple opioid receptor profile in vitro and activity in vivo of the potent opioid antagonist Win 44,441-3. Life Sciences, 33(Suppl. 1), 303-306.

Wasden, R. E., Reid, L. D., & Porter, P. B. (1965). Overnight performance decrements with intracranial reinforcement. Psychological Reports, 16, 653-658.

Wauquier, A., Gilbert, H., Clincke, C., & Franson, J. F. (1983). Parameter selection in a rate free test of brain self-stimulation: Towards an alternative interpretation of drug effects. Behavioural Brain Research, 7, 155-164.

Weber, E., Evans, C. J., & Barchas, J. D. (1983). Multiple endogenous ligands for opioid receptors. Trends in Neuroscience, 6, 333-336.

Weeks, J. R. (1962). Experimental morphine addiction: Method for automatic intravenous injections in unrestrained rats. Science, 138, 143-144.

Weibel, S. L., & Wolf, H. H. (1979). Opiate modification of intracranial self-stimulation in the rat. Pharmacology Biochemistry & Behavior, 10, 71-78.

Wise, R. A. (1980). Action of drugs of abuse on brain reward systems. Pharmacology Biochemistry & Behavior, 13(Suppl. 1), 213-223.

Wise, R. A. (1982a). Neuroleptics and operant behavior: The anhedonia hypothesis. The Behavioral and Brain Sciences, 5, 39-53.

Wise, R. A. (1982b). Hypotheses of neuroleptic action: Levels of progress. The Behavioral and Brain Sciences, 5, 78-87.

Wise, R. A. (1983). Brain neuronal systems mediating reward processes. In J. E. Smith & J. D. Lane (Eds.), Neurobiology of opiate reward mechanisms (pp. 405-437). Amsterdam: Elsevier/North Holland Biomedical Press.

Woolverton, W. L., & Schuster, C. R. (1983). Behavioral and pharmacological aspects of opioid dependence: Mixed agonist-antagonists. Pharmacological Reviews, 35, 33-52.

Yardin, E., Guarini, V., & Gallistel, C. (1983). Unilaterally activated systems in rats self-stimulating at sites in the medial forebrain bundle, medial prefrontal cortex, or locus coeruleus. Brain Research, 266, 39-50.

Young, P. T. (1967). Affective arousal: Some implications. American Psychologist, 22, 32-40.

CHAPTER 20

BRAIN STIMULATION REWARD:
MEASUREMENT AND MAPPING BY PSYCHOPHYSICAL TECHNIQUES AND QUANTITATIVE 2-[14C]DEOXYGLUCOSE AUTORADIOGRAPHY

Ralph U. Esposito,[1] Linda J. Porrino,[2] and Thomas F. Seeger[3]

[1]Laboratory of Psychology and Psychopathology
[2]Laboratory of Cerebral Metabolism
[3]Biological Psychiatry Branch
National Institute of Mental Health
U.S. Public Health Service
Department of Health and Human Services
Bethesda, Maryland 20205

ABSTRACT

Brain stimulation reward is a useful model for the study of the neural mechanisms of reinforcement. A number of methods used to assess the reinforcing qualities of brain stimulation and the effects of drugs of abuse on this behavior are reviewed with emphasis on the relative advantages and disadvantages of each. In addition, the use of the quantitative 2-[14C]-deoxyglucose method as a novel means to map the neural substrates of drug-induced effects on brain stimulation reward is described.

INTRODUCTION

Since its discovery the phenomenon of rewarding brain stimulation (Olds & Milner, 1954) has received intensive study as a means to understand brain mechanisms involved in motivated behavior. Recent advances in neuroanatomy, electrophysiology, and neuropharmacology have indicated an important relationship between certain ascending catecholaminergic pathways and this behavior (Crow, 1976; Fibiger, 1978; German & Bowden, 1974). Regarding the reinforcing properties of drugs of abuse it is noteworthy that the two most widely abused and euphorigenic classes of drugs, the opiates and psychostimulants, exert specific facilitative effects on self-stimulation to these same projection systems (Esposito & Kornetsky, 1978; Wise & Bozarth, 1981). Further studies, therefore, concerning the effects of these agents on brain stimulation reward, in conjunction with other techniques, should lead to important insights concerning the precise site and mechanisms of the reinforcing action of these agents. Conversely, and perhaps of more general significance, these same types of studies will also shed light on the neural substrates of goal-oriented or motivated behavior.

This chapter will briefly review methods used to assess the behavioral effects of drugs on brain stimulation reward and suggest adequate criteria for the design of future studies. Secondly, we will present recent developments concerning the use of quantitative 2-deoxyglucose autoradiography as a novel and unique means to identify the substrate of these drug-induced effects.

METHODS FOR THE DETERMINATION OF DRUG EFFECTS ON BRAIN STIMULATION REWARD

Response Rate and Brain Stimulation Reward

Rate of response is by far the most commonly used measure of the reinforcing value of rewarding brain stimulation. Typically this type of experiment involves a rat lever pressing (in a standard operant chamber) for a fixed intensity of brain stimulation on a continuous reinforcement schedule. The inadequacies of response rate as a measure of the reinforcing value of brain stimulation have been thoroughly discussed in detail elsewhere (Liebman, 1983; Valenstein, 1964), and only the major problems will be reviewed here.

Valenstein and associates have demonstrated on both empirical and logical grounds the inadequacy of response-rate measures. Thus, in rats given a choice between two levers, each activating a different electrode, the rate of responding was not found to correlate significantly with lever preference in a choice situation (Hodos & Valenstein, 1962) nor with measures of resistance to competition from other reinforcers such as food or the avoidance of foot shock (Valenstein & Beer, 1962). With respect to the choice situation in particular, it has been reliably noted that rats will choose "low-rate" septal stimulation over "higher-rate" lateral hypothalamic sites. This demonstration itself indicates that assertions regarding the rewarding value of stimulation to specific brain sites cannot be based on the simplistic equation of increasing response rate with increasing rewarding value. It is important to keep in mind that we know very little about animals' preferred rates of responding for many brain sites and, furthermore, even less about the interactive effects of various drugs on these response patterns.

In addition to the above, more general interpretative problems are encountered when one attempts to measure the effects of drugs on the reinforcing value of brain stimulation. Drug induced changes on rate of responding for brain stimulation are often automatically interpreted as a specific change in the reinforcing value of the stimulation when, in fact, these changes may be due to any number of nonspecific drug effects on attention, arousal level, or various perceptual and/or sensory-motor functions related to the task performance per se. Drug-induced changes may also be related to other important nonspecific factors such as differences in predrug baseline rates of responding. Even if animals are equated in terms of number of responses/minute, important individual differences may still exist. For instance, some animals may actually be straining to meet a particular response rate criterion while others do so with ease. Differences in response rate after drug treatment are difficult to interpret when this type of pretreatment variable is taken into consideration. Thus, taking the drug morphine as an example, one can find studies, using rate of lever pressing as the dependent measure, showing that morphine can either increase, decrease, or have no effect on the rate of self-stimulation, depending upon dose, time of measurement, baseline rate, and pattern of responding, plus a host of other variables such as general sedative or stimulatory effects of the drug (for a review, see Esposito & Kornetsky, 1978; cf. Reid, this volume). From these studies one can draw any preferred conclusion concerning the effects of morphine on rewarding brain stimulation.

Finally, an important methodological problem with rate in drug studies involving brain stimulation reward has been pointed out recently by Liebman (1983). It concerns the fact that a particular dose of a drug may have rather selective effects on high or low stimulation intensities (see Figure 1). It is clear that these important differences are obscured entirely when one examines

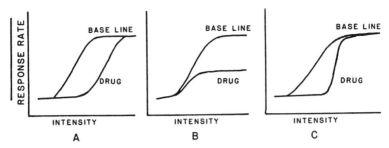

Figure 1: Response rate plotted as a function of stimulus intensity.
A shows a clear drug-induced shift in a rate-intensity function. **B**
shows a selective attenuation of response rate at higher stimulus
intensities, while **C** shows a selective drug-induced attenuation of
rate of responding at lower stimulus intensities. Reprinted with
permission from Liebman, 1983. Copyright 1983 by ANKHO International,
Inc.

the drug's effects at a single intensity, as is the case in many, if not most,
studies employing response rate as the dependent variable. Even if a clear
shift in a rate-intensity function is noted, its interpretation is still
subject to all of the aforementioned ambiguities relating to drug-induced
changes on brain stimulation reward. For these reasons some investigators have
adopted psychophysical methods in order to obtain more valid measures of the
reinforcing effects of brain stimulation.

Psychophysical Techniques and Brain Stimulation Reward

Contemporary psychophysical methods are essentially based on the
systematic approaches to the quantitative analysis of sensory processing set by
certain nineteenth century neurophysiologists, notably von Helmholtz and Weber.
The actual founding of psychophysics, however, can be traced to Gustav Theodor
Fechner, the physician, mathematician, physicist, philosopher, and poet, whose
first book on the subject, modestly entitled Zend-Avesta, ober wher die Dinge
des Himmels und des Jenseits (1851; or On the Nature of the Heavens and the
Nonmaterial World), laid down the essential ideas detailed in the subsequent
Elemente der Psychophysik, (1860) which marked the official beginning of the
field of psychophysics. The general aim of the early psychophysicists was to
find the quantitative relationships between physical events and their "mental"
representation. Although rooted in sensory processes, Fechner and his
scientific followers wanted the general principles of psychophysics to be
applied to other areas so as to eventually achieve a complete, systematic and
quantitative knowledge of the relationship of the physical world to mental
processes. Few would agree that the field of psychophysics has achieved this
goal, but nonetheless psychophysical methodology finally separated psychology
as a field distinct from philosophy and has had a profound positive influence
on experimental psychology with wide application in many areas, particularly in
the area of sensory psychology.

To avoid the problems inherent in rate-dependent studies of brain
stimulation reward, some investigators have adopted the use of classical
psychophysical procedures. These investigators attempt to obtain a more valid
measure of the reinforcing value of brain stimulation by determining the

absolute threshold,[1] generally expressed in terms of current intensity or frequency, necessary to support self-stimulation behavior to any particular brain site. This absolute reinforcing threshold is then used as a baseline against which the effect of various experimental manipulations such as lesions or drug administration can be expressed quantitatively in psychophysical units. This insures the specificity of effects and also permits quantification of the magnitude of any observed changes. Another distinct advantage is that the low stimulus intensities typically employed in these threshold determinations should more accurately reflect drug-induced changes in the excitability of the underlying neural activity with minimal tissue damage. Thus, in general, psychophysical studies of drug effects on brain stimulation reward determine the reinforcing threshold by obtaining a discrete measure of responding over a range of stimulus values, which by definition will maintain responding 50% of the time. An example of such a determination of reinforcing threshold before and after drug administration can be seen in Figure 2. As mentioned, several research groups have employed a variety of psychophysical techniques to obtain accurate estimates of the reinforcing value of brain stimulation and the specific effects of psychoactive drugs thereon. The remainder of the section will critically review some of the most representative of these endeavors, noting the relative advantages and disadvantages of each. These methods were chosen on the basis of their utility and representativeness, while no attempt to review the vast literature concerning drug effects on brain stimulation is intended.

The Two-Lever Reset Method

The method was first introduced by Stein and Ray (1960) who measured reinforcing thresholds for brain stimulation to the posterior hypothalamus and the ventral tegmentum. Typically in this procedure a rat is placed in a chamber with two levers available for responding. A response on one of the levers results in a positively reinforcing brain stimulation with a fixed decrease of intensity in a step-wise manner. Responding at the second lever resets the level of stimulation available at the first lever to its original level. The reinforcement threshold is defined as the average intensity at which reset responses are made (see Figure 3).

Stein (1962) has employed the two-lever procedure to demonstrate the threshold lowering effect of amphetamine, and the potentiation of this effect by imipramine. A dissociation of these effects from simple rate measures was reported by Stein, who noted that amphetamine-induced increases in rate of responding on the "rewarding" lever were most evident after the threshold lowering effect had returned to baseline. Nazzaro, Seeger, and Gardner (1981) have used this procedure in slightly modified form to demonstrate the threshold-lowering effect of morphine on ventral tegmental self-stimulation, as

----

[1]The term absolute threshold indicates the lowest point on a particular stimulus continuum (i.e., electrical intensity or frequency) at which behavior will be maintained 50% of the time. This measurement is not to be confused with the differential threshold which refers to the lowest magnitude of physical change (increment or decrement relative to a standard) on a stimulus continuum required for a subject to detect a difference relative to a standard 50% of the time. In this chapter the term reinforcement threshold will refer to the absolute threshold. It is important to note that the historical use of the term absolute is misleading because due to the subject's variability of response the threshold is not an absolute value but is a statistical approximation.

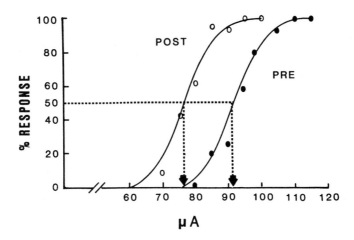

Figure 2: The effects of 4 mg/kg of morphine, administered subcutaneously to a rat, on the reinforcing threshold for brain stimulation reward. The ordinate shows the percent of trials in which the subject responded at each current intensity plotted on the abscissa. Current intensity was systematically varied in alternating ascending and descending series of 10 µA "step-size" increments and decrements, respectively. The data were collected immediately pre- and 10 minutes postinjection. Reinforcement thresholds are specified as the median reinforcing intensity at which the subject responded. Data adapted from Esposito and Kornetsky, 1977.

well as the additive effects of the co-administration of amphetamine and morphine (Seeger & Carlson, 1981). The two-lever procedure represents a significant advancement over the simple rate-dependent free operant method as it generates reliable and stable thresholds, but it is not without disadvantages, both theoretical and practical.

The major theoretical problem with the method is related to the regular descending serial order presentations of the stimuli. The use of descending series may lead to response habituation and thus yield inaccurate or spurious threshold measurements (Engen, 1971). The serial order stimulus presentations may also enable the animal to anticipate the regular decrease in reinforcement value and learn to make reset responses at intensities above the actual reinforcing level, thereby maintaining the stimulation at a preferred suprathreshold level (Valenstein, 1964). Modification of the experimental environment and procedure can partly obviate these limitations. For example, more valid threshold measures may be obtained by using a large number of current steps, such that the magnitude of the current decrement is minimal, or by physically separating the two levers enough to insure that the animal spends a considerable amount of time away from the stimulus lever while resetting the current level. Empirical evaluation of these limitations, however, must await parametric investigations which systematically vary both the initial (i.e., maximal) stimulus intensity as well as the magnitude of the decremental step size. So far, work in this area is limited to one report which indicates that

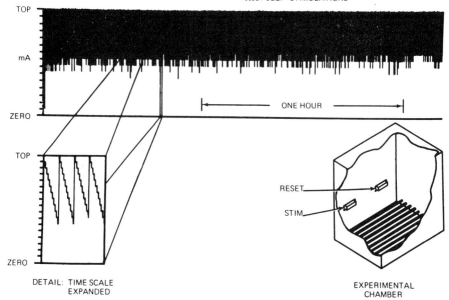

1,270 RESETS

9,531 SELF–STIMULATIONS

DETAIL: TIME SCALE
EXPANDED

EXPERIMENTAL
CHAMBER

Figure 3: Schematic representation of the basic two-lever reset method determining intracranial self-stimulation thresholds in the rat. Level of stimulation current (amplitude) is plotted on the ordinate while experiment time is recorded along the abscissa. Responding on the stimulus in a fixed decremental "step-wise" manner. Response at the reset lever resets the level of stimulation available on the first lever to its original intensity. A measure of the average intensity at which reset responses are made is taken as the estimate of the reinforcement threshold. Reprinted with permission from Stein, 1962. Copyright 1962 by Plenum Press.

variation of the maximal current level does not necessarily result in significant alterations in the reinforcing threshold (Schaeffer & Holtzman, 1979; see also Fouriezos & Nawiesniak, this volume).

In studies involving primates, the requirement of restraint in a chair precludes the physical separation of the levers. In this situation the animals quickly learn to alternate responses in order to keep the stimulus intensity at highly rewarding levels. Gardner (1971) has reported a modification of the two-lever procedure that makes it suitable for studies with primate subjects. This modified technique essentially involves the use of one response manipulandum only and requires the subject to withhold responding for a specified time, as in a modified DRL free-operant schedule, in order to obtain a reset of the stimulus intensity to its original high level. Seeger and Gardner (1979) have used this modified procedure to demonstrate neuroleptic-induced supersensitivity by threshold-lowering effects in the nucleus accumbens. Despite these modifications it must be noted that theoretically the current level at which animals reset the intensity is not the lowest level which will support behavior (i.e., the reinforcement threshold), but rather some preferred level of current intensity. Threshold measures using other methods typically yield lower intensities than the two-lever method (Valenstein, 1964).

Another potential problem with the two-lever reset method can arise with the use of drugs such as amphetamine, for example, that cause nonspecific effects such as disinhibition of responding, stereotypy, response perseveration, and perseverative switching (Evenden & Robbins, 1983). Each of these nonspecific effects could conceivably distort the validity of threshold determination. Behaviorally, however, the more severe nonspecific high dose drug effects are sufficiently detrimental to the operant procedure such that performance of the task tends to become completely erratic, precluding any valid measures. The more subtle confounding factors may be addressed if empirical means are used to assess and separate nonspecific from specific response alterations. For example, Seeger, Carlson, and Nazzaro (1981) attempted to parcellate specific from nonspecific responding by statistical criteria. They recorded the current level at which an animal chose to reset current level and thus generated a reset frequency distribution, taking the mean of this distribution as the reinforcement threshold, while the standard deviation was adopted as a measure of response integrity (i.e., an increasing standard deviation would indicate deterioration of responding). By means of such analysis they were able to detect the specific, low dose (10 mg/kg) threshold-lowering effect of pentobarbital without concurrent response deterioration, as was noted at higher doses (e.g., 20 mg/kg) which produced marked ataxia.

In summary, the two-lever reset technique possesses features which clearly improve on the limitations of purely rate-dependent measures. It produces stable, reliable, and practical measures of relative reinforcement, which can be maximized for resistance to nonspecific confounding effects on performance. Its greatest utility may be in assessing drug effects, both with regard to specificity of action on reward mechanisms and also in its ability to monitor simultaneously the temporal pattern of drug effects, which can provide information concerning the time of onset and duration of action particularly important in those studies involving agonist/antagonist interactions (cf. Fouriezos & Nawiesniak, this volume).

The Post-Reinforcement Pause Method

Huston and Mills (1979) have devised a procedure to determine reinforcement thresholds which capitalizes on certain aspects of schedule control. In their procedure rats lever pressed to self-stimulate on a fixed ratio (FR) schedule, while superimposed on this schedule was another continuous reinforcement (CRF) schedule of reinforcement. The intensity of the reinforcing stimulus on the FR schedule was always kept at a highly rewarding value, while the value (i.e., stimulus intensity) of the CRF component was varied, in ascending and descending steps of 5 μA according to the method of limits, at different FR components. When the CRF value was low, and presumably nonreinforcing, responding was controlled by the FR component and accordingly the cumulative record showed characteristic high response rates and post-reinforcement pauses. At higher levels of CRF reinforcement intensity, this component came to control responding, and the record showed typical patterns of continuous reinforcement. By varying the CRF intensity between these two extremes, Huston and Mills found an intensity at which post-reinforcement pauses (an interresponse interval 3 or more standard deviations above the mean

interresponse time at a given current level) appeared in the record and defined
this as the reinforcement threshold (see Figure 4). Cassens and Mills (1973)
have used this procedure to demonstrate opposite effects of lithium and
amphetamine on intracranial reinforcement thresholds in rats. Amphetamine was
found to lower the threshold while lithium elevated the threshold. In a
follow-up study Cassens, Actor, Kling, and Schildkraut (1981) demonstrated a
marked increase in reinforcing thresholds 24 to 48 hours after cessation of
chronic amphetamine administration, which peaked between 24 to 72 hours. The
post-reinforcement pause method was also used by Kelly and Reid (1977) to
demonstrate the threshold lowering effects of morphine. In their study rats
with lateral hypothalamic implants were given 10 mg/kg of morphine daily for 20
consecutive days and tested on the threshold procedure. Morphine-induced
reductions in the thresholds evidenced no tolerance over the entire testing
period, even though the animals showed clear signs of physical dependence.

The post-reinforcement pause method is ingenious inasmuch as it relies on
classic schedule control patterns to determine a threshold whereas virtually
all other measures use the reinforcing brain stimulation itself both to control
and to maintain responding when determining the reinforcing thresholds. This
reliance on pattern of responding, however, can also present problems,
particularly when trying to assess the effects of drugs which may disrupt
timing or selectively enhance responding at low rates. Another problem with

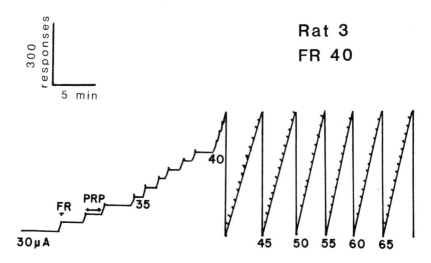

Figure 4: Cumulative record for a rat on a concurrent CRF:FR
schedule. This rat received FR reinforcements of 120 μ A on a FR-40
schedule. Changes in the CRF intensity are indicated along the base
of the curve and are expressed in microamperes (μ A) base to peak.
The post-reinforcement pauses (PRPs) are long and consistent when the
CRF stimulation is low, such as 30 or 35 μ A, but disappear when the
CRF intensity is raised to 60 or 65 μ A. When the PRPs disappear,
the behavior is identical to that of a subject on a simple CRF
schedule of equal reinforcements. Reprinted with permission from
Cassens and Mills, 1973. Copyright 1973 by Springer-Verlag.

the current use of CRF stimuli superimposed on the FR schedule is related to the fact that sub-reward-threshold stimuli delivered to brain sites, which support self-stimulation, possess drive or incentive-induction properties (Coons & Cruce, 1968; Huston, 1971). Thus, considering that drive-inducing stimuli can certainly affect responding, it becomes theoretically impossible to determine if, for example, the appearance of CRF responding is due to summating level of drive-induction or control by reward factors. As in the case with the two-lever method, these theoretical problems do not detract from the method's utility in assessing drug effects, as it does seem to generate stable and reliable effects. Finally, in the early studies employing this method the definition of what actually constituted a post-reinforcement pause was somewhat arbitrary and subjective. For example, Cassens and Mills (1973) noted that a " . . .lower limit of 7 seconds was arbitrarily chosen because this interval was just visually discernible on a cumulative record with a time base of 5 mm/min" (Cassens & Mills, 1973, p. 284). The procedure has since been automated (Cassens, Shaw, Dudding, & Mills, 1975) so that post-reinforcement pauses (PRP) are based upon their relative frequency. A PRP is defined as an interresponse interval 3 or more standard deviations outside the mean interresponse interval at any particular current level of CRF stimulation. On this basis a PRP/FR ratio can be calculated at each current level and a least square regression analysis applied to the resulting proportions as a function of current level in order to determine the line of best fit for the data. The threshold can thus be specified in terms of current intensity at which the proportion of PRP/FR is 0.5. Further refinements in this method have been made by Phelps and Lewis (1982; Lewis & Phelps, this volume). They interfaced a minicomputer (PDP8-Digital) with a constant current stimulator so that the stimulator functions as a voltage follower-regulator with continuous feedback. Instantaneous samples of the resistance (impedance) to the electric current are made and result in voltage adjustments to maintain constant current intensity. Another modification involved a reduction of the usual FR requirement (e.g., FR-40 reduced to FR-15), plus reducing the number of total FR components. These latter adjustments reduce the mean time necessary for threshold determination without affecting the reliability of the measurement. Data on total session time, reinforcement threshold, and average impedance values are collected by the computer and analyzed by a statistical program which summarizes and calculates means and standard errors of the mean and correlates each measure of a subject's performance at each current range tested.

Using this method of analysis Lewis (1981; Lewis & Phelps, this volume) has been able to demonstrate normal age-related changes in motivation and their rejuvenation with amphetamine as assessed by the self-stimulation model. He reported a decline in responding vigorously and reliably at 6 months of age. The decline in behavior was characterized by a decrease in response rate, increased impedance to the stimulating current, and failure to complete the reinforcement threshold procedure described above. Priming, increased current, food deprivation, and reshaping were all ineffective in restoring the behavior. A single dose of d-amphetamine (0.25 to 0.30 mg/kg), however, reinstated the self-stimulation, although thresholds and impedance value were higher than the 6 month values, and priming was required in some cases. It is of interest that rate of responding remained unchanged, arguing against a nonspecific arousal. Microanalysis of the electrode tips in both young and old animals showed no significant differences in size of necrosis around the electrode tips, indicating that the behavioral decline was not likely to be a function of tissue damage or electrode defects. The most parsimonious explanation of these findings is that the amphetamine activated central motivational systems in the aged rats, possibly by a restoration of functioning of age-related functionally declining catecholamine systems. The effect on motivational systems is supported by the finding that all the amphetamine-treated aged rats showed an improved performance in at least two subsequent consecutive sessions without further drug treatment. It is possible that the amphetamine treatment may have aided a motivationally relevant component of reacquisition of the rather demanding threshold procedure. In any case, this study provides age-related information about motivational systems and suggests that the brain self-stimulation thresholds may provide useful information relative to the functional integrity of catecholamine systems which are important for this behavior and show decline (particularly dopaminergic cells) with age (Ordy, Brizee, Kaack, & Hansche, 1978). The full automation of this somewhat complex technique should now permit its wider use.

The Reward-Summation Method

The reward-summation method, designed by Gallistel and associates, has been used along with various modifications and adjunctive manipulations as part of a systematic attempt to measure the fundamental parameters prerequisite to an understanding of the basic psychophysical relationships underlying motivation and reward through use of the self-stimulation model (Gallistel, 1983). In this respect this method has proven to be particularly useful in disassociating performance variables from specific effects on reward.

In the basic paradigm a rat is placed in a start box and receives a train of priming pulses and then runs down an alley to a goal box where a single lever-press response results in the contingent delivery of a train of rewarding brain stimulation pulses. After this discrete trial the lever is retracted, and the animal is placed back in the start box until the initiation of another trial. Over trials the number of rewarding pulses available on the response lever is varied systematically in ascending and descending series (i.e., classical method of limits) through a wide range of values. Running speed in the alley typically was noted to increase precipitously from low to asymptotic speeds at a particular value of reinforcement available on the response lever. This value represents the point on the reward-summation function which can be taken as a measure of the absolute reinforcing threshold. Specific effects on reinforcement threshold are seen as a shift in this "locus of rise" point on the reward-summation function (i.e., running speed plotted against the number of reward pulses in the stimulus train), while performance effects are independently reflected in the asymptotic level of running speed. Performance effects have, in fact, been shown to be quite sensitive to nonspecific factors such as running uphill, administration of muscle relaxants, et cetera, while the reinforcement threshold remained unchanged as assessed by locus of rise (Edmonds & Gallistel, 1974). Utilizing this method Franklin (1978) was able to demonstrate the specific reward-attenuating effect of the relatively selective dopamine antagonist, pimozide, as evidenced by a shift in the locus of rise without a concomitant change in the asymptotic level of running speed (see Figure 5).

The work of Gallistel and associates represents an empirical attempt to develop a psychophysics of intracranial self-stimulation. For instance, Edmonds and Gallistel (1974) and Gallistel, Rolls, and Greene (1969) have provided some empirical data supporting the proposed distinction between the neural circuitry mediating the drive-inducing effects of brain stimulation and that circuitry which mediates the rewarding or reinforcing component of such stimulation on the basis of differential sensitivity to variations in interpulse intervals within the stimulus train. To our knowledge, however, there have been few published investigations of the reinforcing properties of

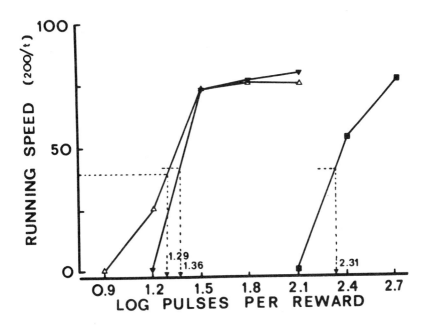

Figure 5: The effect of pimozide on the reward summation function, the curve relating performance (i.e., running speed in an alley) to the number of pulses in the train of reinforcing stimulation. At a dose of 0.2 mg/kg the range is shifted by 1.0 log units (a 10-fold change) to the right of its normal locus, with no decline in the asymptotic level of performance. This indicates that the drug reduced the reinforcing efficacy of the stimulation without impairing the innumerable other processes that translate a reinforcing effect into an observable behavior. Reprinted with permission from Franklin, 1978. Copyright 1978 by ANKHO International, Inc.

drugs of abuse that have used this method, most likely due to the time consuming and performance-demanding nature of the procedure which would lead to practical difficulties in studies of drugs with short duration of action or manifest tolerance or sensitization with repeated administration. However, it would seem that with appropriate modifications useful information could be gained from such investigations. For example, Belluzzi and Stein (1977) could have hypothesized that certain drugs (i.e., psychostimulants) may exert their major facilitative action on the motivational or drive-induction (i.e., behavior activating) properties of intracranial self-stimulation, while other drugs (i.e., opiates) may preferentially affect the drive-reduction or reinforcing aspect of goal-oriented behavior such as self-stimulation. To the extent that psychophysical methods such as these can empirically separate drive induction effects from reward effects they should be extremely useful in future studies attempting a finer dissection of the effects of drugs of abuse and, further, in discerning what drugs of abuse may teach us about the process(es) and substrate(s) of reinforcement.

The Double-Staircase Method

This method, based on a modification of the original procedure as proposed by Cornsweet (1962), has been employed in only one study concerned with the effects of drugs on brain stimulation reward. This study (Marcus & Kornetsky, 1974) represents the sole use of the technique successfully applied to infrahuman subjects and, additionally, was the first psychophysical demonstration of an "acute-onset" (30 minutes postinjection) specific facilitative effect of morphine on rewarding brain stimulation.

For the determination of positive reinforcement thresholds on this procedure, a trial began with the delivery of a noncontingent 0.5 second pulse train. A response (discrete wheel turn) within 7.5 seconds of this stimulus was immediately followed by a contingent stimulus identical in all parameters to the noncontingent stimulus. The response also terminated the trial, so that only one response-contingent stimulus was available on each trial. Failure to respond had no scheduled consequences, and the trial terminated after 7.5 seconds. Thus, the noncontingent stimulus served two functions: (a) It served as a discriminative stimulus for the availability of response-contingent stimulation, and (b) it also served as a comparative stimulus in that it was a predictor of the stimulus amplitude (and hence reinforcement strength) of the contingent stimulus. Trials began on the average of once every 15 seconds and intertrial or "error" responding resulted in a 15 second "time-out" period (see Figure 6).

The amplitude of the stimuli presented on a given trial was selected according to the double-staircase procedure. Briefly, the stimulus intensities were determined by two independent "staircases" alternating with one another. One staircase determined the stimulus intensity presented on odd-numbered trials, while the other staircase determined the intensity on the even-numbered trials. The occurrence of a successful response on trial n, indicating that the stimulus was reinforcing, resulted in a decrease by one step of the intensity on trial n + 2; failure to respond resulted in an increase by one step on trial n + 2. Similarly, the occurrence or nonoccurrence of a response on trial n + 1 determined the intensity on trial n + 3. Step size was selected on the basis of preliminary investigations so as to conform with certain practical and theoretical requirements (Dixon & Massey, 1957). Thresholds were calculated on the basis of the number of responses (or failures) at each intensity level (Dixon & Massey, 1957).

On this procedure morphine administered subcutaneously reliably lowered the reinforcing threshold in all subjects at a dose range of 2 to 8 mg/kg and lasted for a period ranging from 1 to 3 hours postinjection. In terms of psychophysical criteria for drug studies, this study is technically exemplary in several respects. Notably, the use of two interlocking staircases circumvents many commonly encountered problems in other procedures. The threshold determination is independent of rate and/or pattern of responding, and nonspecific responding is controlled for by the time-out component. The quasi-random order of stimulus presentation eliminates the confounding effects of serial order presentations with brain stimulation as well as errors of anticipation or response habituation (Boren & Malis, 1961; Valenstein, 1964). Since the stimuli to be presented are determined on the basis of the subject's responding during the course of the experiment, there is by definition a high density of data points at intensities near the absolute threshold. This increases both the efficiency (e.g., allowing for a maximum information per trial ratio) and the validity of the measurement. The tracking or titration-like feature of the method permits more "on-line" monitoring of drug-induced

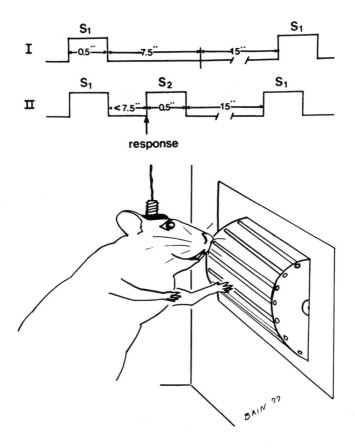

Figure 6: A diagrammatic and pictorial representation of the basic discrete-trial instrumental procedure utilized in the double-staircase and modified method of limits procedures (see text) for determining a reinforcing threshold with brain stimulation reward. **I.** Depicts the sequence of events that occur when a subject does not respond. **II.** Depicts the sequence of events when a subject emits a correct response (i.e., wheel turn within the appropriate time constraint). S_1 represents the noncontingent stimulus which initiates the trial while S_2 represents a stimulus that is delivered contingently upon a subject-emitted correct response. S_2 is identical to S_1 within each trial at a given current intensity throughout the variation of the amplitude parameter. Reprinted with permission from Kornetsky and Bain, 1983. Copyright 1983 by Elsevier/North Holland Biomedical Press.

changes (e.g., onset, magnitude, and duration of blockade) that are critical and other types of drug interactions such as additivity, synergism, or potentiation. The main problem with this technique relates to its practical limitations. Because the procedure does not allow a high density of suprathreshold stimuli, the thresholds tend to "drift" up over daily testing sessions, with some animals showing signs of extinction, thus presenting obvious problems for studies involving chronic drug administration (unpublished observations).

The Modified Method of Limits

In this method animals were trained on the same basic discrete-trial procedure as described above for the double-staircase method (see above and Figure 6). Determination of reward thresholds involved variation of the stimulus intensities according to the classical method of limits. Stimuli were presented in alternating descending and ascending series with a step size of 10 μ A. Ten trials were given in succession at each step size or interval. A descending series was initiated at a previously determined intensity which invariably yielded a contingent response in at least 9 out of 10 trials, and then 10 more successive trials were conducted at the next lowest interval and so on. Five or more responses at a particular intensity were arbitrarily scored as a plus for the interval. Descending series were conducted until minus scores were achieved in two successive intervals. An ascending series was then started at one step size below the lowest intensity in the descending series and continued until a level was reached in which there were at least 9 responses out of 10 trials, whereupon a descending series would be initiated at least one interval above the last intensity used in the ascending series. Threshold was determined by calculating the arithmetic mean ($\bar{x}$) in microamperes of the midpoints between intervals in which the animal made greater than five responses (a plus score) and less than five responses (a minus score). Results could also be plotted as the psychophysical function of responses plotted against stimulus intensity as shown in Figure 7.

Esposito and Kornetsky have employed this method to assess the effects of opiates and other major agents of abuse. With respect to the opiates, morphine was found to produce an immediate (i.e., 15 minutes post subcutaneous injection of 2 to 8 mg/kg) lowering of the reward threshold at a number of catecholamine-opiate-receptor rich sites within the brain (Esposito & Kornetsky, 1977; Esposito, McLean, & Kornetsky, 1979). In contrast, naloxone administered alone was without effect at these same sites (Kornetsky, Esposito, McLean, & Jacobson, 1979; Perry, Esposito, & Kornetsky, 1981). Of particular interest was that these threshold-lowering or reward-enhancing effects showed no evidence of tolerance (Esposito & Kornetsky, 1977). This latter finding has subsequently been replicated by a number of other investigators and has important basic and theoretical implications for our understanding of opiate reward mechanisms (for discussion, see Esposito & Kornetsky, 1978; Kornetsky et al., 1979). An important advantage of this method is sensitivity and, accordingly, it has been able to discriminate between the mixed opiate agonist/antagonists on the basis of their relative euphorigenic or abuse potential. Specifically, the abused agent, pentazocine, was found to lower reward thresholds, while other mixed agonist/antagonists (e.g., cyclazocine, nalorphine) that do not possess abuse potential, but are potent analgesics, did not (Kornetsky & Esposito, 1979). Flexibility is another advantage of this psychophysical procedure inasmuch as it has been able to demonstrate the threshold elevating or reward-attenuating effect of neuroleptics (Esposito, Faulkner, & Kornetsky, 1979; Esposito, Perry, & Kornetsky, 1981) and document the threshold-lowering or reward-enhancing effects of morphine (see above) and the psychostimulants amphetamine and cocaine (Esposito, Motola, & Kornetsky, 1978; Esposito, Perry, & Kornetsky, 1980), independent of the many nonreward-specific actions these drugs possess. Recently, Hubner, Bain, and Kornetsky

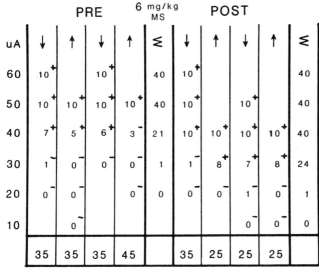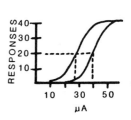

X̄ 37.5 µA   27.5 µA

Figure 7: An example of the data collection procedure followed during the modified method of limits for determination of reinforcing thresholds. Ascending and descending series for PRE and POST drug sessions are indicated by the arrows at the top of each column or series, with the individual series threshold at the bottom of each column. The numbers within the columns represent the number of contingent responses at each intensity. The total number of responses at each intensity is indicated at the right-hand column after each session (PRE & POST). Response as a function of intensity can also be plotted as in the accompanying graph. The data show the threshold-lowering effect of a subcutaneous (6 mg/kg) dose of morphine in a rat. Reprinted with permission from Esposito and Kornetsky, 1977. Copyright 1977 by the American Association for the Advancement of Science.

(1983) have demonstrated a synergistic action of morphine/amphetamine combinations on brain stimulation reward thresholds with this procedure consistent with the "street" users predilection for this drug combination. It is noteworthy that the opiate antagonist, naloxone, was able to block or greatly attenuate the reward-enhancing effectiveness of both amphetamine and cocaine at doses of naloxone which when administered independently do not alter reward thresholds (see Figure 8; Esposito et al., 1980; Kornetsky, Bain, & Reidl, 1981). These latter findings are in agreement with those of Seeger, Nazzaro, and Gardner, who used the two-lever method (see above) and suggest an important dopaminergic-endogenous opiate interaction(s) in the mediation of central reward processes (for detailed discussion, see Esposito, 1984).

Reinforcing-threshold measures derived from this method have also been compared to rate-intensity functions derived from the same placements in the same subject. With few exceptions (e.g., ventral tegmentum), there was little correlation between these two measures at a variety of commonly studied sites

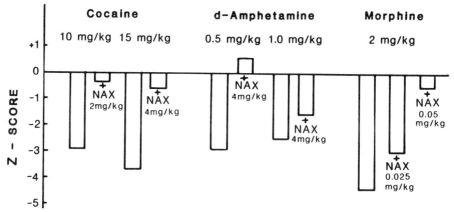

Figure 8: Effects of various combinations of naloxone with cocaine, d-amphetamine, or morphine on brain stimulation reinforcement threshold. Z-scores are based on the mean and standard deviation of threshold changes (POST-PRE) after respective vehicle injections. Z-scores + 2 are considered significantly different. Data are based on the mean Z-score for six subjects with cocaine, four subjects with d-amphetamine, and a typical morphine subject. The naloxone blockade or attenuation of the respective drug effect was observed in all animals. Reprinted with permission from Kornetsky and Wheeling, 1982. Copyright 1982 by Elsevier/North Holland Biomedical Press.

in self-stimulation studies (Payton, Kornetsky, & Rosene, 1983). This method has also been used to differentiate the threshold for brain stimulation reward from the threshold for brain stimulation detection and, additionally, the dose-related differential effect of cocaine on these measures within the same subjects (Kornetsky & Esposito, 1981). The reward threshold was determined in the usual manner, whereas the measurement of the brain stimulation detection threshold simply required varying the initial stimulus (i.e., noncontingent) in a quasi-random manner through a predetermined range of sub-to-suprathreshold (nonreinforcing) intensities according to the procedure of the classical method of constant stimuli while keeping the second or response-contingent stimulus at a highly rewarding value in order to maintain responding (see Figure 9).

Two groups of investigators have employed modified versions of this basic method, essentially varying current frequency rather than amplitude (Porrino & Coons, 1979; Schenk, Williams, Coupal, & Shizgal, 1980). For example, using such frequency variations Schenk et al. (1980) reported variable effects of morphine on self-stimulation in rats with placements in the lateral hypothalamus and dorsal raphe. Varying frequency rather than amplitude has the advantage of controlling for current spread at higher stimulus intensities; however, the use of different frequencies probably incurs the recruitment of different neural populations (Myers, 1971).

The modified method of limits has several distinct practical and theoretical advantages. The procedure is easily acquired and, most importantly for drug studies, places minimal performance demands on the subjects. Reliable and stable baseline thresholds can be obtained within one week, and the procedure, unlike many others, works well at various brain sites. Responding

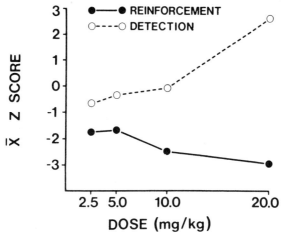

Figure 9: Dose related effects of cocaine on the reinforcing threshold for rewarding brain stimulation and the threshold for brain stimulation detection in the same subjects. The graph shows a clear dissociation between effects on a sensory dimension (i.e., detection) and a reinforcement dimension (see text for details). Data are expressed as Z-scores based on the respective mean and standard deviation of effects of vehicle (saline) injections. (N=4). Adapted with permission from Kornetsky and Esposito, 1981. Copyright 1981 by Elsevier/North Holland Biomedical Press.

is maintained throughout the experimental session with minimal stimulation at low intensities, and specific effects of drugs from diverse classes have been demonstrated.

In sum, there are a number of techniques which attempt to meet the basic criteria for an adequate assessment of drug effects on brain stimulation reward (see Table 1). These basic criteria should be used as guideposts in the

Table 1

Criteria for Adequate Psychophysical Threshold Determination

---

1. Easy to train with minimal performance demands on subject
2. Control for serial order stimulus presentations, response set, and contrast effects
3. Dissociate effects on reward from effects on detection thresholds
4. Maintain responding throughout the session with minimal stimulation at the lowest intensities
5. Yield stable thresholds for chronic studies
6. Have adequate flexibility to assess drugs from different classes
7. Allow sensitivity to dose-response effects, plus agonist/antagonists
8. Possess reliability and validity

---

design of future studies because it is essential to insure <u>specificity</u> of drug effects before attempting the study of the neural substrate of these effects.

.

METABOLIC MAPPING OF THE NEURAL SUBSTRATE OF BRAIN STIMULATION REWARD

In the first part of this chapter, we have focused on ways in which drug effects on brain stimulation reward can be assessed. In parallel, the problem of determining the neural substrates of these actions of psychoactive substances, whether studied alone or in conjunction with brain stimulation reward, has been approached in quite similar fashion. Much of our present knowledge regarding the identity of the pathways that are specifically related to intracranial self-stimulation (ICSS) has been obtained from neuroanatomical tracing methods, electrophysiological recording techniques and studies of the effects of lesions, among others.

The recent development by Sokoloff and colleagues of the 2-$[^{14}C]$deoxyglucose method affords a novel and unique opportunity to map functional neural pathways simultaneously in all anatomical components of the central nervous system. This method, therefore, allows the identification of complex neural circuits that are functionally active during behavioral or pharmacological manipulation. The technique is based on the close relationship between energy metabolism (In the brain glucose is virtually the exclusive substrate for metabolism.) and functional neural activity. By measuring glucose utilization in different regions of the brain, it is possible to estimate the level of functional activity within that structure. The technique makes use of a radioactive labeled analogue of glucose, 2-$[^{14}C]$deoxyglucose, which like glucose is transported into neurons and phosphorylated by hexokinase, but unlike glucose deoxyglucose cannot be further metabolized and is therefore trapped within the cells. Thus, quantitative autoradiography can be used permitting not only the measurement of actual rates of glucose utilization in individual brain regions, but also a pictorial representation of the relative rates of glucose utilization throughout the entire brain. For detailed discussion of the theoretical bases of the radioactive deoxyglucose method and reviews of some of its applications, see Sokoloff (1981; 1982) and Sokoloff et al. (1977).

To date the 2-$[^{14}C]$deoxyglucose method has proved highly useful in determining the sites of actions of pharmacological agents. The method has the particular advantage of allowing the visualization of alterations in metabolic activity throughout the entire brain, thereby making possible the identification of the complex neural circuitry which mediates the complete behavioral response to such pharmacological challenges. Studies with amphetamine, for instance, have shown that at high doses (i.e., those eliciting stereotypic responses) altered metabolic activity was evident throughout the dopaminergic nigrostriatal system and the rest of the extrapyramidal system (Orzi, Dow-Edwards, Jehle, Kennedy, & Sokoloff, 1983; Porrino, Lucignani, Dow-Edwards, & Sokoloff, 1984b; Wechsler, Savaki, & Sokoloff, 1979). In contrast, lower doses (i.e., those which have been shown to lower thresholds for ICSS and to facilitate exploratory behavior) produced changes in glucose utilization that were limited mainly to the dopaminergic mesolimbic system, in particular the nucleus accumbens (Porrino et al., 1984b).

In contrast to these pharmacological studies, early work with the 2-$[^{14}C]$deoxyglucose technique to map the functional pathways activated during brain stimulation reward were not as promising. In these experiments which utilized modifications of the original methodology of Sokoloff and colleagues, rewarding brain stimulation to the medial forebrain bundle, medial prefrontal cortex, or the locus coeruleus produced no consistent pattern of changes in relative rates of glucose utilization when comparisons were made between stimulated and unstimulated sides of the brain (Yadin, Guarini, & Gallistel, 1983).

Work in this laboratory with the fully quantitative 2-[^{14}C]deoxyglucose autoradiographic method at a different stimulation site, however, has yielded quite a different picture. In our studies we assessed changes in functional activity by comparing the actual rates of glucose utilization in various brain regions of rats self-stimulating to the ventral tegmental area (VTA) and passive control rats. We chose the VTA because there is extensive evidence for a significant role for dopamine in the mediation of ICSS, in particular the mesocorticolimbic system which receives its dopaminergic innervation predominantly from cells in the VTA (Clavier & Routtenberg, 1980; Phillips & Fibiger, 1978). In these experiments the standard protocol for the 2-[^{14}C]deoxyglucose technique as developed in this laboratory by Sokoloff and colleagues was followed. On the day of the experiment each rat was lightly anesthetized with halothane/nitrous oxide and implanted with femoral arterial and venous catheters that exited the skin at the nape of the neck. Thus, the animals were free to move and respond in the chamber during the experimental session. After surgery the animals were allowed 3 to 4 hours to recover. Both self-stimulating rats were allowed to begin lever pressing for brain stimulation to the VTA (current parameters: biphasic rectangular wave pulses, 100 Hz, 250 μA, 400 msec train). The procedure for the measurement of glucose utilization was initiated by the intravenous injection of a pulse of 2-[^{14}C]deoxyglucose at 125 μCi/kg. Timed arterial samples were taken for the next 45 minutes. At the end of this time, animals were killed by the intravenous administration of an overdose of sodium pentobarbital. The brains were rapidly removed and frozen in isopentane cooled to -45°C. The blood samples were immediately centrifuged and plasma concentrations of 2-[^{14}C]deoxyglucose were determined by means of liquid scintillation counting and plasma glucose concentrations were assayed as well.

The brains were then cut in 20 μm sections in a cryostat maintained at -22°C. The sections were picked up on glass coverslips and dried on a hot plate. Sections were autoradiographed along with a set of calibrated standards on Kodak OM-1 x-ray film for approximately 12 days. The autoradiographs were analyzed by quantitative densitometry. Optical density measurements for each structure were made in a minimum of four brain sections, both ipsilateral and contralateral to the electrode site. Tissue ^{14}C concentrations were determined from the optical densities and a calibration curve obtained from the densitometric analysis of the standards. Local cerebral glucose utilization (LCGU) in each structure was then calculated from the ^{14}C tissue concentrations, time courses of the plasma 2-[^{14}C]deoxyglucose and glucose concentrations and the appropriate constants according to the operational equation of Sokoloff et al. (1977).

LCGU was calculated in the terminal fields of the VTA and in various sensory and motor areas. There was an intense increase in metabolic activity at the site of stimulation in the VTA extending laterally into the substantia nigra. Discrete fiber activation was evident through the medial forebrain bundle into the diagonal band of Broca rostrally and in the pontine reticular formation caudally. Within the terminal fields of the VTA a very consistent pattern of LCGU changes were found in the self-stimulating animals compared to the unstimulated controls. Bilateral increases in LCGU were found in the nucleus accumbens, lateral septum, mediodorsal nucleus of the thalamus and in the hippocampus. Ipsilateral to the stimulation site, increased LCGU was evident in the medial prefrontal cortex, bed nucleus of the stria terminalis, and within the basolateral and central nuclei of the amygdala, as well as in the locus coeruleus and the medial parabrachial nucleus (Esposito, Porrino, Seeger, Crane, Everist, & Pert, 1984).

These results show that self-stimulation to the VTA is associated with the discrete activation of projection fibers and selective terminal fields of the VTA rather than a diffuse, nonspecific pattern of altered activity throughout the brain. They also show that the $2-[^{14}C]$deoxyglucose method can be quite useful in the analysis of the neural substrates of goal-oriented behavior. In a further experiment we have shown that the pattern of changes in LCGU found in self-stimulating animals is specific to this behavior and not merely the result of the electrical stimulation itself. When glucose utilization in self-stimulating animals was compared to that in animals which received noncontingent electrical stimulation delivered by the experimenter (at rates and current parameters comparable to those of the self-stimulating rats) to VTA placements shown to support self-stimulation, a very different pattern of changes was found (Porrino, Esposito, Seeger, Crane, Pert, & Sokoloff, 1984a). These differences are summarized in Table 2.

Table 2

Significant Changes in Metabolic Activity Following Stimulation of the Ventral Tegmental Area

---

Bilateral	Ipsilateral
SELF-STIMULATION	
nucleus accumbens	medial prefrontal cortex
lateral septum	central amygdala
bed nucleus of the stria terminalis	basolateral amygdala
hippocampus (CA3)	
mediodorsal thalamus	
locus coeruleus	
medial parabrachial nucleus	
dorsal raphe	
EXPERIMENTER-ADMINISTERED STIMULATION	
locus coeruleus	lateral septum
dorsal raphe	mediodorsal thalamus
	hippocampus (CA3)

Note: Projection fields of the ventral tegmental area in which increased glucose utilization was found following intracranial self-stimulation or experimenter-administered stimulation. In bilateral fields, changes were ipsilateral and contralateral to the stimulation site. In ipsilateral fields, increases were confined to the side of stimulation.

We believe that these results can form the basis of future studies in which the effects of drugs such as the psychostimulants and the opiates on the substrates of rewarding brain stimulation can be assessed. Preliminary results of an experiment in which amphetamine (0.5 mg/kg) was administered to animals lever pressing for stimulation to the VTA at current levels one third those used in our earlier work revealed a complex pattern of alterations in metabolic activity which was similar in many areas to those changes seen in animals receiving either drug or stimulation alone. In other areas, however, effects were seen which were unique to this combination of treatments, indicating that the facilitative actions of amphetamine on rewarding brain stimulation may be exerted in areas that are not predicted by the effects of rewarding brain stimulation alone or amphetamine's actions on other behaviors or other measures of reward (Seeger, Porrino, Esposito, Crane, Pert, & Sokoloff, in preparation).

CONCLUSIONS

The 2-[^{14}C]deoxyglucose method can be used to identify pathways underlying goal-oriented behavior and the changes that result in such behavior following the administration of psychostimulants or opiates. This requires first the careful definition and assessment of the behavior to be studied, with methods such as those outlined in the first part of this chapter. The analysis of the substrates of behavioral changes requires the use of the fully quantitative 2-[^{14}C]deoxyglucose autoradiographic technique, which takes into account various factors including plasma glucose levels and other physiological changes that can influence the amount of radioactive label present in the tissue. In this way it is possible not only to make valid comparisons between sites ipsilateral and contralateral to the brain stimulation, but, more importantly, to make valid comparisons between subjects. In summary, the fully quantitative 2-[^{14}C]deoxyglucose method, used with appropriate psychophysical techniques, can form the basis for research directed towards an understanding of the complex patterns of neural activity mediating the behavioral process of reinforcement.

ACKNOWLEDGMENT

We thank Dr. Agu Pert and Dr. Louis Sokoloff for their critical commentary on earlier versions of this manuscript, J. D. Brown for his help in preparing the figures, and Brenda Sandler for her editorial assistance.

REFERENCES

Belluzzi, J. D., & Stein, L. (1977). Enkephalin may mediate euphoria and drive reduction reward. Nature, 266, 556-558.

Boren, J. J., & Malis, J. L. (1961). Determining thresholds of aversive brain stimulation. American Journal of Physiology, 201, 429-433.

Cassens, G. P., Actor, C., Kling, M., & Schildkraut, J. (1981). Amphetamine withdrawal: Effects on the threshold of intracranial reinforcement. Psychopharmacology, 73, 318-322.

Cassens, G. P., & Mills, A. W. (1973). Lithium and amphetamine: Opposite effects on threshold of intracranial reinforcement. Psychopharmacologia, 30, 283-290.

Cassens, G., Shaw, C., Dudding, K. E., & Mills, A. W. (1975). On-line brain stimulation: Measurement of threshold of reinforcement. Behavioral Research Methods and Instrumentation, 7, 145-150.

Clavier, R. M., & Routtenberg, A. (1980). In search of reinforcement pathways: A neuroanatomical odyssey. In A. Routtenberg (Ed.), Biology of reinforcement: Facets of brain stimulation reward (pp. 81-107). New York: Academic Press.

Coons, E. E., & Cruce, J. A. F. (1971). Lateral hypothalamus: Food current intensity in maintaining self-stimulation. Science, 159, 1117-1119.

Cornsweet, T. N. (1962). The staircase method in psychophysics. American Journal of Psychology, 75, 485-491.

Crow, T. J. (1976). Specific monoamine systems as reward pathways: Evidence for the hypothesis that activation of the ventral mesencephalic dopaminergic neurones and noradrenergic neurones of the locus coeruleus complex will support self-stimulation responding. In A. Wauquier & E. T. Rolls (Eds.), Brain-stimulation reward (pp. 211-238). New York: American Elsevier Publishing.

Dixon, W. J., & Massey, F. J. (1957). Introduction to statistical analysis. New York: McGraw Hill.

Edmonds, D. E., & Gallistel, C. R. (1974). Parametric analysis of brain stimulation reward in the rat. III. Effects of performance variables on the reward summation function. Journal of Physiological and Comparative Psychology, 87, 876-883.

Edmonds, D. E., & Gallistel, C. R. (1977). Reward vs. performance in self-stimulation: Electrode specific effects of alpha-methyl-p-tyrosine on reward in the rat. Journal of Comparative and Physiological Psychology, 91, 962-974.

Engen, T., Kling, J. W., & Riggs, L. A. (1971). Experimental psychology (3rd edition). New York: Holt, Rhinehart, and Winston.

Esposito, R. U. (1984). Cognitive-affective integration: Some recent trends from a neurobiological perspective. In H. Weingartner & E. Parker (Eds.), Memory consolidation; Toward a psychobiology of cognition (pp. 15-63). Hillsdale, NJ: Lawrence Erlbaum.

Esposito, R. U., Faulkner, W., & Kornetsky, C. (1979). Specific modulation of brain stimulation reward by haloperidol. Pharmacology Biochemistry & Behavior, 10, 937-940.

Esposito, R. U., & Kornetsky, C. (1977). Morphine lowering of self-stimulation thresholds: Lack of tolerance with long-term administration. Science, 195, 189-191.

Esposito, R. U., & Kornetsky, C. (1978). Opioids and rewarding brain stimulation. Neuroscience & Biobehavioral Reviews, 2, 115-122.

Esposito, R. U., McLean, S., & Kornetsky, C. (1979). Effects of morphine on intracranial self-stimulation to various brain stem loci. Brain Research, 168, 425-429.

Esposito, R. U., Motola, A. H. D., & Kornetsky, C. (1978). Cocaine: Acute effects on reinforcement thresholds for self-stimulation behavior to the medial forebrain bundle. Pharmacology Biochemistry & Behavior, 8, 437-439.

Esposito, R. U., Perry, W., & Kornetsky, C. (1980). Effects of d-amphetamine and naloxone on brain stimulation reward. Psychopharmacology, 69, 187-191.

Esposito, R. U., Perry, W., & Kornetsky, C. (1981). Chlorpromazine and brain-stimulation reward: Potentiation of effects by naloxone. Pharmacology Biochemistry & Behavior, 15, 903-905.

Esposito, R. U., Porrino, L. J., Seeger, T. F., Crane, A. M., Everist, H. D., & Pert, A. (1984). Changes in local cerebral glucose utilization during rewarding brain stimulation. Proceedings of the National Academy of Sciences, 81, 635-639.

Evenden, J. L., & Robbins, T. W. (1983). Increased response switching, perseveration, and perseverative switching following d-amphetamine in the rat. Psychopharmacology, 80, 67-73.

Fechner, G. T. (1851). Zend-avesta, oder uber die dinge des himmels und des jenseits. Leipzig: Voss.

Fechner, G. T. (1860). Elemente der psychophysik. Leipzig: Breitkopf & Hartel.

Fibiger, H. C. (1978). Drugs and reinforcement mechanisms: A critical review of the catecholamine theory. Annual Review of Pharmacology and Toxicology, 18, 37-56.

Franklin, K. B. J. (1978). Catecholamines and self-stimulation: Reward and performance effects dissociated. Pharmacology Biochemistry & Behavior, 9, 813-820.

Gallistel, C. R. (1983). Self-stimulation. In J. A. Deutch (Ed.), The physiological basis of memory consolidation (2nd ed., pp. 270-351). New York: Academic Press.

Gallistel, C. R., Rolls, E. T., & Greene, D. (1969). Neuron function inferred by behavioral and electrophysiological measurement of refractory period. Science, 166, 1028-1030.

Gardner, E. L. (1971). An improved technique for determining brain reward threshold in primates. Behavioral Research Methods and Instrumentation, 3, 273-274.

German, D. C., & Bowden, D. M. (1974). Catecholamine systems as the neural substrate for intracranial self-stimulation: A hypothesis. Brain Research, 73, 381-419.

Hodos, W., & Valenstein, E. S. (1962). An evaluation of response rate as a measure of rewarding intracranial stimulation. Journal of Comparative and Physiological Psychology, 55, 80-84.

Hubner, C. B., Bain, G. T., & Kornetsky, C. (1983). Morphine and amphetamine: effect on brain stimulation reward. Society for Neuroscience Abstracts, 9, 893.

Huston, J. P. (1971). Relationship between motivating and rewarding stimulation of the lateral hypothalamus. Physiology & Behavior, 6, 711-716.

Huston, J. P., & Mills, A. (1971). Threshold of reinforcing brain stimulation. Communications in Behavioral Biology, 5, 331-340.

Kelly, K., & Reid, L. D. (1977). Addictive agents and intracranial stimulation: morphine and thresholds for positive intracranial reinforcement. Bulletin of the Psychonomic Society, 10, 298-300.

Kornetsky, C., & Bain, G. (1983). Effects of opiates on rewarding brain stimulation. In J. E. Smith & J. E. Lane (Eds.), The neurobiology of opiate reward processes (pp. 237-256). Amsterdam: Elsevier/North Holland Biomedical Press.

Kornetsky, C., Bain, G., & Reidl, E. M. (1981). Effects of cocaine and naloxone on brain stimulation reward. The Pharmacologist, 23, 192.

Kornetsky, C., & Esposito, R. U. (1979). Euphorigenic drugs: Effects on the reward pathways of the brain. Federation Proceedings, 38, 2473-2476.

Kornetsky, C., & Esposito, R. U. (1981). Reward and detection thresholds for brain stimulation: Dissociative effects of cocaine. Brain Research, 209, 496-500.

Kornetsky, C., Esposito, R. U., McLean, S., & Jacobson, J. O. (1979). Intracranial self-stimulation thresholds: A model for the hedonic effect of drugs of abuse. Archives of General Psychiatry, 36, 321-330.

Kornetsky, C., & Wheeling, H. S. (1982). Theoretical and methodological issues in the use of animal models of drug abuse. In M. Y. Spreglestein & A. Levy (Eds.), Behavioral models and analysis of drug action (pp. 21-38). Amsterdam: Elsevier/North Holland Biomedical Press.

Lewis, M. J. (1983). Age related decline in brain stimulation reward: Rejuvenation by amphetamine. Experimental Aging Research, 7, 225-234.

Liebman, J. M. (1983). Discriminating between reward and performance: A critical review of intracranial self-stimulation methodology. Neuroscience & Biobehavioral Reviews, 7, 45-72.

Marcus, R., & Kornetsky, C. (1974). Negative and positive intracranial reinforcement thresholds: Effects of morphine. Psychopharmacologia, 38, 1-13.

Myers, R. D. (Ed.) (1963). Methods in psychobiology (Vol. 1). New York: Academic Press.

Nazzaro, J. M., Seeger, T. F., & Gardner, E. L. (1981). Morphine differentially affects ventral tegmental and substantia nigra brain reward thresholds. Pharmacology Biochemistry & Behavior, 14, 325-331.

Ordy, J. M., Brizee, K. R., Kaack, B., & Hansche, J. (1978). Age differences in short-term memory and cell loss in cerebral cortex of the rat. Gerontology, 24, 276-285.

Orzi, F., Dow-Edwards, D., Jehle, J., Kennedy, C., & Sokoloff, L. (1983). Comparative effects of acute and chronic administration of amphetamine on local cerebral glucose utilization in the conscious rat. Journal of Cerebral Blood Flow and Metabolism, 3, 154-160.

Payton, M., Kornetsky, C., & Rosene, D. (1983). Brain stimulation reward: Thresholds versus response rates from various brainstem loci. Society for Neuroscience Abstracts, 9, 977.

Perry, N., Esposito, R. U., & Kornetsky, C. (1981). Effects of chronic naloxone treatment on brain-stimulation reward. Pharmacology Biochemistry & Behavior, 14, 247-249.

Phelps, R. W., & Lewis, M. S. (1982). A multifunctional on-line brain stimulation system. Behavioral Research Methods and Instruments, 14, 323-328.

Phillips, A. G., & Fibiger, H. C. (1978). The role of dopamine in maintaining intracranial self-stimulation in the ventral tegmentum, nucleus accumbens, and medial prefrontal cortex. Canadian Journal of Psychology, 32, 58-66.

Porrino, L. J., & Coons, E. E. (1979). Effects of GABA on stimulation-induced feeding and self-stimulation. Pharmacology Biochemistry & Behavior, 12, 125-130.

Porrino, L. J., Esposito, R. U., Seeger, T. F., Crane, A. M., Pert, A., & Sokoloff, L. (1984a). Metabolic mapping of brain during rewarding self-stimulation. Science, 244, 306-309.

Porrino, L. J., Lucignani, G., Dow-Edwards, D., & Sokoloff, L. (1984b). Correlation of dose-dependent effects of acute amphetamine administration on behavior and local cerebral metabolism in rats. Brain Research, 307, 311-320.

Schaeffer, G. J., & Holtzman, S. G. (1979). Free-operant and auto-titration brain self-stimulation procedures in the rat: A comparison of drug effects. Pharmacology Biochemistry & Behavior, 10, 127-135.

Schenk, S., Williams, T., Coupal, A., & Shizgal, P. (1980). A comparison between the effects of morphine on the rewarding and aversive properties of lateral hypothalamic and central gray stimulation. Physiological Psychology, 8, 372-378.

Seeger, T. F., & Carlson, K. R. (1981). Amphetamine and morphine: Additive effects on ICSS threshold. Society for Neuroscience Abstracts, 7, 974.

Seeger, T. F., Carlson, K. R., & Nazzaro, J. M. (1981). Pentobarbital induces a naloxone-reversible decrease in mesolimbic self-stimulation threshold. Pharmacology Biochemistry & Behavior, 15, 583-586.

Seeger, T. F., & Gardner, E. L. (1979). Enhancement of self-stimulation behavior in rats and monkeys after chronic neuroleptic treatment: Evidence for mesolimbic supersensitivity. Brain Research, 175, 49-57.

Sokoloff, L. (1981). Localization of functional activity in the central nervous system by measurement of glucose utilization with radioactive deoxyglucose. Journal of Cerebral Blood Flow and Metabolism, 1, 7-36.

Sokoloff, L. (1982). The radioactive deoxyglucose method: theory, procedure and applications for the assessment of local glucose utilization in the central nervous system. In B. W. Agranoff & M. H. Aprison (Eds.), Advances in neurochemistry (pp. 1-82). New York: Plenum Press.

Stein, L. (1962). Effects and interactions of imipramine, chlorpromazine, reserpine, and amphetamine on self-stimulation: Possible neurophysical basis of depression. In J. Wortis (Ed.), Recent advances in biological psychiatry (Vol. 4, pp. 297-311). New York: Plenum Press.

Stein, L., & Ray, O. S. (1960). Brain stimulation reward "thresholds" self-determined in rat. Psychopharmacologia, 1, 251-256.

Valenstein, E. S. (1964). Problems of measurement and interpretation with reinforcing brain stimulation. Psychological Review, 71, 415.

Valenstein, E. S., & Beer, B. (1962). Reinforcing brain stimulation in competition with water reward and shock avoidance. Science, 137, 1052-1054.

Wechsler, L. R., Savaki, H. E., & Sokoloff, L. (1979). Effects of d- and l-amphetamine on local cerebral glucose utilization in the conscious rat. Journal of Neurochemistry, 32, 15-22.

Wise, R. A., & Bozarth, M. A. (1981). Brain substrates for reinforcement and drug self-administration. Progress in Neuro-Psychopharmacology, 5, 467-474.

Yadin, E., Guarini, V., & Gallistel, C. R. (1983). Unilaterally activated systems in rats self-stimulating in the medial forebrain bundle, medial prefrontal cortex, or locus coeruleus. Brain Research, 266, 39-50.

CHAPTER 21

A COMPARISON OF TWO METHODS
DESIGNED TO RAPIDLY ESTIMATE THRESHOLDS
OF REWARDING BRAIN STIMULATION

George Fouriezos & Edward Nawiesniak

School of Psychology
University of Ottawa
Ottawa, Ontario, Canada K1N 6N5

ABSTRACT

Four experiments evaluated the relative merits of two procedures for rapidly estimating thresholds of rewarding brain stimulation. In the first method termed autotitration, rats earned brain stimulation by pressing a lever, and the stimulation became progressively weaker in pulse frequency with continued responding. The depression of a second lever restored the stimulation to its original strength. In the second protocol or timed method, rats worked through the same descending sequence of frequencies and eventually quit responding but, here, they had no control over resets of stimulation; resets were automatically triggered at timed intervals by the equipment. Experiment 1 showed that autotitration consistently produced higher reset thresholds than the threshold estimates of the timed method. The second experiment showed that autotitration's reset thresholds climbed when the stimulation sequence began at twice the customary frequency but that thresholds derived from the timed method remained at control levels with this double-frequency test. Reset thresholds from autotitration were found in Experiment 3 to be strongly influenced by changes in only the first frequency of the sequence, but this manipulation had no effect on timed-method estimates. Finally, the last experiment illustrated how autotitration might miss or seriously underestimate the effect of a pharmacological treatment. Together, these data suggest that resets made in autotitration are influenced by the value of the reinforcer made available immediately after the reset but that the alternative, timed method, is free of this problem.

INTRODUCTION

Two somewhat intertwined objectives prompt the study of drug effects on intracranial self-stimulation. One aim is to learn the neurochemical nature of components of the brain's reward circuitry. By inspecting the effects of compounds with well-documented, relatively specific neurochemical actions, psychopharmacologists hope to identify the neurotransmitters or neuromodulators at the various stages of the circuit. A second concern is to use self-stimulation as a model or an assay for the abuse liability of psychoactive substances. The rationale here is that some compounds may possess abuse potential via their interaction with central reward circuits. Such interactions might be revealed or screened by assessing the ability of drugs to lower the threshold for rewarding brain stimulation.

Threshold estimation is a time-consuming endeavor when conventional procedures are used. It involves measuring the behavioral vigor displayed in earning each of several values of a stimulation variable such as pulse frequency or current amplitude. A threshold estimate is derived by determining either the lowest stimulation value that reliably produces a just noticeable departure from no responding or one that elicits a constant but moderate level of behavior. To assess a drug effect, the procedure is repeated following injection of each of several doses of the compound. The time required to perform these assessments becomes a serious obstacle when drugs with short-lived actions are tested because such drugs cannot be trusted to sustain plateaus of effect for the 15 minutes or so needed to obtain one estimate.

To reduce the time required to estimate self-stimulation thresholds, some investigators have recently re-introduced the Stein and Ray (1960) self-determined "threshold" method. Here, rats are tested in a chamber containing two levers. The depression of one lever triggers a brief train of brain stimulation. Continued responding earns weaker and weaker stimulation; in most paradigms it is the current intensity that drops with successive stimulations. The second lever delivers no stimulation. Its depression instead resets the intensity of the available stimulation to the original suprathreshold value. The rat may then return to the first lever and run through the descending sequence again. The current when the reset occurs is deemed to be the threshold. Each excursion through the sequence takes a fraction of a minute; the speed in amassing data thus allows the assessment of short-acting compounds, provides a finer resolution to time-course studies, and enables testing a greater number of subjects. The reader is referred to Schaefer, Baumgardner, and Michael (1979) for a recent description of control circuitry.

The autotitration method has seen extensive use in psychopharmacological experiments. Its earliest (Stein, 1962; Stein & Ray, 1960) and most frequent application involved catecholamine manipulations (Schaefer & Holtzman, 1979; Schaefer & Michael, 1980; Seeger & Gardner, 1979; Zarevics & Setler, 1979), but it has also been used to examine the role of GABA in reward (Nazzaro & Gardner, 1980; Zarevics & Setler, 1981) and to investigate the effects of morphine on self-determined thresholds (Nazzaro, Seeger, & Gardner, 1981).

Despite its recent popularity the autotitration technique has not been validated; indeed, at least six cautionary notes about its use or concerning the interpretation of the self-determined thresholds have appeared. Stein (1961) noted that rats tested in autotitration reset at higher currents than those necessary to sustain responding; thus self-determined estimates of threshold were higher than those obtained by more conventional procedures. A similar, possibly related problem was noted by Gardner (1971) who found that his Rhesus monkeys would reset at higher and higher currents with experience in the task. (Rats, however, were free of this problem.) Gardner's solution was to impose a time-out of up to 5 seconds after a depression of the reset lever. A task- or effort-dependence of autotitration reset-thresholds was noted by Neill and Justice (1981; Neill, Gaar, Clark, & Britt, 1982) who found that the distribution of reset currents shifted up when a barrier that partially separated the stimulation and reset levers was removed. Valenstein (1964) raised two concerns. In addition to the fear that the method may lack general applicability--some positive brain sites, because of the low rates or the seizures they engendered, were poor candidates for evaluation by autotitration--Valenstein's main concern was that the demonstrated ability of a drug, such as amphetamine, to reduce self-determined thresholds might incorrectly be interpreted as a facilitation of reward. The alternative was that amphetamine potentiated perseverative tendencies for reasons independent of any action on reward circuitry, and the resulting persistent pressing of the stimulation lever would artificially drive down the self-determined thresholds. Finally, in his thorough review of techniques designed to distinguish between drug effects on reward and those on general performance, Liebman (1983) noted that chlorpromazine has not always been found to increase reset thresholds (Schaefer & Michael, 1980) and that picrotoxin has been reported to decrease (Nazzaro & Gardner, 1980) and to increase (Zarevics & Setler, 1981) reset thresholds. Sufficient conceptual concerns and empirical discrepancies surround autotitration to justify its re-evaluation as a useful research tool.

Derived from autotitration, a second method was introduced by Leith and Barrett (1980, 1981; Leith, 1983) which shares autotitration's speed of data acquisition. Like autotitration this method features a rapid progression through a descending sequence of currents, but unlike autotitration the rats in this second method are not permitted to depress a reset lever nor does their behavior in any way promote a reset. Instead, resets to the initial current occur under the control of programming equipment; in the Leith and Barrett method and in the "timed" method of this report, trials are started (the equipment resets) at fixed intervals of time.

This paper describes an evaluation of these two approaches to rapid estimation of reward thresholds. The first experiment examined long-term stability of the estimates, and the next two challenged the robustness of the estimates with alterations in the sequence of rewarding stimuli. The final experiment tested the prediction derived from the results of earlier tests that autotitration may fail to detect some genuine drug effects.

EXPERIMENT 1

This experiment was designed to compare thresholds obtained from the timed and autotitration paradigms. Five measures from each rat were taken using both methods in five consecutive days in the first and last weeks of the 6-week protocol. (Experiments 2, 3, and 4, described below, were conducted in the intervening weeks.) Thus in addition to a comparison of the two methods, this experiment provided an assessment of within- and between-session reliability with a determination of long-term stability of the measures.

Method

Subjects

Under sodium pentobarbital anesthesia (60 mg/kg, intraperitoneally) five male Long-Evans rats weighing between 340 and 620 g at surgery were stereotaxically provided with a chronic, monopolar stimulating electrode (0.25 mm diameter.) aimed at the lateral hypothalamus. The heads were fixed in the plane of de Groot (1959) and the stainless steel, Formvar-insulated electrodes were directed with the following coordinate sets: 1.0 mm caudal to bregma (C), 1.5 mm lateral to midline (L), and 8.0 mm below dura (V) (n = 1); 1.0C, 1.0L, 8.0V (n = 1); and 0.4C, 1.7L, 8.0V (n = 3). A wire wrapped around four skull screws served as the current return.

Apparatus

The floor of the wooden test chambers measured 30 x 36 cm and the walls were 38 cm high. Two Lehigh Valley rodent manipulanda were located opposite each other centered on the 30 cm walls. The levers extended 25 mm into the boxes and their top surfaces were 4 cm above the 13 mm grid floor.

A constant-current generator (Mundl, 1980) provided stimulation pulses that were continuously adjustable to 1 mA. Although the pulses were always monophasic, the unit incorporated a low resistance shunt to ground between pulses to prevent a temporal accumulation of charge at the electrode. The current was adjusted and monitored by reading the voltage drop across a 1 kohm resistor in series with the current return.

The remaining stimulation variables were controlled by a pulse generator that automatically advanced through a programmed sequence of pulse frequencies. This unit controlled both the autotitration and the timed paradigms, and it accumulated the following data: a running total of the delivered stimulations, the number of resets made, the time spent at each frequency, and the number of responses made in earning the eight stimulations at each step.

Paradigms

Figure 1 represents a cumulative record (with the stepper pen traveling down) to illustrate the similarities and differences between the present implementations of the autotitration and timed reset methods. In both methods rats pressed a stimulation lever to deliver a 0.5 second train of 0.1 msec cathodal pulses. All responses were counted but only those occurring after trains were delivered could reinitiate a stimulation train. Current intensities, individually selected in preliminary training sessions for each rat, remained unchanged throughout all testing; in these studies the frequency of pulses in the train decreased with repeated responding. Pulse frequencies followed a descending series with shifts from one frequency to the next occurring after every eight stimulations. The sequence followed approximately a 0.1 log unit progression and the standard or baseline sequence was 100, 80, 63, 50, 40, 32, 25 . . .Hz continuing for a total of 16 steps. The first five steps of this standard sequence are represented by the horizontal bands (labeled 100, 80, 63, et cetera) in Figure 1. The resets to the initial frequency, whether triggered by machine or by rat, were signaled by a brief tone.

The chief difference between the paradigms was in triggering resets to the initial frequency. In the timed method they occurred under timer control at 1 minute intervals without regard to the behavior of the rat. This is shown in the left-hand panel of Figure 1 as the vertical resets of the stepper pen occurring well after responding has ceased which, in turn, is represented by the horizontal trace of the recorder. In the autotitration method the second lever was active; its depression restored the stimulation to the initial frequency (Figure 1; right-hand panel).

Training

Rats were given at least 3 days recovery after surgery before screening for self-stimulation and training in the timed method. Immediately following the machine-produced resets, rats were shaped or primed to self-stimulate. Currents were initially adjusted to obtain self-stimulation performance over most of each minute-long, inter-reset interval. Shaping and priming were

TIMED RESETS   AUTOTITRATION

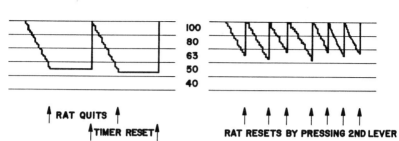

↑ RAT QUITS ↑
↑TIMER RESET↑   **RAT RESETS BY PRESSING 2ND LEVER**

Figure 1: Comparison of methods: representation of a cumulative
record with time running left to right and stepper traveling down.
In autotitration rats earn eight 0.5 second trains of pulses at 100
Hz, then eight at 80 Hz, then 63 Hz, etc. Stimulation may be reset
by the rat to 100 Hz at any time by depression of another lever;
resets are indicated by vertical rises of trace to top of 100 Hz
band. In the timed method the rat cannot reset. The rat can obtain
reinforcements by pressing the stimulation lever or it can quit
responding as is shown by the horizontal tracks of the recorder pen.
Here, resets are controlled by a timer adjusted to reset at 1 minute
intervals.

occasionally omitted, and these omissions became more frequent as the session
progressed. Once the rat demonstrated proficiency in this paradigm as
indicated by repeatedly quitting at about the same frequency and by rapidly
returning to the stimulation lever upon tone signaled resets, the current was
reduced so that quitting occurred at 50 or 40 Hz (4th or 5th steps). This
training session lasted about 2 hours.

The rats were then trained in the autotitration paradigm. Initially,
shaping was used to draw the rat to the reset lever after it had quit
responding on the stimulation lever. Several reset responses were manually
reinforced with brain stimulation at the beginning of this training: The number
of rewarded resets was reduced to one or two after about 10 shuttles between
the levers; rewards for resets were intermittently omitted over the next 30
shuttles or so; and, finally, they were omitted altogether. This training
session, too, lasted about 2 hours.

Finally, the rats were given daily training sessions in both paradigms for
at least 6 days. These sessions lasted 20 minutes and their order of
presentation was reversed daily. Minor re-adjustments in current were made at
this stage, but each rat received the full 6-day training at the final current.
These currents ranged from 160 to 250 µA across subjects, and they remained
unchanged for the remainder of the tests.

Procedure

Rats were tested for 5 consecutive days in both paradigms during Week 1
and again in Week 6. Both daily sessions lasted 25 minutes; the first 10
minutes constituted a warm up period when no data were collected and the last
15 minutes yielded five threshold estimates. The 3 minutes devoted to each

estimate were partitioned as a 2-minute trial followed by 1 minute used to retrieve data. Although no new data were amassed during retrieval, this process did not interfere with the ongoing testing; that is, from the rat's perspective, this third minute was no different from the previous 2 minutes. The two methods were presented in opposite orders from day to day and about 2 hours separated them.

Data Analysis

In the majority of autotitration implementations, estimates of threshold are derived by noting the value of the stimulation when the reset is made. In our version we obtained such measures by counting the number of stimulations earned and of resets made in a 2-minute period. Their ratio gave the average number of stimulations per reset, and because each frequency was offered for eight stimulation trains, division of the ratio by 8 yielded the average number of steps per reset. This value was used to interpolate the frequency at which the resets were made; this latter value is termed reset frequency (F_{RST}) in this paper.

In the timed method the rates of responding for each frequency through the sequence were used to interpolate the frequency corresponding to a rate of 0.5 responses per second; we refer to this value as required frequency (F_{REQ}). The theoretical justification of this and of related procedures has been presented elsewhere (Gallistel, Shizgal, & Yeomans, 1981).

Although we wished to use identical analytic methods in the two paradigms, this proved to be impossible. Rats in autotitration rarely drop to rates low enough to permit interpolation, and when tested in the timed method, they do not reset. Moreover, noting the frequency offered when the machine performed the reset would have been misleading because, after having quit at a given frequency, rats in the timed method often emitted anticipatory responses just before the reset. These anticipatory responses usually advanced the pointer to the next frequency. Although unequivocal quitting might have occurred at one frequency, the one available at the machine-produced reset may have been one or two steps lower.

Results and Discussion

The data from these baseline determinations are illustrated in Figure 2. Three features are immediately apparent. First, there seems to be more within-session variability in the timed method than in autotitration. This, we think, is partly an artifact of our fixed trial duration of 2 minutes. In autotitration 2 minutes sufficed for about 6 to 10 resets (see Figure 1). Although individual resets may have been widely scattered, allowing this many passes through the sequence renders stability across trials to the average point of reset calculation. In contrast the 2-minute trial in the timed method permits exactly two passes. Based on fewer passes, the individual F_{REQ}s are less likely to be anchored near each other. Both methods offer acceptable within-session variability; with five replications per point, standard errors of the mean would be about one third of the magnitude of the shown confidence limits.

Second, both threshold estimates appear to be higher in Week 6 than in Week 1. Day to day fluctuation seems acceptable but the long-term change is substantial. An inspection of baseline data of the experiments performed during the intervening weeks revealed that the climb was gradual. Thus, both

Figure 2: Comparison of reset frequencies (F_{RST}; autotitration; filled circles) and required frequencies (F_{REQ}; timed method; open circles). Each symbol represents the geometric mean and 0.95 confidence interval of five threshold estimates taken daily over the five days of Week 1 and Week 6. With rare exception (Rat E-1, for example) autotitration resets are made at frequencies higher than those where rats quit responding when tested in the timed method.

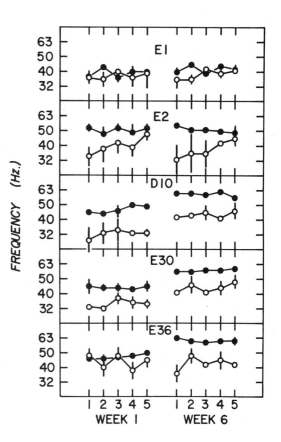

paradigms might be trusted in within-subject designs provided that control conditions interpose experimental ones. The comparisons of experimental results to control tests performed days earlier, such as in assessment of irreversible lesions, would not be recommended; between-subject designs would be preferred in evaluating permanent or long-lasting challenges.

The third feature is that autotitration gave F_{RST}s that were consistently higher than the timed method's F_{REQ}s (binomial test, $P = Q = 0.5$, $p < 0.001$). Thus these rats reset at stimulation values higher than those values where they quit responding, a finding that replicates Stein's (1961) observation that rats tested in autotitration do not reset upon arriving at a nonreinforcing stimulation. Instead, they reset at values that would be revealed to be suprathreshold by a more conventional paradigm.

EXPERIMENT 2

Methods of threshold estimation should yield stable measures under a variety of manipulations assuming, of course, that the manipulations do not genuinely alter the "true" threshold. One such manipulation we investigated was changing the strength and number of suprathreshold values in the descending progression before the usual point of resetting or quitting. The gradient of descent was psychophysically maintained; each new frequency was still 0.1 log unit less than the prior one. However, the frequency to which the rat or timer reset--as was the entire sequence--was double the customary one.

Method

The five rats were given four sessions daily on the 5 days of Week 2. Two of the sessions were control runs, one in each paradigm, that were identical to those described in Experiment 1. That is, we used the sequence 100, 80, 63, 50 . . .Hz. The test sessions contained three additional steps inserted at the beginning thus: 200, 160, 125, 100, 80, 63 . . .Hz. The four combinations of paradigm (autotitration or timed) and condition (double or control) were randomly ordered with the provision that no order was repeated for any particular rat.

Results and Discussion

The four daily sessions generated five estimates each; these measures were averaged and the effect of the double-frequency progression was expressed by the ratio of the test-data geometric mean to control-data geometric mean. Each rat provided two such ratios daily, one from autotitration and the other from the timed method. The geometric means and 95% confidence intervals averaged over the five animals are depicted in Figure 3.

Doubling the frequencies on the sequence had little or no effect on F_{REQ}s of the timed method as indicated by the inclusion of the control (1.0) level by the 0.95 confidence intervals. In contrast, the F_{RST}s of autotitration were

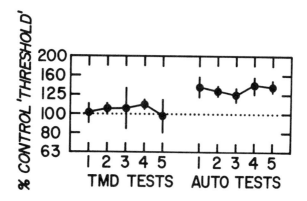

Figure 3: Effect of double frequency. Geometric means and 0.95 confidence intervals averaged across subjects (n = 5) and replications (r = 5). Data express the effect of starting rats at 200 Hz pulse frequency as percentage of threshold estimate obtained with the usual 100 Hz initial frequency. Both timed and autotitration tests were held on Days 1 to 5 (abscissa) of Week 2; they are shown separately for clarity. Double-frequency starts had little or no effect on threshold estimates made by timed method but the autotitration measures were higher under this condition.

strongly affected. Rats reset at frequencies 30% greater, a little more than one full step in our sequence, when the progression was doubled.

Such an effect on autotitration was not seen, however, by Schaefer and Holtzman (1979) who examined the effect of adding or subtracting 12 to 36 μA to their starting currents which ranged from 103 to 176 μA. The present challenge was relatively greater; that this experiment doubled initial frequencies while the Schaefer and Holtzman starting currents were altered by about 20% may account for the difference. Furthermore, Schaefer and Holtzman (1979) employed pulse durations of 2 msec. From strength-duration data on lateral hypothalamic self-stimulation (Matthews, 1977), 2 msec pulses are roughly 9 times more effective than 0.1 msec pulses, and we suspect that equivalent currents (1 mA for 0.1 msec pulses) probably excite the entire bundle of reward-related neurons; increases in current beyond 1 mA are poorly compensated by reductions in frequency, suggesting that a ceiling of pulse effectiveness is reached by currents this high or their equivalents. Thus, whereas Schaefer and Holtzman (1979) did increase the strength of their pulses, the increase in current might not have sufficiently altered the rewarding value of the initial stimulation. Their conclusion that rats in autotitration are not simply resetting after emitting a constant number of responses is undoubtedly correct; the point made here, however, is that our observed changes in autotitration thresholds may be reconciled with the stability seen by Schaefer and Holtzman (1979) by considering whether the change in stimulation effectively altered the rewarding value of the initial frequency or current.

There are two possible accounts for the shifts seen in autotitration. One is that doubling the frequencies engendered a genuine but subtle contrast effect that was detected only by autotitration. We believe this explanation is incorrect for the following three reasons. First, the manipulation of adding three levels of suprathreshold stimulation at the top of the sequence is unlikely to give rise to a real contrast effect. Contrast might have been produced if the gradient of the progression were steeper, but in this experiment the gradient had been strictly defended. Second, contrast effects are not seen when a conventional paradigm is used to document refractory periods and conduction times for the fibers supporting self-stimulation (Bielajew & Shizgal, 1982). When rats are tested with each stimulation value available for a full minute, the insertion of additional frequencies at the beginning of a determination does not influence the frequency threshold (C. Bielajew, personal communication). Third, if the contrast effect had been genuine, then the timed method would have detected it as well. The timed method is sensitive to pharmacological treatments that affect self-stimulation threshold such as injection of d-amphetamine (see Experiment 4 of this report) and the neuroleptic alpha-flupenthixol (Corbett, Stellar, Stinus, Kelley, & Fouriezos, 1983). Similarly, it readily detects changes in orthogonal stimulation variables such as current intensity and train duration by showing compensatory shifts in F s (unpublished observations). If a genuine contrast effect had been there to be detected, then both methods should have revealed it.

The alternative explanation for the autotitration shifts is to propose that an immediate history of higher than usual stimulation causes rats to reset earlier than they do with the customary sequence. The results of Experiment 1 showed that autotitration resets occurred at frequencies that were still rewarding. This experiment shows that the point of reset thence rises if higher level stimulation is made available after the reset response. These data lead to the notion that the decision of when to reset might be based upon a relative judgment. Instead of assessing the value of currently earned

- 455 -

stimulation for its own merit, rats in autotitration might be comparing the delivered stimulation to that offered immediately after the reset response. For example, 63 Hz may be worth earning when resets restore the stimulation to 100 Hz; 63 Hz might not, however, compare as favorably when the rat can reset the stimulation to 200 Hz. The possibility that this sort of relative assessment occurs in the timed method is precluded because there the rats have no control over resets. The sole decision confronting them is whether to take the offered stimulation. The possibility that autotitration methods suffer this contaminant was tested directly in the following experiment.

EXPERIMENT 3

The argument to this point is that the reset response is not guided by an absolute decision (Is this stimulation worth earning?) but rather is based on a relative judgment (Is it worth working for given what's available immediately after a reset?). If a relative judgment does indeed guide resets, then it should be possible to change the point of resetting by altering the standard used for comparison to the present stimulation. The autotitration points of reset did rise, in Experiment 2, in reaction to adding three steps to the top of the sequence, a manipulation which effectively would have doubled the standard if the standard was the first frequency made available after the reset. In addition to altering the initial frequency, however, the manipulation of Experiment 2 suffers the confound of increasing the distance between the initial stimulus and the usual point of reset. Experiment 3 removed the confound; here, the customary sequence was employed except that only the first frequency, normally 100 Hz, was replaced by others. The remainder of the sequence (80, 63, 50, 40 . . .Hz) was left intact.

The prediction was that if relative assessments guided resetting responses and if the standard used was the first value following the reset, then the point of reset would rise when the 100 Hz starting frequency was replaced by higher initial values (125 or 160 Hz). Moreover, the power of the standard might work in both directions. If the initial frequency was reduced to 80 or 63 Hz (and followed by the normal remainder of the sequence), then the point of reset would drop because the standard would now be lower than normal. In other words, the prediction was that there would be a positive correlation between the initial frequency and the point at which the rats in autotitration reset.

Method

Each rat received four sessions daily for 4 days in Week 3 following the protocol established in Experiments 1 and 2. A test session and control session were held for each paradigm, and these control sessions were identical to the control tests described above. The test sessions featured substitution of the usual starting frequency of 100 Hz with one of these initial frequencies--160, 125, 80, and 63 Hz. The paradigm and condition were randomized with respect to within-day order of presentation, and a unique order of substitutes across days was administered to each rat.

Results and Discussion

Figure 4 shows the effect of altering only the initial frequency on F_{REQ}s of the timed method and on F_{RST}s of autotitration. The method outlined in Experiment 2 of calculating and depicting these data was used. Rats tested in

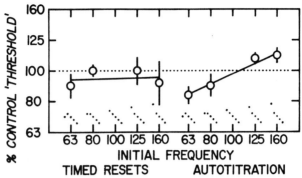

Figure 4: Changes in initial frequency. Geometric means and 0.95 confidence intervals of five rats' threshold-estimate averages which, in turn, were based on five determinations. These data are expressed as percentage of control (100 Hz) starting frequency. Abscissa indicates the frequency that replaced the customary 100 Hz and the insets just above the abscissa reflect the progression of pulse frequency. (These insets are not to be read against this ordinate.) The lines represent best fitting linear regressions. Changes in the starting frequency had no systematic effect on estimates of threshold using the timed method. In contrast, reset frequencies reliably tracked the initial frequency in autotitration tests.

the timed method showed no consistent effect of altered initial frequencies. They quit at about the same frequencies regardless of the value of the top frequency. These same rats, however, demonstrated resetting in the autotitration paradigm that closely followed changes in the initial frequency. Not only did they reset above their usual points when offered initial frequencies above 100 Hz, but they also reduced their points of reset when the initial frequency was dropped below the usual value. The correlation between initial frequency and F_{RST} was 0.98. These results provide compelling evidence that rats tested in autotitration make comparative assessments of the stimulation's value relative to the stimulation available immediately after the reset.

Note that the data shown for the initial frequencies of 63 and 80 Hz in autotitration were based on four instead of five rats. One rat when confronted with the 63 Hz starting frequency ceased to reset altogether. The rat completed only two of the five trials; in both it advanced the frequency to 25 Hz, a frequency that was less than half its usual point of reset. It did complete all five trials when the sequence started at 80 Hz, but its behavior appeared disorganized here as well. On several occasions it quickly turned to the reset lever and without pressing it rapidly returned to the stimulation lever even though it had driven the stimulation well below values that it worked for in other tests. Despite the fact that the rat reliably self-stimulated in autotitration and in the timed method for frequencies of 80 and 63 Hz, its resetting behavior was completely disrupted when these values were used as initial frequencies in autotitration. Apart from providing adequate justification for the exclusion of this rat's data from the 63 and 80 Hz conditions, this profound disruption of behavior produced by altering only the initial frequency in the sequence dramatically highlights the importance of that initial stimulus in controlling when the rat resets in the autotitration paradigm.

EXPERIMENT 4

Despite the problem that autotitration resets are based upon relative assessments, it may be argued that the paradigm nonetheless retains some usefulness. As long as F_{RST}s are documented with sequences that are never changed—with standards that remain fixed—then it does not matter that resets are guided by comparisons of the currently obtained stimulation to the reset value; reliable estimates of threshold will emerge. Consider, however, the following. Autotitration was originally developed for drug testing. Without evidence to the contrary, the influence of a drug such as cocaine or amphetamine is thought to affect all values of stimulation equally. For a very wide range of values, there is no reason to believe that the ability of a stimulant to enhance the per-pulse effectiveness differs as a function of pulse frequency. Consider a control run in the autotitration paradigm. As discussed above, frequency of the currently administered stimulation is compared to the initial frequency. At some point the obtained stimulation is deemed to compare poorly to the frequency available immediately after reset and the reset response is made. Now consider a test with the rat injected with an agent that potentiates a downstream synaptic effect of the stimulation; a re-uptake blocker is a good example. Once again a comparison is made; this time it is the currently earned stimulation, with the effect potentiated by the drug, that is compared to the standard, with the effect also potentiated by the drug. If the effects of the standard and the currently earned stimulation have both been potentiated to the same degree, then the relative standing of the frequency where resetting normally occurred will not have changed. Thus, despite the genuine effect, autotitration may fail to detect it. In other words, autotitration may fail in the very domain, psychopharmacology, for which it was originally introduced.

Obviously, an extreme case is presented above. Such extremes are unlikely to occur when one considers the results of Experiment 2. There the entire sequence was doubled but the F_{RST}s rose by only 30%. The relevance of this result becomes clear if the double frequency is treated as an analogy to a drug experiment; if odd pulses are imagined to be the original ones and if even pulses are imagined to represent an agonist's contribution, then it must be concluded that autotitration did indeed detect the contribution of the electronic agonist but did not measure it faithfully.

In this experiment we compared the ability of the two methods to detect the threshold-lowering effect of amphetamine. If the argument presented above is correct, that is if the ability of an agonist to potentiate all stimulation by roughly equal degrees poses a problem for autotitration, then the magnitude of amphetamine's effect in autotitration should consistently be less than that measured by the timed method.

Method

Rats received daily test sessions over the 5 days of Week 4 and Week 5. Each test lasted 33 minutes, not including a warm-up period of about 5 minutes. Three baseline determinations were made in the first 9 minutes, the rat was injected at the start of the next 9-minute period, and five threshold estimates were taken in the last 15 minutes of the session. Amphetamine (d-amphetamine sulphate; 0.5 mg/kg in saline) was injected intraperitoneally on Days 1, 3, and

5 and saline was injected on Days 2 and 4 of each week. Three rats were tested in autotitration on Week 4 followed by timed-method tests in Week 5 while the other two rats had the reverse order of tests.

Results and Discussion

Figure 5 shows in detail the results of these drug tests. (Figure 6 summarizes these details by grouping the data from all subjects without regard to the order of test paradigm.) The data from the three rats which received the autotitration assessments first, followed by the timed evaluations in the

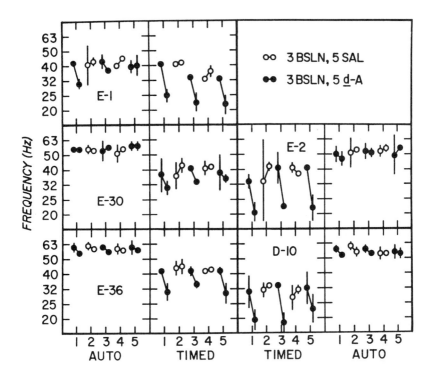

Figure 5: Detailed results in d-amphetamine tests. Rats in left half underwent drug tests first using autotitration on Week 4 and then with the timed method on Week 5. Rats E-2 and D-10 on right received opposite order of testing. Each pair of linked symbols shows, first, three preinjection thresholds and, second, five postinjection estimates. Filled symbols represent amphetamine tests (Days 1, 3, and 5) and open symbols depict saline injections (Days 2 and 4). Autotitration tests (left and right extremes) failed to measure any effect of d-amphetamine (0.5 mg/kg, intraperitoneally) in four of the cases but a diminishing effect was seen in Rat E-1. The timed-method tests (inner panels) revealed substantial and consistent drops in threshold after amphetamine injections.

next week, are shown in the left half of Figure 5 while the results from Rats
E-2 and D-10, which experienced the opposite order, are depicted in the right
half. The left member of each pair of linked symbols shows the preinjection
estimate of threshold while the second member shows the postinjection result.
Filled circles represent amphetamine tests and the open circles are saline
tests. Except in the first test for rat E-1, the autotitration method failed to
detect a threshold-lowering effect of amphetamine. This is seen clearly in the
far right-hand panels for rats E-30 and E-36 and again in the far left panels
for Rats E-2 and D-10. In marked contrast to the lack of effect witnessed by
autotitration, the timed method revealed strong and consistent drops in
threshold after amphetamine administration in the same animals. The results
from E-1 are especially instructive; this rat showed a modest drop in reset
threshold with the first drug test in autotitration, but the magnitude of the
effect was reduced in the second test and altogether absent in the third. This
pattern follows the dynamics of tolerance; but tolerance cannot explain the
resumption of the drug effect when E-1 was subsequently tested with the timed
method in the following week, nor can such an explanation account for the
consistent lack of effect measured by autotitration regardless of autotitration
preceding or following the timed tests.

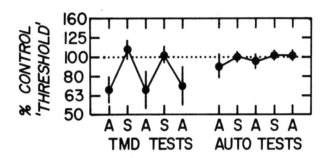

Figure 6: Summary of the Amphetamine Tests. The data shown in Figure
5 are collapsed and expressed as geometric means and 0.95 confidence
intervals of preinjection baseline tests. Amphetamine (A) tests were
administered on Days 1, 3, and 5 while saline (S) was injected on
Days 2 and 4. The timed method measured a consistent decrease in
required frequency produced by amphetamine injections whereas the
autotitration technique appears to have missed the drug effect.

CONCLUSION

The results of these experiments suggest that rats tested with the
autotitration method press the reset lever when the stimulation fails to meet
some internal criterion <u>relative</u> to the stimulation available at the beginning
of the sequence. This conclusion is consistent with, but not exclusively
supported by, the results of Experiment 1 and 2 which demonstrated, first, that
autotitration resets occurred at values of stimulation that were still
reinforcing and, second, that rats reset at even higher stimulation values when
the sequence began at twice its customary value. Better support for the notion
was found in Experiment 3 wherein the first frequency of the series--the one
that may be viewed as the most immediate consequence of a reset response--was
found to strongly influence resetting; there it was shown that reset thresholds

rose and fell, faithfully following the first frequency. The fourth experiment provided the strongest support for a relative comparison guiding resetting by showing that autotitration greatly underestimated the magnitude of amphetamine's threshold-lowering effect. In marked contrast the timed method, which is a simple modification of the autotitration protocol, demonstrated an acceptable stability throughout Experiments 1 to 3 and was sensitive to the amphetamine effect in Experiment 4.

Neill and his colleagues (Neill, Gaar, Clark, & Britt, 1982; Neill & Justice, 1981) have shown that the distribution of reset intensities collected in an autotitration paradigm can be shifted towards higher currents (i.e., rats reset earlier in the sequence) by removing a barrier that partially separates the stimulation and reset levers. They suggested that the decision to reset is influenced by the effort required to make the reset response. With the partition in place, the greater effort required to move to the reset lever biases staying at the stimulation lever; when the barrier is eliminated, the rats leave the stimulation lever earlier in the descending sequence of currents. Obviously, a method that produces shifts in estimates of threshold as a result of altered task requirements is of limited utility in assessing the influence of a drug on central reinforcement mechanisms. It denies to the psychopharmacologist the possibility of distinguishing a selective effect on reinforcement from a general debilitation produced by the drug. Together, autotitration's compliance to task demands and its underestimation of a drug effect seriously mitigate its recommendation for further use. The simple modification of transferring control of resets from the rat to the machine apparently rectifies these shortcomings without sacrificing the speed of data acquisition.

ACKNOWLEDGMENTS

We thank Dr. Catherine Bielajew for critical reading of earlier drafts of this paper. This project was supported by Ontario Mental Health Foundation Grant 808 and Natural Sciences and Engineering Research Council of Canada Grant A7886 to the first author.

REFERENCES

Bielajew, C., & Shizgal, P. (1982). Behaviorally derived measures of conduction velocity for rewarding medial forebrain bundle stimulation. Brain Research, 237, 107-119.

Corbett, D., Stellar, J. R., Stinus, L., Kelley, A., & Fouriezos, G. (1983). Time course of alpha-flupenthixol action explains "response artifacts" of neuroleptic action on brain stimulation reward. Science, 222, 1251-1252.

de Groot, J. (1959). The rat brain in stereotaxic coordinates. Amsterdam: N. V. Noord-Hollandsche Uitgevers.

Gallistel, C. R., Shizgal, P., & Yeomans, J. S. (1981). A portrait of the substrate for self-stimulation. Psychological Review, 88, 228-273.

Gardner, E. L. (1971). An improved technique for determining brain reward thresholds in primates. Behavior Research Methods and Instrumentation, 3, 273-274.

Leith, N. J. (1983). Effects of apomorphine on self-stimulation responding: Does the drug mimic the current? Brain Research, 277, 129-136.

Leith, N. J., & Barrett, R. J. (1980). Effects of chronic amphetamine or reserpine on self-stimulation responding: Animal model of depression? Psychopharmacology, 72, 9-15.

Leith, N. J., & Barrett, R. J. (1981). Self-stimulation and amphetamine: Tolerance to d and l isomers and cross tolerance to cocaine and methylphenidate. Psychopharmacology, 74, 23-28.

Liebman, J. M. (1983). Discriminating between reward and performance: A critical review of intracranial self-stimulation methodology. Neuroscience and Biobehavioral Reviews, 7, 45-72.

Mundl, W. J. (1980). A constant current stimulator. Physiology & Behavior, 24, 991-993.

Nazzaro, J., & Gardner, E. L. (1980). GABA antagonism lowers self-stimulation thresholds in the ventral tegmental area. Brain Research, 189, 279-283.

Nazzaro, J. M., Seeger, T. F., & Gardner, E. L. (1981). Morphine differentially affects ventral tegmental and substantia nigra brain reward thresholds. Pharmacology Biochemistry & Behavior, 14, 325-331.

Neill, D. B., Gaar, L. A., Clark, A. S., & Britt, M. D. (1982). "Rate-free" measures of self-stimulation and microinjections: Evidence toward a new concept of dopamine and reward. In B. G. Hoebel & D. Novin (Eds.), The neural basis of feeding and reward (pp. 289-297). Brunswick, ME: Haer Institute.

Neill, D. B., & Justice, J. B., Jr. (1981). An hypothesis for a behavioral function of dopaminergic transmission in nucleus accumbens. In R. B. Chronister & J. F. DeFrance (Eds.), The neurobiology of the nucleus accumbens (pp. 338-347). Brunswick, ME: Haer Institute.

Schaefer, G. J., Baumgardner, D. G., & Michael, R. P. (1979). Constant-current, biphasic titrating stimulator for brain self-stimulation. Physiology & Behavior, 22, 1217-1219.

Schaefer, G. J., & Holtzman, S. G. (1979). Free-operant and auto-titration brain self-stimulation procedures in the rat: A comparison of drug effects. Pharmacology Biochemistry & Behavior, 10, 127-135.

Schaefer, G. J., & Michael, R. P. (1980). Acute effects of neuroleptics on brain self-stimulation thresholds in rats. Psychopharmacology, 67, 9-15.

Seeger, T. F., & Gardner, E. L. (1979). Enhancement of self-stimulation behavior in rats and monkeys after chronic neuroleptic treatment: Evidence for mesolimbic supersensitivity. Brain Research, 175, 49-57.

Stein, L. (1961). Inhibitory effects of phenothiazine compounds on self-stimulation of the brain. Diseases of the Nervous System 22(Suppl.), 1-5.

Stein, L. (1962). Effects and interactions of imipramine, chlorpromazine, reserpine, and amphetamine on self-stimulation: Possible neurophysiological basis of depression. In J. Wortis (Ed.), Recent advances in biological psychiatry (pp. 288-308). New York: Plenum Press.

Stein, L., & Ray, O. S. (1960). Brain stimulation reward "thresholds" self-determined in rat. Psychopharmacologia, 1, 251-256.

Valenstein, E. S. (1964). Problems of measurement and interpretation with reinforcing brain stimulation. Psychological Review, 71, 415-437.

Zarevics, P., & Setler, P. E. (1979). Simultaneous rate-independent and rate-dependent assessment of intracranial self-stimulation: Evidence for the direct involvement of dopamine in brain reinforcement mechanisms. Brain Research, 169, 499-512.

Zarevics, P., & Setler, P. E. (1981). Effects of GABAergic drugs on brain stimulation reward as assessed by a 'threshold' method. Brain Research, 215, 201-209.

CHAPTER 22

A MULTIFUNCTIONAL ON-LINE BRAIN STIMULATION SYSTEM:
INVESTIGATION OF ALCOHOL AND AGING EFFECTS

Michael J. Lewis[1] and Richard W. Phelps[2]

[1]Department of Psychology
Howard University
Washington, District of Columbia   20059
and
[2]Cortex Corporation
Wellesley, Massachusetts

ABSTRACT

A multifunctional on-line brain stimulation system designed for brain stimulation reward (BSR) research is described. This microcomputer-based system provides programs which permit determination of BSR thresholds, BSR response rates, and brain resistance. Studies using this system to investigate the reinforcing effects of ethanol and the effects of aging on BSR are discussed.

INTRODUCTION

Brain Stimulation Reward (BSR) has been used to investigate the reinforcing effects of drugs from early after its discovery by Olds and Milner (1954). Olds himself and his collaborators (Olds, 1958; Olds, Killam, & Bach-y-Rita, 1956; Olds, Killam, & Eiduson, 1957) did some of the earliest research examining the effects of several drugs on BSR (e.g., pentobarbital, chlorpromazine, and LSD). Since this early work there has been quite extensive research on the effects of many drugs of abuse on BSR. This work has been thoroughly reviewed at several junctures (e.g., Esposito & Kornetsky, 1978; Miller, 1960; Stein, 1968; Wise, 1978; Wise & Bozarth, 1981). There have been considerably fewer reports on the effects of ethanol (ETOH) on BSR. ETOH is undoubtedly the most abused substance, yet the physiological and neurochemical bases of its reinforcement, as well as other major phenomena, remain a mystery.

There has been relatively little research on the effects of ETOH on BSR. The previous research showed highly variable effects of ETOH. At low doses response rate has been reported to increase (Carlson & Lydic, 1976; Vrtunski, Murray, & Wolin, 1973), whereas with moderate to high doses only depression of response was found by these authors. These authors examined only lateral hypothalamic (LH) loci. Earlier research (St. Laurent, 1972; St. Laurent & Olds, 1967) found that ETOH only reduced response rate at these sites; however, ETOH could still enhance BSR responding at subcortical telencephalic placements such as the septal area. Still another report (Routtenberg, 1981) indicates that ETOH has no effect on BSR even at high doses if animals were primed (given noncontingent stimulation) sufficiently at the beginning of the BSR session.

It is apparent from the variable effects reported by these few studies that the effects of ETOH on BSR are not clear and require more extensive research. Recent research in our laboratory has examined the effects of ETOH on BSR at LH and ventral tegmental brain sites with the discovery of new

- 463 -

effects of ETOH. This research has focused on BSR threshold as well as response rate at these sites and employed a multifunctional, microcomputer-based BSR system. The system has also been employed to examine both opioid agonists and antagonists, psychostimulants, and age-related declines in motivation. This system and the method for determining threshold will be discussed in detail in the first part of this chapter. We will then discuss our research with it on the rewarding effects of ETOH, on the age-related changes in BSR performance, and on the rejuvenating effects of psychostimulants on the performance of aged individuals.

MULTIFUNCTIONAL BSR SYSTEM

Measurement of electrical brain stimulation reward threshold using psychophysical methods presents a significant problem. The subject's behavior (usually lever pressing) is controlled by the reinforcing stimulation for which the threshold is to be found. Many experimenters have tried to avoid this problem by measuring animal response rate using suprathreshold stimulation and inferring changes in threshold from changes in rate. If a rate measure is used, however, it is not possible to discriminate between the reward-relevant effects of the experimental treatment and its effects on motor responses.

Alternative methods (e.g., Huston & Mills, 1971; Marcus & Kornetsky, 1974; Valenstein & Meyers, 1964) determine threshold with less reliance on rate of response. Huston and Mills (1971) measure BSR threshold with a psychophysical procedure based on the observation that performance under a fixed-ratio (FR) schedule is different from that under a continuous reinforcement (CRF) schedule (Ferster & Skinner, 1957). In this procedure rats lever press for rewarding stimulation on an FR schedule and, concurrently, on a CRF schedule, using a single lever. This combined schedule is fixed at a suprathreshold level, which maintains the lever-pressing response at any CRF current intensity.

An animal performing on a simple FR schedule exhibits postreinforcement pauses (PRP; Ferster & Skinner, 1957). As CRF current intensity is increased from zero on a CRF-FR schedule, FR pauses become shorter and eventually disappear. The rat's performance shifts from that which is characteristic of an FR schedule (many PRPs) to that which is characteristic of a CRF schedule (no PRPs). Decreasing the CRF current intensity causes the pauses to reappear. Threshold is determined by appearance or disappearance of these pauses as the CRF current intensity is varied. Huston and Mills (1971) reported that threshold determination was independent of the size of the FR and of the suprathreshold FR current intensity.

The definition of a PRP has been a problem using this threshold technique. Huston originally defined a PRP as the interval just visually discernible on the cumulative recorder. Cassens and Mills (1973) defined it as an interval greater than 7 seconds, but not more than 3 minutes. Cassens, Shaw, Dudding, and Mills (1975) devised a rate-independent definition; a PRP was defined as an interval greater than the mean CRF interresponse interval (IRI) plus three standard deviations. Thus, a PRP was relative to the CRF IRI. This provided a rate-independent means of determining the PRP and, hence, threshold.

The system we have developed employs the same rate-independent concept for determining thresholds. A fixed number of FR reinforcements are presented at each CRF current level. Threshold is defined as the current level that produces PRP half of the time--a PRP/FR ratio of 0.50. Threshold is determined by evaluating PRP/FR ratios over a CRF current range and then by

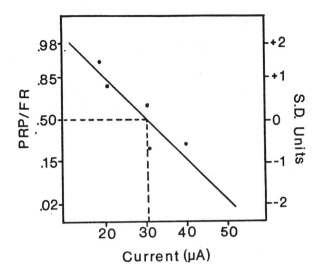

Figure 1: Post reinforcement pauses per fixed-ratio reinforcement (PRP/FR) as a function of current intensity. From Cassens, Dudding, and Mills, 1975.

interpolating the current value at a PRP/FR of 0.50 (see Figure 1).

Threshold determination using this system is reliable and independent of an animal's rate of response. This is essential for many physiological and psychopharmacological BSR experiments. One drawback to previous threshold determinations using this method is the requirement of approximately 2 hours for a single BSR session. Another drawback is that occasionally threshold cannot be determined because of either floor or ceiling effects with the PRP/FR ratio. The PRP/FR ratio can either be 0 or 1.0 for all CRF current levels; thus, no threshold determination, the z-pause, has been developed. With this method it is assumed that with virtually every FR there is a PRP of some duration. The mean PRP interval at each CRF current level is compared with the mean IRI (i.e., during CRF responding). This also results in a rate-independent measure of threshold. No floor or ceiling effects result and, thus, threshold can always be determined.

The principal reason for the development of this system is the need for a reliable, more flexible, and inexpensive computerized BSR threshold system that permits faster threshold determination over a variety of experimental situations. The microcomputer-based system we have developed (Phelps & Lewis, 1982) accomplishes these goals.

<h2 style="text-align:center">Components of the BSR System</h2>

Constant Current Stimulator

Constant electrical current is required for most BSR threshold methods. Wayner, Peterson, and Florczyk (1972) and Emde and Shipton (1970) described such stimulators. Mills and his collaborators (Cassens et al., 1975) designed a constant-current stimulator based on a modification of a system described by Wayner et al. (1972). Constant current is maintained by voltage varying as a function of brain resistance (impedance) in the circuit. Voltage is monitored by the use of FET instrumentation amplifier in the stimulator. The stimulator functions as a voltage follower-regulator with continuous feedback. Instantaneous samples of resistance (impedance) to the stimulating current are made and result in voltage adjustment to maintain a constant current intensity. The stimulator which we have developed is of basic design but modified slightly for better current regulation over a broader resistance range. Current regulation was empirically determined through extensive testing of the design over several years (Lewis & Phelps, in preparation). The components of this stimulator and its operation are described in detail in Phelps and Lewis (1982).

Microcomputer

The microcomputer used in the BSR system is a Cromemco Model Z-2D with 48-K bits of random access memory. Computer peripherals include two 5-inch floppy disk drives, a D+7A board with multiple analog and digital input/output channels, an oscilloscope, and a printer terminal.

Software

The software is written in Cromemco 16-K bit, disk-extended BASIC and Z80 assembly language. Programs for equipment calibration, schedule presentation, data storage, and analysis are all in BASIC. Cross-compatible communication between programming languages provides the ease and flexibility of BASIC programming while meeting the real-time demands of the stimulator operation and current monitoring with an assembly language program. Thus, modification of the experimental paradigm or schedule parameters is easily accomplished as changes in experiment procedures are indicated.

The computer software consists of seven separate programs which permit several types of basic functioning to the system. The primary functions of these programs permit operation of the constant current stimulator, detection of operant responses and their time parameters, training of animals, collection of data, and statistical analysis of data. A detailed discussion of the software and the microcomputer components has been published (Phelps & Lewis, 1982).

BSR Parameter and Methods

The system provides several measures of an animal's performance. Key measures are used to provide data on three parameters of BSR performance. These are BSR threshold, response rate, and brain impedance.

BSR threshold is calculated using the PRP/FR ratio method described above. In addition, threshold is determined by the two-pause method; this second method defines threshold as the CRF current level that results in a mean PRP 2 standard deviations greater than the mean CRF IRI. This measure is an alternative way of calculating BSR threshold. With both methods the equation of the best fitting line for CRF current is calculated using a least squares regression analysis (see Figure 1). Threshold is determined by interpolating the CRF current that corresponds with a PRP/FR ratio of 0.05 or a z-pause of 2.

BSR response rate is determined by dividing the total number of responses by the time required to complete the predetermined CRF current levels. This measure is an overall measure of response to stimulation both above and below threshold. In addition, response rate is usually measured during the first CRF current level. Since we usually employ a descending series of CRF current intensities, this provides a measure of response to suprathreshold intensities which is comparable to other studies using only response rate.

Brain impedance to the stimulating current is also determined. This parameter reflects differences in electrical potential at the site of stimulation when all other sources of resistance in the circuit are constant. Bipolar platinum electrodes (0.3 mm in diameter) are used to stimulate discrete brain sites, and the impedance measure reflects instantaneous changes in electrical potential across the electrode tips. Brain resistance is sampled several hundred times during each stimulation and an average of these values constitutes our impedance parameter. Measurement of impedance occurs at the beginning of each session and periodically throughout the operant session to a 30 microampere (μA) current. This provides a measure of brain impedance which is common to all animals and thus permits comparison across animals and brain loci. Impedance measures to all of the FR and CRF current intensities are also sampled throughout each session.

Although the physiological basis of our impedance measure is not understood, it appears to be fairly constant between BSR sessions and may provide a good correlate of brain activity during behavior.

Brain Stimulation and Training Procedures

Using standard stereotaxic procedures rats are surgically implanted with one or more electrodes aimed at specific brain sites. Subjects are tested in an operant chamber with a single lever at one end. Above the cage a mercury swivel commutator permits the animal free movement while connected to the stimulation apparatus. Each lever press produces a 0.2 second train of 100 Hz biphasic rectangular pulses of 1.0 millisecond duration (Current intensity varies as previously discussed.). After recovery from surgery each animal is shaped to press a lever for BSR on a continuous reinforcement schedule. The rat then acquires the response on a FR-15 schedule of reinforcement using the method of Huston (1968). This procedure involves decreasing CRF current intensities gradually while maintaining FR current intensities at suprathreshold intensities. This added training requires a longer period of time to train each animal but provides more information about reward behavior and the effects of various pharmacological and other experimental manipulations.

The length of time to complete an operant session is variable depending upon (a) the rate of lever pressing by the animal, (b) the number of CRF current intensities tested, and (c) the need to descend or to both descend and ascend the CRF intensity range. We typically use four CRF intensities. Animals with implants at several positive brain sites (e.g., lateral hypothalamus) typically complete a session in approximately 15 to 20 minutes.

USES OF THE BSR SYSTEM

This system has been used to determine BSR threshold, rate of response, and brain resistance in various brain sites, including the lateral hypothalamus, medial forebrain bundle, and locus coeruleus. Extensive research

(Lewis & Phelps, in preparation) using animals implanted with platinum electrodes has shown performance as observed by the three parameters of BSR remains quite constant from day to day over the several weeks required for most of our experiments. Previous research with animals implanted with stainless steel electrodes showed that the threshold and impedance measures were more variable and tended to increase over time. Changing to platinum electrodes eliminated this problem. Histological evidence and microscopic examination of used electrodes indicated that after many testing sessions stainless steel electrode tips were eroded with passage of electrical current. This was probably the reason for the instability in BSR performance. Such erosion was not observed with platinum electrodes even after quite extensive testing over a period of more than one year.

Effects of ETOH on BSR

The positive reinforcing effects of ethanol (ETOH) undoubtedly play a significant role in its abuse. Consumption of alcoholic beverages produces positive affective states which reward drinking behavior. Laboratory experiments of these effects in animals, however, typically encounter considerable difficulty. Two types of experimental paradigms are commonly employed to investigate the rewarding effects of substances of abuse, self-administration, and BSR. We have chosen the latter paradigm because it is the one which permits a more direct evaluation of behavioral parameters with specific brain mechanisms.

Adult male albino rats were used as subjects. All were implanted with single electrodes aimed at either the lateral hypothalamus (LH) or mesencephalic ventral noradrenergic bundle (VNB). The latter is a site which is within an ascending norepinephrine pathway described by Ungerstedt (1971) and Jacobowitz (1978). It lies posterior to the mesencephalic nuclei which give rise to forebrain dopamine terminal. Training procedures for all animals were as described above. After stable performance was attained, all rats received three intraperitoneal injections of saline and ETOH (0.1, 0.25, 0.50, 0.75, and 1.50 g/kg, 30% v/v) 5 to 10 minutes before BSR sessions.

BSR threshold was reduced by the 0.25, 0.5, and 0.75 g/kg ETOH doses at the LH site (see Figure 2). This enhancement of BSR appeared dose dependent over this range. The 1.50 g/kg produced no significant effect on threshold at the lateral hypothalamus, although there was a trend towards a reduction in threshold. Threshold was not affected at the ventral noradrenergic bundle at doses up to 0.75 g/kg. The 1.50 g/kg dose so disrupted performance at the ventral noradrenergic bundle that threshold could not be determined despite frequent priming.

Overall BSR response rate was unchanged at the 0.10., 0.25, and 0.50 g/kg doses at both brain sites (see Figure 3, panel B). It was, however, significantly reduced at the 1.50 doses at both brain loci. The 0.75 dose showed no significant difference from saline baseline, although most VNB animals showed a slight reduction in rate at this dose. Closer inspection of individual data showed that response rate during the first CRF current level was increased by 0.25 and 0.50 doses in many LH animals (see Figure 3, panel A), although statistical significance was not attained. This lack of significance was due to high variability which was generally seen with the response rate measure.

Figure 2: Effects of five doses of ETOH on BSR threshold expressed as the percentage of baseline. Numbers above each bar are absolute threshold values in microamperes. Vertical lines within each bar are the S.E.M. Asterisks indicate significant differences from baseline (p < 0.05).

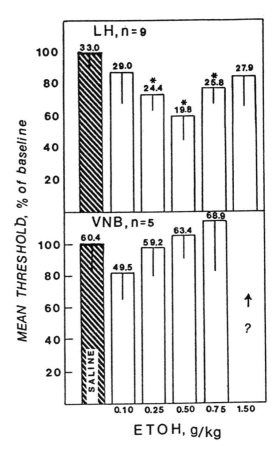

Brain impedance generally declined slightly at all doses of ETOH over values found after saline injection. It failed, however, to show a dose dependent decline. While the meaning of this measure remains unknown and given the considerable research (for a review, see Ingram, 1982) on ETOH effects on cell membranes, it is not unreasonable to speculate that these changes may have to do with alteration of these membranes or their functioning.

ETOH's lowering of BSR threshold is in disagreement with Carlson and Lydic (1976), who found that doses 0.9 and 1.2 g/kg increased threshold while a dose of 0.6 g/kg did not affect threshold but did slightly increase response rate. While many procedural details seem to differ between their research and ours, the most notable was threshold determination. Their method of determining threshold was simply to determine the current intensity which would support a rate of 15 responses per minute. This procedure is highly rate dependent and is not likely to be sensitive to reinforcing doses of ETOH which may also have depressant effects.

The differential effects of ETOH on BSR between lateral hypothalamus and ventral noradrenergic bundle sites is an interesting finding. These data suggest that ETOH may produce reinforcement via neural activity at specific

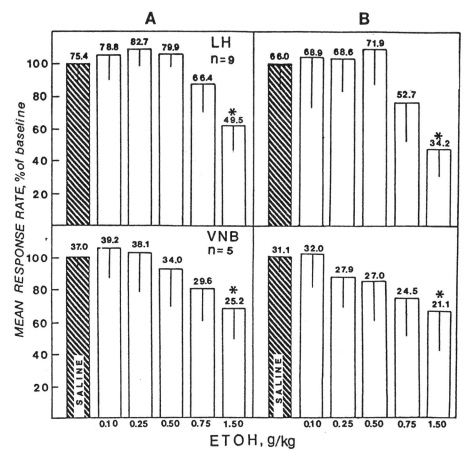

Figure 3: Effects of five doses of ETOH on BSR response rate during the first 300 responses (**A**) and the entire operant session (**B**). Values are expressed as the percentage of baseline. Numbers shown above each bar are absolute response rates in responses per minute. Vertical lines within each bar are the S.E.M. Asterisks indicate significant differences from baseline (p < 0.05).

brain sites. The lateral hypothalamus contains a heterogeneous group of ascending and descending fiber tracks including the monoamines norepinephrine, dopamine, and serotonin. The ventral noradrenergic bundle contains diffuse ascending noradrenergic fibers and other neurotransmitters including ascending and descending serotonergic neurons (Jacobowitz, 1978). In addition, this region contains enkephalin neurons (Uhl, Kuhar, Goodman, & Snyder, 1979).

Previous research (Lewis, 1980; 1981b) in our lab found that the opiate antagonist naloxone increases BSR performance at lateral hypothalamic sites. These data suggest that ETOH and opiates produce their reinforcing effects by different brain systems. This hypothesis is supported by recent data from our lab (Lewis, Andrade, Reynolds, & Phelps, in preparation) which show that naloxone does not affect either the threshold lowering effects of low doses of ETOH on LH BSR or the rate suppressing effects of high doses of ETOH at this site. Our most recent data, while preliminary, show that low doses of ETOH lower BSR threshold at sites in the A10 nucleus of the mesencephalon (which gives rise to limbic and cortical dopamine fibers) and in the medial septal area near the nucleus accumbens, also. Further research with a range of ETOH doses at these sites as well as at other key brain areas (e.g., locus coeruleus and hippocampus) is necessary to determine if the mediation of ETOH reinforcement is site-specific.

Currently, we are investigating the effects of chronic ETOH administration at varying doses. In particular, we want to determine whether the threshold lowering effects of low doses of ETOH and the rate suppressing effects of high doses of ETOH show tolerance. More importantly, we want to determine whether there is a threshold lowering effect of high doses of ETOH after tolerance develops to its depressant effects. If we and others can, indeed, confirm these findings, we will have made a major step in unraveling a major mystery about ETOH and its abuse.

In conclusion, we feel that these data show that ETOH is similar to other substances of abuse in enhancing BSR performance when given in low to moderate doses. BSR threshold was reduced at the lateral hypothalamic brain sites at low doses. It is interesting to note that ETOH did not reliably increase response rate at these doses. Higher doses suppressed response rate at both sites. It is also interesting that no dose of ETOH lowered BSR threshold or increased response rate in animals self-stimulating at the ventral noradrenergic bundle sites. These data suggest that ETOH effects may best be determined by measuring BSR threshold as the same measure of reward at specific brain sites.

Aging Effects on BSR and Amphetamine Rejuvenation

A number of physiological and biochemical changes occur with aging. While all bodily systems show such changes, those of the central nervous system probably play a particularly important role in behavioral changes occurring during aging. Shrinkage of the brain (Dayan, 1971) and loss of cortical cells (Brody, 1976) are among an increasing number of observed changes found in elderly persons (for a review, see Dayan, 1971; Smith & Sethi, 1977). Experimental animals exhibit a similar loss of cells with aging (Ordy, Brizzee, Kaack, & Hansche, 1978). Associated with these are declines in behavior, especially learning (for a review, see Arenberg & Robertson-Tchabo, 1977) and memory (for a review, see Craik, 1977).

Decreased activity, disturbances or alterations of sleep, and reduced sexual behavior (for a review, see Elias & Elias, 1977) have been reported and suggest a possible decrease in motivation. Such a decline may underlie other well-known changes in behavior (e.g., decline in learning and memory). The research from our laboratory (Lewis, 1981a) which is discussed in this section shows that there is a decline in brain stimulation reward (BSR), a potent motivational behavior, in aged rats. Moreover, it was found that amphetamine, a potent psychomotor stimulant, had a rejuvenating effect on BSR behavior in aged rats.

BSR has long been considered a biobehavioral method to investigate motivation. It has been shown to act as a reinforcer for operant behavior in much the same way that food acts as a reinforcer for food-deprived individuals (Olds & Milner, 1954). Furthermore, BSR has been shown to interact with normal motivational systems (e.g., hunger: Margules & Olds, 1962 and sex drive: Caggiula & Hoebel, 1966). Moreover, it is widely believed that BSR involves direct stimulation of neural systems controlling normal motivational states (for a review, see Gallistel, 1973). It is, therefore, appropriate to study the relationship of BSR to aging behavioral processes.

Randomly bred male albino rats were implanted with single electrodes and trained as previously discussed. In the first series of experiments, all animals were implanted and trained at approximately 6 months of age. All animals were vigorous responders and showed stable thresholds between 25 and 50 microamperes.

BSR performance declined with age. This is shown in the first two panels of Figure 4. This is most apparent from the fact that threshold at 15 to 20 months could not be determined because the animals failed to complete enough of the current levels. Impedance levels could, however, be determined during the initial responding, and they were higher at 15 to 20 months in comparison to 6 to 8 month levels. Mean response rate of the first CRF current level in two of three sessions at 15 to 20 months declined also over the rate at 7 to 8 months.

The effects of priming, increased CRF and FR current, food deprivation, and reshaping are shown in Figure 3. These individual procedures were all ineffective in increasing the number of FRs completed by the animals at 15 to 20 months. Combination of these variables did increase significantly the number of FRs completed (see Figure 5); however, this increase was not sufficient to complete all the CRF current intensities of the BSR program which are required for determination of threshold. The combination which generally produced the largest increase in the number of responses was priming and increased current, although individual differences existed as to which of the combinations proved best for a given animal.

Injection of 0.25 to 0.30 mg/kg of amphetamine at 5 to 30 minutes before the BSR session increased responding in all animals (see Figure 5). Priming was sufficient to initiate responding in 3 of 11 rats. Priming and some reshaping to the bar were required for three rats. Five animals responded without either procedure. Using similar procedures during the BSR session, injection of amphetamine 6 to 24 hours before testing did not increase responding (see Figure 5).

Figure 4 (center panel) shows that threshold and impedance levels were higher after amphetamine injection than 6 to 8 month values. Mean response rate of the first CRF current level and overall rate were unchanged. All animals showed (see Figure 4, right panel) an unexpected residual enhancement of BSR in at least two subsequent sessions after the last amphetamine injection. Three of the animals completed the BSR program in five sessions. In all of these tests, priming was given if necessary to initiate responding. Figure 4 shows that threshold levels and impedance in these subsequent tests were elevated over 6 to 8 month values. Response rate at the first CRF current level and overall rate declined slightly, but not significantly in comparison to the rate under amphetamine. Both were unchanged in comparison to 6 to 8 month rates.

Microscopic analysis of the histology showed no indication of sizable necrosis around electrode tips. All animals were found to have the tips of the

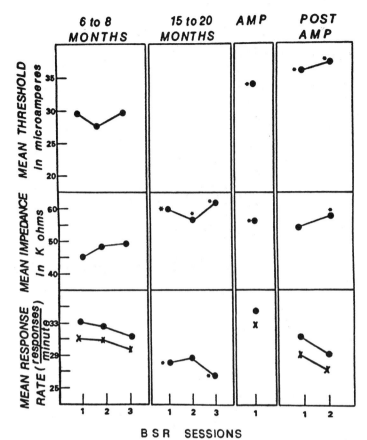

B S R   SESSIONS

Figure 4: Changes in BSR parameters during aging. Mean threshold
values require completion of all CRF intensities within 90 minutes.
Mean impedance was measured at 30 μA of current for all animals.
Mean response rate was calculated based on the performance during (a)
first CRF-FR current intensity (●), (b) entire operant session (**X**).
BSR sessions during 6 to 8 and 15 to 20 month periods were undrugged
operant sessions selected to represent characteristic performance
during these periods. Asterisks indicates p < 0.05 in comparison to
6 to 8 month values. Reprinted from Lewis, 1981a. Copyright 1981 by
Beech Hill Publishing.

electrodes terminating in the lateral hypothalamus medial forebrain bundle
area. The tissue near the electrode tips appeared no different from that of
younger animals which had exhibited high response rates for stimulation at this
brain site.

An age-related decline in BSR is a phenomenon which we have often observed
in our laboratory. Animals with implants in the lateral hypothalamus as well
as other brain sites sometimes stop responding. This may occur at any age;

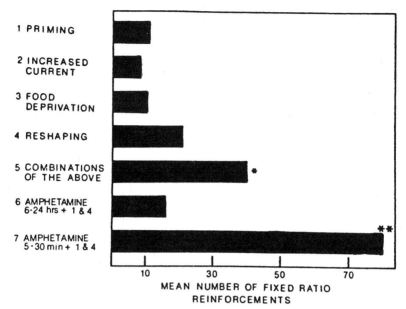

Figure 5: Effects of various manipulations upon the mean number of responses during BSR sessions as indicated by the number of FR reinforcements in 15 to 20 month old rats. The "combination" indicates the use of more than one priming, increased current, food deprivation, and reshaping in a BSR session. One asterisk indicates p < 0.05 in comparison to priming, increased current, food deprivation, shaping and amphetamine (6 to 24 hours). Two asterisks together indicate p < 0.05 in comparison to all others. Reprinted from Lewis, 1981a. Copyright 1981 by Beech Hill Publishing.

however, these animals rarely turn to BSR behavior or respond to priming, reshaping, food deprivation, increased current, some combination of these procedures, or drugs. These procedures were found to be relatively ineffective in restoring BSR produced increments in responding; however, some improvement was seen with a combination of manipulations. The fact that amphetamine reinstated the BSR behavior indicates that the observed decline was probably not a function of some necrosis of tissue under the electrode tip or that the electrode was in some way defective.

The enhancement of BSR behavior by amphetamine has often been observed (for a review, see Wauquier, 1976). Cassens and Mills (1973) report that amphetamine lowers BSR threshold using a similar procedure to that employed here. We have confirmed this observation with amphetamine many times in our laboratory in younger rats. Amphetamine has also been reported to improve motivational behavior in elderly patients (Clark & Manikar, 1979). The results of the current study are consistent with these reports.

Amphetamine may have also rejuvenated brain motivational systems in aged rats. This hypothesis seems possible in light of previous research on neurochemical changes associated with aging and biochemical effects of amphetamine. While many brain neurotransmitter alterations occur with aging, a major and relatively consistent effect appears to be a decline in the activity of catecholamines, particularly in dopamine areas (for a review, see McGeer & McGeer, 1976). In addition, there is a loss of neurons in the substantia nigra where striatal dopamine tracts originate and shrinkage of tissue in the dopamine-rich striatum with aging (McGeer, McGeer, & Suzuki, 1977). Amphetamine's effects on brain neurochemical systems is primarily on dopamine and norepinephrine where it is known to release the stored neurotransmitter from the presynaptic neuron and to block the re-uptake into neurons (Glowinski & Axelrod, 1966; for a review, see Cassens & Mills, 1973). The net effect is to potentiate noradrenergic and dopaminergic neurotransmission. Hence, it is conceivable that amphetamine could have enhanced the functioning of declining catecholamine systems in the aged rats.

The importance of catecholamines, dopamine in particular, in BSR has been shown in a large number of reports (for reviews, see German & Bowden, 1974; Wise, 1978). If catecholamines are indeed highly vulnerable to aging, then a decline in BSR behavior is to be expected in old rats. The fact that amphetamine administered shortly before the BSR session but not 6 to 24 hours before the session enhanced performance on the day of injection and on subsequent sessions suggests that probable BSR and amphetamine interacted to effect brain motivation systems. Dopamine, an apparent common neurochemical substrate of both BSR and amphetamine, may decline with aging as discussed above but may be rejuvenated by them. This hypothesis is supported by Marshall and Berrios (1979) who found that the age-related decline in swimming behavior in rats was "rejuvenated" by administration of the dopamine-receptor stimulant apomorphine and of the dopamine precursor L-DOPA.

While not conclusive, this longitudinal study indicates that there is an age-related decline in motivation and that this decrease may be due to decline in brain dopamine systems. A replication of this age-related decline in BSR has been completed in a study investigating cocaine's effects on aged performance. In a different group of randomly bred rats implanted at 6 months of age, an age-related decline in BSR performance was observed. We compared the effects of cocaine, another dopamine agonist, with amphetamine in improving BSR performance in aged rats. Doses of 0.5, 1.0, and 5.0 mg/kg (intraperitoneally) of cocaine or amphetamine were administered to 18 to 20 month old rats who failed to complete BSR operant sessions. Both drugs enhanced BSR performance with all animals completing the operant session at the 1.0 and 5.0 mg/kg doses. Only amphetamine produced this effect at the 0.5 mg/kg dose. BSR threshold was found to be significantly higher under these drug doses than the original 6-month values (undrugged animals). These data replicate the results of the first experiment and further implicate dopamine and/or other catecholamines in the enhancement of the BSR.

A cross-sectional study of the effects of aging on BSR has recently been completed. Two groups of F-344 NIA rats 6 to 8 months and 18 to 20 months of age were implanted with bipolar platinum electrodes aimed at the medial forebrain bundle. All animals were then shaped for lateral hypothalamic BSR and trained on the computer-controlled system. Surprisingly, there was no difference on the performances of both age groups. Continued testing involving two to three BSR sessions per week showed a decline in performance (e.g., failure to complete the BSR session and lower initial BSR rate) in the older group at 23 1/2 to 26 months. The younger group showed no decline during this period. Both groups received the same number of operant sessions with current intensities within the same range. These data show an age-related decline in BSR performance in rats implanted and trained at very different ages and complement the previous longitudinal data showing an age-related decline in BSR. Publication of this research is in preparation.

While these data are far from conclusive concerning the role of dopamine and/or and/or norepinephrine on age-related changes in BSR performance, they are strongly suggestive, particularly in light of some of the other data we have gathered recently. Dopamine antagonism either by large doses (2.0 mg/kg, intraperitoneally) of the receptor blocker haloperidol or by intracerebral injection of the catecholamine neurotoxin 6-hydroxydopamine produced age-like deficits in BSR performance. Both manipulations produced lower response rate, increased impedance and prevented completion of all CRF current intensities, and thus BSR threshold determination. We have also found that enhancement of serotonin activity by fenfluramine injection fails to enhance BSR performance in aged F-344 rats. Further research on the role of catecholamines in aging is planned using more specific neurotransmitter agonists and other brain sites.

As with the reinforcing effects of ETOH, aging effects on brain motivational mechanisms may be investigated by using BSR. The multifunctional computerized system described in this chapter, we believe, provides a powerful research tool for such studies. The method for determining BSR threshold is quite sensitive and stable. Measurement of it along with the ability to also measure operant response rate and brain impedance provides multiple parameters for understanding brain reward mechanisms and how substances of abuse affect them.

REFERENCES

Arenberg, D., & Robertson-Tchabo. (1977). Learning and aging. In J. E. Birren & K. W. Schaie (Eds.), Handbook of the psychology of aging. New York: Van Nostrand Reinhold.

Brody, H. (1976). An examination of cerebral cortex and brain stem aging. In R. D. Terry and S. Gerhson (Eds.), Aging: Neurobiology of aging. New York: Raven Press.

Caggiula, A. R., & Hoebel, B. G. (1966). "Copulation-reward site" in the posterior hypothalamus. Science, 153, 1284-1285.

Carlson, R. H., & Lydic, R. (1976). The effects of ethanol upon threshold and response rate for self-stimulation. Psychopharmacology, 50, 61-64.

Cassens, G., & Mills, A. (1973). Lithium and amphetamine: Opposite effects on threshold of intracranial reinforcement. Psychopharmacologia, 30, 283-290.

Cassens, G., Shaw, C., Dudding, K., & Mills, A. (1975). On-line brain stimulation: Measurement of threshold of reinforcement. Behavior Research Methods and Instrumentation, 7, 145-150.

Clark, A. N. G., & Manikar, G. D. (1979). D-amphetamine in elderly patients refractory to rehabilitation procedures. Journal of the American Geriatric Society, 27, 174-177.

Craik, F. I. M. (1977). Age differences in human memory. In J. E. Birren & K. W. Schaie (Eds.), Handbook of the psychology of aging. New York: Van Nostrand Reinhold.

Dayan, A. D. (1971). Comparative neuropathology of aging studies on the brain of 47 species of vertebrates. Brain, 94, 31-44.

Elias, M. F., & Elias, P. K. (1977). Motivation and activity. In J. E. Birren & K. W. Schaie (Eds.), Handbook of the psychology of aging. New York: Van Nostrand Reinhold.

Emde, J. W., & Shipton, H. W. (1970). A digital controlled constant current stimulator. Electroencephalography and Clinical Neurophysiology, 29, 310-313.

Esposito, R. U., & Kornetsky, C. (1978). Opioids and rewarding brain stimulation. Neuroscience & Biobehavioral Reviews, 2, 115-122.

Ferster, M., & Skinner, B. (1957). Schedule of reinforcement. New York: Appleton-Century-Croft.

Gallistel, C. R. (1973). Self-stimulation: The neurobiology of reward and motivation. In J. A. Deutsch (Ed.), The physiological basis of memory. New York: Academic Press.

German, D. C., & Bowden, D. M. (1974). Catecholamine systems as the neural substrate for intracranial self-stimulation: A hypothesis. Brain Research, 73, 381-419.

Glowinski, J., & Axelrod, J. (1966). Effects of drugs on the disposition of H^3 - norepinephrine in the rat brain. Pharmacological Review, 18, 775-785.

Huston, J. (1968). Reinforcement reduction: A method for training ratio behavior. Science, 159, 444.

Huston, J. P., & Mills, A. W. (1971). Threshold of reinforcing brain stimulation. Communications in Behavioral Biology, 5, 331-340.

Ingram, L. O. (1982). Effect of alcohol on membranes. In National Institute on Alcohol Abuse and Alcoholism, Biomedical processes and consequences of alcohol use (Alcohol and Health Monograph 2, pp. 3-27). Washington, DC: U.S. Government Printing Office.

Jacobowitz, D. M. (1978). Monoaminergic pathways in the central nervous system. In M. A. Lipton, A. DiMascio, & K. F. Killam (Eds.), Psychopharmacology: A generation of progress (pp. 119-129). New York: Raven Press.

Lewis, M. J. (1980). Naloxone suppression brain stimulation reward in the VNB but not in MFB. Society for Neuroscience Abstracts, 6, 367.

Lewis, M. J. (1981a). Age-related decline in brain stimulation reward: Rejuvenation by amphetamine. Experimental Aging Research, 7, 225-234.

Lewis, M. J. (1981b). Effects of naloxone on brain stimulation reward threshold in the VNB and MFB. Society for Neuroscience Abstracts, 7, 165.

Marcus, R., & Kornetsky, C. (1974). Negative and positive intracranial reinforcement thresholds: Effects of morphine. Psychopharmacologia, 38, 1-13.

Margules, D. L., & Olds, J. (1962). Identical "feeding" and "rewarding" systems. Science, 135, 374-375.

Marshall, J. F., & Berrios, N. (1979). Movement disorders of aged rats. Reversal by dopamine receptor stimulation. Science, 206, 477-479.

McGeer, E., & McGeer, P. L. (1976). Neurotransmitter metabolism in the aging brain. In R. D. Terry & S. Gerhson (Eds.), Aging: Neurobiology of aging. New York: Raven Press.

McGeer, E., McGeer, P. L., & Suzuki, J. S. (1977). Aging and extrapyramidal function. Archives of Neurology, 34, 33-35.

Miller, N. E. (1960). Motivating effects of brain stimulation and drugs. Federation Proceedings, 19, 846-854.

Olds, J. (1958). Self-stimulation experiments and differentiating reward systems. In H. H. Jasper, L. D. Proctor, R. S. Knighton, W. C. Noshay, & R. T. Costello (Eds.), Reticular formation of the brain (pp. 671-687). Boston: Little & Brown.

Olds, J., Killam, K. F., & Bach-y-Rita, P. (1956). Self-stimulation of the brain used as a screening method for tranquilizing drugs. Science, 124, 265-266.

Olds, J., Killam, K. F., & Eiduson, S. (1957). Effects of tranquilizers on self-stimulation of the brain. In S. Garratini & V. Ghetti (Eds.), Psychotrophic drugs (pp. 235-243). New York: Elsevier.

- 477 -

Olds, J., & Milner, P. (1954). Positive reinforcement produced by electrical stimulation of septal area and other regions. Journal of Comparative and Physiological Psychology, 47, 419-427.

Ordy, J. M., Brizzee, K. R., Kaack, B., & Hansche, J. (1978). Age differences in short-term memory and cell loss in the cortex of the rat. Gerontology, 24, 276-285.

Phelps, R., & Lewis, M. J. (1982). A multifunctional on-line brain stimulation system. Behavior Research Methods and Instrumentation, 14, 323-328.

Routtenberg, A. (1981). Drugs of abuse and the endogenous reinforcement system: The resistance of intracranial self-stimulation behavior to the inebriating effects of ethanol. New York Academy of Sciences, 362, 60-66.

Smith, B. H., & Sethi, P. K. (1977). Aging and nervous system. Geriatrics, 18, 109-115.

Stein, L. (1968). Chemistry of reward and punishment. In D. H. Efron (Ed.), Psychopharmacology: A review of progress, 1957-1967 (pp. 105-123). Washington, DC: U.S. Government Printing Office.

St. Laurent, J. (1972). Brain centers of reinforcement and the effects of alcohol. In B. Kissin & H. Begleiter (Eds.), Biology of alcoholism (pp. 85-106). New York: Plenum Press.

St. Laurent, J., & Olds, J. (1967). Alcohol and brain centers of positive reinforcement. In R. Fox (Ed.), Alcoholism - Behavioral research, therapeutic approaches (pp. 80-101). New York: Springer/Verlag.

Uhl, G., Kuhar, M. J., Goodman, R. R., & Snyder, S. H. (1979). Histochemical localization of the enkephalins. In E. Usdin, W. E. Bunney, Jr., & N. S. Kline (Eds.), Endorphins in mental health research (pp. 74-83). New York: Oxford University.

Ungerstedt, U. (1971). Stereotaxic mapping of the monoamine pathways in the rat brain. Acta Physiologica Scandinavica, 82(Suppl. 367), 1-48.

Valenstein, E., & Meyers, W. (1964). Rate independent test of reinforcing consequences of brain stimulation. Journal of Comparative and Physiological Psychology, 57, 52-60.

Vrtunski, P., Murray, R., & Wolin, L. R. (1973). The effect of alcohol on intracranially reinforced response. Quarterly Journal of Studies on Alcohol, 34, 718-725.

Wauquier, A. (1976). The influence of psychoactive drugs on brain self-stimulation in rats: A review. In A. Wauquier & E. T. Rolls (Eds.), Brain-stimulation reward (pp. 123-170). Amsterdam: Elsevier/North Holland.

Wayner, M. J., Peterson, R., & Florczyk, A. (1972). A constant device for brain stimulation. Physiology & Behavior, 8, 1189-1191.

Wise, R. A. (1978). Catecholamine theories of reward: A critical review. Brain Research, 152, 215-247.

Wise, R. A., & Bozarth, M. A. (1981). Brain substrates for reinforcement and drug self-administration. Progress in Neuro-Psychopharmacology, 5, 467-474.

CHAPTER 23

COMBINED MICROINJECTION AND BRAIN STIMULATION REWARD METHODOLOGY
FOR THE LOCALIZATION OF REINFORCING DRUG EFFECTS

Chris L. E. Broekkamp

Organon International BV
P.O.B. 20
5240 OH
Oss, The Netherlands

Abstract

The evidence for the following conclusions is discussed with emphasis on methodological issues related to the technique of local injections into brain tissue:

(1) The enhancing effect of morphine on self-stimulation rate seems to be mediated by receptors in the area of the dopamine containing cell-groups A_9-A_{10}.

(2) The enhancing effect of amphetamine on self-stimulation rate seems to be mediated by receptors in the nucleus accumbens and caudate nucleus.

(3) A depressant effect of morphine seems to be mediated by receptors in the nucleus Raphe Pontis.

(4) Interpretation of such results, obtained with local injections, is more reliable when information is available on dose dependency, on latency and duration of effects, on effects in brain areas surrounding the sensitive site, on pharmacological characteristics of the effect, and on the question whether unilateral or bilateral injections are required.

Introduction

The reinforcing effect of certain drugs of abuse could be caused by an action on one or a few circumscribed areas in the brain. Work based on such a proposition has yielded encouraging results for morphine, amphetamine, and cocaine (Bozarth & Wise, 1981; Goeders & Smith, 1983; Hoebel, Monaco, Hernandez, Aulisi, Stanley, & Lenard, 1983; Phillips & LePiane, 1980; Phillips, Mora, & Rolls, 1981). The evidence for this notion has been obtained with the technique of intracerebral microinjection. This technique enables us to link modified physiological activity in a particular brain area with specific changes in behavior, thus providing insight into the function of that area or into the behavioral significance of a drug action in that area. This technique has several pitfalls. Some of the pitfalls and methods to avoid them were previously reviewed by Routtenberg (1972). The major problem arises from diffusion to areas other than the one meant to be influenced by the injected substance. Also, interpretative problems arise from the high local concentration of the applied substance. This may cause nonspecific effects such as local anesthesia or irritation. With proper control procedures these uncertainties about the significance of data obtained with intracerebral injections can be largely removed. This will be illustrated in the following discussion on local injections of opiates and amphetamines and their effects on intracranial self-stimulation and other behaviors. Intracranial self-stimulation was used in such studies since it provides a stable baseline for determining the intensity and the duration of an effect from local drug injections. The method should provide a set of data that can later be used to guide experiments more directly concerned with the measurement of a reinforcing effect from a local injection.

Locally Applied Morphine on Self-Stimulation

Morphine, when given systemically, has a complex action on self-stimulation. It depresses self-stimulation for 1 to 2 hours and then enhances it (Adams, Lorens, & Mitchell, 1972; Lorens & Mitchell, 1973). Low doses can enhance self-stimulation without initial depression (Gerber, Bozarth & Wise, 1981; Glick & Rapaport, 1974), and the enhancement is particularly strong after repeated morphine treatments (Adams et al., 1972; Lorens & Mitchell, 1973).

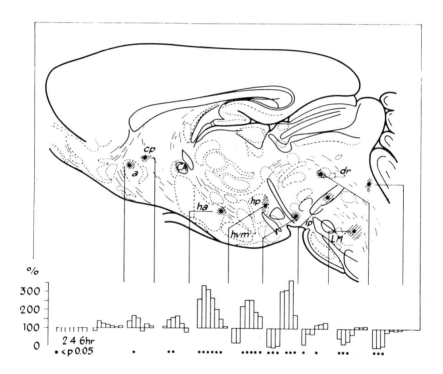

Figure 1: The effects of 5 µg (or 2 x 2.5 µg) morphine into different areas of the brain on hypothalamic self-stimulation. Median effects are given as percentage of the preinjection baseline rates. Reprinted with permission from Broekkamp, van den Bogaard, Heynen, Rops, Cools, and van Rossum, 1976. Copyright 1976 by Elsevier Biomedical Press.

Long ago, Tatum, Seevers, and Collins (1927) suggested that the biphasic effects of opiates on behavior reflect actions on different systems in the brain. By exploring the brain with local, bilateral morphine injections in a variety of sites, it was found that injections into a certain site resulted in an enhancement of self-stimulation and that injections into another site produced a depression of self-stimulation with mixed effects from intermediate areas (see Figure 1). Apparently the locally injected morphine spreads over a large area and this complicates the picture, but the results are consistent with the idea that there exists an area mediating the excitation near the ventral tegmental area or caudal hypothalamus and an area mediating the depression within the pontine mesencephalon or a more caudal area. With a lower dose of 1 µg on each side, injections into the ventral tegmental area were more effective in inducing an immediate enhancement than injections into the caudal hypothalamus, and this indicates that the dopamine-containing cell bodies at A_9-A_{10} represent the site where morphine acts to enhance self-stimulation (see Figure 2; Broekkamp, Phillips, & Cools, 1979a). An important question is to what extent this effect results from a local action and not from diffusion to other brain regions.

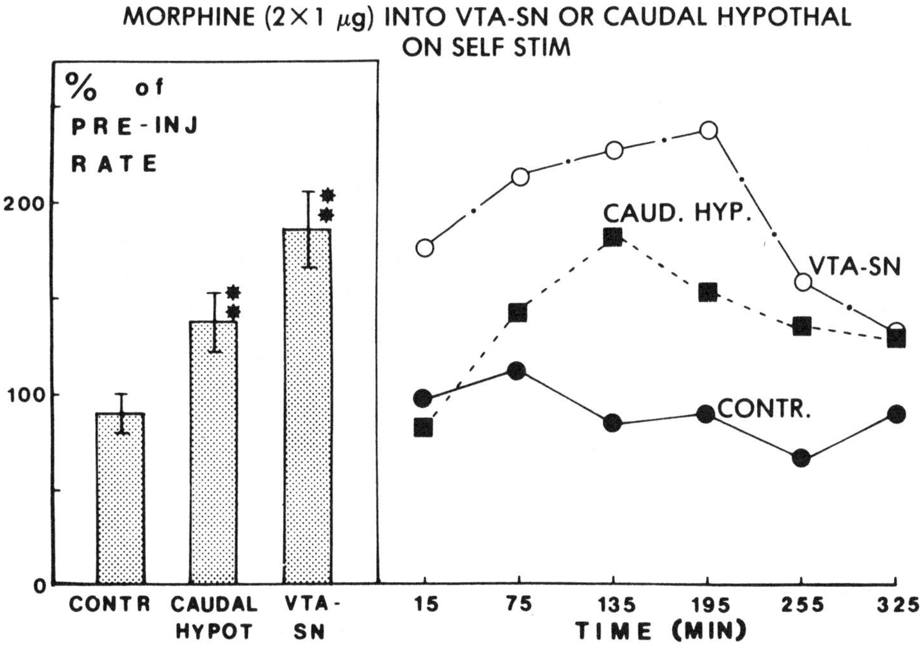

MORPHINE (2×1 µg) INTO VTA-SN OR CAUDAL HYPOTHAL ON SELF STIM

Figure 2: Effects of self-stimulation of 2 x 1 µg morphine into the caudal hypothalamic area and into the ventral tegmental-substantia nigra area (VTA-SN). Bars on the left indicate the overall effect. Graphs on the right show the effect over time. Standard errors of the mean are presented for the overall data as well as statistical significance (** : $p < 0.05$). Groups: ●, controls; ■, caudal hypothalamus; ○, VTA-SN. Reprinted with permission from Broekkamp, Phillips, and Cools, 1979a. Copyright 1979 by ANKHO International, Inc.

It is not sufficient to refer to data on diffusions of dyes, local anesthetics, or radioactively labeled chemicals (Albert & Madryga, 1980; Routtenberg, 1972), because compounds with different chemical and physical properties have widely different diffusion properties. This is elegantly illustrated by the work of Herz and Teschemacher (1971) on the analgesic effects of a series of opiates in rabbits after intraventricular injection. From their findings it could be concluded that a more lipophilic opiate such as fentanyl spreads rapidly through brain tissue and also quickly leaves the brain. Thus, for intracerebral studies where limited spread and an extended duration of action is wished, one should select a hydrophilic compound (e.g., Britt & Wise, 1983).

Another reason not to rely on observed spread of a labeled compound is the uncertainty about the detection threshold for visualization in comparison to the threshold for a pharmacological effect. If an effect is mediated by concentrations that cannot be visualized, such diffusion data are inconclusive. Therefore the safest way to exclude mediation of an effect by areas neighboring the injection site is to actually inject the drug into the surrounding areas or into the cerebral ventricle and to demonstrate that (1) higher doses are needed, (2) a smaller effect is obtained, or (3) a longer latency for an effect is observed. This worked reasonably well for morphine and the A_9-A_{10} site for self-stimulation enhancement (Broekkamp et al., 1979a): Animals were tested

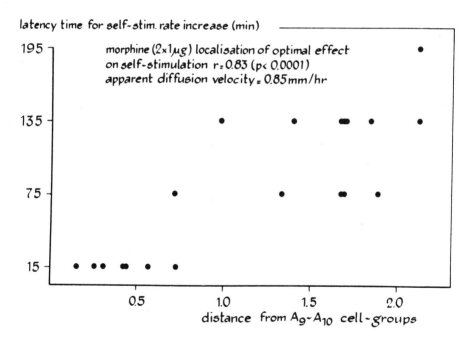

Figure 3: Scatter diagram illustrating the latency for an increase in self-stimulation by local injections of 2 x 1 μg morphine HCl and the distance (in mm) between the infused site and a point located in the middle of the A_9-A_{10} area. Reprinted with permission from Broekkamp, 1976.

for self-stimulation each hour for a 15-minute period following the microinjection of morphine into the A_9-A_{10} area or surrounding structures. Despite the high variance a coherent picture emerged. The latency for the occurrence of an increase to at least 150% of the baseline was correlated significantly with the distance from the center of the dopamine-cell conglomerate A_9-A_{10} (see Figure 3). The slope of the regression line indicated a diffusion speed for morphine through brain tissue of 0.9 mm/hour. This figure was also obtained by Herz and Teschemacher (1971), who derived it from the latency for analgesia after intraventricular injections.

The other crucial question in relation to the local morphine effect is whether nonspecific effects related to a high local concentration are involved. Controls with local anesthetics or excitant substances can provide useful information, but the best way to address this problem is to investigate the pharmacological properties of the effect with other agonists and/or antagonists. The pharmacological characteristics of an effect from local application should not have unexplainable aspects different from the known characteristics of effects mediated by similar receptors. For example, in order to meet this requirement for pharmacological consistency of an opiate effect, one should be able to obtain a similar effect with an endorphin or an enkephalin. Indeed the stabilized enkephalin analog D-Ala^2-Met^5-enkephalinamide also enhances self-stimulation when injected bilaterally into the morphine sensitive site (Broekkamp, et al., 1979a). This is useful information because, from a chemical point of view, the compound is entirely different from morphine and will have different nonspecific effects. Support for pharmacological consistency is also provided by the observation that the local effect of morphine can be antagonized by systemic treatment with naloxone (Broekkamp et al., 1979a). Several other behaviors have been shown to be influenced by injections of opiates into the dopamine cell area. Stereotypy, circling, and locomotor activity increase after β-endorphin or D-Ala-Met-enkephalinamide infusions into this area (Broekkamp, Phillips, & Cools, 1979b; Iwamoto & Way, 1977; Joyce, Koob, Strecker, Iversen, & Bloom, 1981). Similar microinjections induce place preference in a conditioning paradigm (Phillips & LePiane, 1980, 1982), and self-administration is supported by microinjections into the ventral tegmental area (Bozarth & Wise, 1981). All these effects were antagonized by an opiate antagonist. Reports on effects with unmodified leucine or methionine enkephalins into the A_9-A_{10} area are lacking. Enkephalin doses as high as 50 to 200 µg into the ventricle were required to depress lever pressing for food by rats (Belluzzi & Stein, 1977). It is relevant to point out here that local injections with natural transmitters provide special problems. This will be discussed separately after this section.

From the data reviewed above, it emerges that the opiate effects in the A_9-A_{10} area are well established and have adequate controls. Results obtained with self-stimulation behavior and additional data with locomotor activity made it easier to establish the importance of this area for the mediation of opiate reward with techniques such as place-preference conditioning or local self-administration (Bozarth & Wise, 1981, 1983; Phillips & LePiane, 1980; Wise & Bozarth, 1981).

We should remain alert for the possibility that other sites contribute to the reinforcement by opiates in man. The behavior depressant effect in man and animals has not been investigated explicitly for its role in opiate reward. A direct test for reinforcement related to opiate depression will be possible now that more precise information is available on the site in the brain where opiates depress behavior of rats. Behavioral depression or akinesia was measured by placing the experimental animals in abnormal postures and observing the duration of maintenance of such postures (for details of the method, see Dunstan, Broekkamp, & Lloyd, 1981). With local injections it was found that a site identical to or near the nucleus raphe pontis mediates akinesia induced by morphine (Broekkamp, LePichon, & Lloyd, 1984). A comparison of bilateral injections confirmed that the sensitive site is in the midsagittal plane (see Figure 4). More work on the pharmacological properties of this effect is needed in order to rule out nonspecific drug effects.

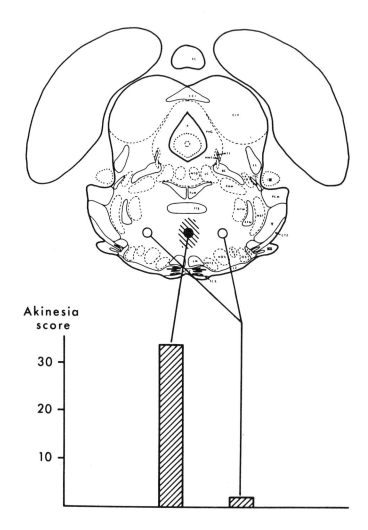

Figure 4: Coronal section illustrating infusion sites for comparing akinesia response to local morphine after bilateral (2 x 5 µg/0.5 µl) or midline infusion (10 µg/ µl).   Reprinted with permission from Broekkamp, LePichon, & Lloyd, 1984. Copyright 1984 by Elsevier Scientific Publishers.

Locally Applied Natural Transmitter: An Intermezzo

Not many reports are available describing effects with natural transmitters after intracerebral injections, and when effects are demonstrated, they invariably occur at doses in the microgram range (Garrigou, Broekkamp & Lloyd, 1981; Leibowitz, 1978; Leibowitz & Brown, 1980). This is a much higher concentration than endogenously present. Part of the reason is that natural compounds are vulnerable to endogenous enzymes which makes it difficult for them to diffuse through membranes and reach the receptor unmodified. For example, dopamine has an effect in the nucleus accumbens only in rats pretreated with the monoamine oxidase inhibitor nialamide (Pijnenburg & van Rossum, 1973). Despite the evidence for rapid metabolism, critics often still feel that the concentrations required are too high to be of physiological relevance. In considering this problem it is important to realize that the endogenous transmitter is packaged in a high concentration in synaptic vesicles which are discharged directly over the postsynaptic receptors. In view of this it is more likely that when "physiological" transmitter concentrations in locally applied solutions have any effect, this is mediated by presynaptic receptors inhibiting the release of the endogenous transmitter rather than by a direct postsynaptic effect.

Locally Applied Amphetamine on Self-Stimulation

Systemic dexamphetamine increases self-stimulation. This is evident not only by lever pressing rate enhancement for brain stimulation but also on measures more directly related to the reward value of brain stimulation (Atrens, Von Vietinghoff-Reisch, Der-Karabetian, & Masliyah, 1974; Liebman & Butcher, 1974; Phillips & Fibiger, 1973; Zarevics & Setler, 1979). This effect of amphetamine has been linked to an effect in the nucleus accumbens and nucleus caudatus (Broekkamp, Pijnenburg, Cools, & van Rossum, 1975). Control experiments ruled out the possibility that the anterior hypothalamus was involved or that the ventricular system transported the locally applied drug elsewhere. The latency for the self-stimulation enhancement was less than one minute. In contrast to the akinesia-inducing effect of morphine, amphetamine was most effective after bilateral injections. Pharmacological consistency is supported by experiments showing that the dopamine-receptor blocker haloperidol has opposite effects when applied into the same area (Broekkamp & van Rossum, 1975). In addition, there is an obvious substrate for the amphetamine effect available in the form of a rich innervation of dopamine containing terminals in the nucleus accumbens and caudate nucleus. The relevance for amphetamine reward has been clearly demonstrated by local self-administration experiments wherein the nucleus accumbens proved to be a sensitive brain area (Hoebel et al., 1983).

Other Drugs of Potential Abuse and Brain Stimulation

The technique of combining brain stimulation and local injections can also be used in research on brain systems involved in the addiction potential of benzodiazepines. For this type of drug, it is better to use aversive brain stimulation which is strongly influenced by benzodiazepines (Bovier, Broekkamp, & Lloyd, 1982). It is probably also the aversion antagonizing effect of benzodiazepines which makes them drugs of potential abuse. A soluble and potent benzodiazepine is available for local infusions (Pieri et al., 1981; Shibata, Kataoka, Gomita, & Ueki, 1982), and the newly developed benzodiazepine antagonists allow control for pharmacological specificity of local effects

(Bonetti et al., 1982; Czernik et al., 1982).

Conclusions

The technique of local injections combined with brain self-stimulation at a steady rate enables the collection of information concerning the sensitive brain areas possibly involved in mediating reinforcing effects of drugs of abuse. In this chapter the sensitive sites for self-stimulation effects of morphine and dexamphetamine are discussed. It is illustrated that with the local injection technique and self-stimulation attention can be paid to the following issues:

-Is there a dose dependent effect?

-What is the duration of action and latency of onset?

-Should the area be influenced in both hemispheres or is unilateral injection sufficient?

-Can the effect of a low dose be linked to a particular brain site? Have injections into surrounding brain tissue a smaller effect or an effect after a longer latency?

-Is there a pharmacological consistency? This can be studied by using other agonists and antagonists for the receptor under investigation.

-Is there a physiological consistency? This can be studied by using transmitter metabolism inhibitors or transmitter reuptake inhibitors.

This information enables a more rapid and reliable advance with more elaborate techniques aimed to measure reinforcing effects directly.

References

Adams, W. J., Lorens, S. A., & Mitchell, C. L. (1972). Morphine enhances lateral hypothalamic self-stimulation in the rat. Proceedings of the Society for Experimental Biology and Medicine, 140, 770-771.

Albert, D. J., & Madryga, F. J. (1980). An examination of the functionally effective spread of 4 μl of slowly infused lidocaine. Behavioral and Neural Biology, 29, 378-384.

Atrens, D. M., Von Vietinghoff-Reisch, F. Der-Karabetian, A., & Masliyah, E. (1974). Modulation of reward and aversion processes in the rat diencephalon by amphetamine. American Journal of Physiology, 226, 874-880.

Belluzzi, J. D., & Stein, L. (1977). Enkephalin may mediate euphoria and drive-reduction reward. Nature, 266, 556-558.

Bonetti, E. .P., Pieri, L., Cumin, R., Schaffner, R., Pieri, M., Gamzu, E. R., Muller, R. K., & Haefely, W. (1982). Benzodiazepine antagonist RO 15-1788: Neurological and behavioral effects. Psychopharmacology, 78, 8-18.

Bovier, Ph., Broekkamp, C. L. E., & Lloyd, K. G. (1982). Enhancing GABAergic transmission reverses the aversive state in rats induced by electrical stimulation of the periaqueductal grey region. Brain Research, 248, 313-320.

Bozarth, M. A., & Wise, R. A. (1981). Intracranial self-administration of morphine into the ventral tegmental area in rats. Life Sciences, 28, 551-555.

Bozarth, M. A., & Wise, R. A. (1983). Neural substrates of opiate reinforcement. Progress in Neuro-Psychopharmacology and Biological Psychiatry, 7, 569-575.

Britt, M. D., & Wise, R. A. (1983). Ventral tegmental site of opiate reward: Antagonism by a hydrophilic opiate receptor blocker. Brain Research, 258, 105-108.

Broekkamp, C. L. E. (1976). The modulation of rewarding systems in the animal brain by amphetamine, morphine and apomorphine. (Doctoral thesis, University of Nijmegen) Druk: Stichting Studentenpers Nijmegen.

Broekkamp, C. L. E., LePichon, M., & Lloyd, K. G. (1984). Akinesia after locally applied morphine near the nucleus raphe pontis. Neuroscience Letters, 50, 313-318.

Broekkamp, C. L. E., Phillips, A. G., & Cools, A. R. (1979a). Facilitation of self-stimulation behavior following intracerebral microinjections of opioids into the ventral tegmental area. Pharmacology Biochemistry & Behavior, 11, 289-295.

Broekkamp, C. L. E., Phillips, A. G., & Cools, A. R. (1979b). Stimulant effects of enkephalin microinjection into the dopaminergic A10 area. Nature, 278, 560-561.

Broekkamp, C. L. E., Pijnenburg, A. J. J., Cools, A. R., & van Rossum, J. M. (1975). The effect of microinjections of amphetamine into the neostriatum and the nucleus accumbens on self-stimulation behavior. Psychopharmacology, 42, 179-183.

Broekkamp, C. L. E., van den Bogaard, J. H., Cools, A. R., Heynen, H. J., Rops, R. H., & van Rossum, J. M. (1976). Separation of inhibiting and stimulating effects of morphine on self-stimulation behavior by intracerebral microinjections. European Journal of Pharmacology, 36, 443-446.

Broekkamp, C. L. E., & van Rossum, J. M. (1975). The effect of microinjections of morphine and haloperidol into the neostriatum and the nucleus accumbens on self-stimulation behavior. Archives Internationales de Pharmacodynamie et de Therapie, 217, 110-117.

Czernik, A. J., Petrack, B., Kalinsky, H. J., Psychoyos, S., Cash, W. D., Tsai, C., Rinehart, R. K., Granat, F. R., Lovell, R. A., Brundish, D. E., & Wade, R. (1982). CGS 8216: Receptor binding characteristics of a potent benzodiazepine antagonist. Life Sciences, 30, 363-372.

Dunstan, R., Broekkamp, C. L., & Lloyd, K. G. (1981). Involvement of caudate nucleus, amygdala or reticular formation in neuroleptic and narcotic catalepsy. Pharmacology Biochemistry & Behavior, 14, 169-174.

Garrigou, D., Broekkamp, C. L., & Lloyd, K. G. (1981). Involvement of amygdala in the effect of antidepressants on the passive avoidance deficit in bulbectomised rats. Psychopharmacology, 74, 66-70.

Gerber, G. J., Bozarth, M. A., & Wise, R. A. (1981). Small-dose intravenous heroin facilitates hypothalamic self-stimulation without response suppression in rats. Life Science, 28, 557-562.

Glick, S. D., & Rapaport, G. (1974). Tolerance of the facilatory effect of morphine on self-stimulation of the medial forebrain bundle in rats. Research Communications in Chemical Pathology & Pharmacology, 9, 647-652.

Goeders, N. E., & Smith, J. E. (1983). Cortical dopaminergic involvement in cocaine reinforcement. Science, 221, 773-775.

Herz, A., & Teschemacher, H. (1971). Activities and sites of antinociceptive action of morphine-like analgesics and kinetics of distribution following intravenous, intracerebral and intraventricular application. Advances in Drug Research, 6, 79-119.

Hoebel, B. G., Monaco, A. P., Hernandez, L., Aulisi, E. F., Stanley, B. G., & Lenard, L. (1983). Self-injection of amphetamine directly into the brain. Psychopharmacology, 81, 158-163.

Iwamoto, E. T., & Way, E. L. (1977). Circling behavior and stereotypy induced by intranigral opiate microinjections. Journal of Pharmacology and Experimental Therapeutics, 203, 347-359.

Joyce, E. M., Koob, G. F., Strecker, R., Iversen, S. D., & Bloom, F. E. (1981). The behavioral effects of enkephalin analogues injected into the ventral tegmental area and globus pallidus. Brain Research, 221, 359-370.

Leibowitz, S. F. (1978). Paraventricular nucleus: A primary site mediating adrenergic stimulation of feeding and drinking. Pharmacology Biochemistry & Behavior, 8, 163-175.

Leibowitz, S. F., & Brown, L. L. (1980). Histochemical and pharmacological analysis of noradrenergic projections to the paraventricular hypothalamus in relation to feeding stimulation. Brain Research, 201, 289-314.

Liebman, J. M., & Butcher, L. L. (1974). Comparative involvement of dopamine and noradrenaline in rate-free self-stimulation in substantia nigra, lateral hypothalamus and mesencephalic central gray. Nauyn-Schmiedeberg's Archives of Pharmacology, 284, 167-194.

Lorens, S. A., & Mitchell, C. L. (1973). Influence of morphine on lateral hypothalamic self-stimulation in the rat. Psychopharmacologia, 32, 271-277.

Phillips, A. G., & Fibiger, H. C. (1973). Dopaminergic and noradrenergic substrates of positive reinforcement: Differential effects of d- and l-amphetamine. Science, 179, 575-577.

Phillips, A. G., & LePiane, F. G. (1980). Reinforcing effects of morphine microinjection into the ventral tegmental area. Pharmacology Biochemistry & Behavior, 12, 965-968.

Phillips, A. G., & LePiane, F. G. (1982). Reward produced by microinjection of (D-Ala[2]), Met[5]-enkephalinamide into the ventral tegmental area. Behavioral Brain Research, 5, 225-229.

Phillips, A. G., Mora, F., & Rolls, E. T. (1981). Intracerebral self-administration of amphetamine by rhesus monkeys. Neuroscience Letters, 24, 81-86.

Pieri, L., Schaffner, R., Scherschlicht, R., Polc, P., Sepinwall, J., Davidson, A., Mohler, H., Cumin, R., Daprada, M., Burkard, W. P., Keller, H. H., Muller, R. K. M., Gerold, M., Pieri, M., Cook, L., & Haefely, W. (1981). Pharmacology of midazolam. Arzneimittel Forschung, 31, 2180-2201.

Pijnenburg, A. J. J., & van Rossum, J. M. (1973). Stimulation of locomotor activity following injection of dopamine into the nucleus accumbens. Journal of Pharmacy and Pharmacology, 25, 1003-1005.

Routtenberg, A. (1972). Intracranial chemical injection and behavior: A critical review. Behavioral Biology, 7, 601-641.

Shibata, K., Kataoka, Y., Gomita, Y., & Ueki, S. (1982). Localization of the site of the anticonflict action of benzodiazepines in the amygdaloid nucleus of rats. Brain Research, 234, 442-446.

Tatum, A. L., Seevers, M. H., & Collins, K. H. (1927). Morphine addiction and its physiological interpretation based on experimental evidence. Journal of Pharmacology and Experimental Therapeutics, 36, 447-475.

Wise, R. A., & Bozarth, M. A. (1981). Brain substrates for reinforcement and drug self-administration. Progress in Neuro-Psychopharmacology and Biological Psychiatry, 5, 467-474.

Zarevics, P., & Setler, P. E. (1979). Simultaneous rate-independent and rate-dependent assessment of intracranial self-stimulation: Evidence for the direct involvement of dopamine in brain reinforcement mechanisms. Brain Research, 169, 499-512.

CHAPTER 24

ADDICTION RESEARCH CENTER INVENTORY (ARCI):
MEASUREMENT OF EUPHORIA AND OTHER DRUG EFFECTS

Charles A. Haertzen and John E. Hickey

NIDA Addiction Research Center
c/o Francis Scott Key Medical Center
Baltimore, Maryland 21224

Abstract

This paper reviews the evolution of the Addiction Research
Center Inventory (ARCI) into a viable instrument for determining the
subjective effects of drugs. Primary focus is on item selection,
scale development, the development of short forms for different
objectives, and the use of the ARCI as a diagnostic tool. The
importance of items and scales of euphoric content in the ARCI is
highlighted.

The item selection process for both the 550 item inventory and
the additional 50 items dealing with classical withdrawal symptoms is
described. Discussion of scale development begins with the
construction of the empirical scales which distinguished a given drug
from placebo and continues through the development of drug-specific
scales, those scales that can distinguish between drugs.

The clinical scales, which discriminate between groups, are
briefly discussed with emphasis on the appropriate use of the
psychopathology scales. In terms of test validity, the effective use
which has been made of the drug orientated ARCI short forms and
selected scales is discussed in some detail with relevant comment
regarding the utility of the total ARCI.

Introduction

One of the primary reasons for developing the Addiction Research Center
Inventory (ARCI) was to measure the subjective effects of a large variety of
drugs. Since July of 1958 when the first ARCI was given to an opiate addict,
the ARCI has been applied to evaluate the effects of dozens of different
psychoactive compounds. A large percentage of the reports on the ARCI are in
volumes published by the Committee on Problems of Drug Dependence. The ARCI
has received some attention both in the U.S.A. and abroad as it has been
translated into German (Battig & Fischer, 1967), French (Pichot, 1964), Spanish
(Meketon & Perea, 1967), and Swedish (Sjoberg, 1969b).

Interest in the development of the ARCI as an instrument to measure drug
effects, psychopathology, and personality was stimulated by a number of
findings. On the negative side, established tests such as the Minnesota
Multiphasic Personality Inventory (MMPI) were not uniformly effective in

showing drug effects. Thus, it revealed changes for LSD (Belleville, 1956) but not for morphine or pentobarbital (Haertzen & Hill, 1959). In contrast, Beecher (1959) and associates uncovered subjective effects of opiates and other drugs in both opiate addicts and normal subjects with adjective check lists. The utility of several different adjective check lists had been affirmed in other studies of drugs or in studies of stimulating social factors (Clyde, 1960; Nowlis & Nowlis, 1956). Adjective check lists have continued to be used to detect the effects of drugs (Cameron, Specht, & Wendt, 1967; McNair, Lorr, & Droppelman, 1971) and the effects of social factors (Datel, Gieseking, Engle, & Dougher, 1966).

In the 1950 era the LSD questionnaire developed by Abramson (Abramson, Jarvik, Kaufman, Kornetsky, Levine, & Wagner, 1955) was used at the Addiction Research Center for showing acute effects of LSD and other hallucinogens as well as tolerance and cross tolerance to them (Isbell, Belleville, Fraser, Wikler, & Logan, 1956). A preliminary questionnaire developed by Belleville to show the effects of a marijuana compound (dimethylheptyl derivative called CA 101 or SKF-5390) showed a large variety of significant changes (Haertzen, Hill, & Belleville, 1963).

The idea of including indicators of psychopathology and personality in the ARCI was stimulated by theories and findings in the 1950s and before which related drug effects to these determinants. In the 1920s Kolb (1925) came to the conclusion that psychopaths were more likely to obtain euphoria from opiates. The elevation of opiate addicts on the Psychopathic Deviate scale of the MMPI seemed consistent with the Kolb conclusion (Hill, Haertzen, & Glaser, 1960). Also, addicts felt euphoric from opiates whereas normals did not (Beecher, 1959). It was characteristic of the 1950s to speculate about the similarity of psychopathology such as schizophrenia and the psychotomimetic effects of LSD, mania, and drug euphoria or about the possible causes of delirium tremens (Haertzen, 1964; Hoch & Solomon, 1952; Isbell, Fraser, Wikler, Belleville, & Eisenman, 1955; Savage, 1955). More recently the discovery of endorphins has served as fuel for speculations and studies of possible pathophysiology of those with mental disorders and of treatment of these (Feinberg, Pegeron, & Steiner, 1983). In the 1950s Eysenck implicated both psychopathology and personality as determinants of drug effects or drugs affecting personality. Thus, according to Eysenck (1957), central nervous system depressants such as alcohol and barbiturates should increase cortical inhibition, decrease cortical excitation, and thereby produce extraverted behavior patterns.

By simultaneously using items which were believed to reflect psychopathology, personality, and drug effects, it was thought that the study of the interrelation of these variables and the effects of drugs would be expedited. The original study with the ARCI partially permitted some analysis of interrelationships of personality and drug effect dimensions, because the MMPI (Hathaway & McKinley, 1951), the California Personality Inventory (CPI; Gough, 1957), Guilford-Zimmerman Temperament Survey (Guilford & Zimmerman, 1949), and the Sixteen Personality Factor Questionnaire (16 P.F.; Cattell, 1957) were included under a no-drug condition (Haertzen & Miner, 1965).

Item Selection

In selecting a new set of items, there can be no guarantee that valid items will be included, especially in the area of psychopathology, as it has been demonstrated that expert judges have misconceptions about how psychopathological types will answer questions (Gough, 1954). Granting the limitations imposed by judgment, it is thought that the method of generating original items, of classifying the items into content areas, of requiring consensus among the authors to accept an item, and of editing of accepted items led to the ultimate validity of the item pool for the various objectives. Validity of the scales is probably related to use of a large number of subjects and to the methods of scale construction.

The primary means of generating items consisted of having opiate addicts respond to a 200 item sentence completion test when they were under a no-drug condition and when they were under the influence of drugs such as morphine, LSD, pentobarbital, chlorpromazine, a marijuana-like compound (1'-2'-dimethylheptyl cannabinol, SKF-5390), and placebo (Haertzen, Hill, & Belleville, 1963). Sentence completion stems consisted of phrases such as "I feel _____ " and "My appetite is _____." The huge corpus of possible items was initially reduced to about 3300 and then to 550 through a judgment process. The list also included MMPI items. If Hill, Haertzen, or Belleville thought that an item was worthy of further consideration, it was checked and committed to a card. At this stage items were categorically eliminated from consideration if the names of drugs were mentioned except in the case of alcohol, cigarettes, and coffee. This exclusion was followed because it was our intent to use the test on many different populations including those who did not use drugs.

Items were classified according to the categories in Table 1. To prevent exclusion of items in content areas, items were judged for acceptability only within a common subcategory. Content of a particular category is generally larger than the table suggests as some categories are potentially very broad. For example, items indicative of euphoria or anxiety which are broad dimensions were classified under other categories such as attitudes toward people. In contrast with the content of personality tests, many items of the ARCI concern alterations in motivation and mood, in sensation and perception, and in reportable physiological processes (Haertzen, Hill, & Belleville, 1963). Selected items were edited through consideration of the Thorndike-Lorge word counts (1944) so that the most difficult word in an item was below the sixth grade level. Items were predominantly phrased in the present tense rather than the past tense because drug effects were more commonly found on items that were phrased in the present tense. The final form of the ARCI contained 550 items including 30 items which were repeated exactly or in logically opposite form. The repeated items were used to form a Carelessness scale to evaluate the validity of responses in individual subjects (Haertzen & Hill, 1963). The original 550 items (Hill, Haertzen, & Belleville, 1958) have been retained to the present time. All of the 39 basic recommended scales can be scored with this set of items.

The middle 1960s permitted the testing of subjects undergoing opiate withdrawal (Haertzen & Hooks, 1969; Haertzen, Meketon, & Hooks, 1970). Since no sentence completion tests were given to subjects under any withdrawal condition, including opiates, it seemed desirable to include some classic withdrawal symptoms described chiefly by Himmelsbach (1941). For this reason 50 additional questions were added. In this set of items, rules about using drug names and Thorndike-Lorge word count criteria were suspended. It may be parenthetically noted that most drug names occurred infrequently in print or not at all. The added part is called Supplemental Questionnaire Number 4. It need not be given to subjects who are not drug abusers. The use of drug names may give clues about the possible purpose of the test.

Table 1

Classification of ARCI Items

			N[a]
1. General Information	a. Family		16
	b. Law		3
2. Interests and Drives	a. Interests in activity now		20
	b. Energy		15
	c. General interests (occupation)		20
	d. Appetite		10
	e. Sex		23
	f. Sleep		7
3. Sensation and Perception	a. Hearing		6
	b. Internal sensations		10
	c. Kinesthetic sensations		7
	d. Pain		7
	e. Smell		2
	f. Taste		6
	g. Time		4
	h. Touch		4
	i. Vision		17
	j. Temperature		5
4. Bodily Symptoms and Processes	a. Head		7
	b. Nose and lungs		4
	c. Body image		2
	d. Muscular coordination		10
	e. Mouth, throat, stomach		10
	f. Heart		2
	g. Nerves		4
	h. Skin		2
	i. Speech		5
	j. Extremities		6
	k. Neck		1
	l. Excretion and genitals		5
	m. Eyes		7
	n. Ears		6
5. Feelings and Attitudes	a. Ability		
		1) general discouragement or confidence	18
		2) concentration	15
		3) memory	2
		4) specific skills	3
		5) maturity	5
		6) social expression	15
	b. Reactions toward the test		11
	c. Attitudes toward people		45
	d. Attitudes toward institutions		4
	e. Content of thought		7

```
        f. Character traits
             1) empathy, sympathy                        7
             2) control, patience, hostility            44
             3) personal appearance                      5
             4) impulsiveness vs. planning              19
        g. Schizophrenia
             1) affect                                  10
             2) loss of interest                         5
             3) idea of things being changed             4
             4) ideas of reference, mind reading         5
             5) hallucinations                           6
             6) supernatural powers                      2
             7) feeling of being abused                 20
             8) suspicion                                3
             9) weird experiences                       15
            10) general characteristics                 15
        h. Expression                                    7
        i. Fears
             1) fears                                   11
             2) anxiety                                  6
             3) nervousness                             13
             4) "bothered by..."                         6
             5) pain                                     3
        j. Guilt
             1) guilt                                    8
             2) worry                                   15
             3) depression                              10
        k. Mood
             1) state of feeling                        12
             2) euphoria                                14
             3) depression                               7
             4) excitement                              12
        l. Interpersonal relations:                     20
             much overlap with other categories
        m. Orientation                                   8
        n. Philosophy of life                           10
                                                        ---
                                     Total              550
```

Note: a, N = number of items. Table 1 was originally adapted from a
dissertation (Haertzen, 1961). A complete list of items for
each category is also given.

Scale Development

Scale development on the ARCI has gone through many phases. Several
hundred scales have been constructed for the ARCI, but 39 scales are
recommended including the Carelessness scale (Haertzen, 1974a). Scale
development on the ARCI was influenced by the empiricism associated with the
MMPI (Hathaway & McKinley, 1951) and California Personality Inventory (CPI;
Gough, 1957) but also by the factor analytic methodology associated with tests
such as the Guilford-Zimmerman Temperament Survey (Guilford & Zimmerman, 1949)
and Sixteen Personality Factor Questionnaire (16 P.F.; Cattell, 1957),
Cattell's theories of causation (Cattell, 1952, 1957; Haertzen, 1966a), and
Eysenck's (1950) criterion analysis (Haertzen, 1962, 1969b). In addition
Martin and colleagues developed an amphetamine scale based on dose-effect

relationships (Martin, Sloan, Sapira, & Jasinski, 1971). Other investigators have also developed scales (Cole, Orzack, Beake, Bird, & Bar-tal, 1982; Resnick, Kestenbaum, & Schwartz, 1977).

The first set of published scales were empirical drug scales that applied to drugs included in the initial ARCI drug study (Hill, Haertzen, Wolbach, & Miner, 1963a, 1963b). The full item content for each scale is listed in the Appendix for ready reference. The drugs or conditions included in the study included no-drug, placebo, amphetamine, pentobarbital, chlorpromazine, alcohol, LSD, and pyrahexyl. More than one dose of some drugs was given. In the empirical scale development phase, we were interested in the question of whether the drug-placebo differences in responses on items would be maintained under cross validation. Hence, the sample of 100 subjects was divided into two equal parts for a test group and a cross validation group. A so-called significant scale for a particular drug consisted of those items which differentiated responses for a drug condition from a placebo condition at the 0.05 level or less for both the test group and cross validation group. LSD at a 1.5 μg/kg oral dose yielded the greatest number of significant changes. There were 67 items which met the cross validation criterion. LSD produced a huge assortment of changes from anxiety and difficulty in thinking to perceptual changes and hallucinations.

A second type of empirical scale is called a marginally significant scale and consisted of those remaining items which differentiated a placebo condition and drug condition using an N of 100. There were a total of 174 items in the combined significant and marginally significant LSD scales. Studies showed that the correlations between responses for the significant items were higher than that between the marginally significant items (Haertzen, 1966a). However, in spite of the fact that the differentiations of drugs and placebo were greater on individual items of the significant scale, the differentiations using total scores for significant and marginally significant scales were comparable (Hill, Haertzen, Wolbach, & Miner, 1963a). Therefore, if empirical scales are used, it is advisable to obtain just a score for the combined total. The significant scale items, however, may be considered under some circumstances as a short scale (Angrist, Rotrosen, & Gershon, 1974; Battig & Fischer 1965, 1966, 1968; Ehlers, 1966; Gold, Pottash, Sweeney, & Kleber, 1979, 1980a, 1980b).

The content of empirical scales overlaps with pattern or group variability drug scales which measure the more specific effects of various drugs. This is true in terms of items of euphoric content. Recently a naive subject rated ARCI items for euphoric content. When the overlap of items selected was determined for empirical scales, Benzedrine and Morphine scales were found to be high in euphoric content while the Chlorpromazine scale was very low (one item). Between these two extremes were scales for pyrahexyl, pentobarbital, LSD, and alcohol showing decreasing but measurable levels of euphoria. This variation in euphoric content on empirical scales is consistent with the findings of Hill, Haertzen, Wolbach, and Miner (1963a). Similarly when the overlap of items was determined for the more drug specific scales, euphoria items were found to be most concentrated in the Morphine-Benzedrine (MBG) scale and least in Chlorpromazine (CS) scale, which is consistent with the findings of Haertzen (1966b).

Empirical drug scales have the virtue of showing the variety of changes produced by a drug. The chief disadvantage is that empirical scales show general as well as more specific effects of a drug. Items which refer to feeling different or weird or to having a dry mouth or a lump in the throat are general effects. Empirical scales are less powerful for differentiating drugs than the pattern scales to be mentioned (Haertzen, 1966b).

Group Variability Scales and Drug Correction Scales

Some of the second set of scales called the group variability or drug correction scales are recommended (Haertzen, 1974a). Group variability refers to the pattern of the percentage of true responses found for opiate addicts for the various drugs mentioned (Haertzen, 1966b). Figure 1, upper panel, gives an example of a group variability pattern for the question 201 "I feel anxious and upset." It will be noted that the maximum true percentage was obtained for the highest dose of LSD of 1.5 µg/kg and that the second highest percent was obtained for the low dose of 1.0 µ g/kg of LSD. This pattern is referred to as the LG pattern, L is for LSD and G is for group variability. The recommended scale is called LSD. Items in the pattern include anxiety, restlessness, and perceptual changes (see Appendix, Scale 5 in List 116). The items contained in the LSD short form will be presented later.

In the pattern indicated by item 3, "I feel as if I would be more popular with people today" (see Figure 1, lower panel), it can be seen that the maximum percentages of true responses were found for Benzedrine and morphine. Relative to placebo, modest increases in true responses were found for other drugs except chlorpromazine. In this pattern called MBG, M is for morphine, B is for Benzedrine, and G is for group variability. The items which correlate highly with the MBG pattern suggest well being, euphoria, and optimal functioning.

The third common pattern is PCAG and refers to the common effects of pentobarbital, chlorpromazine, and alcohol. The marker for this pattern is item 66 "I feel drowsy" (see Figure 2, upper panel). The three drugs in the pattern name produced the highest effect. Morphine and pyrahexyl had a modest but significant effect on this item also. Items in this category suggest sedation, sluggishness, and low motivation.

A fourth pattern for Benzedrine (see Figure 2, lower panel) is marked by item 548 "Answering these questions was very easy today." Benzedrine produced a strong effect relative to other drugs such as LSD, pentobarbital, and alcohol. Feeling of intellectual efficiency or wakefulness are most specific to amphetamine (BG).

Several other patterns were found. The symptom of itching is relatively specific for morphine (MG; Haertzen, 1966b). A need to urinate and a high feeling similar to that produced by alcohol are specific to alcohol (AG). A feeling of excitement is common to LSD and amphetamine and to a lesser extent to morphine (Ex).

Scales were constructed to represent these various patterns. Simply stated these group variability marker patterns were correlated with the patterns for all other items and then factor analyzed by the diagonal (Fruchter, 1954) or profile method (Haertzen, 1963b). Items were selected which correlated highly with a pattern and showed some differentiation of drugs.

Space does not permit a full description of some of the remaining scales (Haertzen, 1965a, 1965b, 1970; Haertzen & Meketon, 1968; Sharp, Fuller, & Haertzen, 1967) nor of the methods used to reduce the vast number of scales. The number of scales were reduced from 200 to 39 by discriminant function

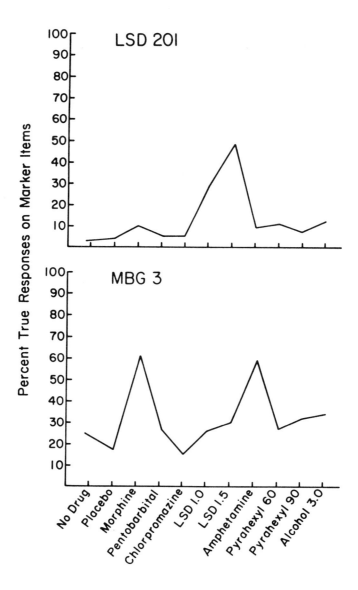

Figure 1: Percentage of "true" responses on ARCI items 201 (upper panel) and 3 (lower panel). The treatment conditions are listed on the abscissa. The drugs and routes of administration were morphine (20 mg, im), pentobarbital (200 mg, im), chlorpromazine (Day 1, 25 mg, oral, qid; Day 2, 50 mg, oral, qid; Day 3, 75 mg, oral at 8 a.m. only), LSD-25 (1.0 µg/kg, oral), LSD-25 (1.5 µg/kg, oral), pyrahexyl (60 mg, oral), pyrahexyl (90 mg, oral), and alcohol (3.0 ml/kg of 30% alcohol). See Appendix, ARCI column for guide to items.

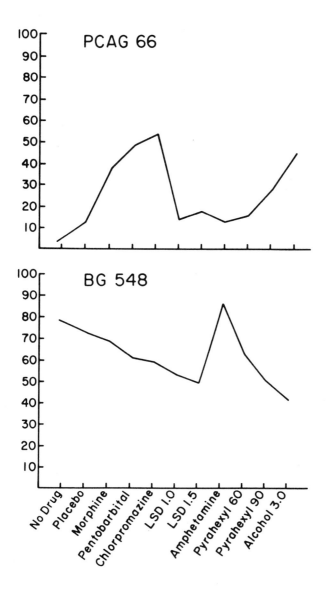

Figure 2: Percentage of "true" responses on ARCI items 66 (upper panel) and 548 (lower panel). The treatment conditions are listed on the abscissa. See Figure 1 caption for drugs and routes of administration. See Appendix, ARCI column for guide to items.

analyses (Haertzen, 1974a). Table 2 presents the names of the 38 recommended scales with the exception of the Carelessness scale. There are drug scales covering the effects of narcotic antagonists and of opiate and alcohol withdrawal and so forth along with factor analytic scales such as Impulsivity and Reactivity, and clinical scales such as Psychopathy and Social Withdrawal.

Clinical Scales

Some brief attention needs to be given to the clinical scales. The development of these scales required the use of clinical groups such as alcoholics (Haertzen & Fuller, 1967), criminals (Haertzen & Panton, 1967), other opiate addicts (Haertzen, Meketon, & Hooks, 1970), the mentally ill (Haertzen, Long, & Philip, 1964), and normal subjects contributed by Grupp (Haertzen, 1974a). Additional groups such as neurotics would have been desirable.

The clinical scales were developed through a modification (Haertzen, 1974a) of Eysenck's criterion analysis (Eysenck, 1950). Criterion analysis consists of selecting items which differentiate criterion conditions in a manner similar to that defined by the correlation of responses to an individual difference factor or scale, holding criterion conditions constant. A good scale via criterion analysis is one in which the pattern of differentiation between a pair of criterion conditions agrees with the pattern of correlations between the response to an item and a whole scale. The Alcohol Withdrawal scale (AWS) is the best scale according to this definition (Haertzen, Hooks, & Hill, 1966).

One of the principal clinical scales is the Psychopathy scale (Haertzen, 1974a). The original form of the scale (Haertzen & Panton, 1967) and the revised form (Haertzen, 1974a) highly differentiated alcoholics, opiate addicts, and criminals from the mentally ill and normal subjects. In a fairly recent study of alcoholics, opiate addicts, and normal subjects, the Psychopathy scale differentiated the groups better than the MMPI scales including Pd or the newly developed scales for the Psychopathic State Inventory (Haertzen, Martin, Hewett, & Sandquist, 1978). Ottomanelli (1973, 1977, 1978; Ottomanelli & Halloran, 1982) has used the Psychopathy scale in a variety of treatment oriented studies.

Scoring

The ARCI answer sheet is in true-false format. In scoring all scales except Carelessness, one point is given for each response which agrees with the scoring direction on a scale (Haertzen, 1974a). In some studies items for a particular subject were excluded when the response under placebo was in accord with the scoring on a scale (Rosenberg, Wolbach, Miner, & Isbell, 1963). This procedure is not recommended for several reasons. The scale length differs for each individual. It denies the possibility that scores on a scale can go down as well as up. Others have used linear scales or multiple choices (Battig & Fischer, 1965). The principal disadvantage of the multiple choice format is that standard T-scores cannot be found. The principal advantage of multiple choice format is realized in item analyses because more powerful parametric tests can be used. A large N is frequently needed to achieve significance at the item level when chi square is used on true-false responses.

In most studies raw scores are used. In statistical analyses some

Table 2

List of 38 Recommended Scales

No.	Abbr.	Full Name	Mean Raw Score Total	Standard Deviation Within Groups
101	Re	Reactivity #2	34.96	22.14
2	GDP	General Drug Predictor	15.48	7.623
102	Pyp	Psychopath #2	37.79	6.568
10	MBG	Morphine-Benzedrine GV	19.27	7.363
108	SoW	Social Withdrawal	15.54	5.611
111	Con	Self-Control	31.94	4.371
127	Mal	Maladjustment #2	34.83	5.243
125	GDE	General Drug Effect #3	16.11	4.904
123	Tir	Tired	7.156	2.457
29	Imp	Impulsive Factor Analytic	25.50	5.458
143	Int	Interests	16.21	4.732
115	Taste	Taste	1.238	1.798
4	PCAG	Pent, CPZ, Alc GV	12.77	5.813
7	AG	Alcohol GV	5.213	2.049
11	MG	Morphine GV	13.90	4.968
12	BG	Benzedrine GV	21.33	5.522
17	CS	Chlorpromazine Specific	17.43	3.901
19	Ex	Excitement GV	11.77	3.875
21	LSD	LSD Drug Correction	10.97	3.397
47	IT	Infrequent True	11.02	9.190
48	IF	Infrequent False	6.422	3.202
52	Mar	Marijuana	15.17	2.584
55	AWS	Alcohol Withdrawal Specific	31.72	16.62
87	Ef	Efficiency #3	29.92	8.967
106	Pop	Popularity	28.19	7.534
112	Cr	Critical	36.21	6.639
122	Weak	Weak	14.99	3.954
129	Dr	Drunk	6.081	2.398
136	Com	Competitive	39.97	5.165
145	Proj	Projection	20.46	5.627
153	NAnt	Narcotic Antagonist	18.33	7.961
161	ChrO	Chronic Opiate	6.868	3.038
163	SimO	Simulated Opiate	11.73	7.506
191	WOW	Weak Opiate Withdrawal	27.15	8.037
199	WOWs	Most significant WOW	18.16	3.149
207	SOW	Severe Opiate Withdrawal	17.86	10.13
220	AW	Alcohol Withdrawal greater than SOW	59.21	7.506
223	Hum	Sense of Humor	17.93	4.051

Note: GV means Group Variability; Pent means pentobarbital; Alc means Alcohol; CPZ means chlorpromazine. The mean for the total is based on the average raw scores from sums for the mentally ill (conditions 26, 27), normal (28), alcoholic (86, 87, 88), criminal (94), and opiate addicts (170, 173) (see Clinical Scales and Scoring). The standard deviation within groups is based on the within-conditions variance of the above conditions. These condition numbers are given in the manual (Haertzen, 1974).

transformation such as a log transformation may make variation under placebo and drugs more comparable. This is true for scales such as PCAG in which the distribution of scores is skewed with many low scores under the placebo condition. On empirical scales (Hill, Haertzen, Wolbach, & Miner, 1963a) and group variability scales (Haertzen, 1966b), a normalized T-score transformation is provided. This transformation tends to equalize variance under different drug conditions. The ARCI manual gives a T-score transformation that assumes a normal distribution (Haertzen, 1974a). This transformation is recommended for reporting averages. Table 2 presents the average raw scores and within conditions standard deviations for the five clinical groups used for standardization purposes. To make scores on one scale comparable to scores on another scale, the scores are converted to T-scores. Using this derived T-score, the average for the standardization sample is set at 50 and the standard deviation is set at 10. The raw scores are converted to T-scores by the formula:

$$T_i = 50 + (X_i - Mean_i) \times \frac{10}{SD_i}$$

where X_i is the raw score of a subject on the ith scale. $Mean_i$ is the average raw score of standardization on sample on the ith scale. SD_i is the standard deviation within for the ith scale. For example, the T-score of a raw score of 59 on Reactivity is

$$T_{Re} = 50 + (59 - 34.96) \times \frac{10}{22.14} = 50 + 10.86 = 61$$

The manual also gives corrected T-scores which correct for variation on scales such as the Psychopathy scale. This transformation should be used only for making drug or clinical diagnoses. Averages based on corrected T-scores are not recommended because the effect of corrections is extremely large.

In reporting results, uncorrected averages for groups are recommended as this form permits comparisons of magnitude and change using variability estimates based on the standardization sample. Difference scores, though useful as an adjunct, obscure the position of a sample on a scale. Percentage or ratio scores based on a placebo reference point are not recommended as the scales are not ratio scales.

To obtain significance between drugs, statistics for groups rather than individuals are recommended. For example, in one study it was noted that monotonic increases in PCAG as a function of the dose of pentobarbital were found in all five subjects, but that significance was obtained in only two subjects (Griffiths, Bigelow, Liebson, & Kaliszak, 1980). It was added that a group analysis would have been more sensitive to such effects. Using the same type of analysis, no significant effects from secobarbital were found in each of six subjects (Stitzer, Griffiths, Bigelow, & Liebson, 1981). Using group statistics, dose effects have been found for secobarbital (Jasinski, 1973).

Alternate Forms

The main focus of use of the ARCI has been with short forms or whole single scales. Martin (1967) and Jasinski, Martin, and Hoeldtke (1971) used items from PCAG (scale 452), MBG (scale 453), and LSD (scale 454) in their short form (Haertzen, 1974a). These items are presented in the Appendix. In the typical Addiction Research Center study of acute drug effects, the short form is given, but it is supplemented by other ratings in the Single-Dose Questionnaire such as liking of a drug, adjective check lists, similarity with common drugs, and physiological measures such as pupillary diameter (Jasinski, 1977; Martin, Jasinski, Haertzen, Kay, Jones, Mansky, & Carpenter, 1973a). To determine the degree of equivalency of drugs, drugs are usually given in multiple doses to determine dose effects or by different routes to study the mode of administration. Also some standard drug in the same class as an experimental drug is included. Observations are taken at hourly intervals. The paper by Henningfield, Johnson, and Jasinski, in this volume illustrates the variety of scales used to measure these parameters. Thus, for example in a study by Martin et al., (1973a), subcutaneously administered morphine and methadone were about equally potent. However, subcutaneously administered methadone is about twice as strong as orally administered methadone. Methadone was regarded as having a longer duration of action than morphine. MBG or euphoric effects in these drugs were regarded as having a shorter latency to onset than pupil diameter.

Chronic and withdrawal effects of 100 mg of oral methadone were also evaluated. Thus, during the chronic phase tolerance occurs for euphoria (MBG), but sedative-like effects (PCAG) increase. Another laboratory using a lower maintenance dose has found that euphoria (MBG) manifests itself when a high dose of hydromorphone is administered (McCaul, Stitzer, Bigelow, & Liebson, 1981, 1982, 1983). During withdrawal from methadone, lethargy, weakness, and tiredness (PCAG) increase as do the classic opiate withdrawal symptoms (WOW, SOW). Euphoria (MBG) and other indicators of efficiency (Ef) decrease. As compared with withdrawal under morphine or heroin (Haertzen & Hooks, 1969), withdrawal on methadone is more prolonged.

Classification of drug effects is possible using the full ARCI (Haertzen, 1974a, 1974b). Space does not permit a full description of the diagnostic system of the ARCI. Briefly, the system involves converting raw scores on 38 scales into corrected T-scores. An index of similarity between these scores and standard profiles as for drugs or withdrawal conditions is calculated based on differences squared between the test profile and the standard drug profiles. Classification is based on the lowest sum of differences squared. Correctness of the classification is contingent on the dose level and the number of subjects used in the sample. Correct classifications are most possible with a high dose. Distinctions are probably blurred at lower doses because of a general drug effect. Effects of sampling have not been determined with all drugs, but an N of about 10 for morphine has been found adequate to achieve correct hits.

In this system of classification, the magnitude of differences squared are partially a function of the sample size. If the hypothesis of a study is to determine whether a drug is producing a new pattern, a much larger N than 10 is required.

Separate diagnostic systems are applicable for making clinical and drug diagnoses. The actual scales involved for clinical and drug diagnoses do not overlap to a great degree. It should be added here that a computer is necessary to convert raw scores into corrected T-scores and to do the differences-squared analysis. A program is available for the Apple II+.

Although this writer considers classifications of drugs based on the total ARCI to be most robust, many distinctions among drugs can be made with the short form which includes MBG, PCAG, and LSD scales if adequate doses are given (Fischman & Schuster, 1980, 1981; Jasinski, Martin, & Hoeldtke, 1971; Martin, et al., 1971; McClane & Martin, 1976). However, additional distinctions may be possible if scales for opiate withdrawal (SOW), efficiency (Ef) or amphetamine effects (BG or A), drunkenness (Dr), excitement (Ex), and morphine effects (MG) are included. The short form called ARCI List 116 covers these areas. This list has been used by Cole and his group (Cole, Orzack, Beake, Bird, & Bar-tal, 1982; Cole, Pope, LaBrie, & Pioggia, 1978; Orzack, Cole, Pioggia, Beake, Bird, Lobel, & Martin, 1982). The items are presented in the Appendix with the direction of scoring.

Table 3 gives an estimate of the patterns for different drugs. The elevations shown for Ef and SOW are estimates since these scales were not included in most studies. Generally a range of -- to ++ is adequate. However, the range of withdrawal symptoms is extremely large; modest levels of withdrawal may suggest dysphoria. Probably the average for a group should be at least a standard deviation from the control value before it is considered as withdrawal. The average T-scores of drugs are presented in the ARCI manual (Haertzen, 1974a).

Stimulants such as amphetamine and cocaine are placed on top of the table. Both of these drugs (Fischman & Schuster, 1980; Haertzen, 1966b, 1974a; Resnick, Kestenbaum, & Schwartz, 1977; Van Dyke, Jatlow, Ungerer, Barash, & Byck, 1978) as well as other drugs in the stimulant class such as d-methamphetamine, l-ephedrine, dl-phenmetrazine, methylphenidate (Martin et al., 1971) and diethylpropion (Jasinski, Nutt, Griffith, 1974) had an effect on Efficiency or equivalents of it (e.g., BG or the Martin A scale). The MBG effect of stimulants occurs regularly. Procaine did not have an MBG effect (Fischman, Schuster, & Rajfer, 1983) though it did produce a slight "high" effect. An LSD effect from amphetamine has not been consistently found (Henningfield & Griffiths, 1981). In the Martin et al. (1971) study of stimulants, it was only at the highest dose that LSD scores exceeded those of placebo. Cocaine did produce LSD effects at higher doses (Fischman & Schuster, 1980; Fischman, Schuster, Resnekov, Schick, Krasnegor, Fennell, & Freedman, 1976). In simulations of cocaine, LSD-like effects are evident (Haertzen, 1974a). Simulations require that subjects answer the questions as they have felt while under the influence of a drug. Simulations are done under a no-drug state.

The MBG effect is marked for opiates. These effects have been extensively reviewed (Jasinski, 1977). The PCAG effect of opiates is not great but can be shown if the N is sufficiently large (Haertzen, 1966b). The patterns for partial opiate agonists range from being quite similar to opiates to drifting toward narcotic antagonists at higher doses. A shift towards narcotic antagonists is indicated by a decrease in Efficiency and an increase in PCAG and LSD effects (Jasinski & Mansky, 1972; Jasinski, Martin, & Hoeldtke, 1970). This shift was found for pentazocine. The pattern of effects shown for opiates is for the immediate effects. From 12 to 72 hours after the administration of morphine, methadone, or buprenorphine, the PCAG effect is evident (Jasinski, Pevnick, & Griffith, 1978). The simulated effects of opiates are similar to the acute effects. Surprisingly, subjects also ascribe euphoria to the chronic phase (Haertzen, 1974a). Tolerance to MBG occurs during chronic administration

Table 3

Drug Effect Patterns on Selected Scales

	Ef	MBG	PCAG	LSD	SOW
Stimulants--amphetamine, cocaine	+	++	0	0+	0
Opiates--heroin, morphine, methadone	0	++	0+	0	0
Partial opiate agonists-- pentazocine, nalbuphine	-	+	+	+	0
Marijuana	-0	++	0+	+	0
Barbiturates--pentobarbital, secobarbital	0-	+	++	0	0
Minor tranquilizers--diazepam	0-	+0	++	0	0
Alcohol	-	+	++	0	0
Major tranquilizers-- chlorpromazine	-	0	++	0	0
Narcotic antagonists-- nalorphine, cyclazocine	-	0	++	+	+
Hallucinogens--LSD	-	+	0	++	+
Others--scopolamine	--	0	++	+	+
Inactive--zomepirac, loperamide, bupropion		0	0	0	
Opiate withdrawal--morphine, heroin, methadone	--	-	++	+	+++
Alcohol withdrawal	--	-	++	+	++
Simulated barbiturate withdrawal	--	-	++	++	+++
Simulated alcohol withdrawal	--	--	++	++	+++
Simulated opiate withdrawal	--	-	++	++	+++
Simulated pep pill come down	--	-	++	++	++
Simulated cocaine come down	--	-	++	++	++

Note: Ef = Efficiency or BG (Benzedrine group variability)
      MBG = Morphine-Benzedrine group
      PCAG = Pentobarbital, chlorpromazine, and alcohol group
      LSD = LSD group or drug correction
      SOW = Strong opiate withdrawal

(Haertzen & Hooks, 1969; Martin et al., 1973a). Interestingly, acupuncture increases euphoria or MBG (Toyama & Heyder, 1981; Toyama, Popell, Evans, & Heyder, 1980).

The characteristics of effects of marijuana-like compounds is less certain. Subjective effects have been found in various studies (Hollister & Gillespie, 1973, 1975; Hollister, Overall, & Gerber, 1975; Kiplinger, Manno, Rodda, & Forney, 1971; Manno, 1970). Interpretation is hampered by the fact that the marijuana scales were not supplemented with other scales such as MBG. Pyrahexyl, a weak marijuana-like compound, produced a PCAG effect (Haertzen, 1966b). LSD-like effects have been found for THC (Hollister & Gillespie, 1975; Isbell, Gorodetsky, Jasinski, Clausen, Spulak, & Korte, 1967; Isbell & Jasinski, 1969; Jasinski, Haertzen, & Isbell, 1971). Valid assays of LSD and delta-9-THC were possible using Abramson's psychotomimetic scale and the ARCI General Drug Effect scale but not on the ARCI Marijuana or LSD scales. On the last two scales, the drugs could not be distinguished. THC and LSD were different on pupil diameter and knee jerk (Isbell & Jasinski, 1969). In a recent study (Boren, personal communication), THC, nabilone, and marijuana cigarettes produced euphoria; PCAG effects were found for marijuana cigarettes and nabilone but not THC. LSD effects were increased for THC and nabilone. Using simulations in opiate addicts, the profile of marijuana effects was indicative of euphoria (MBG), Efficiency, and Excitement but not PCAG or LSD (Haertzen, 1974a). In simulations of marijuana effects, normals who have not used marijuana overdramatized symptoms (Fabian & Fishkin, 1982).

Barbiturates, minor tranquilizers, and alcohol have some effects in common by being high on PCAG, intermediate on MBG, and low on Efficiency (Cole, Orzack, Beake, Bird, & Bar-tal, 1982; Fraser & Jasinski, 1977; Haertzen, 1966b; Jasinski, 1973; McClane & Martin, 1976). A small group of alcoholics showed an MBG effect from alcohol, but they failed to show a PCAG effect with alcohol and pentobarbital up to a dose of 400 mg oral (Henningfield, Chait, & Griffiths, 1984); they showed a PCAG effect at 600 mg of pentobarbital. Alcohol effects have been found in normal, alcoholic and heroin addicts (Battig & Fischer, 1965, 1966, 1968; Henningfield et al., 1983; Hill et al., 1963a). Buspiron (dopaminergic anti-anxiety drug) had sedative but no euphoric effects (Cole, Orzack, Beake, Bird, & Bar-tal, 1982).

Major tranquilizers differ from barbiturates by not producing euphoria (Haertzen, 1966b). In normal subjects 75 mg of oral chlorpromazine had little effect (Davis, Evans, & Gillis, 1968). In another study of normals, a PCAG effect was shown with 100 mg (Stitzer, Griffiths, Bigelow, & Liebson, 1981). It is of some interest to note that the effects of lithium were most similar to chlorpromazine. Lithium also reduced euphoria feelings on MBG (Jasinski, Nutt, Haertzen, Griffith, & Bunney, 1977).

Narcotic agonist-antagonists produced a strong effect on the LSD and the Strong Opiate Withdrawal scales (Haertzen, 1974a, 1974b; Jasinski & Mansky, 1972; Jasinski, Martin, & Haertzen, 1967). It should be remembered here that withdrawal is characterized by symptoms of anxiety, tension, cognitive difficulty, and tiredness as well as by symptoms such as cramps that are more specific to withdrawal (Haertzen & Hooks, 1969; Haertzen, Meketon, & Hooks, 1970; Himmelsbach, 1941). Opiate withdrawal and narcotic antagonists are quite distinguishable (Haertzen, 1974a). Narcotic antagonists such as naloxone or naltrexone which are devoid of agonist activity do not have effects on these scales (Martin, Jasinski, & Mansky, 1973b). However, in one study naltrexone produced a slight MBG effect (Gritz, Schiffman, Jarvik, Schlesinger, & Charuvastra, 1976). This result could be considered tentative because the subjects disclaimed a drug effect.

LSD is different from narcotic antagonists in showing some euphoria and excitement. Euphoria is more evident at lower doses. Psychotomimetic effects may occur at lower doses (Haertzen, 1966b; Isbell & Jasinski, 1969; Rosenberg, Isbell, & Miner, 1963; Rosenberg, Wolbach, Miner, & Isbell, 1963). LSD produced a very large range of changes (Martin & Sloan, 1977). Mescaline, psilocybin, psilocin (Martin & Sloan, 1977), and DOM (Angrist, Retrosen, & Gershon, 1974) produced effects like LSD.

Scopolamine has effects most similar to narcotic antagonists (Haertzen, 1974a). Scopolamine as well as the narcotic antagonists are different from opiate withdrawal chiefly on the differences in the magnitude of withdrawal symptoms. Scopolamine produced some symptomatic changes, such as blurred vision, which are much greater than other drugs. The larger print on the inventory was helpful in this respect, but subjects at the highest dose frequently required the examiner to read and to record responses.

Little has been done with antidepressants. The effects of bupropion were similar to those of placebo and were different from amphetamine (Miller & Griffith, 1983) on MBG, BG, LSD, and PCAG. Miller and Griffith cite studies with rats and monkeys which indicate bupropion has some similarity with stimulants.

Some other drugs which are inactive according to ARCI scales are zomepirac (Johnson & Jasinski, 1982; Johnson, Jasinski, & Kocher, 1983) and loperamide (Jaffe, Kanzler, & Green, 1981). Placebo effects have been found on the first trial relative to later trials (Haertzen, 1969a). MBG decreased under placebo over weeks (Gritz, Schiffman, Jarvik, Schlesinger, & Charuvastra, 1976).

Opiate and alcohol withdrawal reduced efficiency and increased PCAG and opiate and alcohol withdrawal symptoms by a great margin (Haertzen & Fuller, 1967; Haertzen & Hooks, 1969; Martin et al., 1973a). It will be noted that opiate withdrawal symptoms for simulated withdrawal for alcohol, barbiturates, and opiates were very strong (Haertzen, 1974a), especially when the simulation occurs after a no-drug condition (Haertzen & Hooks, 1971). The pattern shown in Table 3 does not fully indicate the distinctiveness of withdrawal types. The profiles of actual and simulated alcohol-withdrawal deviate so much from the standards that alcohol withdrawal becomes a needed additional standard. In studies of alcohol or barbiturate withdrawal, the alcohol withdrawal scale should also be included.

The similarity of classifications based on subjective reports in humans and animals has been noted in several ways. Thus, internal stimuli which account for drug discrimination in animal studies has been likened to the occurrence of subjective experiences (Colpaert, 1978, this volume; Shannon & Holtzman, 1976). Overton and Batta (1979) suggest that drugs may be more sharply distinguished in animals by the discrimination model than in man by subjective reports with the ARCI. More human experimentation needs to be done to see if humans can sharpen their discriminations. Using the self-administration model, Griffiths and Balster (1979) found concordance between conclusions derived from subjective report and self-administration. The occurrence of euphoria probably accounts for some of the concordance as animals are more likely to self-administer those drugs which produce an MBG effect in man (Schuster, Fischman, & Johanson, 1981).

MBG effects, as for opiates, are in substantial agreement with other indicators of reinforcement such as liking when drugs are administered acutely. However, during chronic administration of opiates, MBG effects are first attenuated and then disappear (Haertzen & Hooks, 1969; Martin et al., 1973a; Schuster et al., 1981). Opiate addicts, nevertheless, attest that they would like to take the drug every day (Martin & Fraser, 1961). Similarly on an Appetite Rating scale in which subjects are asked to rate their current appetite (from absolute necessity to refusal of the drug if it were offered) or projected appetite for the experimental drug (morphine or heroin), appetite for the experimental drug increased during the course of the chronic phase (Haertzen & Hooks, 1969). During the phase of increasing doses of methadone, opiate addicts rode an exercise bicycle to supplement their methadone dose with Dilaudid. This behavior was extinguished in some subjects when they obtained 100 mg of methadone orally (Martin et al., 1973a). During opiate withdrawal opiate addicts significantly agreed to ARCI Q 587 "A shot of morphine or heroin would help to settle my system" (Haertzen, Meketon, & Hooks, 1970). At this phase MBG was below the normal no-drug state. During withdrawal of morphine or heroin, the appetite for these experimental drugs decreased (Haertzen & Hooks, 1969). This decrease is interpreted as indicating that they disparaged the amount or quality of the drug given during withdrawal.

Depending on the drug, linear acute-dose effects and time-related effects have been found with MBG, with liking a drug, and with getting high from it. On the other hand appetite for "more of a drug right now" is curvilinear with respect to dose. That is, subjects recognized a satiation effect even with opiates. Projected appetite (how much appetite for a drug is likely to occur on other days) is dose related. It is possibly more immune to a time effect; subjects may retain an idea of an appetite for a desired drug even after the effect has worn off. Feeling that a drug has utility (to settle one's system) is correlated with the severity of opiate withdrawal or is dependent on the level of the disturbance (withdrawal).

Liking of the acute effects of a drug is more indicative of a general drug effect than might be expected considering other criteria. That is, liking of drug effects in acute experiments occurs even for drugs such as barbiturates (McClane & Martin, 1976) which have no great appeal for opiate addicts in a no-drug condition (Haertzen & Hooks, 1969; Haertzen, Hooks, & Ross, 1981). There is some comparative basis for liking pentobarbital, since subjects liked both diazepam and pentobarbital, but they chose pentobarbital over diazepam in a choice situation (Griffiths, Bigelow, & Liebson, 1981; Griffiths, Bigelow, Liebson, & Kaliszak, 1980). Some drugs are liked to some degree under acute administration but not under chronic administration. This is true for orally administered propoxyphene, codeine, and morphine (Fraser, Kay, Gorodetzky, Yeh, & Dewey, 1978). It was speculated that the change in liking was due to the accumulation of nor-metabolites. Opiate addicts liked cyclazocine or nalorphine when moderate doses were given (Martin, Fraser, Gorodetzky, & Rosenberg, 1965), but in chronic studies subjects would not tolerate nalorphine at a dose above 130 mg (Isbell, 1956) and did not show drug-seeking behavior upon withdrawal of cyclazocine (Martin et al., 1965).

Liking for varied drugs after acute administration may suggest that the frame of reference or baseline for the rating of liking is indefinite or floats depending on the drug. It would be interesting to alter the baseline for rating of liking a drug by having subjects rate the experimental drug against standards such as heroin, marijuana, or alcohol. Such ratings have not been tried. If a reference were made to heroin, it is postulated that the degree of liking for barbiturates, minor tranquilizers, and narcotic antagonists would be significantly downgraded. Also a rating of drug liking obtained a day after the drug administration may provide an estimate which reflects perceived advantages or disadvantages of a drug. Changes in liking ratings during chronic administration, as for opiates, may be due to other factors such as nor-metabolites (Fraser et al., 1978).

Ratings of liking, high, or MBG reveal the transitory nature of drug effects. In contrast measures of addiction which refer to past experiences with a drug or which imply a diagnosis of addiction appear to be more resistant to drug effects (Haertzen, 1978; Haertzen & Hooks, 1969). The strength of the verbal habit for a drug, marked by a tendency to associate many drug relevant words or experiences with a drug, is regarded as more malleable in those subjects who have not had extensive experience with it. Opiate addicts given chronic methadone developed a verbal habit for it. Furthermore, the habit was maintained after withdrawal was completed (Haertzen, Hooks, & Pross, 1974).

As indicated, a considerable portion of work has been devoted to showing drug similarity to characterize drug effects. Scales have been used for a variety of other experimental purposes. Thus, the Weak Opiate Withdrawal scale has been used to follow the treatment efficacy of agents to reduce opiate withdrawal. For example, following clonidine administration, methadone-abstinence symptoms were reduced within 120 minutes (Gold, Pottash, Sweeney, & Pottash, 1980a; Kleber, Gold, & Riordan, 1980). In another study clonidine suppressed autonomic signs more than morphine (Jasinski, Haertzen, Henningfield, Johnson, Makhzoumi, & Miyasato, 1982). However, morphine was more effective in reducing the subjective discomfort of withdrawal. In delaying the onset of withdrawal symptoms after placebo substitution, acetylmethadol (LAAM) had a longer duration of action than methadone since withdrawal symptoms on the ARCI withdrawal scale and a symptom check list arose at 36 hours for methadone but not for acetylmethadol (Jaffe, Schuster, Smith, & Blachley, 1970).

Buprenorphine has also been proposed as an opiate detoxification agent and as a maintenance drug (Jasinski, 1982). It has virtue as a maintenance drug because it is long acting and produces very little physical dependence (Jasinski, Pevnick, & Griffith, 1978). As a detoxification agent it reduces withdrawal symptoms of morphine or methadone. However, withdrawal symptoms ascribed to methadone arose again when buprenorphine was discontinued at a time when methadone withdrawal symptoms would be expected to still be present (Jasinski, Henningfield, Hickey, & Johnson, 1983). Opiate withdrawal scales are predictive of the probability of staying in treatment in opiate addicts volunteering for treatment. That is, the stronger the opiate withdrawal symptoms, the shorter the stay (Meketon, 1967).

In an experiment designed to see if opiate addicts would reduce their methadone intake via self-administration, the amount of self-administered methadone varied with a pretreatment dose of methadone. MBG or euphoria scores were greater in those given a 30 mg pretreatment dose of methadone than for those given placebo. There were no differences on the ARCI Weak Opiate Withdrawal scale, but there were differences on the symptom scale devised by the Behavioral Pharmacology Research Unit (BPRU) staff (McLeod, Bigelow, & Liebson, 1982). In another experiment by the same group, those subjects informed of a dose-reduction schedule experienced fewer symptoms with a dose reduction on a BPRU symptom scale than those who were blind to the dose-reduction schedule (Stitzer, Bigelow, & Liebson, 1982).

Evidence for conditioned opiate-abstinence symptoms was found using an ARCI opiate withdrawal scale. Opiate addicts who were shown opiate related stimuli such as the word heroin, an injection of drugs, or a stoned addict subsequently showed greater opiate withdrawal symptoms. On the other hand abstinence symptoms did not increase following exposure to neutral stimuli such as sugar (Teasdale, 1973). Further replication is needed because in an analogous procedure no withdrawal effects were found on the Weak Opiate Withdrawal scale but skin temperature was reduced (Ternes, O'Brien, Grabowski, Wellerstein, & Hayes, 1979) and heart rate increased (Sideroff & Jarvik, 1980). Opiate addicts gave an immediate emotional response to drug-related argot words as measured by pupil diameter (Bernick, Altman, & Mintz, 1972).

Changes in mood or feelings as measured by the ARCI are induced by stress factors. College students who were currently under some stress-producing situation obtained greater Reactivity scores (Haertzen, 1974a). College students decreased in MBG (euphoria) and increased in tiredness (PCAG) following the viewing of "Christmas in Appalachia," which is a depressing film showing poverty in that area (Cowan, Kay, Neidert, Ross, & Belmore, 1979, 1980). Scores from other scales from the Profile of Mood States (POMS) such as Depression-Rejection and scales devised by Cowan et al. (1980) for Joylessness increased also. Sleep deprivation increased scores on PCAG and LSD and reduced scores on MBG and BG. Cocaine nullified the 24 hour sleep deprivation effect on MBG and BG (Fischman & Schuster, 1980). Motivational factors affect scores in drug experiments (Sice, Levin, Levine, & Haertzen, 1975).

Emphasis in this paper has been on drug oriented scales and the significance of elevations on these scales for classifying drugs, characterizing drug effects, and rating the abuse potential of drugs. Many studies have been devoted to relating personality and psychopathology to drug abuse (see review by Haertzen, 1978). Psychopathy has been found to be one of the more important nonspecific correlates of drug abuse (Hill, Haertzen, & Glaser, 1960). The degree of psychopathy is correlated with follow-up criteria of drug abuse such as unemployment and arrest records (Ottomanelli, 1977). However, primary measures of psychopathy have been immune to the acute, chronic, or withdrawal effects of drugs such as opiates (Haertzen & Hooks, 1973; Martin, Jasinski, Haertzen, Kay, Jones, Mansky, & Carpenter, 1973a). This may be due to restricted opportunity on closed experimental wards or to the characteristics of psychopathy scales. That is, most psychopathy items, as for example in the MMPI, refer to past behavior. It is hoped that some psychopathy scales from the Psychopathic State Inventory which measures psychopathy as a state will be more susceptible to the measurement of psychopathic episodes (Haertzen, Martin, Ross, & Neidert, 1980; Kay, 1980; Martin, Hewett, Baker, & Haertzen, 1977). Unpublished studies by Monroe, Mathews, and Haertzen of drug abusers in a therapeutic community revealed that several indicators of psychopathy such as hypophoria (depression) reduced with progress in treatment. Within the context of experimental drug studies, only modest attempts have been made to correlate personality or psychopathology with drug effects or to drug-taking behavior. Kolb (1925) thought that psychopaths were more likely to obtain euphoria from opiates. Recent studies have shown the relevance of some characteristics believed to be indicative of psychopathic states in predicting drug-taking behavior. In an experimental drug study, subjects who chose amphetamine over placebo were more egocentric and had a greater desire to become high (de Wit, Johanson, & Uhlenhuth, 1983). Individual differences other than psychopathy have predicted drug-taking behavior. Anxious and depressed subjects were more likely to elect to receive amphetamine in a choice situation (Uhlenhuth, Johanson, Kilgore, & Kobasa, 1981).

These relatively recent studies to develop a more precise understanding of the relationship of psychopathology to drug choice, drug effects, and treatment outcomes represent an important direction for future use of the ARCI or other tests. It is hoped that such work will sharpen the prediction of drug effects and/or drug-taking behavior and contribute to the development of more effective treatment interventions.

References and Selected Bibliography

Abramson, H. A., Jarvik, M. E., Kaufman, M. R., Kornetsky, C., Levine, A., & Wagner, M. (1955). Lysergic acid diethylamide (LSD-25): I. Physiological and perceptual responses. Journal of Psychology, 39, 3-60.

Angrist, B., & Gershon, S. (1979). Variable attenuation of amphetamine effects by lithium. American Journal of Psychiatry, 136, 806-810.

Angrist, B., Rotrosen, J., & Gershon, S. (1974). Assessment of tolerance to the hallucinogenic effects of DOM. Psychopharmacologia, 36, 203-207.

Battig, K., & Fischer, H. (1965). Personlichkeitsmerkmale, subjectives Selbstempfinden und psychomotische Leistung unter Alkohol-einflusz bei jungen, nicht Alkohol gewohnten Individuen. (The effects of alcohol on personality traits, subjective states and psychomotor performance in young subjects not used to the effects of alcohol.) Zeitschrift fur Praventivmedizin, 10, 386-396.

Battig, K., & Fischer, H. (1966). Haben rezeptfreie Analgetica und Placebos eine verschiedene Wirkung auf das subjektive Selbstempfinden, die Personlichkeitslage und die psychomotorische Leistung? (Have nonprescription analgesics and placebos a different action on subjective states, personality traits, and psychomotor performance?) Schweizerische Medizinische Wochenschrift, 96, 570-575.

Battig, K., & Fischer, H. (1967). Complete German translation of the Addiction Research Center Inventory. Obtainable from Dr. C. A. Haertzen, NIDA, Addiction Research Center, Francis Scott Key Medical Center, Bldg. C, 4940 Eastern Avenue, Baltimore, Maryland, 21224 or from Dr. K. Battig, Eidg. Technische Hochschule, Institut fur Hygiene und Arbeitsphysiologie, Clausiusstrasze 25, Zurich 6, Switzerland.

Battig, K., & Fischer, H. (1968). Die Suggerierbarkeit bei der psychischen Wirkung von Pharmaka. (Suggestibility in the psychological action of drugs.) Schweizerische Medizinische Wochenschrift, 98, 898-904.

Beecher, H. K. (1959). Measurement of subjective responses. New York: Oxford University Press.

Belleville, R. E. (1956). MMPI score changes induced by lysergic acid diethylamide. Journal of Clinical Psychology, 12, 279-282.

Bernick, N., Altman, F., & Mintz, D. L. (1972). Pupil responses of addicts in treatment to drug culture argot: II. Responses during verbalization of visually presented words. Psychonomic Science, 28, 81-82.

Biehl, B. (1979). Studies of clobazam and car-driving. British Journal of Clinical Pharmacology, 7, 85S-90S.

Biehl, B., Fuhrmann, J., & Seydel, U. (1969). Auswirkungen der gleichzeitigen Einnahme von Alkohol und vitaminhaltigen Fruchtsaften auf psychologische Testleistungen und die Blutalkoholkonzentration. (The effect of simultaneous administration of alcohol and fruit juice containing vitamins on psychological test performance and blood alcohol levels.) Zeitschrift fur Experimentelle und Angewandte Psychologie, 16, 402-419.

Cameron, J. S., Specht, P. G., & Wendt, G. R. (1967). Effects of two meprobamate-amphetamine combinations on moods, emotions, and motivations. Journal of Psychology, 67, 169-181.

Cattell, R. B. (1952). Factor analysis. New York: Harper & Brothers.

Cattell, R. B. (1957). The Sixteen Personality Factor Questionnaire (rev. ed.). Champaign, IL: Institute for Personality and Ability Testing.

Clark, S. C., Jasinski, D. R., Pevnick, J. S., & Griffith, J. D. (1976). Azidomorphine: Subjective effects and suppression of morphine abstinence. Clinical Pharmacology and Therapeutics, 19, 295-299.

Clyde, D. J. (1960). Self ratings. In L. Uhr & G. Miller (Eds.), Drugs and behavior (pp. 583-586). New York: John Wiley & Sons.

Cole, J. O., Orzack, M. H., Beake, B., Bird, M., & Bar-tal, Y. (1982). Assessment of the abuse liability of buspirone in recreational sedative users. Journal of Clinical Psychiatry, 43, 69-75.

Cole, J. O., Pope, H. G., LaBrie, R., & Ionescu-Pioggia (1978). Assessing the subjective effects of stimulants in casual users. Clinical Pharmacology and Therapeutics, 24, 243-252.

Colpaert, F. C. (1978). Theoretical review: Discriminative stimulus properties of analgesic drugs. Pharmacology Biochemistry & Behavior, 5, 401-408.

Cowan, J. D., Kay, D. C., Neidert, G. L., Ross, F. E., & Belmore, S. M. (1979). Drug abusers: Defeated and joyless. In L. S. Harris (Ed.), Problems of drug dependence. 1979 (National Institute on Drug Abuse Research Monograph 27, pp. 170-176). Washington, DC: U.S. Government Printing Office.

Cowan, J. D., Kay, D. C., Neidert, G. L., Ross, F. E., & Belmore, S. M. (1980). Defeated and joyless: Potential measures of change in drug abuser characteristics. Journal of Nervous and Mental Disease, 168, 391-399.

Datel, W. E., Gieseking, C. F., Engle, E. O., & Dougher, M. J. (1966). Affect levels in a platoon of basic trainees. Psychological Reports, 18, 271-285.

Davis, K. E., Evans, W. O., & Gillis, J. S. (1968). The effects of amphetamine and chlorpromazine on cognitive skills and feelings in normal adult males. In W. O. Evans & N. S. Kline (Eds.), The psychopharmacology of the normal human (pp. 126-161). Springfield, IL: Charles C. Thomas. (Also as report #92, Institute of Behavioral Science, University of Colorado, June 1967.)

de Wit, H., Johanson, C. E., McCracken, S., & Uhlenhuth, E. H. (1983). The effects of two non-pharmacological variables on drug preference in humans. In L. S. Harris (Ed.), Problems of drug dependence, 1982 (National Institute on Drug Abuse Research Monograph 43, pp. 251-257). Washington, DC: U.S. Government Printing Office.

de Wit, H., Johanson, C. E., & Uhlenhuth, E. H. (1983, June). Comparison of subjects who consistently chose amphetamine (Choosers, N =11) and subjects who consistently chose placebo (non-choosers, N = 11). Presented at the meeting of the Committee on Problems of Drug Dependence, Lexington, KY.

de Wit, H., Johanson, C. E., & Uhlenhuth, E. H. (1984). Drug preference in humans: Lorazepam. In L. S. Harris (Ed.), Problems of drug dependence, 1983 (National Institute on Drug Abuse Monograph 49, pp. 227-232). Washington, DC: U.S. Government Printing Office.

Ehlers, T. (1966). Alkoholbedingte Motivationsanderungen und Unfallgefahrdung. (Alcohol induced motivational changes and accident proneness.) Zeitschrift fur Experimentelle und Angewandte Psychologie, 13, 1-18.

Eisenberg, H. A. (1983). A cross-reference to the Addiction Research Center Inventory. Mimeographed, Portland State University, Portland, OR.

Eisenberg, H. A. (1974). Scale membership and scoring for the Addiction Research Center Inventory. Mimeographed, Portland State University, Portland, OR.

Evans, M., Chadd, M. A., Evans, C. M., Fry, D. M., & Robson, P. J. (1983). Administration of meptazinol to opiate-dependent patients. Postgraduate Medical Journal, 59, 78-84.

Eysenck, H. K. (1950). Criterion analysis--An application of the hypothetico deductive method to factor analysis. Psychological Review, 57, 38-53.

Eysenck, H. K. (1957). The dynamics of anxiety and hysteria. New York: Frederick A. P. Praeger.

Fabian, W. D., & Fishkin, S. M. (1982). Attentional absorption in marijuana and alcohol intoxication. Submitted to the American Psychological Association. Reference paper: Fabian, W. D., Jr. & Fishkin, S. M. (1981). A replicated study of self-reported changes in psychological absorption with marijuana intoxication. Journal of Abnormal Psychology, 6, 546-553.

Feinberg, M., Pegeron, J. P., & Steiner, M. (1983). The effect of morphine on symptoms of endogenous depression. In L. S. Harris (Ed.), Problems of drug dependence, 1982 (National Institute on Drug Abuse Research Monograph 34, pp. 245-250). Washington, DC: U.S. Government Printing Office.

Fischman, M. W., & Schuster, C. R. (1980). Cocaine effects in sleep deprived humans. Psychopharmacology, 72, 1-8.

Fischman, M. W., & Schuster, C. R. (1981). Acute tolerance to cocaine in humans. In L. S. Harris (Ed.), Problems of drug dependence, 1980 (National Institute on Drug Abuse Research Monograph 34, pp. 241-242). Washington, DC: U.S. Government Printing Office.

Fischman, M. W., Schuster, C. R., & Rajfer, S. (1983). A comparison of the subjective and cardiovascular effects of cocaine and procaine in humans. Pharmacology Biochemistry & Behavior, 18, 711-716.

Fischman, M. W., Schuster, C. R., Resnekov, L., Krasnegor, N. A., Schick, J. F. E, Fennell, W., & Freedman, D. X. (1976). Cardiovascular and subjective effects of intravenous cocaine administration in humans. Archives of General Psychiatry, 33, 983-989.

Fraser, H. F., & Jasinski, D. R. (1977). The assessment of the abuse potentiality of sedative/hypnotics (depressants): Methods used in animals and man. In W. R. Martin (Ed.), Drug addiction I: Morphine, sedative/hypnotic and alcohol dependence (pp. 589-612). New York: Springer-Verlag.

Fraser, H. F., Kay, D. C., Gorodetzky, C. W., Yeh, S. Y., & Dewey, W. L. (1978). Evidence for the importance of n-dealkylation in opioid pharmacology. Drug and Alcohol Dependence, 3, 1-22.

Fruchter, B. (1954). Introduction of factor analysis. New York: D. Van Nostrand.

Gold, M. S., Pottash, A. L. C., Sweeney, D. R., & Kleber, H. D. (1979). Clonidine detoxification: A fourteen-day protocol for rapid opiate withdrawal. In L. S. Harris (Ed.), Problems of drug dependence, 1979 (National Institute on Drug Abuse Research Monograph 27, pp. 226-232). Washington, DC: U.S. Government Printing Office.

Gold, M. S., Pottash, A. L. C., Sweeney, D. R., & Kleber, H. D. (1980a). Efficacy of clonidine in opiate withdrawal: A study of thirty patients. Drug and alcohol dependence, 6, 201-208.

Gold, M. S., Pottash, A. L. C., Sweeney, D. R., & Kleber, H. D. (1980b). Opiate withdrawal using clonidine. Journal of the American Medical Association, 243, 343-346.

Gough, H. G. (1954). Some common misconceptions about neuroticism. Journal of Consulting Psychology, 18, 287-292.

Gough, H. G. (1957). California Psychological Inventory Manual. Palo Alto, CA: Consulting Psychologist Press.

Griffith, J. D., Carranza, J., Griffith, C., & Miller, L., (1983). A comparison of bupropion and amphetamine for abuse liability. In L. S. Harris (Ed.), Problems of Drug Dependence, 1982 (National Institute on Drug Abuse Monograph 43, pp. 373). Washington, DC: U.S. Government Printing Office.

Griffiths, R. R., & Balster, R. L. (1979). Opioids: Similarity between evaluations of subjective effects and animal self-administration results. Journal of Pharmacology and Therapeutics, 25, 611-617.

Griffiths, R. R., Bigelow, G. E., & Liebson, I. A. (1981). Human preference comparison of pentobarbital, diazepam, and placebo. In L. S. Harris (Ed.), Problems of drug dependence, 1980 (National Institute on Drug Abuse Research Monograph 34, pp. 220-225). Washington, DC: U.S. Government Printing Office.

Griffiths, R. R., Bigelow, G. E., & Liebson, I. A. (1983). Differential effects of diazepam and pentobarbital on mood and behavior. Archives of General Psychiatry, 40, 865-873.

Griffiths, R. R., Bigelow, G. E., Liebson, I. A., & Kaliszak, J. E. (1980). Drug preference in humans: Double-blind choice comparison of pentobarbital, diazepam and placebo. Journal of Pharmacology and Experimental Therapeutics, 215, 649-661.

Gritz, E. R., Schiffman, S. M., Jarvik, M. E., Schlesinger, J., & Charuvastra, V. C. (1976). Naltrexone: Physiological and psychological effects of single doses. Clinical Pharmacology and Therapeutics, 19, 773-776.

Guelfi, J. D., Brun, J. P., & Dreyfus, J. F. (1983). French Translation of Addiction Research Center Inventory (ARCI). Paris: Therapharm Recherches.

Guilford, J. P., & Zimmerman, W. S. (1949). The Guilford-Zimmerman Temperament Survey. Beverly Hills, CA: Sheridan Supply.

Haddox, V. G., Jacobson, M. D., & Selden, R. W. (1972). Development of an instrument for assessing addict rehabilitation success. Paper presented at the meeting of the American Psychological Association.

Haertzen, C. A. (1961). A test of a basic assumption of causation in factor analytic theory: Changes in correlation between responses and changes in factor composition following the administration of LSD. Unpublished doctoral dissertation, University of Kentucky.

Haertzen, C. A. (1962). Criterion analysis of seven drug scales. Paper presented at the meeting of the Midwestern Psychological Association, Chicago.

Haertzen, C. A. (1963a). An Appendix of Addiction Research Center Inventory (ARCI) Scales: Temporary Report. NIMH Addiction Research Center, Lexington, KY.

Haertzen, C. A. (1963b). Method for direct determination of inverted factor loadings. Psychological Reports, 12, 399-402.

Haertzen, C. A. (1964). On the Addiction Research Center Inventory scores of former addicts receiving LSD, and untreated schizophrenics. Psychological Reports, 14, 483-488.

Haertzen, C. A. (1965a). Addiction Research Center Inventory (ARCI): Development of a general drug estimation scale. Journal of Nervous and Mental Diseases, 141, 300-307.

Haertzen, C. A. (1965b). Subjective drug effects: A factorial representation of subjective drug effects on the Addiction Research Center Inventory. Journal of Nervous and Mental Diseases, 140, 280-289.

Haertzen, C. A. (1966a). Changes in correlation between responses to items of the Addiction Research Center Inventory produced by LSD-25. Journal of Psychopharmacology, 1, 27-36.

Haertzen, C. A. (1966b). Development of scales based on patterns of drug effects, using the Addiction Research Center Inventory (ARCI). Psychological Reports, 18, 163-194.

Haertzen, C. A. (1969a). Contrast effect on subjective experience in drug experiments. Psychological Reports, 24, 69-70.

Haertzen, C. A. (1969b). Implications of Eysenck's criterion analysis for test construction: Is the MMPI Schizophrenia scale a criterion for schizophrenia? Psychological Reports, 24, 3.

Haertzen, C. A. (1970). Subjective effects of narcotic antagonists. Cyclazocine and nalorphine on the Addiction Research Center Inventory (ARCI). Psychopharmacologia, 18, 366-377.

Haertzen, C. A. (1974a). An overview of Addiction Research Center Inventory scales (ARCI): An appendix and manual of scales (DHEW Publication No. (ADM) 74-92). Rockville, MD: National Institute on Drug Abuse.

Haertzen, C. A. (1974b). Subjective effects of narcotic antagonists. In M. C. Braude, L. S. Harris, E. L. May, J. P. Smith & J. E. Villarreal (Eds.), Narcotic antagonists (pp. 383-398). New York: Raven Press.

Haertzen, C. A. (1978). Clinical psychological studies. In W. R. Martin, & H. Isbell (Eds.), Drug addiction and the U. S. Public Health Service, DHEW Publication No. (ADM) 77-434, (pp. 155-168). Rockville, MD: National Institute of Drug Abuse.

Haertzen, C. A. (1983). Measurement of subjective drug effects with the Addiction Research Center Inventory. Paper presented in a symposium held by The American Psychological Association, Anaheim, CA.

Haertzen, C. A., & Fuller, G. (1967). Subjective effects of acute withdrawal of alcohol as measured by the Addiction Research Center Inventory (ARCI). Quarterly Journal of Studies on Alcohol, 28, 454-467.

Haertzen, C. A., & Hill, H. E. (1959). Effects of morphine and pentobarbital on differential MMPI profiles. Journal of Clinical Psychology, 15, 434-437.

Haertzen, C. A., & Hill, H. E. (1963). Assessing subjective effects of drugs: An index of carelessness and confusion for use with the Addiction Research Center Inventory (ARCI). Journal of Clinical Psychology, 19, 407-412.

Haertzen, C. A., Hill, H. E., & Belleville, R. E. (1963). Development of the Addiction Research Center Inventory (ARCI): Selection of items that are sensitive to the effects of various drugs. Psychopharmacologia, 4, 155-166.

Haertzen, C. A., Hill, H. E, & Monroe, J. J. (1968). MMPI scales for differentiating and predicting relapse in alcoholics, opiate addicts and criminals. International Journal of the Addictions, 3, 91-106.

Haertzen, C. A., & Hooks, N. T., Jr. (1968). Effects of adaptation level, context and face validity on responses to self-report psychological inventories. Psychological Record, 18, 339-349.

Haertzen, C. A., & Hooks, N. T., Jr. (1969). Changes in personality (MMPI) and subjective experience (ARCI) throughout a cycle of addiction to morphine. Journal of Nervous and Mental Disease, 148, 606-614.

Haertzen, C. A., & Hooks, N. T., Jr. (1971). Contrast effects from simulation or subjective experiences: A possible standard for behavioral modification. British Journal of Addiction, 66, 225-227.

Haertzen, C. A., & Hooks, N. T., Jr. (1973). Dictionary of drug associations to heroin, Benzedrine, alcohol, barbiturates, and marijuana. Journal of Clinical Psychology, 29, 115-164.

Haertzen, C. A., Hooks, N. T., Jr., & Hill, H. E. (1966, December). Prediction of subjective responses to drugs. Proceedings of the American College of Neuropsychopharmacology, San Juan, Puerto Rico.

Haertzen, C. A., Hooks, N. T., Jr., & Pross, M. (1974). Drug associations as a measure of habit strength for specific drugs. Journal of Nervous and Mental Disease, 158, 189-197.

Haertzen, C. A., Long, R., & Philip, P. (1964, November). A survey of mental hospital patients on the Addiction Research Center Inventory (ARCI): A comparison of post addicts and mental patients. Paper presented at the meeting of the Kentucky Psychological Association, Louisville, KY.

Haertzen, C. A., Martin, W. R., Hewett, B. B., & Sandquist, V. (1978). Measurement of psychopathy as a state. Journal of Psychology, 100, 201-214.

Haertzen, C. A., Martin, W. R., Ross, F. E., & Neidert, G. L. (1980). Psychopathic State Inventory (PSI): Development of a short test for measuring psychopathic states. International Journal of the Addictions, 15, 137-146.

Haertzen, C. A., & Meketon, M. J. (1968). Opiate withdrawal as measured by the Addiction Research Center Inventory (ARCI). Diseases of the Nervous System, 29, 450-455.

Haertzen, C. A., Meketon, M. J., & Hooks, N. T., Jr. (1970). Subjective experiences produced by the withdrawal of opiates. British Journal of Addiction, 65, 245-255.

Haertzen, C. A., & Miner, E. J. (1965). Effect of alcohol on the Guilford-Zimmerman scales of extraversion. Journal of Personality and Social Psychology, 1, 333-336.

Haertzen, C. A., & Panton, J. (1967). Development of a "psychopathic" scale for the Addiction Research Center Inventory (ARCI). International Journal of the Addictions, 2, 115-127.

Haertzen, C. A., Fuller, G., Hooks, N. T., Jr., Monroe, J. J., & Sharp, H. (1968). Nonsignificance of membership in Alcoholics Anonymous in hospitalized alcoholics. Journal of Clinical Psychology, 24, 99-103.

Haertzen, C. A., Hill, H. E., Wikler, A., & Wolbach, A. B. (1961). Evaluating subjective effects of six drugs by means of an especially designed inventory. Paper presented at the meeting of the Midwestern Psychological Association, Chicago.

Hathaway, S. R., & McKinley, J. C. (1951). Minnesota Multiphasic Personality Inventory manual (Rev. Ed.). New York: Psychological Corporation.

Henningfield, J. E., Chait, L. D., & Griffiths, R. R. (1983). Cigarette smoking and subjective response in alcoholics: Effects of pentobarbital. Clinical Pharmacology and Therapeutics, 33, 806-812.

Henningfield, J. E., Chait, L. D., & Griffiths, R. R. (1984). Effects of ethanol on cigarette smoking by volunteers without histories of alcoholism. Psychopharmacologia, 82, 1-5.

Henningfield, J. E., & Griffiths, R. R. (1981). Cigarette smoking and subjective response: Effects of d-amphetamine. Clinical Pharmacology and Therapeutics, 30, 497-505.

Hill, H. E., Haertzen, C. A., & Belleville, R. E. (1958). The Addiction Research Center Inventory (ARCI) Test Booklet. Lexington, KY: NIMH Addiction Research Center.

Hill, H. E., Haertzen, C. S., & Glaser, R. (1960). Personality characteristics of of narcotic addicts as indicated by the MMPI. Journal of General Psychology, 62, 127-139.

Hill, H. E., Haertzen, C. A., Wolbach, A. B., & Miner, E. J. (1963a). The Addiction Research Center Inventory: Appendix I. Items comprising empirical scales for seven drugs. II. Items which do not differentiate placebo from any drug condition. Psychopharmacologia, 4, 184-205.

Hill, H. E., Haertzen, C. A., Wolbach, A. B., & Miner, E. J. (1963b). The Addiction Research Center Inventory: Standardization of scales which evaluate subjective effects of morphine, amphetamine, pentobarbital, alcohol, LSD-25, pyrahexyl and chlorpromazine. Psychopharmacologia, 4, 167-183.

Himmelsbach, C. K. (1941). The morphine abstinence syndrome, its nature and treatment. Annals of Internal Medicine, 15, 829-839.

Hoch, P. E., & Solomon, G. (1952). Experimental induction of psychosis. In P. B. Cobb (Ed.), The biology of mental health and disease (pp. 539-547). New York: Harper & Brothers.

Hollister, L. E., & Gillespie, H. K. (1973). Delta-8- and delta-9-tetrahydrocannabinol: Comparison in man by oral and intravenous administration. Clinical Pharmacology and Therapeutics, 14, 353-357.

Hollister, L. E., & Gillespie, H. K. (1975). Action of delta-9-tetrahydrocannabinol. Clinical Pharmacology and Therapeutics, 18, 714-719.

Hollister, L. E., Overall, J. E., & Gerber, M. L. (1975). Marijuana and setting. Archives of General Psychiatry, 32, 798-801.

Isbell, H. (1956). Attempted addiction to nalorphine. Federation Proceedings, 1, 442.

Isbell, H., Belleville, R. E., Fraser, H. F., Wikler, A. & Logan, C. R. (1956). Studies on lysergic acid diethylamide: I. Effects in former morphine addicts and development of tolerance during chronic intoxication. Archives of Neurology and Psychiatry, 76, 468-478.

Isbell, H., Fraser, H. F., Wikler, A., Belleville, R. E., & Eisenman, A. J. (1955). An experimental study of the etiology of "rum fits" and delirium tremens. Quarterly Journal Studies Alcohol, 16, 1-33.

Isbell, H., Gorodetzky, C. W., Jasinski, D. R., Claussen, U., Spulak, F. V., & Korte, F. (1967). Effects of (-)-Δ^9-Transtetrahydrocannabinol in man. Psychopharmacologia, 11, 184-188.

Isbell, H., & Jasinski, D. R. (1969). A comparison of LSD-25 with (-)-Δ^9-Transtetrahydrocannabinol (THC) and attempted cross tolerance between LSD and THC. Psychopharmacologia, 14, 115-123.

Jaffe, J. H., Kanzler, M., & Green, J. (1981). Abuse potential of loperamide: Adaptation of established evaluative methods to volunteer subjects. In L. S. Harris (Ed.), Problems of Drug Dependence, 1980 (National Institute on Drug Abuse Research Monograph 34, pp. 232-240). Washington, DC: U.S. Government Printing Office.

Jaffe, J. H., Schuster, C. R., Smith, C. R., & Blachley, P. H. (1970). Comparison of acetylmethadol and methadone in the treatment of long-term users. Journal of the American Medical Association, 211, 1834-1836.

Jasinski, D. R. (1973). Assessment of the dependence liability of opiates and sedative hypnotics. In L. Goldberg & F. Hoffmeister (Eds.), Bayer-Symposium IV-Psychic Dependence (pp. 160-170). New York: Springer-Verlag.

Jasinski, D. R. (1974). Narcotic antagonists as analgesics of low dependence liability-theoretical and practical implications of recent studies. In Yearbook of drug abuse (pp. 37-48). New York: Behavioral Publications.

Jasinski, D. R. (1977). Assessment of the abuse potentiality of morphine like drugs (methods used in man). In W. R. Martin (Ed.), Drug addiction I: Morphine, sedative/hypnotic and alcohol dependence (pp. 197-258). New York: Springer-Verlag.

Jasinski, D. R. (1982). Buprenorphine as a pharmacologic treatment modality for narcotic addicts. Presented in a symposium on buprenorphine held by the American Society for Pharmacology and Experimental Therapeutics, Louisville, Kentucky, August 1982. The Pharmacologist, 24, 89.

Jasinski, D. R., Carr, C. B., & Griffith, J. D. (1975). Etorphine in man. 1. Subjective effects and suppression of morphine abstinence. Clinical Pharmacology and Therapeutics, 17, 267-272.

Jasinski, D. R., Carr, C. B., Gorodetzky, C. W., Griffith, J. D., & Kullberg, M. P. (1974). Progress report from the clinical pharmacology section of the Addiction Research Center. Committee on problems of Drug Dependence, 88-115. Springfield, VA: National Technical Information Service.

Jasinski, D. R., Haertzen, C. A., Henningfield, J. E., Johnson, R. E., Makhzoumi, H. M., & Miyasato, K. (1982). Progress Report of the NIDA Addiction Research Center. In L. S. Harris (Ed.), Problems of drug dependence, 1981 (National Institute on Drug Abuse Research Monograph 41, pp. 45-52). Washington, DC: U.S. Government Printing Office.

Jasinski, D. R., Haertzen, C. A., & Isbell, H. (1971). Review of the effects in man of marijuana and tetrahydrocannabinols on subjective state and physiologic functioning. Annals of the New York Academy of Sciences, 191, 196-205.

Jasinski, D. R., Henningfield, J. E., Hickey, J. E., & Johnson, R. E. (1983). Progress report of the National Institute on Drug Abuse Addiction Research Center, 1982. In L. S. Harris (Ed.), Problems of drug dependence, 1982. (National Institute on Drug Abuse Research Monograph 43, pp. 92-98). Washington, DC: U.S. Government Printing Office.

Jasinski, D. R., & Johnson, R. E. Abuse potential of chlordiazepoxide. The Pharmacologist, 132, 24, 133.

Jasinski, D. R., & Mansky, P. A. (1972). Evaluation of nalbuphine for abuse potential. Clinical Pharmacology and Therapeutics, 13, 78-90.

Jasinski, D. R., Martin, W. R., & Haertzen, C. A. (1967). The human pharmacology and abuse potential of N-allylnoroxymorphone (naloxone). Journal of Pharmacology and Experimental Therapeutics, 157, 420-426.

Jasinski, D. R., Martin, W. R., Hoeldtke, R. D. (1970). Effects of short- and long-term administration of pentazocine in man. Clinical Pharmacology and Therapeutics, 11, 385-403.

Jasinski, D. R., Martin, W. R., & Hoeldtke, R. D. (1971). Studies of the dependence-producing properties of GPA-1657, profadol, and propiram in man. Clinical Pharmacology and Therapeutics, 12, 613-649.

Jasinski, D. R., Martin, W. R., & Sapira, J. D. (1968a). Antagonism of the subjective, behavioral, pupillary, and respiratory depressant effects of cyclazocine by naloxone. Clinical Pharmacology and Therapeutics, 9, 215-222.

Jasinski, D. R., Martin, W. R., & Sapira, J. D. (1968b). Progress report on the dependence-producing properties of GPA-1657, profadol hydrochloride (CI-572), propiram fumarate (Bay-4503) and dexoxadral. Paper presented at 30th meeting, Committee on Problems of Drug Dependence, Indianapolis.

Jasinski, D. R., Nutt, J. G., & Griffith, J. D. (1974). Effects of diethylpropion and d-amphetamine after subcutaneous and oral administration. Clinical Pharmacology and Therapeutics, 16, 645-652.

Jasinski, D. R., Nutt, J. G., Haertzen, C. A., Griffith, J. D., & Bunney, W. E. (1977). Lithium: Effects on subjective functioning and morphine-induced euphoria. Science, 195, 582-584.

Jasinski, D. R., Clark, S. C., Griffith, J. D., & Pevnick, J. S. (1977). Therapeutic usefulness of propoxyphene napsylate in narcotic addiction. Archives of General Psychiatry, 34, 227-233.

Jasinski, D. R., Pevnick, J. S., & Griffith, J. D. (1978). Human pharmacology and abuse potential of the analgesic buprenorphine. Archives of General Psychiatry, 35, 501-516.

Johnson, R. E., & Jasinski, D. R. (1982). Abuse potential of zomepirac. Paper presented at American Society for Pharmacology and Experimental Therapeutics, Louisville, KY.

Johnson, R. E., Jasinski, D. R., & Kocher, T. R. (1983). Abuse potential of zomepirac (Zomac)R. Journal of Clinical Pharmacology and Therapeutics, 34, 386-389.

Kay, D. C. (1980). The search for psychopathic states in alcoholics and other drug abusers. In W. E. Fenn (Ed.), Phenomenology and treatment of alcoholism, (pp. 269-304). Jamaica, NY: Spectrum Publications.

Kiplinger, G. F., Manno, J. E., Rodda, B. E., & Forney, R. B. (1971). Dose-response analysis of the effects of tetrahydrocannabinol in man. Clinical Pharmacology and Therapeutics, 12, 650-657.

Kleber, H. D., Gold, M. S., & Riordan, C. E. (1980). The use of clonidine in detoxification from opiates. Bulletin on Narcotics, 32, 1-10.

Kolb, L. (1925). Pleasure and deterioration from narcotic addiction. Mental Hygiene, 9, 699-724.

Manno, J. L. (1970). Clinical investigations with marihuana and alcohol. unpublished doctoral dissertation, University of Indiana.

Martin, W. R. (1966). Assessment of the dependence producing potentiality of narcotic analgesics. In C. Radouco-Thomas & L. Lasagna (Eds.), International encyclopedia of pharmacology and therapeutics (Vol. 1, pp. 155-180). Glasgow: Pergamon Press.

Martin, W. R. (1967). Clinical evaluation for narcotic dependence. In New Concepts in pain and its clinical management. Philadelphia: F. A. Davis.

Martin, W. R. (1973). Assessment of the abuse-potentiality of amphetamines and LSD-like hallucinogens in man and its relationship to basic animal assessment programs. In L. Goldberg & F. Hoffmeister (Eds.), Bayer-Symposium IV, psychic dependence (pp. 146-155). New York: Springer-Verlag.

Martin, W. R. (1974). Drug abuse--the need for a rational pharmacologic approach. In Yearbook of drug abuse (pp. 1-15). New York: Behavioral Publications.

Martin, W. R., & Fraser, H. F. (1961). A comparative study of physiological and subjective effects of heroin and morphine administered intravenously in postaddicts. Journal of Pharmacology and Experimental Therapeutics, 133, 388-399.

Martin, W. R., Fraser, H. F., Gorodetzky, C. W., & Rosenberg, D. E. (1965). Studies of the dependence-producing potential of the narcotic antagonist 2-cyclopropylmethyl-2'hydroxy-5, 9-dimethyl-6, 7-benzomorphan (cyclazocine, WIN-20, 740, ARC II-C-3. Journal of Pharmacology and Experimental Therapeutics, 15, 426-436.

Martin, W. R., Hewett, B. B., Baker, A. J., & Haertzen, C. A. (1977). Aspects of the psychopathology and pathophysiology of addiction. Drug and Alcohol Dependence, 2, 185-202.

Martin, W. R., Jasinski, D. R., Haertzen, C. A., Kay, D. C., Jones, B. E., Mansky, P. A., & Carpenter, R. W. (1973a). Methadone--a reevaluation. Archives of General Psychiatry, 28, 286-295.

Martin, W. R., Jasinski, D. R., & Mansky, P. A. (1973b). Naltrexone, an antagonist for the treatment of heroin dependence. Archives of General Psychiatry, 28, 784-791.

Martin, W. R., & Sloan, J. W. (1977). Pharmacology and classification of LSD-like hallucinogens. In W. R. Martin (Ed.), Drug addiction II (pp. 305-368). New York: Springer-Verlag.

Martin, W. R., Sloan, J. W., Sapira, J. D., & Jasinski, D. R. (1971). Physiologic, subjective and behavioral effects of amphetamine, methamphetamine, ephedrine, phenmetrazine, and methylphenidate in man. Clinical Pharmacology and Therapeutics, 12, 245-258.

McCaul, M. E., Stitzer, M. L., Bigelow, G. E., & Liebson, I. A. (1981). Acute effects of oral methadone in methadone maintenance subjects. Paper presented at the American Psychological Association Convention held in Los Angeles, CA.

McCaul, M. E., Stitzer, M. L., Bigelow, G. E., & Liebson, I. A. (1982). Physiological and subjective effects of hydromorphone in postaddict volunteers. In L. S. Harris (Ed.), Problems of drug dependence, 1981 (National Institute on Drug Abuse Research Monograph 41, pp. 301-308). Washington, DC: U.S. Government Printing Office.

McCaul, M. E., Stitzer, M. L., Bigelow, G. E., & Liebson, I. A. (1983). Intravenous hydromorphone: Effects in opiate-free and methadone maintenance subjects. In L. S. Harris (Ed.), Problems of drug dependence, 1982 (National Institute on Drug Abuse Research Monograph 43, pp. 238-244). Washington, DC: U.S. Government Printing Office.

McClane, T. K., & Martin, W. R. (1976). Subjective and physiologic effects of morphine, pentobarbital, and meprobamate. Clinical Pharmacology and Therapeutics, 20, 192-198.

McLeod, D. R., Bigelow, G. E., & Liebson, I. A. (1982). Self-regulated opioid detoxification by humans: Effects of methadone pretreatment. In L. S. Harris (Ed.), Problems of drug dependence, 1981 (National Institute on Drug Abuse Research Monograph 41, pp. 232-238). Washington, DC: U.S. Government Printing Office.

McNair, D. M., Lorr, M., & Droppelman, L. F. (1971). EITS Manual for the profile of mood states. San Diego, CA: Educational and Industrial Testing Service.

Meketon, M. J. (1967). Exploring motivation within a total institution for drug addicts. Unpublished doctoral dissertation, University of Kentucky.

Meketon, M. J., & Perea, E. (1967). Partial Spanish translation of the Addiction Research Center Inventory. Lexington, KY.

Meyer, R. E., Altman, J. L., McNamee, B., & Mirin, S. M. (1976). A behavioral paradigm for the evaluation of narcotic antagonists. Archives of General Psychiatry, 33, 371-377.

Miller, L., & Griffith, J. (1983). A Comparison of bupropion, dextroamphetamine, and placebo in mixed-substance abusers. Psychopharmacology, 80, 199-205.

Nakano, S., Gillespie, H. K., Hollister, L. E. (1978). A model for evaluation of antianxiety drugs with the use of experimentally induced stress: Comparison of nabilone and diazepam. Clinical Pharmacology and Therapeutics, 23, 54-62.

Nowlis, V., & Nowlis, H. H. (1956). Description and analysis of mood. Annals of the New York Academy of Science, 65, 345-355.

Nutt, J. G., & Jasinski, D. R. (1974). Methadone-naloxone mixtures for use in methadone maintenance programs: I. An evaluation in man of their pharmacological feasibility; II. Demonstration of acute physical dependence. Clinical Pharmacology and Therapeutics, 15, 156-166.

O'Brien, C. P., & Minn, F. L. (1980). Evaluation of withdrawal symptoms following zomepirac administration. Journal of Clinical Pharmacology, 20, 397-400.

Orzack, M. H., Cole, J. L., Ionescu-Pioggia, Beake, B. J., Bird, M. P., Lobel, M., & Martin, M. D. (1982). A comparison of some subjective effects of prazepam, diazepam and placebo. In L. S. Harris (Ed.), Problems of drug dependence, 1981 (National Institute on Drug Abuse Research Monograph 41, pp. 309-317). Washington, DC: U.S. Government Printing Office.

Ottomanelli, G. A. (1973). The MMPI as a predictor of outcome in a methadone maintenance program. Unpublished doctoral dissertation, School of Education, New York University.

Ottomanelli, G. A. (1977). MMPI and Pyp prediction compared to base rate prediction of six-month behavioral outcome for methadone patients. British Journal of Addictions, 72, 177-186.

Ottomanelli, G. A. (1978). Patient improvement, measured by the MMPI and Pyp, related to paraprofessional and professional counselor assignment. International Journal of the Addictions, 13, 503-507.

Ottomanelli, G. A., & Halloran, G. (1982). Patient expectations and participation in a polydrug treatment program: A replicated field study. International Journal of the Addictions, 17, 1289-1311.

Overton, D. A., & Batta, S. K. (1979). Investigation of narcotics and antitussives using drug discrimination techniques. Journal of Pharmacology and Experimental Therapeutics, 211, 401-408.

Pevnick, J. S. (1981). Abuse of pentazocine (P) combined with tripelennamine (T): An interaction of psychopharmacological and societal factors. Federation of American Societies of Experimental Biology.

Pevnick, J. S., Haertzen, C. A., & Jasinski, D. R. (1978). Abrupt withdrawal from therapeutically administered diazepam. Archives of General Psychiatry, 35, 995-998.

Pichot, P. (1964). French Translation of the Addiction Research Center Inventory. NIMH Addiction Research Center. Can be obtained from Dr. Pichot at Hospital Sainte Anne, 1 Rue Canabnis, Paris (14) France.

Platt, J. J., & Labate, C. (1976). Heroin addiction theory, research and treatment. [Note: The book contains a review of the ARCI on pp. 331-336.] New York: John Wiley & Sons.

Resnick, R. B., Kestenbaum, R. S., & Schwartz, L. K. (1977). Acute systemic effects of cocaine in man: A controlled study by intranasal and intravenous routes. Science, 195, 696-698.

Rosenberg, D. E., Isbell, H., & Miner, E. J. (1963). Comparison of a placebo, N-dimethyltryptamine, and 6-hydroxy-N-dimethyltryptamine in man. Psychopharmacologia, 4, 39-42.

Rosenberg, D. E., Isbell, H., Logan, C. R., & Miner, E. J. (1964). The effect of N, N-dimethyltryptamine in human subjects tolerant to lysergic acid diethylamide. Psychopharmacologia, 5, 217-227.

Rosenberg, D. E., Wolbach, A. B., Miner, E. J., & Isbell, H. (1963). Observations on direct and cross tolerance with LSD and d-amphetamine in man. Psychopharmacologia, 5, 1-15.

Savage, C. (1955). Variations in ego feeling induced by d-lysergic acid diethylamide (LSD-25). Psychoanalytic Review, 42, 1-16.

Schuster, C. R., Fischman, M. W., & Johanson, C. E. (1981). Internal stimulus control and subjective effects of drugs. In T. Thompson, & C. E. Johanson (Eds.), Behavioral pharmacology of human drug dependence. (National Institute on Drug Abuse Research Monograph 37, pp. 116-129). Washington, DC: U.S. Government Printing Office.

Shannon, H. E., & Holtzman, S. G. (1976). Evaluation of the discriminative effects of morphine in the rat. Journal of Pharmacology and Experimental Therapeutics, 198, 54-65.

Sharp, H., Fuller, G. B., & Haertzen, C. A. (1967). Acute alcohol withdrawal scales on the Addiction Research Center Inventory. Current Conclusions, July 11, 1-13.

Sice, J., Levin, J. J., Levine, H. D., & Haertzen, C. A. (1975). Effects of personal interactions and setting on subjective drug responses in small groups. Psychopharmacologia, 43, 181-186.

Sideroff, S. I., & Jarvik, M. E. (1980). Conditioned responses to a videotape showing heroin-related stimuli. International Journal of the Addictions, 15, 529-536.

Sjoberg, L. (1969a). Alcohol and gambling. Psychopharmacologia, 14, 284-298.

Sjoberg, L. (1969b). A Swedish translation of the ARCI alcohol scale. Obtainable from L. Sjoberg, Universitetet i Stockholm, Drottninggatan 95 A, Stockholm VA Sweden.

Stitzer, M., Bigelow, G. E., & Liebson, I. A. (1981). Granting dose increases to methadone maintenance patients: Effects on symptomatology and drug use. In L. S. Harris (Ed.), Problems of drug dependence, 1980 (National Institute on Drug Abuse Research Monograph 34, pp. 387-393). Washington, DC: U.S. Government Printing Office.

Stitzer, M. L., Bigelow, G. E., & Liebson, I. A. (1982). Comparison of three outpatient methadone detoxification procedures. In L. S. Harris (Ed.), Problems of drug dependence, 1981 (National Institute on Drug Abuse Research Monograph 41, pp. 239-245). Washington, DC: U.S. Government Printing Office.

Stitzer, M. L., Griffiths, R. R., Bigelow, G. E., & Liebson, I. A. (1981). Human social conversation: Effects of ethanol, secobarbital and chlorpromazine. Pharmacology Biochemistry & Behavior, 14, 353-360.

Teasdale, J. D. (1973). Conditioned abstinence in narcotic addicts. International Journal of the Addictions, 8, 273-292.

Ternes, J. W., O'Brien, C. P., Grabowski, J., Wellerstein, H., & Jordan-Hayes, J., (1979). Conditioned drug responses to naturalistic stimuli. In L. S. Harris (Ed.), Problems of drug dependence, 1979 (National Institute on Drug Abuse Research Monograph 27, pp. 282-288). Washington, DC: U.S. Government Printing Office.

Thorndike, E. L., & Lorge, I. (1944). The teacher's workbook of 30,000 words. New York: Bureau of Publications, Teacher's College, Columbia University.

Toyama, P., & Heyder, C. (1981). Acupuncture induced mood changes reversed by the narcotic antagonist naloxone. Journal of Holistic Medicine, 3, 46-52.

Toyama, P. M., Popell, C., Evans, J., & Heyder, C. (1980). Acupuncture and moxibustion in the management of rheumatoid arthritis. Stress, 1, 19-24.

Uhlenhuth, E. H., Johanson, C. E., Kilgore, K., & Kobasa, S. C. (1981). Drug preference and mood in humans: Preference for d-amphetamine and subject characteristics. Psychopharmacology, 74, 191-194.

Van Dyke, C., Jatlow, P., Ungerer, J., Barash, P. G., & Byck, R. (1978). Oral cocaine: Plasma concentration and central effects. Science, 200, 211-213.

Watkins, D. C. (1972). The effects of hypnotic suggestions on the alcohol withdrawal syndrome. Unpublished doctoral dissertation, Temple University.

Wikler, A. (1964). Survey of research on alcohol at the National Institute of Mental Health, Addiction Research Center, In Proceedings of the 26th International Congress on alcohol and alcoholism, Stockholm, 1960. Stockholm: Swedish Congress Committee by Eklunds and Vasatryck.

Yanagita, T. Japanese Translation of selected ARCI Scales.

Yanagita, T., Inanaga, K., Kato, N., & Ueyama, M. (1980). Subjective effects of Afloqualone (HQ-495), a muscle relaxant, in healthy volunteers -- A measure of psychological dependence-producing properties of drugs. Japanese Journal of Clinical Pharmacology and Therapeutics, 11, 181-195.

Appendix

Items From Addiction Research Center Inventory Short Form (List 116)

Scale 1 OW: Opiate Withdrawal [ARCI Scale #459]

TRUE

ARCI	List 116	
599	1	I have sneezing spells
590	3	I feel cold all over
79	15	My face feels hot
578	16	I feel as if I have the flu
378	20	Something is making me break out in goose pimples
111	28	Some parts of my body ache
479	29	My eyes are watering more than usual
29	38	I am unusually restless
552	45	I have been getting cramps
582	49	My nose has been running
566	51	I have lost weight within the last week
592	55	I have spells of shaking and trembling
9	61	I feel weak
584	66	I have not been keeping up with my personal appearance
289	67	My mouth is watering more than usual
571	68	I feel physically ill
511	70	I feel like yawning
182	71	I feel so miserable that other people must be aware of it
424	73	I feel as if I had taken a laxative
591	80	I have been feeling some pain in my muscles or joints
573	88	My skin feels damp and clammy

FALSE

491	27	I am sure I will sleep well tonight

Scale 2 MBG: Morphine-Benzedrine Group [ARCI #463]

TRUE

ARCI	List 116	
396	2	I would be happy all the time if I felt as I feel now
98	12	I am in the mood to talk about the feeling I have
384	19	I am full of energy
319	21	I would be happy all the time if I felt as I do now
325	26	Things around me seem more pleasing than usual
102	33	I feel less discouraged than usual
218	34	I fear that I will lose the contentment that I have now
91	41	I feel as if something pleasant just happened to me
77	44	Today I say things in the easiest possible way
345	57	I feel so good that I know other people can tell it
190	60	I feel more clear-headed than dreamy

168	63	I can completely appreciate what others are saying when I am in this mood
3	72	I feel as if I would be more popular with people today
279	75	I feel a very pleasant emptiness
407	78	I feel in complete harmony with the world and those about me
2	92	I have a pleasant feeling in my stomach
614 of SQ9	94*	I feel high (Note: This scale [ARCI #463] is exactly like ARCIScale #453 with the exception that #463 contains SQ9 item #614.)

*"I feel high" is probably a good euphoria item, but it also should be a more general drug effect item.

Scale 3 MG: Morphine Group [ARCI #460]

TRUE

ARCI   List 116

457	17	My nose itches
603 of SQ9	30	I have been scratching myself
604 of SQ9	37	I have had some pins and needles sensations
21	42	I have a sentimental feeling
443	48	I would like to sit and think
92	79	I have a peculiar craving for ice cream or something cold
541	86	My speech is not as loud as usual
611 of SQ9	90	I have been dozing occasionally for seconds or minutes

Scale 4 Ex: Excitement [ARCI #461]

TRUE

ARCI   List 116

354	10	I feel like joking with someone
484	13	I notice that my heart is beating faster
278	18	Some parts of my body are tingling
602 of SQ9	22	I feel more excited than sluggish
265	46	A thrill has gone through me one or more times since I started the test
429	54	I feel more excited than dreamy
376	64	My hands feel light
401	69	My head feels light
504	74	I feel now as I have felt after a very exciting experience
499	85	I feel an increasing awareness of bodily sensations

FALSE

605 of SQ9	52	I feel more dreamy than lively

Scale 5   LSD: LSD Drug Correction [ARCI #454]

TRUE

ARCI	List 116	
209	4	My hands feel clumsy
267	8	I have a weird feeling
390	11	I have an unusual weakness of my muscles
278	18	Some parts of my body are tingling
201	23	I feel anxious and upset
160	36	I have a disturbance in my stomach
265	46	A thrill has gone through me one or more times since I started the test
96	62	I notice my hand shakes when I try to write
499	85	I feel an increasing awareness of my bodily sensations
164	89	It seems I'm spending longer than I should on each of these questions

FALSE

30	14	My movements are free, relaxed, and pleasurable
319	21	I would be happy all the time if I felt as I do now
72	40	I feel very patient
66	83	I feel drowsy

Scale 6   PCAG: Pentobarbital, Chlorpromazine, Alcohol Group [ARCI #452]

TRUE

ARCI	List 116	
452	7	I feel dizzy
54	32	I feel like avoiding people, although I usually do not feel this way
475	35	My speech is slurred
219	47	I have a feeling of just dragging along rather than coasting
463	50	People might say that I am a little dull today
76	56	My head feels heavy
11	58	I am not as active as usual
86	82	It seems harder than usual to move around
66	83	I feel drowsy
513	84	I am moody
166	87	I feel sluggish

FALSE

384	19	I am full of energy
265	46	A thrill has gone through me one or more times since I started the test
429	54	I feel more excited than dreamy
190	60	I feel more clear-headed than dreamy

Scale 7 Dr: Drunk [ARCI #462]

TRUE

ARCI   List 116

330		5	I can hardly control my speech
601	of SQ9	6	When I stand up, I feel unsteady
452		7	I feel dizzy
613		25	Big words seem harder to pronounce
478		24	My mind can be described as slow rather than blank
462		31	I have a high feeling which is similar to that produced by alcohol
475		35	My speech is slurred
76		56	My head feels heavy
528		59	My head feels as it does during a hangover
607	of SQ9	65	My handwriting is not as easy to read as usual
401		69	My head feels light
608	of SQ9	76	My hands seem somewhat clumsy
609	of SQ9	77	I would have some difficulty threading a needle
610	of SQ9	81	It is somewhat harder to walk in a straight line
612	of SQ9	91	I feel drunk

FALSE

257		9	I would have no trouble walking a chalk line
10		39	I believe I could stay awake all night driving a car
81		43	I seem to be very much aware of the little things that people do
606	of SQ9	53	My sense of balance is very good
190		60	I feel more clear-headed than dreamy
283		93	My movements seem no faster than usual

CHAPTER 25

OPERANT ANALYSIS OF HUMAN DRUG SELF-ADMINISTRATION: MARIHUANA, ALCOHOL, HEROIN AND POLYDRUG USE

Nancy K. Mello and Jack H. Mendelson

Harvard Medical School - McLean Hospital
115 Mill Street
Belmont, Massachusetts 02178

ABSTRACT

The evolution of operant procedures to study human drug self-administration in clinical research ward settings is described. The advantages and limitations of several techniques developed between 1965 and 1984 are discussed. Illustrative data from studies of alcohol, marihuana, heroin, and polydrug self-administration are summarized. The advantages of objective operant behavioral measures of drug acquisition, in contrast to anecdotal or retrospective reports, for evaluating new pharmacotherapies for the treatment of drug abuse are described. The importance of direct observation of drug use patterns and drug effects on behavioral and biological variables under controlled clinical research ward conditions is emphasized.

INTRODUCTION

Although the examination of drug self-administration patterns in human subjects is a relatively recent development, the value of this approach for the study of substance abuse has now been amply demonstrated in many laboratories. Advances in techniques for the analysis of behavior have been paralleled by an expansion of and refinement in the type of questions asked. This review will discuss some dependent variables that can be studied in a human drug self-administration paradigm. These issues will be considered in the context of a quasi-historical review of some operant procedures developed in our laboratory and their advantages and limitations. Finally, selected data obtained on patterns of alcohol, heroin, marihuana, and multiple-drug self-administration will be described.

DEPENDENT VARIABLES IN HUMAN DRUG SELF-ADMINISTRATION

Since 1965, we have studied the self-administration of a number of abused drugs in human volunteers with a history of drug use or addiction (Mello & Mendelson, 1965). Multidisciplinary studies have been conducted on an inpatient clinical research ward, and each subject has been observed before, during, and after a period of self-regulated drug intoxication. Drug self-administration was observed over several days or weeks. This approach permits study of an encapsulated sequence of the basic behavioral disorder, drug abuse, under clinical research ward conditions.

Our objective has been to study natural or relatively unconstrained drug use patterns and to correlate these with a number of biological and behavioral variables. We have attempted to devise situations where drug self-administration would simulate drug use patterns in the natural environment as closely as possible. Two general categories of dependent variables can be examined in such studies: drug-effect variables and patterns of drug self-administration.

Drug-Effect Variables

The pharmacological actions of drugs are defined by effects on many aspects of behavioral and biological function. Studies of physiological responses to drugs may include examination of many systems such as neuroendocrine hormones, plasma lipid levels, and sleep EEG (Mendelson, 1964, 1970; Mendelson, Kuehnle, Ellingboe, & Babor, 1974a; Mendelson & Mello, 1976, 1984a; Mendelson, Mello, & Ellingboe, 1978; Mendelson, Rossi, & Meyer, 1974b). Behavioral studies may explore drug-related changes in subjective states, perceptual and cognitive function, social interaction, and objective measures of performance (Mello & Mendelson, 1978). Another drug-effect variable is the fine-grain analysis of operant responding, including interresponse time analysis. Many other examples of drug-effect variables could be listed. However, our main point is to distinguish between drug-effect variables and patterns of drug self-administration.

Patterns of Drug Self-Administration

The pattern of drug self-administration is itself an important dependent variable which may be central to our understanding of human substance abuse. Basic and human behavioral pharmacology have repeatedly shown that the schedule of drug reinforcement--the dose and frequency of drug availability--influences the effects of drugs on behavior (Kelleher, Goldberg, & Krasnegor, 1976). By observing an individual's drug self-administration pattern, we can study the self-imposed schedule of reinforcement. However, this is only possible if the individual determines his or her own pattern of drug use.

Examination of the self-imposed pattern of drug use may assist in the identification of factors which contribute to the maintenance of drug abuse. The diversity of individuals with drug abuse problems and the fact that no single psychological, social, or biological factor appears to predict drug abuse suggest that it may be more productive to try to determine how drug abuse is maintained than to focus exclusively on etiological factors (for review, see Mello, 1983). Moreover, as we study the self-administration of different drugs under similar conditions, we hope to be able to compare use patterns across drugs. Eventually, this type of analysis should help to identify some commonalities and differences in the determinants of patterns of heroin abuse, alcohol abuse, marihuana and tobacco use, stimulant and hallucinogen abuse, et cetera. If an analysis of drug use patterns can reveal commonalities which transcend particular drug effects, such information might generalize to future forms of drug abuse as well. Although we cannot now predict the type of tomorrow's drug abuse problems, some form of substance abuse seems almost inevitable. Clarification of factors that maintain drug self-administration should facilitate the development of more effective intervention procedures.

The pattern of drug self-administration can be operationally defined by the following measures:

(1) <u>Number</u> of drug self-administration occasions
     (per hour, 'per day; per week),
(2) Drug <u>dose</u> per occasion, and
(3) <u>Interval</u> between drug self-administration occasions--
     the distribution of drug doses over a 24-hour period.

Although it could be argued that drug use also affects the subsequent pattern of drug self-administration and that this also should be classed as a drug-effect variable, we believe a distinction between drug use patterns and drug effects has both conceptual and methodological advantages.

This approach to the study of human drug self-administration and the questions posed are different from studies which attempt to manipulate human drug use patterns by varying the conditions necessary for drug acquisition. It has been demonstrated that manipulation of conditions such as response-cost, the time of drug availability, or the dose of drug available can change both the amount and frequency of drug use (Babor, Mendelson, Greenberg, & Kuehnle, 1978; Bigelow, Griffiths, & Liebson, 1976; Griffiths, Bigelow, & Liebson, 1976a; Mello, McNamee, & Mendelson, 1968; Pickens, Cunningham, Heston, Eckert, & Gustafson, 1977;). The generality of these relationships across drugs as well as between man and animal models has been repeatedly demonstrated (Griffiths, Bigelow, & Henningfield, 1980).

Since the use patterns of several drugs have been shown to be modified by manipulation of acquisition variables, these studies may have implications for social controls of drug use (e.g., hours of drug availability, taxation, price; Popham, Schmidt, & de Lint, 1975). However, the identification of common controlling variables does not suggest that the use patterns of different drugs are identical. Rather, use patterns appear to be quite different depending upon the pharmacological action and the rate of absorption and disposition of the particular drug.

Limitations of Drug Self-Administration Studies

One disadvantage of the study of spontaneous drug self-administration patterns is that precise time-dose-response relationships between the various drug-effect variables cannot be established since drug dose, frequency, and inter-dose intervals will vary on an unpredictable basis. Yet, this variability constitutes the drug self-administration pattern which is our primary dependent variable.

One alternative is to ignore drug self-administration patterns and to focus instead on drug-effect variables. The most efficient way to do this is to use a <u>programmed</u> drug administration regimen in which fixed drug doses are administered every four to six hours. This permits precise dose-time correlations with whatever drug-effect variable has been selected for study.

Programmed drug administration is the traditional method used to examine the basic pharmacological effects of drugs. The pioneering studies of drug effects conducted at the Lexington Addiction Research Center employed programmed drug administration with only one exception (Wikler, 1952). The first studies of the effects of chronic alcohol intoxication in alcoholics were conducted in a programmed administration paradigm (Mendelson, 1964).

It is evident that programmed dose paradigms are useful for asking different types of questions than drug self-administration paradigms. However, there are also other factors which may limit the utility of a programmed dosage paradigm, even for the study of drug-effect variables. When the consequences of programmed alcohol administration and spontaneous self-regulated alcohol consumption were compared in eight alcoholic subjects, it was found that biological drug-effect variables varied markedly between the two alcohol administration conditions (Mello & Mendelson, 1970). Each subject served as his own control during a 20 day spontaneous alcohol administration paradigm and 20 days of programmed alcohol administration. Programmed alcohol administration was associated with greater toxicity (e.g., gastritis, vomiting) during intoxication than spontaneous drinking. Subjects were able to tolerate higher doses of alcohol during the spontaneous self-administration paradigm and distributed alcohol consumption to achieve higher peak blood alcohol levels than were measured during programmed alcohol administration. The severity of alcohol withdrawal signs and symptoms after cessation of drinking was markedly greater after spontaneous drinking than after programmed alcohol administration, even in those subjects who drank equivalent quantities of alcohol in each condition.

We concluded that the pattern of drinking was more critical than the duration of drinking as a determinant of biological reactions to alcohol intoxication and withdrawal. These data seemed to justify our pursuit of self-determined patterns of drug self-administration both as a primary dependent variable and as the most sensitive and reality-concordant baseline against which to correlate biological as well as behavioral drug-effect variables.

TECHNIQUES TO STUDY HUMAN DRUG SELF-ADMINISTRATION

Operant techniques to study human drug self-administration have developed in parallel with those used in basic behavioral pharmacology and are derived from concepts and procedures for the experimental analysis of behavior (Skinner, 1938, 1953). Operant procedures have been shown to produce orderly sequences of responding which provide an objective index of the relative reinforcing consequences of various drugs (or competing reinforcers such as money) at any point in time. It is possible to directly observe the amount and frequency of drug self-administration and the behavioral consequences of drug intoxication without reliance upon retrospective self-reports.

Drug acquisition in real life involves engaging in a variety of behaviors, since drugs are not available without some expenditure of effort or money. Consequently, it seems realistic to require performance on an operant task to obtain drugs in a clinical research setting. The nature of the task can vary from performance on a relatively simple schedule of reinforcement to complex procedures which concurrently assess variables such as timing behavior or memory function. When we designed our first operant paradigm to study alcohol self-administration by alcoholics, we thought it necessary to use a very simple task so that subjects could perform and earn alcohol irrespective of their intoxication level (Mello & Mendelson, 1965). We anticipated that if alcohol reinforcement was made contingent upon successful performance of a complex discrimination task, the subject would not be able to sustain his initial performance as he became progressively more inebriated. Of course, this would preclude examination of behavior to acquire alcohol and would only yield data on the effects of alcohol on some aspect of perceptual or cognitive function, which was not the primary goal. Subsequently, we learned that behavioral tolerance for alcohol permits alcohol addicts to perform very complex tasks with accuracy, even when blood alcohol levels exceed 250 mg/dl (Mello, 1973).

Study of drug acquisition using operant techniques permits examination of a wide range of behavioral variables (e.g., time, duration, and pattern of operant work for the drug); the rate of operant work (assessed by both analog --cumulative recorder--measures and quantitative interresponse time measures); the time and number of drug purchases; and the effects of each successive drug use occasion on both rate and duration of operant responding. The effects of drug use on operant response patterns and choices between alternative reinforcers (e.g., marihuana vs. money or alcohol vs. marihuana) can also be examined. Such data provide direct measures of performance capacity and permit inferences about drug effects or intervening variables such as "motivation," sometimes postulated to affect performance.

Alcohol Acquisition on Multiple Schedules

There are a variety of ways to examine human drug self-administration, and the technical aspects of the behavioral procedures define and limit the type of data acquired. It may be of some historical interest to review the types of operant procedures developed in our laboratory and comment on their advantages and limitations. The first machine designed for the study of alcohol self-administration in alcoholic subjects is shown in Figure 1 (Mello & Mendelson, 1965). The subject could select whether to work for alcohol or for money reinforcement and could work at the machine at any time.

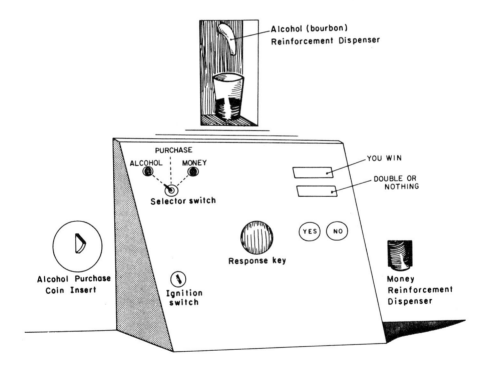

Figure 1: Operant manipulandum used to study alcohol self-administration by alcoholic subjects. Reprinted from Mello, 1972. Copyright 1972 by Plenum Press.

The subjects' task was to press the center response key which was trans-luminated with a number of colored stimulus lights associated with a series of simple schedules of reinforcement. These schedules occurred in an irregular sequence and included: fixed ratios of 60, 120, 240, 360; fixed intervals of 1, 2, and 3 minutes; extinction of one minute; and differential reinforcement of no responding. Subjects were told to press the translucent response key in order to make the key color change as often as possible, since reinforcement occurred only when the colors changed. Upon completion of the response requirement, 10 ml of bourbon or three nickels were directly dispensed, and the key color and schedule changed. The value of a single alcohol or money reinforcement was equated, and subjects could use money earned to buy alcohol. In an effort to make the task more interesting, a gambling contingency was added. When reinforcement became available, subjects could choose to take that reinforcement or to try for double-or-nothing by pressing the yes or no key at the right of the operant panel.

Subjects worked at the operant task for alcohol for 14 days. After seven days when subjects' response behavior failed to come under control of the various schedules of reinforcement, explicit verbal descriptions of the schedule requirements associated with the various colored lights were provided. Subjects still failed to respond under schedule control, except for one component--differential reinforcement of no responding. When that particular stimulus light appeared on the response key, subjects usually left the room. This behavior was adventitiously reinforced since the light associated with another schedule came on during their absence.

Rates of operant responding and time spent working at the machine were unimpaired by alcohol intoxication. Subjects maintained relatively high blood alcohol levels (200 to 300 mg/dl) throughout the period of alcohol access. Subjects usually worked for 1.5 to 2 oz of alcohol before removing the glass. Each glass removal shut off the machine for a period of 10 minutes. An immediate alcohol reinforcement was consistently preferred to money reinforcement, even though money could be used to buy an equivalent amount of alcohol at any time.

Despite the ease of working at this simple operant task, subjects complained continually about the machine. They were bored, and they did not gamble (double-or-nothing) except on rare occasions. Distaste for the machine was illustrated by the fact that one subject incorporated distorted thoughts and perceptions about the operant instrument in his hallucinatory experiences and delusional ideations during alcohol withdrawal.

Negative reactions to the task did not prevent subjects from working for alcohol. However, since response behavior did not come under control of any of the operant schedules of reinforcement provided, these data suggested that analysis of drug effects on schedule control, in the usual sense, would be very difficult in alcoholic subjects. Subsequently, we have used a simple fixed ratio or fixed interval schedule rather than multiple schedules for drug acquisition studies.

Alcohol Acquisition With Observing Response Procedures

An additional 14 subjects were studied under comparable experimental conditions over a 7-day period of alcohol availability (Mello et al., 1968). The machine shown in Figure 1 was modified so that the subjects' task was to press the response key whenever a light of 500 msec duration appeared (i.e., an observing response). The light onset occurred at irregular intervals which ranged between 2.5 and 10 seconds. Errors of omission or of commission resulted in the loss of all accumulated points. Alcohol and money acquisition were contingent upon completion of a fixed ratio of 16 (FR-16) or 32 (FR-32) consecutive responses to the signal light.

Although differences in response-cost did not change the amount of alcohol earned per session (as defined by removal of the receptacle glass), the average blood alcohol levels maintained by the FR-16 group were almost twice as high as in the FR-32 group. Subjects required to work twice as hard for alcohol tended to drink half as much. Individual blood alcohol levels were highly variable within and between days, and no subject earned all the alcohol potentially available.

Subjects complained vociferously about the demands of the operant task and pounded the machine in frustration after an omission or commission error. However, they were able to perform at all levels of intoxication, and the accuracy of performance was unrelated to blood alcohol levels. Most subjects did not work for money, and only five subjects gambled (double-or-nothing) with any consistency. The occurrence of gambling was also unrelated to blood alcohol levels. These data suggest that risk taking as defined by this task cannot be predicted on the basis of intoxication. The accuracy of performance at blood alcohol levels which averaged 200 mg/dl testifies to the behavioral tolerance for alcohol developed by alcohol addicts.

Alcohol Acquisition Using a Simulated Driving Machine

Figure 2 shows a driving machine that was developed to study group drinking behavior (Mendelson et al., 1968). The subjects' task was to steer a model automobile and keep it on the moving road on a revolving drum. Each time the auto touched a metal contact on the road, a point was registered. After 120 points were earned, 10 ml of bourbon was automatically dispensed into a common reservoir. Since the subjects could earn about 60 points per minute or 3600 points per hour, the maximum amount of alcohol that could be earned each hour was about 300 ml or 10 oz. Each subject had an ignition key and could work at the machine at any time. Each subject could also withdraw as much alcohol from the reservoir as he wished at any time by activating the ignition switch. The total time each subject worked, the number of 10 ml alcohol reinforcements earned, and the amount of alcohol each subject withdrew were automatically recorded. Subjects were permitted to work at the driving machine to earn alcohol for a period of 30 days.

Subjects took turns working at the driving machine and their ability to perform was not discernibly impaired, even at blood alcohol levels over 200 mg/dl. No subject drank continuously throughout the 30-day period, and no subject drank as much alcohol as was available. Subjects spontaneously terminated drinking episodes on several occasions; four of these occasions were correlated with stressful situations on the ward. There were seldom clearly definable events which accompanied resumption of drinking by these subjects. All subjects showed discernible increases in anxiety and agitation during intoxication and appeared far more depressed and anxious when they terminated drinking than when they initiated a subsequent drinking episode. Two subjects drank more than one fifth of bourbon per day on an average and maintained blood alcohol levels that fluctuated between 50 and 250 mg/dl. A third subject drank during three separate episodes of 8, 6, and 7 days respectively. A fourth subject became agitated, depressed, and assaultive and left the study after three days of drinking.

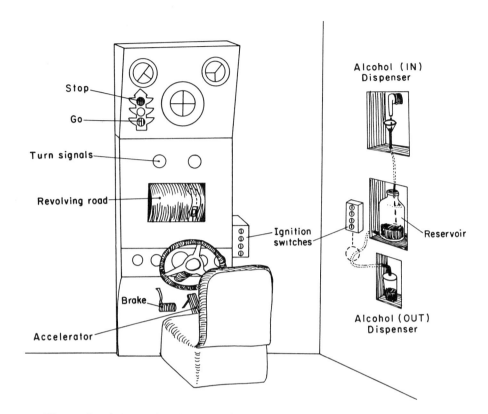

Figure 2: Schematic diagram of an operant apparatus used to study alcohol self-administration by alcoholic subjects. Each subject could activate the instrument by placing his key in the appropriate ignition switch located at the right of the revolving road. The modified driving machine had a steering wheel, brake, and accelerator which controlled the movement of a model automobile on the revolving road drum. Periodically, signals to stop, go, or turn appeared on the panel above the revolving road. Points were earned only for keeping the car on the road. Every 120 points earned resulted in 10 ml of alcohol being directly dispensed from the alcohol IN dispenser into the group reservoir. Each subject had a key to one of the four ignition switches located to the right of the reservoir. Any subject could withdraw alcohol from the group reservoir by placing his key in the ignition switch. Alcohol was dispensed into a glass underneath the OUT dispenser and would flow for as long as the ignition switch was activated. Reprinted from Mendelson, Mello, and Solomon, 1968. Copyright 1968 by Williams and Wilkins.

These subjects evolved a stable pattern of group interaction and maintained their mutually defined roles in relation to alcohol acquisition. One subject consistently removed more from the group alcohol reservoir than he contributed, and another consistently contributed more than he removed. The free-loader appeared to be the leader of the group. Another subject contributed an amount of alcohol to the group reservoir approximately equivalent to the amount that he withdrew. This machine was considerably more acceptable to the subjects than the machine shown in Figure 1. Subjects perceived the driving machine as more of a game than a performance task.

Alcohol Acquisition Using a Portable Operant Manipulandum (FR-1000)

Relocation of our laboratory to Washington prevented further studies with these instruments and necessitated the development of a non-automated, portable instrument shown in Figure 3 (Mello & Mendelson, 1972). While new automated instruments were being constructed, these simple hand-held manipulanda permitted study of operant work-contingent drinking patterns in alcoholic men. Subjects could work for alcohol or for cigarettes by depressing a button which activated a mechanical counter inside the box. Subjects could earn one ounce of alcohol or one cigarette within about 5 minutes of performance on a fixed ratio-1000 schedule of reinforcement. Points earned were exchanged for color-coded tokens each day.

Tokens could be used to buy alcohol or cigarettes directly dispensed from an apparatus shown in Figure 4. To activate the dispenser, the subject turned on an ignition switch with a coded ignition key which told the programming circuitry who was activating the dispenser and when. After the subject set a

OPERANT MANIPULANDUM

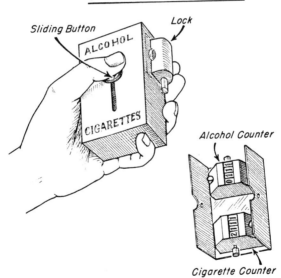

Figure 3: Operant manipulandum used to study alcohol self-administration by alcoholic subjects. Reprinted from Mello, 1972. Copyright 1972 by Plenum Press.

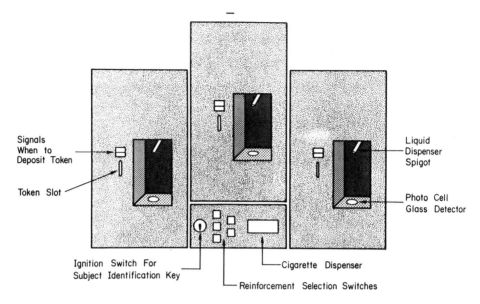

SCHEMATIC DIAGRAM OF ALCOHOL AND CIGARETTE DISPENSER PANEL

Figure 4: Schematic diagram of an alcohol and cigarette dispenser. Subjects could use poker chips earned at a simple operant task to purchase one of three types of alcohol (vodka, bourbon, or gin) or cigarettes. To activate the dispenser, the subject first turned on the ignition switch which automatically informed the circuitry of his identity and the time. He then selected which type of reinforcer he wanted and deposited a colored poker chip in the token slot when the signal light came on. A photocell had to be interrupted--by the drinking glass--before the liquid was dispensed and the signal light illuminated.

glass receptacle over the photocell, a signal light came on indicating that the dispenser would receive tokens. One ounce of alcohol was dispensed into the glass for each token deposited. The circuitry recorded the time of purchase, the number of purchases, and the subjects' identification numbers. Subjects could also buy alternative reinforcers, such as 15 minutes of television time.

The major disadvantage of the portable manipulandum was that it was not possible to analyze time, duration or rate of operant work since responses could not be recorded by the programming circuitry. However, the manipulandum proved to be tamper proof and yielded reliable data on drinking patterns, as described in a later section of this review. The manipulandum was also used to study marihuana self-administration patterns in young men (Mendelson et al., 1974b) and heroin self-administration by heroin addicts (Meyer & Mirin, 1979).

Alcohol Acquisition Using a Titrated Delayed Matching-To-Sample Task

The behavioral tolerance for alcohol shown by alcoholics in several studies persuaded us that it was possible to combine work-contingent alcohol acquisition with the assessment of drug-effect variables in addition to operant performance. Consequently, we designed and constructed an operant system that could be used to evaluate various aspects of perceptual or cognitive function. Each response panel was located in a separate operant booth, and six subjects could work simultaneously at their individual machines in relative privacy.

There has been considerable debate about whether alcohol directly affects short-term memory function. One way to evaluate this question was to use a titrated delayed matching-to-sample procedure. The operant response panel is shown in Figure 5 (Mello, 1973). The subjects' task was to select the comparison key which contained a picture identical to that which had previously appeared on the sample key. Short-term memory was defined as the interval between the offset of a picture on the sample key and the onset of pictures on four comparisons keys. Attention to the sample stimulus was insured by requiring the subject to make an observing response (FR-10) to turn on the sample stimulus. The subject then pressed the sample key until the picture projected on it went off. After a delay interval elapsed, four pictures were projected on the comparison keys. Selection of one of the comparison keys ended the trial. The length of the delay interval increased with each correct match trial and decreased with each incorrect trial in 4 second increments. The possible delay intervals ranged from 0 to 6 minutes. The matching-to-sample stimuli included pictures of the ward staff, movie stars and political figures, household objects, liquor and cigarette labels, nude figures, trigrams and abstract geometric designs—a total of 120 stimulus sets in several different sequences.

SCHEMATIC DIAGRAM OF RESPONSE PANEL

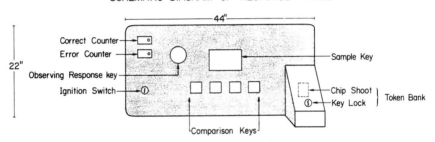

SEQUENCE OF EVENTS IN A MATCHING TO SAMPLE TRIAL

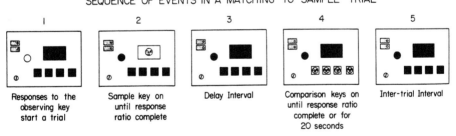

Figure 5: Apparatus used to study alcohol self-administration and the effects of alcohol on short-term memory function in alcoholic subjects. Reprinted from Mello, 1973. Copyright 1973 by Plenum Press.

In order to encourage the subject to perform as well as possible, completion of four correct trials was required to earn a single token. Correct trials were indicated on the "correct" counter at the upper left of the panel. However, if four error trials occurred before completion of four correct trials, each counter reset to zero and the subject was required to begin accumulating correct trials again in order to earn tokens to buy alcohol. After completion of four correct trials, a single token was directly dispensed into the token bank shown on the right of the operant panel. The bank was clear plastic, and the subject could see the number of tokens he had earned at any time. Each subject had the only key to his token bank and could remove tokens to purchase alcohol whenever he wished from the dispenser shown in Figure 4.

All subjects maintained high blood alcohol levels, and performance for alcohol was sustained throughout a 12-day period of alcohol access. Alcohol had no discernible effect on "short-term memory" defined operationally by the interval between sample stimulus offset and comparison stimulus onset. Subjects were able to match correctly at the longest delay intervals even when blood alcohol levels exceeded 300 mg/dl. Subjects with a history of alcoholic "blackouts" performed as well as subjects who had never experienced blackouts during intoxication. The conclusion that alcohol does not impair "short-term memory" and that the alcoholic "blackout" probably cannot be accounted for by an alcohol-specific disruption of memory (Mello, 1973) has been confirmed in other laboratories (for review, see Mello & Mendelson, 1978).

This machine was probably the most powerful tool we have developed for assessing both alcohol acquisition behavior and the effects of alcohol on cognitive function. Subjects found the task challenging and interesting, perhaps because a continuously changing array of visual stimuli was provided. Since subjects were highly motivated to acquire alcohol, they appeared to perform at the limit of their capacity. Unfortunately, a de-emphasis on intramural research by the National Institute on Alcohol Abuse and Alcoholism during the early 1970s prevented further studies with this instrument. However, this study demonstrated the feasibility of asking questions related to drug effects in combination with questions about drug self-administration patterns.

Drug Acquisition on a Second-Order Schedule of Reinforcement

After return of the laboratory to Boston in 1974, we again developed a simple hand-held operant manipulandum for the study of drug acquisition patterns. The manipulandum was about the size of a pack of cigarettes and weighed about 198 grams. The prototype manipulandum was attached to a movable cable which could be connected to coded terminals permitting subjects to work at the operant task in their individual bedrooms or in a central day room. Subsequently, the manipulandum was modified to be completely portable.

A schematic drawing of the portable manipulandum is shown in Figure 6. Each response transmits a radio frequency signal on a discrete band which activates the programming and recording circuitry in an adjacent room. Points earned are registered on a central panel, and subjects always have a record of their earnings. Unlike the portable manipulandum shown in Figure 3, operant response patterns are automatically recorded by the programming circuitry, and both rate of response and interresponse times can be measured. Each manipulandum is color coded and labeled with the subject's number to permit easy identification by the ward staff and to discourage subjects from exchanging manipulanda.

Figure 6: Portable operant manipulandum used to study heroin, marihuana, and alcohol self-administration. Each response transmits a radio frequency signal to the programming circuitry.

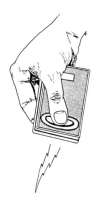

Subjects were required to press the button on the manipulandum on a fixed interval one-second schedule of reinforcement (FI-1 sec). Only the first response after one second elapsed was recorded as a point by the programming circuitry. A signal light flashed each time an effective response was made. Subjects could earn one purchase point for 300 effective responses on an FI-1 second schedule or for 5 minutes of sustained operant work. This schedule is designated as a second-order FR-300 (FI-1 sec:S).

The prices of different drugs or money reinforcers are assigned a purchase-point cost which can be adjusted to reflect the current price prevailing in the Boston area. One advantage of a time-based schedule is that price can easily be translated into time required at the operant task. Whenever a subject elects to purchase a drug, the points spent are immediately deducted from the accumulated reinforcement points. Subjects are allowed to work on the operant task at any time, and a record of their point accumulation is continuously available.

We have used this simple procedure to study alcohol, marihuana, and heroin self-administration (Mello, Mendelson, & Kuehnle, 1978, 1982; Mello, Mendelson, Kuehnle, & Sellers, 1981; Mendelson, Babor, Kuehnle, Rossi, Bernstein, Mello, & Greenberg, 1976a; Mendelson, Kuehnle, Greenberg, & Mello, 1976b, 1976c). The manipulandum and the task are well tolerated by subjects, and they have not been able to tamper with or destroy the device. Subjects are able to perform the operant task while talking, reading, watching television, and eating. Although the manipulandum can be used with any schedule of reinforcement, we have continued to employ an FI-1 second schedule to permit comparisons across successive studies with different samples of drug users.

In summary, our experience with these several operant drug-acquisition procedures suggests the following general conclusions. Subjects will accept complicated and challenging procedures which maintain their interest (e.g., Figure 5). If acquisition of a meaningful reinforcer (drugs or money) is contingent upon accurate performance, subjects will usually perform to the limit of their capacity. Severe intoxication produces surprisingly little performance impairment in alcohol addicts because of behavioral tolerance. The extent to which comparable behavioral tolerance occurs with other classes of abused drugs remains to be determined. However, it does appear feasible to study alcohol and drug self-administration patterns with a task that simultaneously assesses some drug-effect variable.

A task which requires minimal attention or effort to perform, such as the simple second-order schedule procedure we currently use, is also accepted by subjects. This task yields reliable data on drug self-administration patterns as well as rates of operant responding. The relative ease of construction and maintenance of a portable manipulandum must be balanced against the complexities of construction and maintenance of a device which involves coded filmstrips, special recording procedures, and continual adjustment as did the machine shown in Figure 5. The most realistic compromise is probably to use a simple procedure to study drug self-administration patterns and to assess cognitive and perceptual variables separately in a situation where relatively larger amounts of drug are provided as a reinforcer for accurate performance. Unfortunately, there have been very few studies in which accurate performance is reinforced with a consequence that is significant for the subject. This failure to establish contingent relationships between accuracy and reinforcers has contributed to the numerous inconsistencies in data on the behavioral effects of alcohol (for review, see Mello & Mendelson, 1978).

The importance of using a mechanical dispenser for most drug reinforcers cannot be over-emphasized. The machine is consistently neutral and cannot encourage or discourage drug purchase. Although staff can be trained to dispense drugs without comment, it is impossible to insure that some attitude about further drug use by an intoxicated individual is not conveyed. There is no way to evaluate the extent to which the attitude of a human drug-dispenser may have influenced the basic datum--drug self-administration patterns. Alcohol, marihuana and tobacco cigarettes, and any drug that can be given in capsule form can be automatically dispensed. Intravenously administered drugs, such as heroin, are an obvious exception. Staff-supervised heroin administration under limited drug availability conditions is necessary for patient safety.

PATTERNS OF ALCOHOL, MARIHUANA, POLYDRUG, AND HEROIN SELF-ADMINISTRATION

This section will summarize selected data on alcohol, marihuana, polydrug and heroin self-administration and illustrate the application of several of the techniques previously described. In each of these studies, volunteer subjects lived on a clinical research ward for several weeks. Behavioral studies were conducted simultaneously with physiological, biochemical, and neuroendocrine studies designed to examine the biological effects of chronic drug use. Subjects were observed during a drug-free baseline, a period of drug self-administration, and a post-drug baseline period. An own-control design is essential for human drug self-administration studies, since the use of "normal" control groups in the conventional sense is precluded by medical and ethical considerations. A control group consisting of "occasional drug users" is usually ill advised since such subjects are not sufficiently drug tolerant to permit meaningful comparisons with heavy users or drug addicts.

Alcohol Self-Administration

A number of stereotypic beliefs about alcoholics often appear in the clinical literature despite accumulating evidence to the contrary. One persistent belief is that the alcohol addict has a predictable and invariant drinking pattern--to drink as much as possible. This stereotype is linked to the concept of "craving," usually defined as a loss of control over drinking, with the implication that each time an alcoholic starts to drink he is compelled to continue until he reaches a state of severe intoxication. The circularity inherent in this reasoning is evident (i.e., craving is defined by the behavior it is invoked to explain). Empirical observations of alcoholics allowed to self-administer alcohol have not supported this view (for review, see Mello, 1975).

Two groups of four subjects were allowed to work for alcohol and cigarettes for periods of 30 and 62 consecutive days, respectively (Mello & Mendelson, 1972). The portable operant manipulandum shown in Figure 3 was used, and a fixed ratio of 1,000 responses was required to earn a single token which could be used to buy one cigarette or one ounce of bourbon from the automated dispenser shown in Figure 4. Subjects were able to earn one token in about 5 minutes of rapid performance or the equivalent of about 12 ounces of alcohol in an hour. The task could easily be performed while watching television, eating, drinking, or talking. Each subject had a color-coded manipulandum and an identical colored token to prevent exchanges between subjects. The volume of alcohol and the number of cigarettes purchased by each subject were recorded by the programming circuitry and checked against the number of colored tokens in the dispenser. Blood alcohol levels were measured at 8 a.m., 4 p.m., and 12 midnight each day.

The earning and spending patterns of a typical subject during the pre-alcohol baseline, alcohol availability, and the alcohol withdrawal periods are shown in Figure 7. The pattern of earning and spending for cigarettes is shown in the top row. The pattern of earning and spending for alcohol is shown in the middle row. Daily mean blood alcohol levels are shown in the bottom row. Partial withdrawal signs (e.g., tremor and gastritis) are indicated as asterisks. The type and duration of alcohol withdrawal signs and symptoms are shown at the right of the middle row.

Each subject could work for points for alcohol during the last day of the pre-alcohol baseline period. The number of points earned that day usually was sufficient to sustain a period of drinking of 3 to 6 days. Throughout the remainder of the drinking period, there was a clear dissociation between periods of earning and spending. Subjects alternated between working to earn points for alcohol and spending points earned for a work-free drinking spree. This pattern persisted throughout the 30- and 62-day alcohol-available periods and was strikingly similar in all subjects. Fluctuations in the average blood alcohol levels correlated roughly with the pattern of spending for alcohol. Subjects sustained relatively high blood alcohol levels averaging between 130 and 200 mg/dl for periods up to 62 days. No subject drank all the alcohol available, and all subjects tolerated the discomfort of withdrawal symptoms during the intermittent periods of self-imposed abstinence. These abstinent periods were unexpected in view of the relatively trivial performance requirement involved. Intoxication did not impair the subjects' ability to work at this simple task.

Although all subjects showed a dissociation between working and drinking, subjects worked and drank at different times. Some member of the group was always working, while others were drinking. It is unlikely that the observed behavior represented satiation for alcohol, since other subjects given alcohol with no operant work requirement sustained blood alcohol levels which averaged above 200 mg/dl for periods of 14 to 20 days (Mello & Mendelson, 1972), Similarly, the decrease in operant work for cigarettes did not reflect decreased interest in smoking since subjects attempted to acquire free cigarettes from staff throughout the study.

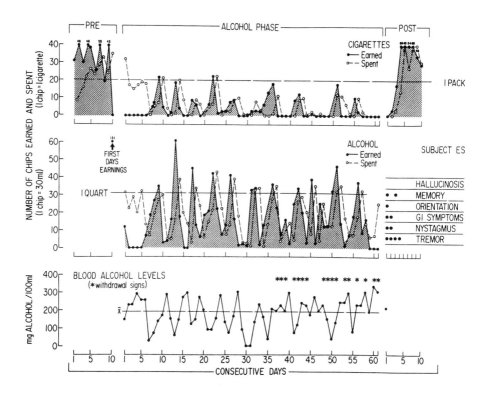

Figure 7: Earning and spending pattern of a single subject working for cigarettes during a 10-day baseline period, for both cigarettes and alcohol during a 62-day alcohol-available period, and for cigarettes during a 10-day withdrawal period. Subjects worked to earn tokens to buy alcohol and cigarettes by pressing a button on a portable operant box (fixed ratio = 1000). Tokens earned for alcohol were not interchangeable with tokens earned for cigarettes. Patterns of earning (filled circles, shaded area) and spending (open circles) for cigarettes are shown in top row. Patterns of earning (filled circles, shaded area) and spending (open circles) for alcohol are shown in the middle row. Subjects were allowed to work for alcohol tokens during the last 24 hours of the baseline period, and these tokens could be spent after 8 a.m. on the first day of the drinking period. Tokens earned during this period are shown at arrow as First Days Earnings. Reprinted from Mello and Mendelson, 1972. Copyright 1972 by the American Psychosomatic Society.

These men described themselves as periodic spree drinkers. The observed pattern of discordant working and drinking was probably more comparable to their real world experience than a stable alcohol intake permitted by an unlimited supply. Since the subjects determined their pattern of alcohol self-administration, it is reasonable to assume that this was their preferred or accustomed pattern. This technique appeared to result in an adequate

- 540 -

simulation of normal drinking patterns by chronic alcoholic individuals in a clinical research ward context. A similar alternation between working and drinking has also been reported by Nathan and co-workers in alcoholics who worked at a comparably simple task (photo cell interruption) for points that could be converted into alcohol (Nathan, O'Brien, & Lowenstein, 1971; Nathan, Titler, Lowenstein, Solomon, & Rossi, 1970).

Marihuana Self-Administration

A number of multidisciplinary studies of marihuana self-administration have been conducted in our laboratory (Mendelson et al., 1974a, 1974b, 1976a). Biological studies of marihuana effects examined in an operant drug self-administration paradigm have included studies of the effects of marihuana on CNS structure (Kuehnle, Mendelson, Davis, & New, 1977), on cardiac and pulmonary function (Bernstein, Kuehnle, & Mendelson, 1976; Goldenheim, Mendelson, Mello, Tilles, & Bavli, 1985), and on reproductive function in men (Mendelson et al., 1974a, 1974b, 1978) and women (Mendelson & Mello, 1984a, 1984b; Mendelson, Mello, Ellingboe, Skupny, Lex, Griffin, & Bavli, 1984). Behavioral studies have examined the effects of marihuana on mood, memory, and social interactions (Mendelson et al., 1976a). In addition to studies of the pattern of marihuana self-administration, the hypothesis that marihuana induces an "amotivational" syndrome was also examined (Mendelson et al., 1976b; Mendelson & Mello, 1984b). Among the effects often ascribed to marihuana are apathy, lethargy and indolence, diminished "drive" and ambition, and decreased productivity and goal directedness.

Marihuana self-administration patterns were examined in 12 casual and 15 heavy users allowed to work for marihuana for 21 consecutive days. "Motivation" was inferred from time spent at the operant task working for marihuana and for money. Subjects worked on a second-order FR-300 (FR-1 sec:S) schedule at the portable operant manipulandum shown in Figure 6. One marihuana cigarette cost 6 purchase points or 30 minutes of sustained operant work. Each marihuana cigarette contained approximately 1 gm of marihuana (1.8 to 2.3% THC). Subjects could also work for money at the cost of 50 cents per 6 points or 30 minutes of sustained operant work. Points earned could be exchanged either for marihuana or for money.

All subjects smoked some marihuana every day. Casual marihuana smokers smoked an average of 2.6 cigarettes per day, and heavy marihuana users smoked an average of 5.7 cigarettes per day. However, both groups showed a linear increase in marihuana smoking over the 21 day period of marihuana availability. On the final day of marihuana availability, the casual users smoked an average of 5.8 cigarettes and the heavy users smoked an average of 14.3 cigarettes (Mendelson et al., 1976b).

All subjects worked longer at the operant task and earned far more points than were required to buy the quantity of marihuana they actually smoked. The heavy user group worked between 6.7 and 14.4 hours per day even though 2.2 to 3 hours of work were required for the 4.3 to 6 cigarettes usually smoked per day. Throughout the period of marihuana use, heavy users worked up to an average of 10 hours each day. The casual marihuana users worked between 5 and 11 hours each day even though the number of cigarettes smoked (2 to 3 per day) required only 1 to 1.5 hours of operant work. No subject stopped operant work even when he smoked 10 or more marihuana cigarettes per day. Moreover, periods of maximal operant work coincided with periods of maximal marihuana smoking (i.e., between 4 p.m. and 12 midnight each day).

Subjects worked more for money than for marihuana, and the dollars saved far exceeded dollars spent on marihuana by both the casual and the heavy marihuana users. At the conclusion of the study, the heavy user group had saved an average of $242.38 (± $19.22 S.E.M.) and the casual users had saved an average of $233.17 (± $26.31 S.E.M.). These earnings reflected sustained operant work and savings during the period of marihuana availability. Since both casual and heavy marihuana users worked for both money and marihuana reinforcement during a period of unrestricted marihuana smoking, these data appear to argue strongly against simplistic descriptions of marihuana effects on motivation (Mendelson et al., 1976b).

Subjects also worked at the operant task at far higher rates of responding than were required. Only the first response after an interval of one second had elapsed was counted as an effective response by the programming circuitry. The response requirements were carefully explained to the subjects but most reported they preferred to respond at a comfortable rate. In most instances this resulted in the emission of approximately 600 responses for each purchase point earned, when 300 responses distributed over 5 minutes would have sufficed. A rate of 120 responses per minute (two responses per second) was typical. Sustained high rates of operant responding by casual and heavy marihuana users during the period of active marihuana smoking are also inconsistent with the notion that marihuana induces an "amotivational" syndrome.

POLYDRUG USE: MARIHUANA, ALCOHOL, AND TOBACCO

Operant procedures for the examination of single drug self-administration patterns can also be extended to study the concurrent self-administration of two or more drugs. Polydrug use appears to be an increasingly frequent drug use pattern, according to clinical and epidemiological studies (Benvenuto, Lau, & Cohen, 1975; Bourne, 1975). The possible combinations of abused drugs appear almost infinite and defy any effort at simple categorization. However, survey data suggest that marihuana is often used in combination with alcohol (Carlin & Post, 1971; Goode, 1969; Grupp, 1972; Tec, 1973), and alcohol is perhaps the most commonly used and abused recreational drug available today. Tobacco use frequently accompanies alcohol use, and it has been shown that alcohol availability increases cigarette smoking in alcoholics (Griffiths, Bigelow, & Liebson, 1976b) and social drinkers (Mello, Mendelson, Sellers, & Kuehnle, 1980a).

The way in which alcohol and marihuana interact and influence concurrent use patterns has long been a subject of speculation. However, there is a prevailing impression that the combined use of marihuana and alcohol leads to a subjective enhancement of the positive or euphorigenic properties of marihuana (Hollister, 1976; Manno, Manno, Kiplinger, & Forney, 1974). Since the combined effects of alcohol and marihuana are thought to be facilitory, we were interested in exploring the effects of concurrent access to marihuana and alcohol. We were interested in learning whether concurrent access to marihuana and alcohol had led to an increase, a decrease, or no change in use patterns of these drugs. On the basis of data demonstrating that alcohol induced an enhancement of tobacco use, we postulated that marihuana and alcohol use would be increased under concurrent access conditions (Mello et al., 1978).

Sixteen adult male volunteers with a history of concurrent alcohol and marihuana use were studied in groups of four on a clinical research ward. Patterns of drug use during 10 days of concurrent access to marihuana and alcohol were compared with successive 5-day periods when only alcohol or only marihuana was available. Two groups were studied in the alcohol first sequence, and two groups were studied in the marihuana first sequence. A drug free control period preceded and followed the 20-day period of spontaneous drug self-administration.

Drug use patterns were assessed by performance on the simple operant task used in studies of marihuana self-administration described previously. Subjects could earn money (50 cents) or marihuana (a 1-gm cigarette containing 1.8 to 2.3% THC) by working at the operant task on an FR-300 (FI-1 sec:S) schedule of reinforcement for 30 minutes. Alcohol (1 ounce) was available as wine, beer, or distilled spirits for 15 minutes of operant work. Subjects could work for only one type of reinforcer at a time, and points were not interchangeable between categories.

The major finding of this study was that concurrent access to alcohol and marihuana resulted in a significant <u>decrease</u> in alcohol consumption in comparison to a 5-day period when only alcohol was available. Fourteen of the 16 subjects studied decreased alcohol use when marihuana was also available ($p < 0.01$), and the magnitude of the decrease in drinking was significant for seven subjects ($p < 0.05$).

During the 10-day period of alcohol and marihuana access, subjects gradually increased marihuana smoking and this increase was significant ($p < 0.001$) as evaluated by a trend analysis. However, this increase cannot be attributed to the concurrent availability of alcohol, since a similar trend was seen in our previous study of casual and heavy marihuana use under comparable experimental conditions (Mendelson et al., 1976b, 1976c). Although 12 subjects smoked more marihuana when alcohol was also available ($p < 0.05$), the magnitude of this increase was statistically significant in only two instances.

Figure 8 illustrates the most common drug use pattern observed: a slight increase in marihuana use and a decrease in alcohol use during the period of concurrent marihuana and alcohol availability. This subject smoked an average of 5 cigarettes per day during the baseline period of marihuana availability. He was also a heavy drinker and consumed an average of 20 drinks per day during the baseline period of alcohol availability. Peak blood alcohol levels ranged between 50 and 140 mg/dl during the hours of maximum drinking. When both alcohol and marihuana were concurrently available, marihuana smoking increased slightly to an average of 6 cigarettes per day. Alcohol consumption decreased to a mean of 5 drinks per day. Peak blood alcohol levels never exceeded 110 mg/dl during the period of concurrent marihuana and alcohol access.

Subjects usually used alcohol and marihuana together during the period of concurrent availability. Despite the temporal concordance of marihuana and alcohol use, there were no instances of adverse reactions or other evidence of toxic drug interactions as has been reported by others following low acute doses of alcohol and marihuana (Sulkowski & Vachon , 1977).

Only 6 of the 16 subjects studied were consistent tobacco users who smoked an average of 15.9 cigarettes per day. Tobacco use was significantly correlated ($p < 0.05$) with both alcohol and marihuana use. Tobacco use also accompanied alcohol use and marihuana use during the single drug availability period. These data are consistent with previous reports of alcohol-induced increases in tobacco use (Griffiths et al., 1976b) and with survey reports of a high correlation between marihuana and tobacco use (O'Donnell, 1976).

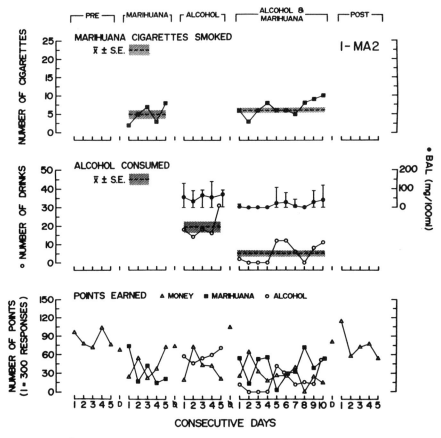

Figure 8: Marihuana and alcohol use and purchase points earned for money and drugs over 34 consecutive days. The successive conditions of drug availability are shown at the top of the figure. The first row shows the number of marihuana cigarettes smoked each day (filled squares). The average number of marihuana cigarettes smoked during each marihuana availability period is indicated by the dotted line and cross hatched area (±S.E.M.). The second row shows the number of alcoholic drinks consumed each day (open circles) and the 24 hour mean and range of blood alcohol levels observed each day (filled circles). The average number of drinks consumed during the 5- or 10-day period is shown as a dotted line and cross hatched area (mean ± S.E.M.). The third row shows the number of purchase points earned for money (open triangles), marihuana (filled squares), and alcohol (open circles). Consecutive days of the study are shown on the abscissa. On the single day (D) immediately following the predrug baseline and preceding the post-drug baseline, an acute combined dose of alcohol and marihuana was given. No drugs were available on the single day (D̸) following the 5-day period of marihuana availability and of alcohol availability. Adapted from Mello, Mendelson, and Kuehnle, 1978.

Data obtained are not consistent with the hypothesis that the simultaneous availability of marihuana and alcohol will lead to a significant increase in the use of both drugs. Only two of the 16 subjects increased consumption of both alcohol and marihuana during the simultaneous access conditions, even though alcohol and marihuana were usually used together. These data suggest the importance of defining conditions under which multiple drug access will result in a depression of the use of one or more drugs, an increase in the use of one or both drugs, or no change in drug use as a function of single or multiple drug access. In future studies it will be important to try to identify the interacting pharmacological and behavioral variables which control patterns of multiple drug use. It will also be necessary to determine the generality of these findings with other groups of heavy drinkers and alcoholic individuals.

HEROIN SELF-ADMINISTRATION

Although opiate self-administration has been studied extensively with animal models (see Johanson & Schuster, 1981; Schuster & Johanson, 1974), there have been relatively few clinical studies of opiate self-administration under controlled research ward conditions. Most of our information about heroin abuse has come from retrospective reports by heroin addicts, usually during a period of drug abstinence. This quasi-anecdotal view has been balanced by the meticulous, empirical studies of the physiological and subjective effects of acute and chronic morphine administration in incarcerated drug addicts who volunteered for research at the Addiction Research Center (ARC) in Lexington, Kentucky (Martin & Isbell, 1978). The long term effects of chronic opiate administration as well as the nature and persistence of the opiate withdrawal syndrome have been examined (for reviews, see Mansky, 1978; Martin & Jasinski, 1969). New therapeutic drugs have been compared with morphine in an effort to predict abuse liability (Jasinski, 1977), and the effects of potential pharmacotherapies for opiate addiction on subjective and physiological reactions to opiates have been evaluated (Martin, 1977; Martin, Jasinski, Haertzen, Kay, Jones, Mansky, & Carpenter, 1973a; Martin, Jasinski, & Mansky, 1973b).

With few exceptions the ARC studies have used a fixed dose opiate administration paradigm. In 1952, Wikler reported the first systematic study in which the dose and frequency of morphine administration was determined by an opiate addict rather than by the investigator. Over a two month period, the subject progressively increased his morphine dose from 30 to 1,000 mg on the last day of morphine availability. During this first simulation of naturalistic opiate use patterns, dreams, fantasies, and subjective drug reactions were studied in clinical interviews (Wikler, 1952). This important study was the beginning of a new approach to the study of drug abuse which has many adherents today--the direct observation of drug self-administration behavior and its consequences (for review, see Krasnegor, 1978).

Methadone Effects on Heroin Self-Administration

During the 1970s, as new pharmacotherapies became available for the treatment of opiate abuse, it became evident that evaluation would be greatly facilitated by the availability of objective and quantifiable measures of drug-seeking behavior. Martin and co-workers (1973a) and Jones and Prada (1975) evaluated the effects of methadone maintenance on operant work for Dilaudid (hydromorphone) in heroin addicts. They reported that some heroin addicts maintained on 50 to 100 mg/day of methadone continued to work for Dilaudid (4 mg/injection, i.v.) for approximately 2.5 months by riding an exercycle 10 miles within one hour. Continued heroin use during methadone maintenance has also been observed clinically.

Naltrexone Effects on Heroin Self-Administration

In 1979, Meyer, Mirin and co-workers reported a series of studies designed to evaluate the efficacy of the long-acting narcotic antagonist, naltrexone, on heroin self-administration by heroin addicts (Meyer & Mirin, 1979). This study demonstrated that it was possible to conduct long term in-patient studies with heroin addict volunteers who were not incarcerated and who were not under any legal or other constraints.

Subjects were allowed to work for heroin on a simple mechanical operant manipulandum similar to that shown in Figure 3. Heroin cost either 300 points or 2100 points per 0.5 mg. Points could be accumulated at about 10,000 per hour. Subjects were allowed to determine the interval between heroin doses and could increase a dose (e.g., from 2.5 to 7.5 mg) by waiting 6 hours rather than taking a smaller dose (2.5 mg) every 2 hours. Although the operant task was relatively simple, the heroin addict subjects rapidly learned how to tamper with the operant manipulanda and advance the counters. They were unrelentingly ingenious in thwarting all efforts to reliably relate operant work for heroin to actual heroin use (Meyer & Mirin, 1979).

Narcotic addicts maintained on naltrexone reported no subjective effects of heroin. In most subjects there was no objective evidence (e.g., myosis, changes in vital signs) that heroin produces physiological effects during naltrexone blockade. These data confirmed the observation of Martin and co-workers that 50 mg of naltrexone produced a total blockade of narcotic effects for a period of 24 hours (Martin, Jasinski, & Mansky, 1973b).

All subjects self-administered significantly more heroin under placebo conditions than under naltrexone blockade. Meyer & Mirin (1979) reported that when naltrexone was administered to informed subjects, there was little experimentation with heroin: Seven of nine subjects sampled heroin an average of 13 times (range 2 to 46) over a 10-day period of heroin availability while maintained on 75 mg/day of naltrexone (p.o.). However, when naltrexone was administered under double blind conditions, each of 22 subjects sampled heroin occasionally. Over a 10-day period of heroin access, 11 subjects took heroin on an average of 15.9 occasions, whereas the other 11 took heroin on an average of 4.3 occasions. Frequency of heroin self-administration among the other members of the group appeared to be the best predictor of heroin-use frequency in any individual (Meyer & Mirin, 1979). It is also possible that the escalating dose schedule used encouraged heroin sampling, since naltrexone-maintained subjects continued to test the antagonist blockade at progressively higher heroin doses.

Despite the effectiveness of the naltrexone blockade, some subjects who sampled heroin frequently during naltrexone maintenance showed respiratory depression and pupillary constriction after the first several heroin doses. Meyer and Mirin (1979) suggested that these autonomic effects were not due to inadequate antagonist blockade but rather were classically conditioned responses which extinguished after repeated blocked heroin injections. The importance of conditioning effects associated with the ritual of heroin self-injection has been clearly demonstrated (Grabowski & O'Brien, 1981; O'Brien, 1976).

The subjective consequences of heroin self-administration observed on the clinical research ward were completely at variance with the euphorigenic, pleasurable effects commonly ascribed to opiate intoxication in retrospective accounts by addicts. Meyer and Mirin (1979) confirmed and extended the previous observations of Wikler (1952) and Haertzen and Hooks (1969) that chronic opiate use is often accompanied by an increase in dysphoria, hypochondriasis and irritability, as well as increased psychopathology, belligerence, negativism, motor retardation, and social isolation. Although it appeared that each heroin injection was associated with a brief elevation in mood, even this transient mood change diminished as a function of chronic drug use (Meyer & Mirin, 1979; Mirin, McNamee, & Meyer, 1976). These data attesting to the dysphoric consequences of chronic heroin use are concordant with data on chronic alcohol intoxication and challenge the notion that drugs are used solely for their rewarding or euphorigenic properties (see Mello, 1977, 1978, 1983). These mood changes associated with chronic heroin use did not occur in subjects maintained on naltrexone for comparable periods. Consequently, the increased psychopathology and dysphoria were probably related to heroin use rather than residence on the research ward.

In the early 1980s, we evaluated the effects of naltrexone on heroin self-administration in comparison to placebo under double blind conditions in a clinical research ward setting (Mello et al., 1981). In order to achieve the primary goals of these studies, it was essential to devise a reliable operant procedure that would yield objective and quantifiable data about drug acquisition. The advantage of direct observation over reliance on retrospective self-reports or predictions of probable behavior by addict subjects is obvious. This design permitted examination of the efficacy and the limitations of this new pharmacotherapy operationally defined by the effect on the amount and frequency of heroin self-administration as well as the behavioral consequences of drug use.

Operant techniques were used to provide an objective and quantitative measure of performance for two alternative reinforcers. Since drugs are not available to most users without some expenditure of effort or money, we compared operant work for heroin with acquisition of an alternative reinforcer, money. The effects of naltrexone on heroin self-administration were measured in terms of duration, rate, and pattern of operant performance for heroin rather than inferred from verbal behavior. The effect of heroin intoxication on operant performance for money was examined in comparison to performance during drug-free conditions. The operant manipulandum shown in Figure 6 proved to be tamper proof and effective for this purpose.

Twelve male heroin addict volunteers lived on a clinical research ward for 34 days. After a 9-day drug-free period, naltrexone or placebo was given and heroin (40 mg/day) was available for 10 days. Subjects could earn money ($1.50) or heroin (10 mg/injection, i.v.) by responding on a second-order schedule of reinforcement (FR-300 [FI-1 sec:S]) for approximately 90 minutes. Subjects were limited to four 10-mg doses of heroin each day for 10 consecutive days for both medical and ethical considerations. Subjects could refuse to take any heroin dose earned but were not allowed to take fractional doses (e.g., 5 instead of 10 mg). Points earned for heroin could not be exchanged for money. However, naltrexone-maintained subjects who worked for heroin points during baseline and then elected not to purchase heroin were allowed to exchange heroin points for money at the end of the study.

Naltrexone effectively suppressed heroin self-administration. The three naltrexone-maintained subjects took only 2 to 7.5% of the total heroin

CUMULATIVE RECORDS OF RESPONDING (FI I SEC)

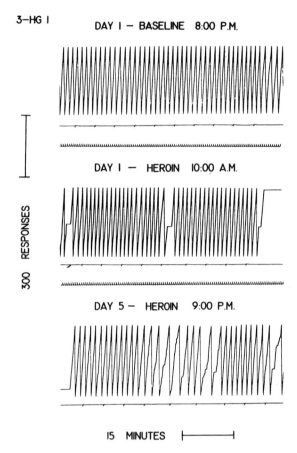

Figure 9: Cumulative records of responses for money and for heroin by a placebo naltrexone subject. Records of responding on an FR-300 (FI-1 sec:S) schedule of reinforcement are shown for the first day of the drug-free condition and for Days 1 and 5 of heroin availability. Cumulative records of responding are a direct read-out of response rates; each response advances the step pen 0.25 mm, and the paper advances at a constant speed of 28 mm/hour. The response pen resets after a fixed number of responses or when the subject changed from working for heroin to money or the converse. Each deflection of the bottom event pen indicates completion of 300 effective responses on the FI-1 second schedule of reinforcement. The top pen codes whether the subject was working for heroin (upward deflections) or money (no deflections). Only money was available on Days 1 to 7 of the drug-free conditions so no code is shown. Reprinted from Mello, Mendelson, Kuehnle, and Sellers, 1981. Copyright 1981 by the Society for Pharmacology and Experimental Therapeutics.

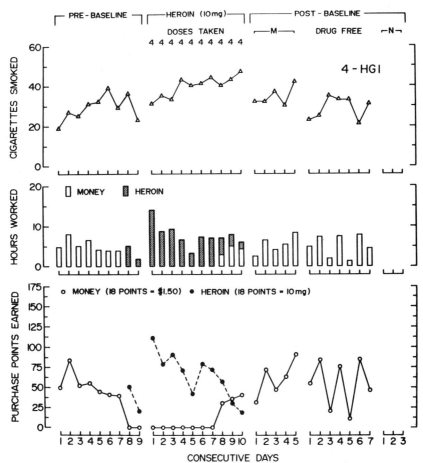

Figure 10: Cigarette smoking patterns of operant earning and spending for money and heroin by a subject assigned to the placebo naltrexone condition. The successive conditions--drug-free baseline (Pre), heroin availability, methadone detoxification (M), drug-free period (Post), and naltrexone maintenance (N)--are shown across the top of the figure. The number of 10-mg doses of heroin taken each day are shown underneath the heroin heading. A maximum of four injections (40 mg/injection) was available each day. The number of tobacco cigarettes smoked each day is shown in the top row. The second row shows the number of hours worked for money (open bars) and heroin (shaded bars) each day throughout the study. The third row shows the number of purchase points earned for money (open circles) and for heroin (filled circles) each day. Acquisition of each purchase point required 300 effective responses on an FI-1 sec schedule of reinforcement (FR-300 [FI-1 sec:S]). On Days 6 and 8 of the pre-heroin base line, blood samples were collected for neuroendocrine studies over 10 consecutive hours. Adapted from Mello, Mendelson, Kuehnle, and Sellers, 1981, and Mello, Mendelson, Sellers, and Kuehnle, 1980b.

available, two subjects stopped heroin self-administration after the first or second injection, and the third subject took a total of three injections over the 10-day period of availability. There were no discernible adverse side effects during 25 consecutive days on naltrexone maintenance. In contrast, the nine placebo naltrexone subjects used 57.5 to 100% of the total heroin available.

Heroin intoxication did not impair operant performance. Heroin users worked longer hours and earned significantly more purchase points during heroin self-administration and subsequent methadone detoxification than during the drug-free period. On the first day of heroin use, subjects worked 10 or more hours at the operant task. Ten days of chronic heroin intoxication were not associated with progressive decreases in operant work. Moreover, heroin intoxication did not compromise the ability of the subjects to titrate their operant work to acquire precisely the amount of heroin they wished to buy. Subjects continually monitored their accumulated points shown on the operant panel and did not earn more points for heroin than it was possible to spend.

A typical cumulative record illustrating that 10 mg of heroin had minimal effects on operant performance is shown in Figure 9. The lack of effect of heroin use on operant performance reflected in total points earned as illustrated in data from individual subjects is shown in Figure 10. These data also show that cigarette smoking increased during the period of heroin use (Mello et al., 1980b), an effect consistently observed with alcohol (Griffiths et al., 1976b; Mello et al., 1980a).

Buprenorphine Effects on Human Heroin Self-Administration

A similar experimental design was used to compare the effects of buprenorphine, an opioid mixed agonist/antagonist, with placebo on operant acquisition of heroin and money studied under double blind conditions (Mello et al., 1982). Buprenorphine combines the salient characteristics of two pharmacotherapies for heroin addiction, because it is both a partial opioid agonist similar to methadone and a potent opioid antagonist similar to naltrexone (Lewis, Rance, & Sanger, 1983). Ten male volunteers with a history of heroin abuse lived on a clinical research ward for 40 days. After a 5-day drug-free period, buprenorphine or placebo was given in gradually ascending doses (0.5 to 8 mg/day, s.c.) over 14 days. Subjects were maintained on 8 mg/day of buprenorphine for 10 days during which they could earn money ($1.50) or heroin (7 or 13.5 mg/injection, i.v.) by responding on a second-order schedule of reinforcement (FR-300 [FI-1 sec:S]) for approximately 90 minutes.

Buprenorphine-maintained subjects took significantly less heroin than subjects maintained on placebo (p < 0.001). Buprenorphine-maintained subjects took only between 2 and 31% of the total amount of heroin available, whereas placebo-maintained subjects took between 93 and 100% of the available heroin.

There were a number of similarities between the operant performance for heroin and money of the subjects studied under placebo buprenorphine and placebo naltrexone maintenance. In both studies subjects showed the capacity to precisely titrate operant work to acquire the desired amount of heroin and then resume working for money. There was no evidence of impairment of operant performance for heroin or for money during heroin intoxication. In fact, there were no significant differences in total operant points earned or in total hours worked during any phase of the study between the placebo group who used heroin and the buprenorphine-maintenance group who did not (Mello et al., 1982).

These points are clearly indicated by data shown in Figure 11. This subject was studied under both buprenorphine-maintenance conditions and placebo-maintenance conditions. It is obvious that maintenance of buprenorphine did not, in and of itself, significantly suppress operant performance for money or for time spent working at the operant task. These data indicate that heroin addicts can perform a simple operant task effectively for long periods of time (6 to 18 hours per day) during heroin intoxication at doses of 21 to 40.5 mg/day (Mello et al., 1982).

SUMMARY AND CONCLUSIONS

Data have been presented to illustrate some ways that operant procedures can be used to study self-administration patterns of a variety of substances. Operant procedures for drug self-administration studies have also been shown to be useful for concurrent examination of a variety of drug-effect variables, especially the effects of drugs on biological systems. Behavioral data were selected to illustrate some clinical research findings which are contrary to conventional wisdom and common expectation. We have seen that alcohol addicts do not maintain a constant pattern of alcohol intake and do not drink all the alcohol available when given unrestricted access to alcohol in a self-administration paradigm. Rather, alcohol addicts tend to alternate periods of alcohol intoxication and operant work, even though periods of abstinence working are accompanied by partial withdrawal symptoms. These data are inconsistent with the notion that alcohol abuse is maintained by either the avoidance of withdrawal signs and symptoms or an uncontrollable "craving" for alcohol (Mello, 1975; Mello & Mendelson, 1972).

Studies of marihuana self-administration are not consistent with the notion that marihuana intoxication produces an "amotivational" syndrome (Mendelson et al., 1976b, 1976c). Rather, subjects worked an average of 10 hours each day while smoking four to six marihuana cigarettes. Most subjects worked while they were smoking marihuana and earned far more money than they spent on marihuana cigarettes.

Similarly, heroin intoxication did not result in sedation and inactivity at doses up to 40 mg/day. Subjects often became more active after a heroin injection. During heroin intoxication subjects worked longer and earned more points than during drug-free or methadone detoxification phases of the study (Mello et al., 1981).

Studies of polydrug use involving alcohol and marihuana indicate that concurrent access to these drugs is not necessarily associated with increased use of alcohol and marihuana as would be predicted from anecdotal accounts and objective data on alcohol and tobacco (Griffiths et al., 1976b). Rather, the simultaneous availability of marihuana and alcohol was associated with a significant decrease in alcohol consumption in comparison to a baseline period when only alcohol was available (Mello et al., 1978).

We conclude that there is no substitute for direct clinical observation of drug use patterns and of the effects of drugs on behavioral and biological variables under controlled conditions. The direct observation of patterns of drug use and assessments of the subjective and objective consequences of drug intoxication have challenged many prevalent assumptions derived from retrospective reports by drug abusers during sobriety (Mello & Mendelson, 1978). It is our contention that direct clinical observation of drug use patterns and associated drug effects in the same individual over time is

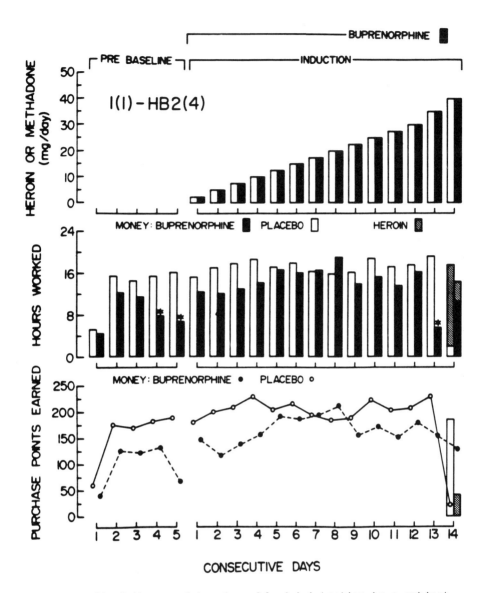

Figure 11: Patterns of heroin self-administration by a subject studied under both buprenorphine maintenance (8 mg/day; filled bars) and placebo maintenance (open bars) conditions. The daily dose of heroin or methadone (mg/day) is shown on the left ordinate. The daily dose of buprenorphine or equal volume placebo control maintenance is shown on the right ordinate. The sequence of conditions (pre-drug baseline, buprenorphine or placebo induction, heroin availability, detoxification with buprenorphine or methadone,

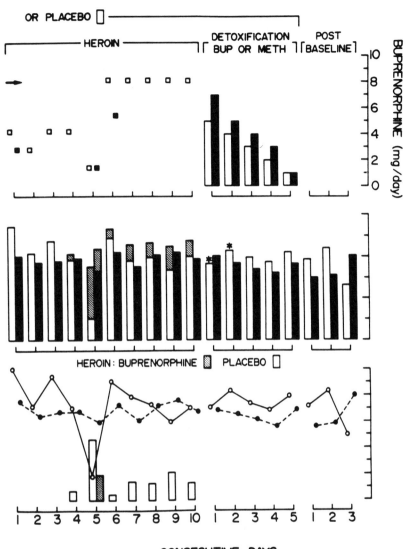

and the post-drug baseline) is shown at the top of the figure.
Consecutive days of the study are shown on the abscissa. Row 2 shows
the hours worked for money under buprenorphine (filled bars) and
placebo (open bars) conditions and hours worked for heroin (shaded
bars) under each condition. The number of purchase points earned for
money and for heroin under buprenorphine and placebo maintenance
conditions are shown in the third row. The consecutive study days
are shown on the abscissa. Adapted from Mello, Mendelson, and
Kuehnle, 1982.

essential to an improved understanding of the behavioral bases of drug abuse. The experimental analysis of drug use patterns is one way to examine factors which maintain and perpetuate drug abuse. The periodicity of drug use and the rate and duration of operant behavior involved in drug acquisition are data which can be measured directly without reliance on alleged intervening variables such as "drug hunger."

On the basis of such information, certain inferences can be made concerning broader questions about the phenomenology of drug abuse. It is of interest to determine if there are consistencies in drug use patterns within the behavior of a single individual or between individuals with comparable drug use histories. Given the diversity of individuals with substance abuse problems, an examination of factors which initiate and maintain periodic substance abuse episodes may prove more productive than a search for origins. A better understanding of how drug self-administration is maintained should permit more effective manipulation of critical maintenance variables and lead to the development of more effective forms of intervention. Both the conceptual and technical aspects of an operant analysis of drug self-administration behavior appear to be optimally designed to facilitate our understanding of how substance abuse is maintained. Comparisons of drug use patterns across addictive disorders may eventually permit identification of some reliable commonalities and differences that in turn will help to clarify the nature of drug-related reinforcers.

ACKNOWLEDGMENTS

Preparation of this review was supported in part by Grants No. K05 DA00101, K05 DA0064, DA02519, and DA02905 from the National Institute on Drug Abuse and AA06252 from the National Institute on Alcohol Abuse and Alcoholism, ADAMHA. Portions of this paper were revised and reprinted with permission from N. Krasnegor (Ed.) (1978), Self-administration of abused substances: Methods for study (National Institute on Drug Abuse Research Monograph 20, pp. 93-127). Washington, DC: U.S. Government Printing Office. We thank Loretta Carvelli for her excellent assistance in preparing this manuscript.

REFERENCES

Babor, T. F., Mendelson, J. H., Greenberg, I., & Kuehnle, J. C. (1978). Experimental analysis of the "happy hour"--effects of purchase price on alcohol consumption. Psychopharmacology, 58, 35-41.

Benvenuto, J. A., Lau, J., & Cohen, R. (1975). Patterns of nonopiate/polydrug abuse: Findings of a national collaborative research project. In Problems of drug dependence. Proceedings of the 37th Annual Scientific Meeting, Committee on Problems of Drug Dependence, (pp. 234-254). Washington, DC: National Academy of Sciences--National Research Council.

Bernstein, J. G., Kuehnle, J. C., & Mendelson, J. H. (1976). Medical implications of marihuana use. American Journal of Drug and Alcohol Abuse, 3, 347-361.

Bigelow, G. E., Griffiths, R. R., & Liebson, I. (1976). Effects of response requirement upon human sedative self-administration and drug-seeking behavior. Pharmacology Biochemistry & Behavior, 5, 681-685.

Bourne, P. G. (1975). Polydrug abuse--status report on the federal effort. In E. Senay, V. Shorty, & H. Alksen (Eds.), Developments in the field of drug abuse: National drug abuse conference (pp. 197-207). Cambridge, MA: Schenkman Publishing.

Carlin, A. S., & Post, R. D. (1971). Patterns of drug use among marihuana smokers. Journal of the American Medical Association, 218, 867-868.

Goldenheim, P., Mendelson, J. H., Mello, N. K., Tilles, D. , & Bavli, S. (1984). Marihuana smoking causes a reduction in single breath carbon monoxide diffusing capacity. American Journal of Medicine, 1985 (in press).

Goode, E. (1969). Marihuana and the politics of reality. Journal of Health and Social Behavior, 10, 83-94.

Grabowski, J., & O'Brien, C. P. (1981). Conditioning factors in opiate use. In N. K. Mello (Ed.), Advances in substance abuse, behavioral and biological research (Vol. 2, pp. 69-121). Greenwich: JAI Press.

Griffiths, R. R., Bigelow, G. E., & Henningfield, J. E. (1980). Similarities in animal and human drug taking behavior. In N. K. Mello (Ed.), Advances in substance abuse, behavioral and biological research (Vol. 1, pp. 1-90). Greenwich: JAI Press.

Griffiths, R. R., Bigelow, G. E., & Liebson, I. (1976a). Human sedative self-administration. Effects of interingestion interval and dose. Journal of Pharmacology and Experimental Therapeutics, 197, 488-494.

Griffiths, R. R., Bigelow, G. E., & Liebson, I. (1976b). Facilitation of human tobacco self-administration by ethanol: A behavioral analysis. Journal of Experimental Analysis and Behavior, 15, 279-292.

Grupp, S. E. (1972). Multiple drug use in a sample of experienced marihuana smokers. International Journal of Addictions, 7, 481-491.

Haertzen, C. A., & Hooks, N. T. (1969). Changes in personality and subjective experience associated with the chronic administration and withdrawal of opiates. Journal of Nervous and Mental Disease, 148, 606-614.

Hollister, L. E. (1976). Interactions of delta-9-tetrahydrocannabinol with other drugs. In E. S. Vesell & M. C. Braude (Eds.), Interactions of drugs of abuse (pp. 212-218). New York: New York Academy of Sciences.

Jasinski, D. R. (1977). Assessment of the abuse potentiality of morphine-like drugs (methods used in man). In W. R. Martin (Ed.), Drug addiction I: Morphine, sedative/hypnotic and alcohol dependence (Handbook of Experimental Pharmacology, Vol. 45, pp. 197-258). Berlin: Springer-Verlag.

Johanson, C. E., & Schuster, C. R. (1981). Animal models of drug self-administration. In N. K. Mello (Ed.), Advances in substance abuse, behavioral and biological research (Vol. 2, pp. 219-297). Greenwich: JAI Press.

Jones, B. E., & Prada, J. A. (1975). Drug seeking behavior during methadone maintenance. Psychopharmacologia, 41, 7-10.

Kelleher, R. T., Goldberg, S. R., & Krasnegor, N. (Eds.). (1976). Control of drug taking behavior by schedules of reinforcement. Baltimore: Williams & Wilkins.

Krasnegor, N. A. (Ed.). (1978). Self-administration of abused substances: Methods for study (National Institute of Drug Abuse Research Monograph 20). Washington, DC: U.S. Government Printing Office.

Kuehnle, J. C., Mendelson, J. H., Davis, K. R., & New, P. F. J. (1977). Computed tomographic examination of heavy marihuana smokers. Journal of the American Medical Association, 237, 1231-1232.

Lewis, J., Rance, M. J., & Sanger, D. J. (1983). The pharmacology and abuse potential of buprenorphine, a new antagonist analgesic. In N. K. Mello (Ed.), Advances in substance abuse, behavioral and biological research (Vol. 3, pp. 103-154). Greenwich: JAI Press.

Manno, J. E., Manno, B. R., Kiplinger, G. F., & Forney, R. B. (1974). Motor and mental performance with marihuana: Relationship to administered dose of delta-9-tetrahydrocannabinol and its interaction with alcohol. In L. L. Miller (Ed.), Marihuana, effects on human behavior (pp. 45-72). New York: Academic Press.

Mansky, P. A. (1978). Opiates: Human psychopharmacology. In L. L. Iversen, S. D. Iversen, & S. H. Snyder (Eds.), Handbook of psychopharmacology (Vol. 12, pp. 95-185). New York: Plenum Press.

Martin, W. R. (Ed.). (1977). Chemotherapy of narcotic addiction. In W. R. Martin (Ed.), Drug addiction I: Morphine, sedative/hypnotic and alcohol dependence (Handbook of Experimental Pharmacology, Vol. 45, pp. 279-318). Berlin: Springer-Verlag.

Martin, W. R., & Isbell, H. (1978). Drug addiction and the U.S. Public Health Service (Department of Health, Education, and Welfare Publication 77-434, pp. 325). Washington, DC: U.S. Government Printing Office.

Martin, W. R., & Jasinski, D. R. (1969). Physiological parameters of morphine dependence in man--tolerance, early abstinence, protracted abstinence. Journal of Psychiatric Research, 7, 9-17.

Martin, W. R., Jasinski, D. R., Haertzen, C. A., Kay, D. C., Jones, B. E., Mansky, P. A., & Carpenter, R. W. (1973a). Methadone--a reevaluation. Archives of General Psychiatry, 28, 286-295.

Martin, W. R., Jasinski, D. R., & Mansky, P. A. (1973b). Naltrexone, an antagonist for the treatment of heroin dependence. Archives of General Psychiatry, 28, 784-791.

Mello, N. K. (1972). Behavioral studies of alcoholism. In B. Kissin & H. Begleiter (Eds.), The biology of alcoholism: Vol. 2, Physiology and behavior (pp. 219-291). New York: Plenum Press.

Mello, N. K. (1973). Short-term memory function in alcohol addicts during intoxication. In M. M. Gross (Ed.), Alcohol intoxication and withdrawal: Experimental studies (pp. 333-334). New York: Plenum Press.

Mello, N. K. (1975). A semantic aspect of alcoholism. In H. D. Cappell & A. E. LeBlanc (Eds.), Biological and behavioral approaches to drug dependence (pp. 73-87). Toronto: Addiction Research Foundation.

Mello, N. K. (1977). Stimulus self-administration: Some implications for the prediction of drug abuse liability. In T. Thompson & K. R. Unna (Eds.), Predicting dependence liability of stimulant and depressant drugs (pp. 243-260). Baltimore: University Park Press.

Mello, N. K. (1978). Control of drug self-administration: The role of aversive consequences. In R. C. Peterson & R. C. Stillman (Eds.), Phencyclidine abuse: An appraisal (National Institute on Drug Abuse Research Monograph 21, pp. 289-308).

Mello, N. K. (1983). A behavioral analysis of the reinforcing properties of alcohol and other drugs in man. In B. Kissin & H. Begleiter (Eds.), The pathogenesis of alcoholism, biological factors (Vol. 7, pp. 133-198). New York: Plenum Press.

Mello, N. K., McNamee, H. B., & Mendelson, J. H. (1968). Drinking patterns of chronic alcoholics: Gambling and motivation for alcohol. In J. O. Cole (Ed.), Clinical research in alcoholism (Psychiatric Research Report 24, pp. 83-118). Washington, DC: American Psychiatric Association.

Mello, N. K., & Mendelson, J. H. (1965). Operant analysis of drinking patterns of chronic alcoholics. Nature, 206, 43-46.

Mello, N. K., & Mendelson, J. H. (1970). Experimentally induced intoxication in alcoholics--A comparison between programmed and spontaneous drinking. Journal of Pharmacology and Experimental Therapeutics, 173, 101-116.

Mello, N. K., & Mendelson, J. H. (1972). Drinking patterns during work-contingent and non-contingent alcohol acquisition. Psychosomatic Medicine, 34, 139-264.

Mello, N. K., & Mendelson, J. H. (1978). Alcohol and human behavior. In L. L. Iversen, S. D. Iversen, & S. H. Snyder (Eds.), Handbook of psychopharmacology, Vol. 12: Drugs of abuse (pp. 235-317). New York: Plenum Press.

Mello, N. K., Mendelson, J. H., & Kuehnle, J. C. (1978). Human polydrug use: Marihuana, alcohol and tobacco. Journal of Pharmacology and Experimental Therapeutics, 207, 922-935.

Mello, N. K., Mendelson, J. H., & Kuehnle, J. C. (1982). Buprenorphine effects on human heroin self-administration: An operant analysis. Journal of Pharmacology and Experimental Therapeutics, 223, 30-39.

Mello, N. K., Mendelson, J. H., Kuehnle, J. C., & Sellers, M. (1981). Operant analysis of human heroin self-administration and the effects of naltrexone. Journal of Pharmacology and Experimental Therapeutics, 216, 45-54.

Mello, N. K., Mendelson, J. H., Sellers, M., & Kuehnle, J. C. (1980a). Effect of alcohol and marihuana on tobacco smoking. Clinical Pharmacology and Therapeutics, 27, 202-209.

Mello, N. K., Mendelson, J. H., Sellers, M. , & Kuehnle, J. C. (1980b). Effects of heroin self-administration on cigarette smoking. Psychopharmacology, 67, 45-52.

Mendelson, J. H. (Ed.). (1964). Experimentally induced chronic intoxication and withdrawal in alcoholics. Quarterly Journal of Studies on Alcoholism, Suppl. 2.

Mendelson, J. H. (1970). Biological concomitants of alcoholism. New England Journal of Medicine, 283, 24-32 & 71-81.

Mendelson, J. H., Babor, T. F., Kuehnle, J. C., Rossi, A. M., Bernstein, J. G., Mello, N. K., & Greenberg, I. (1976a). Behavioral and biological aspects of marihuana use. Annals of the New York Academy of Sciences, 282, 186-210.

Mendelson, J. H., Ellingboe, J., Kuehnle, J. C., & Mello, N. K. (1978). Effects of chronic marihuana use on integrated plasma testosterone and luteinizing hormone levels. Journal of Pharmacology and Experimental Therapeutics, 207, 611-617.

Mendelson, J. H., Kuehnle, J. C., Ellingboe, J., & Babor, T. F. (1974a). Plasma testosterone levels before, during, and after chronic marihuana smoking. New England Journal of Medicine, 291, 1051-1055.

Mendelson, J. H., Kuehnle, J. C., Greenberg, I., & Mello, N. K. (1976b). Operant acquisition of marihuana use in man. Journal of Pharmacology and Experimental Therapeutics, 198, 42-53.

Mendelson, J. H., Kuehnle, J. C., Greenberg, I., & Mello, N. K. (1976c). The effects of marihuana on human operant behavior: Individual data. In M. C. Braude & S. Szara (Eds.) Pharmacology of Marihuana (pp. 643-653). New York: Raven Press.

Mendelson, J. H., & Mello, N. K. (1976). Behavioral and biochemical interrelations in alcoholism. Annual Review of Medicine, 27, 321-333.

Mendelson, J. H., & Mello, N. K. (1984a). Effects of marihuana on endocrine hormones in human males and females. In M. C. Braude & U. P. Ludford (Eds.), Marihuana effects on endocrine and reproductive systems (National Institute on Drug Abuse Research Monograph 44, pp. 97-114). Washington, DC: U.S. Government Printing Office.

Mendelson, J. H., & Mello, N. K. (1984b). Behavioral pharmacology of marihuana use by men and women. In R. Balster & L. Seiden (Eds.), Behavioral pharmacology: The current status (pp. 451-463). New York: Alan R. Liss.

Mendelson, J. H., Mello, N. K., Cristofaro, P., Ellingboe, V., & Benedikt, R. (1985). Acute effects of marijuana on pituitary gonadal hormones during the periovulatory phase of the menstrual cycle. In L. S. Harris (Ed.), Problems of drug dependence, 1984. (National Institute on Drug Abuse Research Monograph 55, pp. 24-31). Washington, DC: U.S. Government Printing Office.

Mendelson, J. H., Mello, N. K., & Ellingboe, J. (1978). Effects of alcohol on pituitary-gonadal hormones, sexual function and aggression in human males. In M. A. Lipton, A. DiMascio, & K. F. Killam (Eds.), Psychopharmacology, A generation of progress (pp. 1677-1691). New York: Raven Press.

Mendelson, J. H., Mello, N. K., & Solomon, P. (1968). Small group drinking behavior: An experimental study of chronic alcoholics. In A. Wikler (Ed.), The addictive states (pp. 399-430). Baltimore: Williams & Wilkins.

Mendelson, J. H., Rossi, A. N., & Meyer, R. E. (Eds.) (1974b). The use of marihuana: A psychological and physiological inquiry. New York: Plenum Press.

Meyer, R. E., & Mirin, S. M. (1979). The heroin stimulus. New York: Plenum Press.

Mirin, S. M., McNamee, H. B., & Meyer, R. E. (1976). Psychopathology, craving and mood during heroin acquisition: An experimental study. International Journal of Addictions, 11, 525-543.

Nathan, P. E., O'Brien, J. S., & Lowenstein, L. M. (1971). Operant studies of chronic alcoholism: Interaction of alcohol and alcoholics. In M. K. Roach, W. M. McIsaac, & P. J. Creaven (Eds.), Biological aspects of alcohol (pp. 341-370). Austin: University of Texas.

Nathan, P. E., Titler, N. A., Lowenstein, L. M., Solomon, P., & Rossi, A. M. (1970). Behavioral analysis of chronic alcoholism: Interaction of alcohol and human contact. Archives of General Psychiatry, 22, 419-430.

O'Brien, C. P. (1976). Experimental analysis of conditioning factors in human narcotic addiction. In R. T. Kelleher, S. R. Goldberg, & N. A. Krasnegor (Eds.), Control of drug taking behavior by schedules of reinforcement (pp. 533-543). Baltimore: Williams & Wilkins.

O'Donnell, J. T. (Ed.). (1976). Young men and drugs: A nationwide survey. (National Institute on Drug Abuse Research Monograph 5). Washington, DC: U.S. Government Printing Office.

Pickens, R., Cunningham, M. R., Heston, L. L., Eckert, E., & Gustafson, L. K. (1977). Dose preference during pentobarbital self-administration by humans. Journal of Pharmacology and Experimental Therapeutics, 203, 310-318.

Popham, R. E., Schmidt, W., & de Lint, J. (1975). The prevention of alcoholism: Epidemiological studies of the effects of government control measures. British Journal of Addiction, 70, 124-144.

Schuster, C. R., & Johanson, C. E. (1974). The use of animal models for the study of drug abuse. In R. J. Gibbins, Y. Israel, H. Kalant, R. E. Popham, W. Schmidt, & R. G. Smart (Eds.), Research advances in alcohol and drug problems (Vol. 1, pp. 1-31). New York: Wiley.

Skinner, B. F. (1938). The behavior of organisms: An experimental analysis. New York: Appleton-Century-Crofts.

Skinner, B. F. (1953). Science and human behavior. New York: MacMillan.

Sulkowski, A., & Vachon, L. (1977). Side effects of simultaneous alcohol and marihuana use. American Journal of Psychiatry, 134, 691-692.

Tec, N. A. (1973). A clarification of the relationship between alcohol and marihuana. British Journal of Addiction, 68, 191-195.

Wikler, A. (1952). A psychodynamic study of a patient during experimental self-regulated re-addiction to morphine. Psychiatric Quarterly, 26, 279-293.

CHAPTER 26

A DRUG PREFERENCE PROCEDURE FOR USE WITH HUMAN VOLUNTEERS

H. de Wit and C. E. Johanson

The University of Chicago
Department of Psychiatry
Drug Abuse Research Center
5841 S. Maryland Avenue
Chicago, Illinois 60637

ABSTRACT

A choice procedure for measuring the reinforcing properties of drugs in humans is described. The use of humans as research subjects is contrasted to the use of laboratory animals in research with psychoactive drugs, and choice measures are contrasted to other measures of reinforcing efficacy. The procedure used in this laboratory is described in detail, and results of several recent studies are summarized. Methodological issues are also discussed.

INTRODUCTION

Laboratory studies of behavior maintained by drugs as reinforcers in animals have gained acceptance as valid experimental models for studying human drug abuse (Thompson & Unna, 1977). This acceptance is based on studies showing that drugs that are abused by humans are also effective reinforcers of behavior in laboratory tests with animals (for reviews see Brady, Griffiths, Hienz, Ator, Lukas, & Lamb, this volume; Johanson & Balster, 1978; Johanson & Schuster, 1981; Weeks & Collins, this volume; Yanagita, this volume). Laboratory animals readily acquire and maintain operant responses when these are followed by delivery of drugs that have high dependence potential in humans (e.g., amphetamine or heroin). In contrast, drugs that are not abused, such as chlorpromazine, do not serve as effective reinforcers in laboratory animals. The study of pharmacological, behavioral, and organismic factors affecting the reinforcing properties of drugs in the laboratory will improve our understanding of factors influencing human drug-taking behavior.

HUMANS AS SUBJECTS

Whereas most studies on the reinforcing properties of drugs have utilized laboratory animals such as rats and monkeys as subjects (Griffiths, Bigelow, & Henningfield, 1980a; Johanson & Schuster, 1981), several researchers have used similar procedures with human subjects. Since work in other areas of behavioral research has shown inter-species generality, it is not surprising that the studies with humans have produced results similar to those with laboratory animals. For example, humans will perform an operant response at a high rate to obtain deliveries of drugs such as pentobarbital (Griffiths, Bigelow, & Liebson, 1976) or alcohol (Mello & Mendelson, 1971, this volume). The patterns of responding observed when a drug is delivered under schedules of intermittent reinforcement are also similar in laboratory animals and humans (Griffiths et al., 1980a) suggesting that the same processes are mediating the behaviors.

There are several distinct advantages to using human subjects in experimental models of drug abuse. First, the inferential steps inherent in generalizing from animal to human drug-taking behavior are avoided. Second, the relation between the subjective effects and the more overt behavioral effects of a drug can be studied in humans. It has often been assumed that certain subjective effects of drugs, such as drug-induced euphoria, are associated with, and may even underlie, the behavior of drug-seeking. This assumption has led some researchers to use only subjective effects of pharmacological agents in humans to predict dependence potential of new, unknown drugs (e.g., Martin & Fraser, 1961). Although there is reason to expect a close relationship between these measures, the association between drug-induced euphoria or any other subjective effect and the behavior of drug-taking must be examined empirically (see Henningfield, Johnson, & Jasinski, this volume; Schuster, Fischman, & Johanson, 1981). It must first be shown that systematic relations exist between drug-induced mood changes and the reinforcing effects of a drug. The further question of whether there is a causal relation between the two actions can only be inferred from the degree of covariance between them under different conditions. Among the possible relations that may exist between subjective effects and behavioral effects of drugs are, for example, that certain drugs are euphorigenic but are not self-administered, while others may be self-administered but produce no euphoria. With yet other drugs, mood alterations other than euphoria, such as decreased anxiety or decreased depression, may form the basis of drug-seeking behavior. Finally, in certain cases the mood-altering effects of a drug may bear no systematic relation at all to whether individuals take it or not. These important relations can only be addressed in behavioral experiments using humans subjects who can report on their internal states.

The use of humans as subjects is also advantageous in the study of individual differences in responsiveness to drugs. Considerable individual differences have been noted in both humans' and animals' tendencies to self-administer drugs. In animal studies these inter-animal differences are often ignored, probably because of the difficulties inherent in studying them. In human subjects, however, these inter-subject differences constitute a rich source of information. A wide range of techniques are available to measure subject differences (e.g., personality tests) and these, combined with a laboratory test of the reinforcing properties of drugs, may reveal important factors underlying drug-taking behavior.

The use of humans as subjects in drug research also has limitations. One of these concerns the amount of control that is attainable over human subjects' current lifestyles and past histories. Animal researchers can arrange that animals within a study have similar pre-experimental histories (e.g., constant supplier, controlled housing and diet conditions, controlled drug and experimental histories). While some aspects of the animals' histories inevitably remain unknown, particularly in the case of monkeys not bred in captivity, the animals' histories can be carefully controlled after arrival in a laboratory. Considerably less control is possible with human subjects, whose diverse experiences, cognitions and current states may influence their behavior in unknown ways, even under highly controlled experimental conditions. Although attempts are made to measure and relate some of these historical variables (e.g., drug use history) to the experimental outcome, these data are limited by their correlational nature. Paradoxically, the variability among individuals' responses that results from the diversity of prior experiences may also lead to the discovery of variables that influence drug-taking behavior simply by increasing the range of factors under study.

Another major limitation of research with human subjects stems from ethical considerations. Clearly, many of the procedures commonly used in animal experiments (e.g., physiological interventions, high drug doses) are not possible with humans, limiting the range of experimental questions that can be addressed using this species. In addition to these procedural limitations, researchers in this area are aware that any exposure to a highly abused drug in an experimental context may entail some risk of subsequent abuse by subjects. This consideration may have practical implications in the experiments such as limiting the range of subjects that can ethically be accepted as well as limiting the frequency with which the drugs can be administered. Thus, ironically, the process of identifying risk factors in individuals may put them at slightly greater risk.

DRUG SELF-ADMINISTRATION PROCEDURES IN HUMANS

Experimenters have used at least two methods to measure the reinforcing properties of drugs in humans. One method uses rate of responding as the dependent variable. In studies using this approach, moderate doses of drugs are made available contingent upon performance of an operant response, such as pushing a button, usually according to a schedule of intermittent reinforcement. The rate of responding is taken as the indicator of the drug's reinforcing efficacy, and the pattern of drug-taking over time can be studied. However, these procedures often entail repeated drug administrations whose frequencies are controlled by the subject. This makes it difficult to determine accurately the quality, magnitude and duration of the drug's direct effects on the organism (e.g., on mood). Rate of responding as a measure of the efficacy of any type of reinforcer has limitations, and this is especially true in the case of drug reinforcers: Factors unrelated to the efficacy of the reinforcer (such as drug effects on the animal's motoric capacity) can influence the rate of responding (Schuster & Johanson, 1975). Methods that employ repeated administrations of drugs in human subjects are also undesirable for ethical reasons.

Preference or choice procedures are a second method that has been used in assessing the reinforcing properties of drugs in humans. These procedures provide a rate-free measure of a drug's reinforcing properties and minimize exposure to the drugs. Typically, subjects initially sample each of two substances on a small number of sampling trials and then choose whichever they prefer on several discrete choice trials. The reinforcing efficacy of a drug is determined by the number of trials it is chosen over a placebo or another drug. Exposure to the drug during sampling is minimized, and the experimenter can arrange to space the trials widely apart (even over days) so that the magnitude and time course of the drug's effects can be accurately monitored.

APPLICATIONS OF HUMAN PREFERENCE TESTS

This laboratory has been testing drug preference in humans for the past 10 years (e.g., de Wit, Johanson, & Uhlenhuth, 1984; de Wit, Johanson, Uhlenhuth, & McCracken, 1983; de Wit, Uhlenhuth, Hedeker, McCracken, & Johanson, 1986a; de Wit, Uhlenhuth, & Johanson, 1985a, 1985b; Johanson & Uhlenhuth, 1977, 1978, 1980a, 1980b). The studies have addressed a variety of questions, including questions about the properties of particular pharmacological agents, about subject variables that influence responses to drugs, and about environmental circumstances that affect responses to drugs. The basic procedure used in these studies will be discussed in the next section, followed by a selection of our findings that will illustrate the applications of the procedure.

Methods

Subjects

In most studies male and female volunteers aged between 21 and 35 are recruited from the university community through newspaper advertisements, posters, and word-of-mouth referrals. About 50% to 75% are students and most of the remainder are faculty or staff associated with the university and hospital. The number of subjects tested in each experiment varies from 12 to 24.

All subjects are carefully screened prior to acceptance into a study. After the initial telephone contact, a screening interview is conducted during which potential subjects complete a battery of psychological tests (e.g., personality tests and a psychiatric symptom checklist) as well as questionnaires pertaining to their medical history and their current and lifetime drug use. A complete psychiatric interview is conducted, and potential subjects with a history of psychosis, major depression, or drug abuse are not accepted. Screening for physical health includes an electrocardiogram and physical examination and, depending on the drug tested, may include further tests.

Prior to participation, subjects sign a consent form which outlines the details of the study and lists the drugs that they might receive. A list of all possible side effects is provided for any drug they might be given. The consent form stipulates that the subject agrees not to take other drugs except his/her normal amounts of coffee and cigarettes before and after taking a capsule for periods of time that are considered safe to prevent drug interactions. In addition, the subject agrees not to drive or operate heavy machinery for 6 hours after capsule ingestion.

Procedure

In each experiment the subjects' relative preference for one of two substances is measured. In most cases the substances compared are a drug and a placebo, but they can also be different doses of one drug or two different drugs. Each experiment consists of seven or nine sessions conducted over a period of 2 or 3 weeks. On each session subjects report to the laboratory between 9 and 10 a.m. to complete pre-drug mood or subjective-effects questionnaires (see below) and to ingest a capsule. Subjects are instructed to note the color of the capsule and to try to associate any drug effects with that color capsule. They are told that the same drug will always be contained in the same color capsule. After taking the capsule, subjects are free to leave the laboratory to resume their normal daily activities, taking with them additional questionnaires to be filled out 1, 3, and 6 hours later. An additional questionnaire is completed at Hour 6 on which subjects indicate how much they liked the drug, whether they noticed any unusual reactions, and what type of drug they thought they had received.

On the first four sessions of each experiment, subjects are given the two substances to sample, once per session, twice in each alternating order. The drug and placebo (or other drug) are contained in color-coded capsules to facilitate future identification, and the colors are varied among subjects to control for color preferences. On the last three to five sessions of each experiment, the procedure is identical except that the subjects are asked to choose between the two different colored capsules. The number of times one substance is chosen over another is taken as an indicator of its reinforcing properties. When the comparison is between a drug and a placebo, it is assumed that the placebo is neutral and that any consistent deviation from chance level of choices of the two substances is due to the drug's reinforcing or aversive properties. When the comparison is between two drugs, preference for one drug may indicate either that one drug has relatively greater positive reinforcing properties or that the other has relatively greater aversive properties.

By allowing subjects to leave the laboratory immediately after taking their capsules on each session, some control over the subjects' behavior is lost, such as in the accuracy of recording the drugs' subjective effects. Nevertheless, the results obtained to date indicate that the method is sensitive and reliable, and that, at least with the subject population currently being tested, subjects complete their questionnaires promptly and candidly. Moreover, mood changes induced by the drugs appear to override normal fluctuations in mood that occur during the course of the day. The subjective-effects measures have proven to be sensitive to differences in the time course and dose of drugs administered and even reflect the changes in mood that occur over the course of the day on sessions when only placebo is administered (e.g., an increase in fatigue in the late afternoon). Thus, despite the relative lack of control of the subjects' behavior (compared to strictly laboratory studies) and despite the myriad other factors that can be presumed to influence mood during the course of the day, the subjective-effects measures appear to be highly sensitive to the drugs' effects. From a practical point of view, the 'outpatient' nature of the procedure entails considerable savings in time and expense for the researcher. From a theoretical point of view, it could be argued that testing the subjects in their normal daily environments increases the validity of the procedure by testing drug responses in a naturalistic setting. This issue will be discussed in greater detail in a later section.

Subjective Effects

The scales used to assess subjective effects include an experimental version of the Profile of Mood States (POMS; McNair, Lorr, & Droppelman, 1971) and a 49-item version of the Addiction Research Center Inventory (ARCI; Haertzen, 1966; Martin, Sloan, Sapira, & Jasinski, 1971; see also Haertzen & Hickey, this volume). The POMS consists of 72 adjectives commonly used to describe momentary mood states. Subjects indicate how they feel at the moment in relation to each of the adjectives on a 5-point scale ranging from not at all (0) to extremely (4). Eight clusters of items have been empirically derived using factor analysis. These clusters, which form the eight subscales of the questionnaire, were given names that best described the clustered adjectives: Anxiety, Depression, Anger, Vigor, Fatigue, Confusion, Friendliness and Elation. Two additional subscales were derived on an intuitive basis from other scales: Arousal = (Anxiety + Vigor) - (Fatigue + Confusion) and Positive Mood = Elation - Depression. Although the POMS was originally developed for use with only a single-administration, researchers in this laboratory pioneered its use with repeated administrations to monitor mood changes over time.

The shortened form of the ARCI consists of 49 true/false items which have been separated into five clusters described as measuring typical drug effects. The Amphetamine (A) and Benzedrine Group (BG) scales measure stimulant-like effects, the Morphine-Benzedrine Group (MBG) scale is thought to reflect drug-induced euphoria, the Pentobarbital-Chlorpromazine-Alcohol Group (PCAG) scale measures sedative-like effects, and the Lysergic-Acid (LSD) scale reflects psychotomimetic effects, often also described as dysphoria (see Haertzen & Hickey, this volume).

Data from these subjective-effects questionnaires can be analyzed using any one of a number of statistical techniques. Most commonly, two- or three-way repeated measures analyses of variance are used, with the factors being Drug (i.e., drugs versus placebo), Hour, and, when comparisons are made among different subject groups, a subject grouping factor (e.g., drug-choosers versus drug non-choosers). The analyses are performed separately on each scale, using the subjects' average scores at each hour on drug and placebo sessions. Data from the sampling sessions only (Sessions 1 to 4) are utilized to minimize expectancy effects which might occur on choice sessions. When significant (p < 0.05) Drug-By-Hour interactions are obtained on any of the subscales, post-hoc tests are conducted to determine the hours at which the drug and placebo scores differ. The data can also be analyzed in other ways. For example, multivariate methods may be used to evaluate a drug's relative effects on different dependence measures (e.g., on different subscales of the mood questionnaires). Analyses may also be performed on difference scores, differences either between pre- and post-drug scores or between placebo and drug session scores. Trend analyses are often useful to describe the time course or dose dependence of a drug's effects. Selection of the appropriate method of analysis depends on the goals of the study and the nature of the data.

Experimental Findings

The choice procedure has been used to evaluate the reinforcing properties of a range of drugs, including stimulants and anorectics as well as tranquilizers and sedatives. The method was first tested with a well-known drug of abuse, d-amphetamine (Johanson & Uhlenhuth, 1980a). Amphetamine is a drug that is reliably self-administered by laboratory animals (Pickens & Harris, 1968). Relative to other drugs, it is a robust reinforcer in many species and under varied environmental circumstances (Johanson & Schuster, 1981). It was therefore not surprising that the majority of human subjects tested in the choice test chose amphetamine (5 mg d-amphetamine) more often than placebo. Subjects (N = 31) chose the drug an average 4 of the 5 choice opportunities. Moreover, amphetamine produced typical, stimulant-like subjective effects and subjects verbally reported liking the drug. Relative to placebo session scores, amphetamine session scores were higher for the Vigor, Elation, Friendliness, Arousal, and Positive Mood subscales of the POMS and lower for the Confusion scale. In subsequent experiments similar results have been obtained with amphetamine and several other stimulant-like drugs. The results of these experiments are summarized in Table 1. Anorectic drugs that produced subjective effects similar to those of amphetamine (e.g., benzphetamine and phenmetrazine) were, on the average, chosen more often than placebo, whereas drugs that produced distinctively different subjective effects (e.g., mazindol and fenfluramine) were chosen as often or less often than placebo.

The procedure has also been used to evaluate the reinforcing properties of the widely prescribed tranquilizer, diazepam (Valium; de Wit et al., 1983,

Table 1

Percent Drug Choice in Experiments With Several Amphetamine-Like
and Non-Amphetamine-Like Anorectic Drugs

Drug	Doses Tested	Percent Choice*	Reference**
A. Drugs with amphetamine-like subjective effects			
d-amphetamine (N = 24)	5, 10 mg	71%	1
benzphetamine (N = 11)	25, 50 mg	71%	2
phenmetrazine (N = 13)	25, 50 mg	63%	2
diethylpropion (N = 10)	25 mg	63%	3
B. Drugs with partially amphetamine-like subjective effects			
phenylpropanolamine (N = 12, 17)	12.5, 25, 50, 75 mg	43%	2
caffeine (N = 18)	100, 300 mg	43%	2
C. Drugs without amphetamine-like subjective effects			
mazindol (N = 12)	0.5, 1.0, 2.0 mg	13%	2
fenfluramine (N = 14)	20 mg	53%	4

Notes: * Percent drug choice is shown for the dose of drug (underlined) at
          which the highest level of choice was obtained.
       ** 1: de Wit, unpublished observations
          2: Chait, unpublished observations
          3: Johanson & Uhlenhuth, 1978
          4: Johanson & Uhlenhuth, 1982

1986a, 1986b; Johanson & Uhlenhuth, 1980b). When tested in laboratory animals,
this and other benzodiazepine drugs have only minimal reinforcing properties
compared to other classes of drugs such as stimulants and opiates. There have
been only occasional reports of animals self-administering benzodiazepines
(Bergman & Johanson, 1985; Griffiths & Ator, 1981; Weeks & Collins, this
volume; cf. Yanagita, this volume). The extent of abuse of these drugs in
humans has been the subject of considerable controversy (Dietch, 1983;
Greenblatt, Shader, & Abernethy, 1983; Rickels, 1981; Woody, O'Brien, &
Greenstein, 1975). While there is concern about the large number of
prescriptions that are written for these drugs, there have been relatively few
documented cases of misuse of these drugs compared to other well-known drugs of
abuse (Marks, 1978). Although physical dependence has been reported in some
cases after prolonged exposure to therapeutic doses of tranquilizers such as
diazepam, the incidence of abuse of benzodiazepines is strikingly low in view
of the large number of people who are exposed to these drugs through
prescription use (Mellinger, Balter, & Uhlenhuth, 1984). Preference for
diazepam has been tested in this laboratory in several studies. Normal

volunteers chose placebo either as often as diazepam or, at higher doses, showed an avoidance of the drug (de Wit et al., 1983; Johanson & Uhlenhuth, 1980b). Whereas lower doses produced negligible subjective effects, the higher doses produced sedation (e.g., decreased Vigor and Arousal and increased Confusion and Fatigue subscale scores of the POMS). Similar results have been obtained with two other benzodiazepines, lorazepam and flurazepam (de Wit et al., 1984, 1985b). Doses of any of these drugs that produced noticeable subjective effects were avoided in the preference test by most of the subjects.

Preferences for several other drugs with sedative properties (e.g., alcohol, pentobarbital) have also been tested using a modified choice procedure in which subjects are tested in a controlled laboratory environment. Results of these studies will be discussed in a later section.

Subject Selection

The results of drug preference tests depend on the subjects who are tested. The appropriateness of a particular subject population in any study depends in part on the experimental question. For example, it has been found subjects with a history of drug abuse are more likely than non-abusing subjects to prefer a drug (such as diazepam) with equivocal reinforcing properties (Griffiths, Bigelow, Liebson, & Kaliszak, 1980b). This may be especially true if the drug shares certain properties with the drugs that these individuals have abused. Thus, these subjects may be appropriate for testing the dependence potential of a new therapeutic agent, particularly if this agent is likely to be prescribed to them and/or if it is believed to have some properties in common with the subjects' known drugs of abuse. However, because of their complex drug use histories, these subjects may be less appropriate in studies designed to assess risks for abuse in the general population or to study individual differences in risk for abuse among drug-naive individuals. For example, our research has shown that normal volunteers do not prefer the tranquilizer diazepam over a placebo, and in fact they avoid it at doses that produced any appreciable subjective effects. This is consistent with epidemiological data from other sources (Mellinger et al., 1984) indicating that the large majority of individuals exposed to benzodiazepines therapeutically or recreationally do not develop patterns of excessive use or abuse of these drugs. Nevertheless, the possibility that some individuals are at risk for dependence on benzodiazepines forms the basis of our investigations with non-drug-abusing subjects.

The drug preference studies in our laboratory have focused on both the behavioral and the subjective responses of non-drug-abusing individuals to identify possible risk factors for abuse. Some studies have utilized a heterogeneous sample of subjects, screened only for age limitations and health for safety reasons, whereas other studies have used individuals who are hypothesized to be a higher-than-average risk for abuse because they possess certain characteristics. The first method may give an indication of the likelihood of abuse in a relatively general or unselected population (taking into account the limitations due to sampling a particular geographic or demographic group and due to the voluntary basis of participation in any experimental study). An advantage of a relatively unselected population is that it provides the variability necessary to study individual differences in responses to the drugs. We have conducted several post-hoc analyses of drug preference studies to explore subject characteristics associated with preferences for or aversions to certain drugs (de Wit, McCracken, Uhlenhuth, & Johanson, 1987a; de Wit, Uhlenhuth, & Johanson, 1986b; de Wit, Uhlenhuth,

Pierri, & Johanson, 1987b; Uhlenhuth, Johanson, Kilgore, & Kobasa, 1981). These analyses have revealed interesting individual differences in subjective response to drugs such as alcohol and amphetamine. For example, subjects who report primarily stimulant-like subjective effects after an acute dose of alcohol (0.5 g/kg) were more likely to show behavioral preference for this drug than subjects who reported predominantly sedative effects from the drug (de Wit et al., 1987b). In another experiment in which preference for amphetamine over placebo was measured, the few individuals who did not prefer the amphetamine in the choice test reported increases in measures of anxiety and depression and no typical stimulant-like effects after ingestion of the drug during sampling sessions (de Wit et al., 1986b). Intuitively logical relations were found in these experiments between the subjective effects of drugs and subjects' behavioral preference (choice). Comparisons can also be made across different drugs to study how drug preferences and aversions can be associated with different subjective effects and with different subject characteristics, depending on the drug.

Other studies have utilized special subject populations hypothesized to be at-risk for abuse. These studies have focused on the "self-medications hypothesis" or the notion that a drug can acquire reinforcing properties through its ability to relieve an aversive state. One subject characteristic hypothesized to be associated with preference for diazepam is anxiety level. The efficacy of benzodiazepines as anxiety-reducing agents is well-known. Thus, assuming that the state of anxiety is an aversive condition, the relief of this state with a drug such as diazepam may be reinforcing in highly anxious subjects. We tested this hypothesis in three groups of anxious subjects (de Wit et al., 1986a, 1987a). One group consisted of subjects who scored high on two standardized anxiety tests (see Speilberger, Gorsuch, & Lushene, 1970; Taylor, 1953) but did not meet criteria for a psychiatric diagnosis. Two groups met criteria for Generalized Anxiety Disorder (APA, 1980). One of these groups consisted of subjects who were sufficiently distressed by their anxiety to desire treatment, whereas the other group was not actively seeking treatment. A control group consisted of subjects who scored within the normal range on anxiety tests. The percent of diazepam choice in each of these groups is summarized in Table 2. The symptomatic subjects did not choose diazepam more often, on the average, than the control subjects. It was found, however, that a small group (N = 4) of the anxious subjects seeking treatment did derive positive effects (i.e., elevated liking scores and apparently positive subjective effects) from the drug and consistently chose it over placebo. Whether these subjects should be considered at-risk for abuse of diazepam or whether their preference in the experiment reflects the genuine therapeutic efficacy of the drug is a question that may be addressed in future research. As important as the finding that certain highly selected subjects did prefer the drug, however, is the finding that the majority of even highly anxious subjects did not choose the drug in preference to a placebo, despite its measurable anxiolytic effects. These findings suggest that the risk for abuse, even for individuals who are most likely to be prescribed these drugs, is low.

Another study examined diazepam preference in older adults. Epidemiological data show that the prescription use of benzodiazepines increases with patients' age (Mellinger et al., 1984). Because high prescription rates are sometimes indicators of excessive or nontherapeutic drug use, the possibility that the reinforcing properties of diazepam increase with age was examined. It was found, however, that subjects aged 40 to 55 years did not exhibit a higher preference for 10 mg diazepam than the control group aged 21 to 35 years.

Table 2

Percent Diazepam Choice in Different Subject Populations

Subject Description	Percent Drug Choice		Reference**
	(5 mg)	(10 mg)	
Normal control (N = 9)	28%	27%	1
Normal control (N = 12)	41%	25%	2
Anxious mood (N = 11)	46%	30%	2
Anxiety disorder (N = 12)	48%	9%	2
Anxiety disorder, seeking treatment (N = 14)	---	42%	3
Older* (N = 11)	47%	38%	4

Notes: * Age 40 to 55 (All remaining subjects were 21 to 35 years of age.)
      ** 1: Johanson & Uhlenhuth, 1980a
         2: de Wit et al., 1986a
         3: de Wit et al., 1987b
         4: de Wit et al., 1986b

Future research of this type may yet reveal subject characteristics which are associated with strong preferences for benzodiazepines or other sedative drugs and allow us to identify patterns of responses that are predictive of risk for abuse. The results with the large majority of subjects tested to date, however, are consistent with epidemiological data and animal self-administration data indicating that, relative to other abused drugs, the risk for dependence on these drugs is low.

The "self-medication hypothesis" has also been investigated in special subject groups with the stimulant amphetamine. In a recent study amphetamine preference was tested in depressed subjects (because of the drug's purported antidepressant properties) and in subjects concerned about being overweight (because of its anorectic properties). We found that neither of these populations showed a stronger preference for amphetamine than a control group (de Wit, unpublished observations).

Thus, the choice procedure can be used with different subject groups to study individual differences in subjective and behavioral responses to drug in a non-abusing population and to test specific hypotheses concerning the basis of non-medical drug use.

Environmental Conditions

Experimental research in behavioral pharmacology over the last 20 years has provided abundant evidence of the importance of environmental variables affecting behavior maintained by drugs as reinforcers. It has been shown that both conditioned and unconditioned contextual factors can increase and decrease responding for drugs across a wide range of drugs, species, and individuals (Johanson, 1975; Young, Herling, & Woods, 1981). In view of these strong environmental influences, results from individual experiments must be interpreted with caution, since they generally employ only one, closely circumscribed set of experimental conditions.

The context in which a drug's effects are experienced may influence whether it is preferred in a choice test. For example, when stimulant drugs are tested in the daytime, outpatient procedure, their subjective effects are consistent with and may even facilitate the subjects' daily activities requiring concentration and alertness. In contrast, sedative-like drugs, some of which may have positive subjective effects in other contexts, are likely to be avoided in the daytime test because they interfere with psychomotor and cognitive performance. Therefore, we adapted our methodology to test preferences for sedative-like drugs in a laboratory-based recreational environment, where outside demands on the subjects' behavior and attention were eliminated. Subjects are tested during the evenings in a comfortable room with a couch, television, games, and movies. They are tested in groups of four and are free to engage in recreational activities of their choice. Under these circumstances preliminary results indicate that a substantial proportion of subjects will choose drugs with sedative properties, such as alcohol (50% to 75% drug choice, depending on experimental conditions) and pentobarbital (45% to 52% drug choice). The level of drug choice appears to be related to both subject characteristics (e.g., drinking history) and aspects of the testing environment (e.g., dose regimen). Preference studies with diazepam under these circumstances are currently in progress. Although direct comparisons of results obtained in the outpatient and laboratory procedures cannot be made, the preliminary findings obtained with ethanol and pentobarbital are consistent with what is expected from other laboratory and epidemiological data. Further data are needed to establish whether the laboratory procedure will provide a valid measure of drug preferences in normal volunteers. It seems likely, however, that a suitable, undemanding context in which to experience the drugs' effects may be a necessary condition for the observation of reinforcement from sedative-like drugs.

Environmental variables have also been shown to attenuate the reinforcing properties of an otherwise highly reinforcing drug, amphetamine. Amphetamine is preferred over placebo when it is administered during the course of normal working days (de Wit et al., 1986b; Johanson & Uhlenhuth, 1980a). However, subjects who were required to take their capsules late in the day (between 4 and 5 p.m.) showed a lower preference (53% drug choice) for 5 mg d,l-amphetamine over placebo than subjects who took the drug between 9 and 10 a.m. (80% drug choice; de Wit et al., 1985a). Some subjects in the afternoon group complained that the drug interfered with their ability to sleep at the normal times, which may have been a reason for the decreased preference. Whatever the reasons, this experiment indicated that a nonpharmacological variable such as time of day of drug administration can influence the drugs efficacy as a reinforcer. Other researchers (Griffiths, Bigelow, & Liebson, 1977) have also shown that self-administration of a drug (i.e., alcohol) which is normally reinforcing in humans can be decreased by an environmental manipulation such as a time-out procedure.

CONCLUSION

In this chapter we have described a drug preference procedure that has been used to test the reinforcing properties of drugs in humans. Some of the advantages as well as the problems with the use of human experimental subjects were discussed, and these were illustrated with examples from this laboratory.

The method can be used to address experimental questions about the pharmacological properties of an unknown drug or about organismic or environmental variables that influence the reinforcing properties of drugs in humans. The method also provides an opportunity to integrate two historically independent approaches to the study of drug dependence, human subjective-effects reports and animal self-administration techniques. Whereas the subjective-effects measures in humans have traditionally been obtained without a concurrent behavioral measure of reinforcement, the animals self-administration experiments have been limited to the measurement of overt behavior. An exploration of the relationship between the internal stimulus properties of a drug and its effects on behavior, in particular its reinforcing effects, using procedures such as the one described here will improve our understanding of the determinants of excessive drug use in humans.

ACKNOWLEDGMENTS

Our thanks to M. Fischman, G. Heyman, and L. Chait for their helpful comments. The research was supported by a grant from the National Institute on Drug Abuse (DA 02812).

REFERENCES

American Psychiatric Association. (1980). Diagnostic and statistical manual of mental disorders, third edition. American Psychiatric Association Washington, DC.

Bergman, J., & Johanson, C. E. (1985). The reinforcing properties of diazepam under several conditions in the rhesus monkey. Psychopharmacology, 86, 108-113.

de Wit, H., Johanson, C. E., & Uhlenhuth, E. H. (1984). Reinforcing properties of lorazepam in normal volunteers. Drug and Alcohol Dependence, 13, 31-41.

de Wit, H., Johanson, C. E., Uhlenhuth, E. H., & McCracken, S. (1983). The effects of two non-pharmacological variables on drug preference in humans. In L. S. Harris (Ed.), Problems of drug dependence, 1982 (National Institute on Drug Abuse Research Monograph 43, pp. 251-257). Washington, DC: U.S. Government Printing Office.

de Wit, H., McCracken, S. M., Uhlenhuth, E. H., & Johanson, C. E. (1987a). Diazepam preference in subjects seeking treatment for anxiety. In L. S. Harris (Ed.), Problems of drug dependence, 1986 (National Institute on Drug Abuse Research Monograph 76, pp. 248-254). Washington, DC: U.S. Government Printing Office.

de Wit, H., Uhlenhuth, E. H., Hedeker, D., McCracken, S., & Johanson, C. E. (1986a). Lack of preference for diazepam in anxious volunteers. Archives of General Psychiatry, 43, 533-541.

de Wit, H., Uhlenhuth, E. H., & Johanson, C. E. (1985a). Drug preference in normal volunteers: Effects of age and time of day. Psychopharmacology, 87, 186-193.

de Wit, H., Uhlenhuth, E. H., & Johanson, C. E. (1985b). Lack of preference for flurazepam in normal volunteers. Pharmacology Biochemistry & Behavior, 21, 865-869.

de Wit, H., Uhlenhuth, E. H., & Johanson, C. E. (1986b). Individual differences in the behavioral and subjective effects of amphetamine and diazepam. Drug and Alcohol Dependence, 16, 341-360.

de Wit, H., Uhlenhuth, E. H., Pierri, J., & Johanson, C. E. (1987b). Individual differences in behavioral and subjective response to alcohol. Alcoholism: Clinical and Experimental Research, in press.

Dietch, J. (1983). The nature and extent of benzodiazepine abuse: An overview of recent literature. Hospital and Community Psychiatry, 34, 1139-1145.

Greenblatt, D. J., Shader, R. L., & Abernethy, D. R. (1983). Current status of benzodiazepines, Parts 1 and 2. New England Journal of Medicine, 309, 354-358 & 410-416.

Griffiths, R. R., & Ator, N. A. (1981). Benzodiazepine self-administration in animals and humans: A comprehensive literature review. In S. I. Szara & J. P. Ludford, (Eds.), Benzodiazepines: A review of research results, 1980 (National Institute on Drug Abuse Research Monograph 33, pp. 22-36). Washington, DC: U.S. Government Printing Office.

Griffiths, R. R., Bigelow, G. E., & Henningfield, J. E. (1980a). Similarities in human and animal drug-taking behavior. In N. K. Mello (Ed.), Advances in substance abuse: Behavioral and biological research (Vol. I, pp. 1-90). Greenwich, CT: JAI Press.

Griffiths, R. R., Bigelow, G., & Liebson, I. (1976). Human sedative self-administration: Effects of interingestion interval and dose. Journal of Pharmacology and Experimental Therapeutics, 197, 488-494.

Griffiths, R. R., Bigelow, G., & Liebson, I. (1977). Comparison of social time-out and activity time-out procedures in suppressing ethanol self-administration in alcoholics. Behavioral Research and Therapy, 15, 329-336.

Griffiths, R. R., Bigelow, G. E., Liebson, I., & Kaliszak, J. E. (1980b). Drug preference in humans: Double-blind choice comparison of pentobarbital, diazepam, chlorpromazine and placebo. Journal of Pharmacology and Experimental Therapeutics, 215, 649-661.

Haertzen, C. A. (1966). Development of scales based on patterns of drug effects using the Addiction Research Center Inventory. Psychological Reports, 18, 163-194.

Johanson, C. E. (1975). Pharmacological and environmental variables affecting drug preference in rhesus monkeys. Pharmacological Review, 27, 343-355.

Johanson, C. E., & Balster, R. L. (1978). A summary of the results of a drug self-administration study using substitution procedures in primates. Bulletin of the Narcotics, 30, 43-54.

Johanson, C. E., & Schuster, C. R. (1981). Animal models of self-administration. In N. K. Mello (Ed.), Advances in substance abuse: Behavioral and biological research, Vol. 2. Connecticut: JAI Press, 219-297.

Johanson, C. E., & Uhlenhuth, E. H. (1977). Drug preference in humans. Paper presented at the 1977 meeting of the American Psychological Association, San Francisco.

Johanson, C. E., & Uhlenhuth, E. H. (1978). Drug self-administration in humans. In N. A. Krasnegor (Ed.), Self-administration of abused sub-stances: Methods of study (National Institute on Drug Abuse Research Monograph 20, pp. 68-85). Washington, DC: U.S. Government Printing Office.

Johanson, C. E., & Uhlenhuth, E. H. (1980a). Drug preference and mood in humans: D-amphetamine. Psychopharmacology, 72, 275-279.

Johanson, C. E., & Uhlenhuth, E. H. (1980b). Drug preference and mood in humans: Diazepam. Psychopharmacology, 71, 269-273.

Johanson, C. E., & Uhlenhuth, E. H. (1982). Drug preference in humans. Federation Proceedings, 233, 228-233.

Marks, J. (Ed.) (1978). The benzodiazepines. Baltimore: University Park Press.

Martin W. R., & Fraser, H. F. (1961). A comparative study of physiological and subjective effects of heroin and morphine administered intravenously in postaddicts. Journal of Pharmacology and Experimental Therapeutics, **133**, 388-399.

Martin, W. R., Sloan, J. W., Sapira, J. D., & Jasinski, D. R. (1971). Physiologic, subjective and behavioral effects of amphetamine, methamphetamine, ephedrine, phenmetrazine and methylphenidate in man. Clinical Pharmacology and Therapeutics, **12**, 245-258.

McNair, D. M., Lorr, M., & Droppelman, L. F. (1971). Profile of mood states (Manual). San Diego, CA: Educational and Industrial Testing Service.

Mellinger, G. D., Balter, M. B., & Uhlenhuth, E. H. (1984). Prevalence and correlates of the long-term use of anxiolytics. Journal of the American Medical Association, **251**, 375-379.

Mello, N. K., & Mendelson, J. H. (1971). A quantitative analysis of drinking patterns in alcoholics. Archives of General Psychiatry, **25**, 527-539.

Pickens, R., & Harris, W. C. (1968). Self-administration of d-amphetamine in rats: Effects of reinforcement magnitude and fixed-ratio size. Psychopharmacologia, **12**, 158-163.

Rickels, K. (1981). Are benzodiazepines overused and abused? British Journal of Clinical Pharmacology, **11**, 715-835.

Schuster, C. R., Fischman, M. W., & Johanson, C. E. (1981). Internal stimulus control and subjective effects of drugs. In T. Thompson & C. E. Johanson (Eds.), Behavioral pharmacology of human drug dependence (National Institute on Drug Abuse Research Monograph **37**, pp. 116-129). Washington, DC: U.S. Government Printing Office.

Schuster, C. R., & Johanson, C. E. (1975). The use of animal models for the study of drug abuse. In R. J. Gibbins, Y. Israel, H. Kalant, R. E. Popham, R. E. Schmidt, and R. B. Smart, (Eds.), Recent advances in alcohol and drug problems (Vol. 1, pp. 1-31). New York: John Wiley and Sons.

Speilberger, C. E., Gorsuch, R. L., & Lushene, R. E. (1970). State-trait anxiety inventory. Test manual for form X. Palo Alto, CA: Consulting Psychologists Press.

Taylor, J. A. (1953). A personality scale of manifest anxiety. Journal of Abnormal and Social Psychology, **48**, 285-290.

Thompson, T., & K. R. Unna (Eds.) (1977). Predicting dependence liability of stimulant and depressant drugs. Baltimore: University Park Press.

Uhlenhuth, E. H., Johanson, C. E., Kilgore, K., & Kobasa, S. C. (1981). Drug preference and mood in humans: Preference for d-amphetamine and subject characteristics. Psychopharmacology, **74**, 191-194.

Woody, G. E., O'Brien, C. P., & Greenstein, R. (1975). Misuse and abuse of diazepam: An increasing common medical problem. International Journal of the Addictions, **10**, 843-848.

Young, A. M., Herling, S., & Woods, J. H. (1981). History of drug exposure as a determinant of drug self-administration. In T. Thompson & C. E. Johanson (Eds.), Behavioral pharmacology of human drug dependence (National Institute on Drug Abuse Research Monograph **37**, pp. 75-89). Washington, DC: U.S. Government Printing Office.

CHAPTER 27

CLINICAL PROCEDURES FOR THE ASSESSMENT OF ABUSE POTENTIAL

Jack E. Henningfield, Rolley E. Johnson, and Donald R. Jasinski

Addiction Research Center
National Institute on Drug Abuse
PO Box 5180
Baltimore, Maryland 21224

ABSTRACT

Procedures are described for assessing the abuse liability of drugs and their potential to produce physiological dependence in human volunteers. Abuse liability of a drug is determined by showing that a drug (a) is psychoactive, (b) produces euphoria, and (c) serves as a reinforcer. The strategies currently used to collect such data include objective assessment of euphoria by use of structured questionnaires and the intravenous drug self-administration paradigm. Dependence potential is determined by the ability of a drug to produce withdrawal when chronic administration is terminated (direct addiction procedure) or to block withdrawal when substituted for a drug known to produce physiological dependence (substitution procedure). Physiological dependence is viewed as a concomitant factor in the abuse potential of a drug, but not the cardinal indicator.

INTRODUCTION

Assessment of abuse potential of drugs is presently pursued at several levels of analysis through many subspecialty areas in pharmacology and psychology as evidenced in this volume. The present chapter is a summary of procedures currently used at the National Institute on Drug Abuse's Addiction Research Center to assess abuse potential using human volunteers as research subjects. The methods are essentially those developed over nearly one half century of clinical research at the Addiction Research Center (Jasinski, 1977) and, more recently, supplemented by the strategies of behavioral pharmacology (Thompson & Johanson, 1980). Studies with opioid drugs using both clinical and behavioral pharmacological procedures have generated a model of substance abuse that is the standard to which other forms of compulsive behavior are compared. The strength of these procedures is that they provide a validated means of quantifying abuse potential, as evidenced by studies involving drugs of previously established liability for abuse (cf. Jasinski, 1977; Jasinski, Henningfield, & Johnson, 1984) and studies of new compounds with suspected potential for abuse (Brady & Lukas, 1984).

Most abused substances share, at least, two measurable properties. First, they serve as reinforcers, as determined from animal and human studies of drug self-administration, and secondly they serve as euphoriants, as determined from human self-report data (Jasinski, 1977; Yanagita, 1980). Additionally, abused drugs may be categorized on the basis of their interoceptive stimulus effects, measured by using psychometric instruments in human subjects (Haertzen & Hickey, this volume) or drug discrimination procedures in animals (Colpaert, this volume; Overton, this volume; Woods, Herling & Young, 1982). Drugs of abuse, notably the opioids and sedatives, produce physiological dependence which may be viewed as a rebound phenomenon that accompanies abrupt abstinence after a period of chronic drug administration (Jaffe, 1980). In this review abuse liability refers to those properties of a drug that are critical to the maintenance of compulsive drug-seeking behavior; dependence potential refers only to the ability of the drug to produce physiological dependence (see also Brady & Lukas, 1984). Currently used procedures for quantifying the subjective effects, reinforcing efficacy, and dependence potential of substances will be summarized.

DEPENDENCE POTENTIAL ASSESSMENT

Procedures for assessing a drug's dependence potential were developed in pioneering studies by Himmelsbach and his coworkers during the 1930s and 1940s (Martin & Isbell, 1978). The fundamental observation was that abrupt termination of morphine administration to a person who had been receiving daily doses of morphine produced a sequence of signs and symptoms that could be quantified. Himmelsbach observed that the intensity of this abstinence syndrome was related to the duration and magnitude of the dosing regimen and that certain signs only occurred after termination of a high dose regimen. Early onsetting (within 24 hours) signs of withdrawal of low to moderate intensity were assigned one point; later onsetting, more severe signs, were assigned three points. Himmelsbach's rating scale, in various forms, remains the cornerstone of most studies of opioid withdrawal in human subjects and in animals. An assumption in the studies by Himmelsbach was that the abuse liability of a drug was measured by its potential to produce physiological dependence. However, as will be discussed below, it was subsequently learned that physiological dependence is not the only indicator of abuse liability.

The strategy used to assess opioid withdrawal has been adopted to study withdrawal from sedatives, alcohol, phencyclidine, and, most recently, benzodiazepines. Current adaptations of these methods include characterization of possible withdrawal effects accompanying termination of chronic use of tobacco and psychomotor stimulants.

In the 1960s, Martin, Haertzen, and their colleagues evaluated the subjective concomitants of opioid withdrawal and showed that subjective withdrawal effects did not necessarily covary with physiological withdrawal effects (Jasinski, 1977). These studies showed that termination of cyclazocine administration to cyclazocine-dependent subjects produced significant withdrawal scores but did not increase subjective discomfort or desire to take the drug (Fraser & Isbell, 1960). Two additional examples of the dissociation between physiologic withdrawal and subjective indices are as follows: First is the finding that buprenorphine administration to opioid-dependent subjects can produce physiological signs of withdrawal without subjective discomfort (Jasinski, Haertzen, Henningfield, Johnson, Makzoumi, & Miyasato, 1982). Second is the finding that clonidine administration during morphine withdrawal blocks physiologic signs without a proportional attenuation of subjective discomfort (Jasinski, Johnson, & Kocher, 1985). Clearly, an important area of study remains the investigations of the relations among the physiological, behavioral and subjective phenomena of drug withdrawal.

Another of Himmelsbach's findings was that administration of either codeine or morphine could reverse the opioid abstinence syndrome at any point in its course. This finding established the principle of cross-dependence and provided the foundation of the substitution strategy to determine which drugs were morphine-like (Himmelsbach & Andrews, 1943). Similar strategies were applied to the measurement and treatment of sedative and alcohol withdrawal in the 1950s; cross-dependence also characterized these drugs.

The procedure initially used by Himmelsbach to study dependence potential was termed the direct addiction procedure. Essentially, volunteers were given gradually increasing doses of the drug and then were maintained for a time (usually a week or more) on a scheduled dosing regimen that maintained relatively high and stable blood levels of the drug. Drug administration was then terminated, and signs and symptoms of withdrawal were measured. Withdrawal effects are rebound phenomena which are generally opposite in direction of those produced as a direct result of drug administration and are presumably due to drug-induced neuroadaptation. For example, opioid-induced constipation may be replaced by diarrhea, and sedative-induced muscle relaxation may be replaced with convulsive activity (Jaffe, 1980). Test compounds can be administered during abstinence to assess their ability to either reverse or attenuate the syndrome. This procedure has been most recently used to evaluate possible withdrawal phenomena following buprenorphine administration to volunteers (Jasinski, Griffith, & Pevnick, 1978).

The most common strategy currently used to evaluate new compounds for efficacy in the treatment of opioid withdrawal is the 24-hour substitution procedure described by Fraser and Isbell (1960). Four doses of morphine (15 mg/dose) are given each day for several days. On test days three of the doses are replaced with either saline or graded doses of the test compound or morphine (as a positive control). Under this dosing regimen saline substitution results in reliable onset of early signs and symptoms of opiate withdrawal. The syndrome is reversed by the return to the morphine dosing regimen at the time of the next normally scheduled dose; however, the syndrome is mild enough that research subjects (moderately paid volunteers) tolerate the procedure and will repeat the experiment, permitting each drug condition to be tested in each subject.

The efficacy of clonidine in the treatment of opioid withdrawal was assessed in a recent study utilizing the 24-hour substitution procedure (Jasinski, Johnson, & Kocher, 1985). As mentioned earlier, when clonidine was substituted for morphine, clonidine reversed the sympathetically mediated signs of withdrawal even more effectively than did morphine (Figure 1, upper frame); however, clonidine did not influence self-reported sickness (Figure 1, lower frame). This finding that physiological signs do not necessarily covary with subjective effects is an important concept in strategies for measuring abuse liability. It also is of clinical relevance, because the subjective effects appear to be more important than the physiological effects in predicting abuse liability.

ABUSE LIABILITY ASSESSMENT

Abuse liability is assessed by procedures that predict the likelihood that drugs will be taken in the nonlaboratory setting. The earliest strategies were those which determined the qualitative nature of the subjective effects of drugs. Drugs shown to produce euphoria and feelings of well being were generally those which were abused, while drugs producing no such effects were

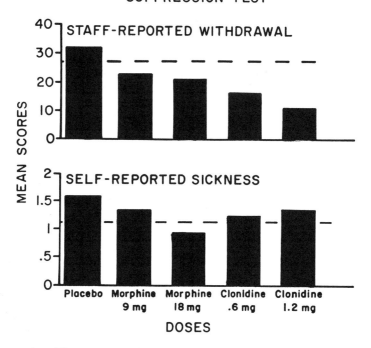

24 HOUR ABSTINENCE SUPPRESSION TEST

Figure 1: Eleven morphine-dependent subjects were given four maintenance doses of morphine each day. On test days these doses were substituted with three doses of morphine, clonidine, or placebo to produce the total daily doses indicated on the abscissa. Mean staff-reported withdrawal scores (including observations such as vomiting and rhinorrhea recorded on the Himmelsbach Scale of opioid withdrawal) are shown in the upper frame. Self-reported sickness scores are shown in the lower frame. Signs (upper frame) and symptoms (lower frame) of withdrawal shown in the figure are mean scores determined 20 to 24 hours following the last maintenance dose of morphine. The dashed line indicates the 95% confidence interval of the mean response to placebo. All doses of morphine and clonidine significantly reduced physiologic signs of withdrawal, whereas only the high dose of morphine reduced subject discomfort. Reprinted with permission from Jasinski, Henningfield, & Johnson, 1984.

not abused (Jasinski, 1977). A more recently developed strategy is to determine the probability that a drug will be voluntarily taken in a laboratory setting by animal and human subjects. Each strategy provides some unique information; however, there is a close correspondence between the predictions resulting from both. For instance, Griffiths and Balster (1979) showed that opioid drugs which serve as reinforcers for animals closely correspond to those drugs that produce morphine-like subjective effects in human subjects (see also, Griffiths, Bigelow, & Henningfield, 1980; Weeks & Collins, this volume).

Quantification of Subjective Effects of Drugs

Unfortunately, there were no generally accepted methods of quantitating subjective effects of drugs early in the twentieth century. The major scientific advance was by Beecher and his colleagues who adapted quantitative bioassay procedures to assess subjective responses to pain stimuli and to the effects of analgesic drugs on such responses (Beecher, 1959). Beecher also established the importance and utility of the crossover design with inclusion of standard and placebo drug control procedures, the double-blind technique, and randomized experimental design to assess subjective drug effects. These pioneers in the assessment of abuse potential of drugs made the following observations that provide the bedrock of current strategies: (a) Drugs produce reproducible transitory psychoactive states, (b) similar states produced by drugs may be used to define drug classes, (c) individuals reliably discriminate drug induced subjective states, (d) the subjective state characteristic of drugs of abuse is one of euphoria, and (e) the nature of the state is related to the propensity to take the drug. A correlate of the observation that abuse liability was not necessarily correlated with physiologic dependence was the observation that it was the subjective effects of drugs that were critical (Jasinski, 1977). The rationale, and even the fundamental scientific strategy used to study abuse liability in humans, was most elegantly described by Isbell (1948):

> Since most people begin the use of drugs and become addicted because the drugs produce effects which they regard as pleasurable, the detection of euphoria is a very important procedure in evaluating abuse liability. The method used is simple: single doses of the drug under test are administered to former drug abusers, and the subjects are unobtrusively watched for a period of 6 hours or more by specially trained observers. For our purposes, euphoria is defined as a series of effects similar to those produced by morphine. These effects are: increased talkativeness, boasting, greater ease in the experimental situation, expression of satisfaction with the effects of the drug, requests for increased doses of the drug, increased motor activity, and, with larger doses, slurring of speech, motor ataxia, and evidence of marked sedation. As many experiments are done as necessary to reach a clear-cut conclusion. The observations are controlled by administering 30 mg of morphine to the same subjects on other occasions. Initially, small subcutaneous doses of the drug under test are used, and if no untoward toxic effects are observed, the dosage is increased progressively in subsequent experiments until evidence of euphoria, roughly equivalent to that produced by 30 mg of morphine is detected or if no evidence of euphoria is detected, the dosage is elevated until further increases would be regarded as dangerous. If euphoria is detected, blind experiments are arranged in which neither the subject nor the observer are aware whether the drug given was morphine or the compound under test. Finally various doses of the drug are administered intravenously.

It is noteworthy that the initial definition of euphoria was judged solely by observed signs, and that the data were exclusively those that could be collected by observers and that the model was based on the effects of morphine.

In recent and ongoing studies at the Addiction Research Center, subjects are tested on a residential research unit, under medical supervision, and formal procedures to protect their rights and welfare (Hickey & Jasinski, note 1). Single doses of drugs are given at sufficient time intervals to eliminate residual drug effects. Drugs are administered according to double-blind procedures. Intervals range from about one hour after short acting drugs such as nicotine to several days after long lasting drugs such as benzodiazepines. Following the drug administration, a variety of physiological, observer-reported (signs or behaviors) and self-reported (symptoms or subjective) effects are assessed at intervals which range from a few seconds to several hours, depending on the time course of drug action.

Typically, the test compound is compared to placebo and to an appropriate positive control (such as morphine in a study of analgesics, or pentobarbital in a study of sedatives). Both the test and control compounds are given at two or more dose levels. A limited number of subjects (usually about 10) participate according to a design whereby every subject is tested under each condition (cross-over or within-subject design). Data are expressed as changes from the pre-drug (baseline) observations and are averaged across subjects. Depending on the temporal pattern, drug effects may be expressed either as peak effect or as the area under the time-action curve for changes in scores.

Self-report measures of subjective drug effects are collected from the subjects using structured questionnaires. The Single-Dose Questionnaire, developed by Fraser and his coworkers (Fraser, Isbell, Martin, Van Horn, & Wolbach, 1961) is among the most elegant psychometric instruments in its simplicity and predictive power. It contains four scales: (a) the first asks whether the drug was felt and thereby determines whether the drug is psychoactive, (b) the second is a 14-item list of substances from which the subject is asked which the administered compound is most like and thereby permits classification (the list includes blank and other), (c) the third is a 14-item list of sensations (including normal and high) that characterizes and quantifies symptoms, and (d) the fourth is a 5-point liking scale which is a measure of euphoria. A similar questionnaire is completed by staff observers.

A variety of drugs have been assessed using the Single-Dose Questionnaire. Figure 2 shows Liking scores obtained following the administration of some of these drugs. As shown in the figure, drugs known to produce widespread compulsive use, such as morphine, d-amphetamine, and pentobarbital, produce dose-related increases in Liking scores. Other substances not known to be abused (e.g., zomepirac, chlorpromazine, or placebo) do not significantly elevate Liking scale scores.

Drug identification responses are also dose-related and a similar effect is also found in animal studies of drug discrimination (Woods, Herling, & Young, 1982). Figure 3 shows that placebo was never identified as drug and that percent of correct drug identification responses for nicotine, nabilone, and diazepam were directly related to drug dose.

Another self-report measure is the Addiction Research Center Inventory (ARCI). The ARCI is a true-false questionnaire with empirically derived scales sensitive to various classes of psychoactive substances (Haertzen, 1974; Haertzen & Hickey, this volume). It contains about 600 items. A 40-item version of the ARCI is used commonly; it contains subsets from three scales: (a) the Morphine-Benzedrine Group (MBG) scale, which reflects feelings of euphoria and well-being; (b) the Pentobarbital-Chlorpromazine-Alcohol Group (PCAG) scale, which reflects sedation and intoxication; and (c) the Lysergic Acid Diethylamide (LSD) specific scale, which may reflect dysphoria and feelings of fear. Scores from the MBG scale usually covary with Liking scale

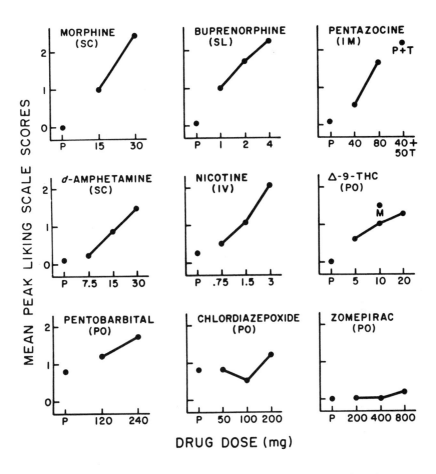

Figure 2: Mean scores on the Liking Scale of the Single Dose Questionnaire from subjects tested at the Addiction Research Center. The number of subjects in each group range from 6 (pentobarbital and chlordiazepoxide) to 13 (d-amphetamine). The high dose of each drug except zomepirac produced significant (p < 0.05) increases in scores above placebo data. The responses are peak responses which occurred after the drug had been given. The time of the peak response ranged from about 1 minute (nicotine) to 5 hours (buprenorphine). Morphine and zomepirac data are from the same group of subjects as are the pentobarbital and chlordiazepoxide data. The P+T point on the pentazocine graph is the score, by the same subjects, to 40 mg pentazocine given in combination with 50 mg tripelennamine (an antihistamine that produced a Liking score of 0.9)--the street combination called "T's and Blue's." The M point on the delta-9-THC graph is the score, from the same subjects, obtained after smoking a marijuana cigarette that contained 10 mg (1% by weight) delta-9-THC. Reprinted with permission from Jasinski, Henningfield, & Johnson, 1984.

DRUG IDENTIFICATION
(SINGLE DOSE QUESTIONAIRE)

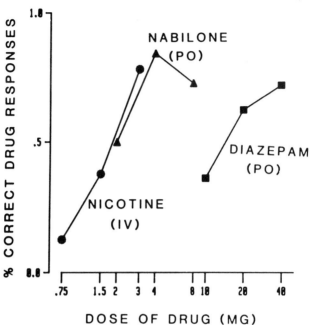

Figure 3: Data are summarized from three different studies involving nicotine (Henningfield, Miyasato, & Jasinski, 1985), diazepam (Jasinski, & Johnson, unpublished observations), and nabilone (Boren, Johnson, & Jasinski, unpublished observations). Percent correct drug identifications of the groups tested are graphed as a function of drug dose (nicotine, n = 8; nabilone, n = 10; diazepam, n = 12).

scores, supporting the notion that this scale reflects euphoric drug effects. Dose-related increases in Liking and MBG scale scores are the cardinal subjective effects of abused drugs and define a drug as a euphoriant.

Verification of self-report data is provided by reports from the trained observers. Observer measures of drug-induced changes in overall subject status include nonstructured reports by trained nurse-research staff and structured questionnaires. The most useful questionnaire is the Observer's Single Dose Questionnaire which is an analogue of the Subject's Single-Dose Questionnaire (described above). Data obtained from trained and vigilant observers parallel those obtained from the subjects' self-reports. Such correspondence between self- and observer-reported data confirmed that self-report data were also reliable and could be objectively quantified and confirmed the premise that subjective drug effects could be objectively assayed (Jasinski, 1981). The use of drug-experienced subjects also enhances the orderliness of the data since such persons have learned to accurately discriminate drug-induced states and do not respond to placebo.

Certain physiological parameters covary with subjective parameters and can also be used to monitor drug activity. Additionally, the physiological data are used to evaluate possible toxic effects of the drugs. Commonly used physiological measures include pupil diameter, heart rate, blood pressure, respiratory rate, oral and rectal temperature. More specialized measures such as electroencephalographic (EEG) responses and changes in neuroendocrine parameters and brain metabolism are also used in certain studies.

From a historical perspective it is interesting to note the changes in the relative role ascribed to what are now termed physiologic and subjective effects of drugs in the phenomenon of drug abuse. In brief, at the beginning of the twentieth century, drug abuse (narcotic addiction) was thought due largely to physiologic processes including immorality and weakness of character. Himmelsbach and colleagues rejected all such mentalistic (subjective) notions and based their studies on observable physiologic consequences of drug taking and drug abstinence. Later, studies by Isbell, Beecher, Frazier, and others showed that subjective responses could be equally valid, if not more important, markers of abuse liability. Subjective responses to drugs are considered the hallmark indicators of abuse potential, and they are now bioassayed with precision comparable to that in physiologic studies. Furthermore, the subjective responses are known to be direct consequences of the activity of pharmacologic agents of specific physiologic loci (e.g., receptors), thus they are no less "physical" than their physiologic concomitants.

Figure 4 provides an example of the data that may be obtained from some of the measures described above. These profiles of pharmacological activity were determined for orally and subcutaneously administered methadone and for subcutaneously administered morphine. As shown in the figure, the drugs differed primarily in their duration of action along certain parameters.

Quantification of Reinforcing Properties of Drugs

A reinforcer is an event that strengthens and maintains behavior leading to its presentation (positive) or removal (negative). By definition, abused drugs are those which serve as reinforcers and thereby maintain drug-seeking behavior. Whether or not reinforcers are pleasant or aversive is an empirical question and is an issue that is not necessarily addressed by procedures for assessing reinforcement. Reinforcing efficacy is directly evaluated in drug self-administration paradigms in which the performance of a specific behavior results in drug administration.

Procedures for the Assessment of Positively Reinforcing Properties of Drugs

In an early study by Wikler, the self-administration behavior was simply the act of preparing a morphine solution, of applying a tourniquet, and of injecting the drug (Wikler, 1952). In animal studies one can arrange for an arbitrary response, such as a lever press, to produce an injection via an implanted cannula (Yokel, this volume) or to present a single dose of a solution which may be consumed orally (Meisch & Carroll, this volume). Mendelson and Mello, at Harvard Medical School, pioneered the adaptation of the drug self-administration methods used with animals to study orally ingested drugs by human subjects (Mendelson & Mello, 1966, this volume). The strategy has since been adapted at several other laboratories (cf. Griffiths, Bigelow, & Henningfield, 1980). Most recently, the strategy has been added to those used at the Addiction Research Center for abuse liability testing.

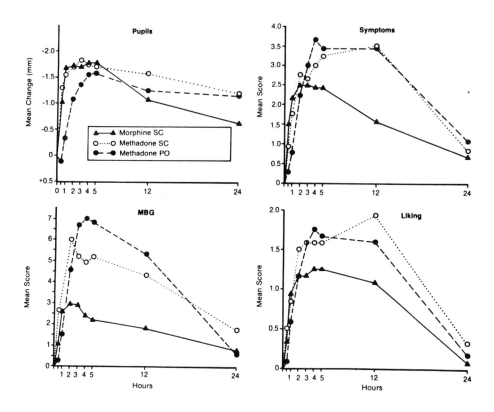

Figure 4: Time-course of morphine sulfate (20 mg/kg, subcutaneous), methadone hydrochloride (20 mg/kg, subcutaneous), and methadone hydrochloride (20 mg/kg, oral), effects on pupillary diameter, opiate symptoms, MBG scale, and subject's Liking. Each point represents the mean of 12 subjects. Reprinted with permission from Martin, Jasinski, Haertzen, Kay, Jones, Mansky, and Carpenter, 1973. Copyright 1973 by The American Medical Association.

At the Addiction Research Center, the intravenous drug self-administration procedure used with animals was explicitly adapted to use with human subjects. Figure 5 shows a schematic of the intravenous drug self-administration paradigm for human subjects. In the initial studies this strategy was utilized to clarify the role of nicotine in cigarette smoking. Pressing a lever produced various levels of nicotine or saline which were delivered via an indwelling forearm catheter to cigarette smokers who were not permitted to smoke during the 3-hour test sessions. The response requirement was 10 lever presses per injection. Injections were about 15 seconds long and were followed by a 1-minute time-out.

In the first seven subjects tested, nicotine maintained orderly patterns of lever-pressing behavior. The patterns resembled those observed when cigarettes are available to cigarette smoking human subjects or when

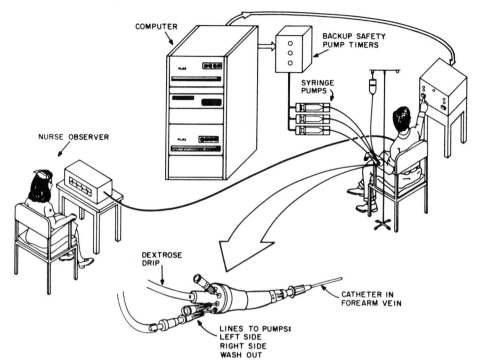

Figure 5: The intravenous drug self-administration paradigm is shown. Prior to the session the subject is equipped with a catheter in a forearm vein. The catheter line is kept patent by a slow intravenous drip. Two different drug solutions can be concurrently provided with the use of a third pump (washout) to push the balance of a dose given from the left or right pumps into the vein.

psychomotor stimulants are available for self-injection by animals. As is discussed in more detail in the chapter by Yokel in this volume (see also the chapter by Meisch & Carroll), demonstration of self-administration behavior is not equivalent to showing that a drug is serving as a reinforcer. In brief, procedures that may be used to demonstrate reinforcing efficacy include (a) substituting saline for drug, (b) providing concurrent access to both drugs and saline, and (c) manipulating drug dose to show that the behavior is sensitive to such manipulations. These procedures are essentially those developed previously in animal drug self-administration studies (Pickens & Thompson, 1968; Yanagita, 1976; Young & Herling, 1983). These procedures are used in the human drug self-administration studies at the Addiction Research Center.

Figure 6 shows acquisition of drug self-administration behavior in a subject without a history of drug abuse. After seven sessions nicotine was replaced with saline. Lever-pressing rates and saline injections increased for three sessions, then decreased to rates below those maintained by nicotine. Such data suggest that the drug itself was necessary for maintenance of the behavior. An additional lever, the operation of which had no scheduled consequence, was available for the subject to press during this study. The

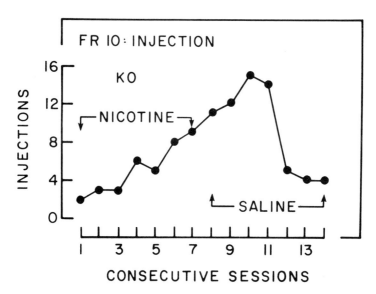

Figure 6: Subject KO was a cigarette smoker without a history of drug abuse. He responded under the simple fixed ratio schedule (FR-10) of nicotine or saline injection. Nicotine was available (1.5 mg nicotine/injection) during seven consecutive sessions; then saline was substituted for an additional seven sessions. Number of injections per session are shown on the ordinate. Reprinted with permission from Henningfield & Goldberg, 1983. Copyright 1983 by ANKHO International, Inc.

subject pressed this lever between 10 and 20 times during the first few sessions and then did not press it any more. This simple procedure demonstrated that injections were necessary for maintenance of lever-pressing behavior.

One of the simplest ways to determine whether or not a drug is serving as a reinforcer is to provide concurrent access to drug and saline and then to alternate the levers which produce either solution. Figure 7 shows the results of this procedure in a subject on the nicotine self-administration study. As shown in the figure, regardless of the lever from which nicotine was obtained, nicotine was consistently preferred to saline. In another study a subject was pretreated with mecamylamine given orally 1 hour before sessions (Henningfield, 1983). As the dose of mecamylamine was increased from 2.5 to 10 mg, nicotine preference to saline decreased. Additionally, postinjection drug liking scores were inversely related to mecamylamine dose.

Finally, in a study by Goldberg and Henningfield (unpublished observations), manipulation of delivered dose for similarly tested human and squirrel monkey subjects produced orderly and similar (across species) changes in behavior. Number of drug injections was inversely related to unit dose, while there was a slight positive relationship between total session drug intake and dose. This sort of compensatory change in the rate of self-administration behavior is typical of that seen when drugs are serving as

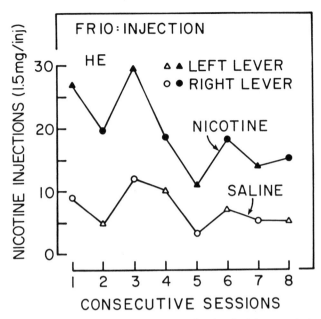

Figure 7: Subject had a history of alcoholism and had been previously tested over a range of nicotine doses. In this study he was given concurrent access to both nicotine (1.5 mg/injection) and saline during 3-hour sessions. Ten responses (FR-10) were required to produce an injection and the levers which were associated with nicotine and saline injections reversed each day. Number of injections per session are shown on the ordinate. As an additional pilot procedure, a mecamylamine capsule was given 1 hour before each session. The mecamylamine doses were: 0 mg, Sessions 1, 3, and 8; 2.5 mg, Sessions 2 and 6; 5 mg, Sessions 4 and 5; 10 mg, Session 7. Mecamylamine attenuated self-reported liking of the nicotine injections and appeared to decrease the rate of nicotine-maintained responding; this may simply have been a trend across sessions. Reprinted with permission from Henningfield & Goldberg, 1983. Copyright 1983 by ANKHO International, Inc.

reinforcers in animal and human subjects (Griffiths, Bigelow, & Henningfield, 1980).

Procedures for the Assessment of Negatively Reinforcing Properties of Drugs

The focus of most abuse potential studies is on the pleasant and the positively reinforcing properties of drugs. However, it is well known that drugs of abuse produce multiple effects which may be both pleasant and aversive. In drug abusing persons, effects considered aversive to non-drug abusers (or effects that were aversive during the drug abuser's initial experience) may become part of the constellation of desired drug effects. For instance, the nausea produced by opioids may be reported as a "pleasant sick"; inability to concentrate, dizziness, and sedation may also be reported as pleasant in the drug abuser (Goldberg, Shannon, & Spealman, 1981; Jasinski, 1977). These effects of drugs may be quantified by their ability to suppress drug-taking behavior (punishing effects) or by their ability to maintain behavior leading to the avoidance of drug administration (negatively reinforcing effects). Such procedures have been developed using animals as subjects (e.g., Goldberg & Spealman, 1982) and were extended to human studies at the Addiction Research Center (Henningfield & Goldberg, 1983).

A subject who self-administered nicotine at a very low rate was tested in a drug avoidance paradigm. Nicotine injections were programmed to be delivered at 15-minute intervals unless the subject blocked the injections by pressing the lever 10 times. As shown in Figure 8, the subject blocked most injections when nicotine was present and took most injections when saline was present. Additionally, ratings of aversive or "bad" effects produced by injections were directly related to avoidance behavior. Additional manipulations in two other subjects showed that the strength of the avoidance behavior was directly related to the dose of nicotine.

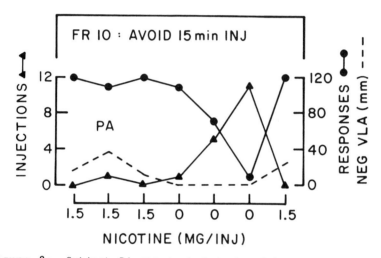

Figure 8: Subject PA was tested during 3-hour sessions on a concurrent schedule in which pressing the right lever (FR-10) produced a nicotine injection and pressing the left lever extinguished the left lever light and avoided the next programmed injection (12 injections were programmed at 15-minute intervals). The dose available was administered once, 15 minutes prior to the start of the session. The subject did not press the right lever. The number of programmed injections and the number of responses (left lever) per session are shown for seven consecutive sessions. The negative Visual Analog Scale scores are the number of mm away from the neutral point on a 100-mm line analogue scale; the instructions on the scale were to place a mark on the line that "indicates the strength of any bad or negative effect which you don't like." The score shown is the mean produced by the first three injections. Reprinted with permission from Henningfield & Goldberg, 1983. Copyright 1983 by ANKHO International, Inc.

DISCUSSION

The strategies which are described in this chapter may be used to evaluate drugs for abuse liability and dependence potential. The theoretical framework underlying such studies is that quantifiable pharmacological properties of drugs determine abuse liability. This theory is not inconsistent with the observation that social, genetic, personality, and other factors are involved in any given instance of substance abuse. Rather, carefully controlled, systematic studies provide a rational means for differentiating substances in accord with the degree to which their pharmacological effects determine their abuse.

It is apparent that techniques developed in studies with human subjects can be adapted to studies with animals (e.g., drug discrimination testing); the converse is also true (e.g., drug self-administration studies). Furthermore, findings from studies with human subjects generally correspond to those obtained with animal subjects, supporting the validity of the methods as well as the biological basis of substance abuse. This cross validation of human and animal findings supports the hypothesis that substances of abuse share common, biologically based mechanisms of action, assessed as euphoriant and reinforcing properties. The ultimate validity of these models of euphoria and reinforcing efficacy will be the extent that they continue to predict and explain the phenomena of drug abuse. An important area of future research will be to further investigate the relationship between subjective drug effects and the properties of drugs as reinforcers.

As is evidenced by the papers in this volume, there are some apparent discrepancies in the evaluation of abuse liability when the results of different methods are compared to one another. For instance, the results of studies involving place preference indicate that drugs known to serve as reinforcers in drug self-administration paradigm may have aversive properties (e.g., ethanol). These findings, however, may not be discrepant at all but may simply reflect the different functional properties of drugs that are measured by the two procedures. The self-administration procedure is a measure of propensity to take a drug while the place preference procedure may reflect the qualitative nature of certain interoceptive effects of drugs.

The notion that drugs of abuse produce both noxious and pleasurable effects is well known. In animal studies, as well, it has been shown that drugs known to serve as reinforcers under certain conditions serve as negative reinforcers and punishers under other conditions (Goldberg & Spealman, 1982; Spealman, 1983; see also, Wise, de Wit, & Yokel, 1976). Observations made from the human studies of intravenous nicotine self-administration may help to resolve these discrepancies. In the human studies it is concurrently possible to assess the reinforcing properties of the drugs, as evidenced by response rate measures, and to assess the degree of noxious and pleasurable effects produced by the drugs (Henningfield, 1983; Henningfield & Goldberg, 1983). Results from an ongoing study suggest that while a drug may be administered at a monotonic rate across a 3-hour session, the subjective effects may change considerably. Typically, liked effects diminished across successive injections (tolerance) while disliked (toxic) effects increased. Following sessions, it was not unusual for a subject to report that he would have taken more injections than he did except that the pleasurable effects of the drug were counterbalanced by noxious effects (e.g., nausea, burning in the arm, dizziness). These data provide direct evidence that a range of subjective drug effects may occur when a drug is serving as a reinforcer and that simple measurement of the nature of the effect may not be a reliable predictor of propensity to take the drug.

Thus, self-administration data may provide a means of quantifying the abuse liability of a drug, while measures of subjective effects (e.g., pleasure inducing or place preference) may be more useful in the descriptive pharmacology of the drug.

The advent of new strategies and the refinement of old strategies for assessing abuse liability and dependence potential have paralleled new concepts underlying the process of drug dependence. The fundamental advance was the finding that drugs of abuse produce orderly changes in mood and feeling (e.g., euphoria), that these effects could be quantified using bioassay-like procedures, and that these changes generally correspond with reinforcing efficacy. Another major conceptual advance was the discovery that physiological dependence was neither necessary nor sufficient to maintain drug-seeking behavior. On the contrary, abuse is maintained by the reinforcing properties of substances, and these properties do not necessarily vary as a function of physiological dependence. Finally, the self-administration paradigm provides a means to quantify the reinforcing properties of substances. Findings from these strategies have blurred the distinction between psychological and physiological dependence--the subjective and reinforcing properties of drugs are clearly a function of physiological alterations in the central nervous system.

REFERENCES

Brady, J. V., & Lukas, S. E. (Eds.) (1984). Report on the assessment of abuse liability and dependence potential (National Institute on Drug Abuse Research Monograph 52). Washington, DC: U.S. Government Printing Office.

Fraser, H. F., & Isbell, H. (1960). Human pharmacology and addiction liabilities phenazocine and levophenalcylmorphan. Bulletin on Narcotics, 12, 15-23.

Fraser, H. F., Van Horn, G. D., Martin, W. R., Wolbach, A. B., & Isbell, H., (1961). Methods for evaluating addiction liability. (A) "Attitude" of opiate addicts toward opiate-like drugs. (B) A short term "direct" addiction test. Journal of Pharmacology and Experimental Therapeutics, 133, 371-387.

Goldberg, S. R., Shannon, H. E., & Spealman, R. D. (1981). Psychotropic effects of opioids and opioid antagonists. In F. Hoffmeister & G. Stille (Eds.), Handbook of experimental pharmacology. (Vol. 55, pp. 269-304). Berlin: Springer-Verlag.

Goldberg, S. R., & Spealman, R. D. (1982). Maintenance and suppression of responding by intravenous nicotine injections in squirrel monkeys. Federation Proceedings, 41, 216-220.

Goldberg, S. R., Spealman, R. D., Risner, M. E., & Henningfield, J. E. (1983). Control of behavior by intravenous nicotine injections in laboratory animals. Pharmacology Biochemistry & Behavior, 19, 1011-1020.

Griffiths, R. R., & Balster, R. L. (1970). Opioids: Similarity between evaluations of subjective effects and animal self-administration results. Clinical Pharmacology and Therapeutics, 25, 611-617.

Griffiths, R. R., Bigelow, G. E., & Henningfield, J. E. (1980). Similarities in animal and human drug taking behavior. In N. K. Mello (Ed.), Advances in substance abuse: Behavioral and biological research. (pp. 1-90). Greenwich, CN: JAI Press.

Haertzen, C. A. (1974). An overview of addiction research center inventory scales (ARCI): An appendix and manual of scales (DHEW Publication No. ADM 74-92). Washington, DC: U.S. Government Printing Office.

Henningfield, J. E. (1983). Measurement issues in cigarette smoking research: Basic behavioral and physiological effects and patterns of nicotine self-administration. In J. Grabowski, & C. S. Bell (Eds.), Measurement issues in tobacco research and treatment (National Institute on Drug Abuse Research Monograph 48, pp. 27-38). Washington, DC: U.S. Government Printing Office.

Henningfield, J. E., & Goldberg, S. R. (1983). Control of behavior by intravenous nicotine injections in human subjects. Pharmacology Biochemistry & Behavior, 19, 1021-1026.

Henningfield, J. E., Miyasato, K., & Jasinski, D. R. (1983). Cigarette smokers self-administer intravenous nicotine. Pharmacology Biochemistry & Behavior, 19, 887-890..

Henningfield, J. E., Miyasato, K., & Jasinski, D. R. (1985). Abuse liability and pharmacodynamic characteristics of intravenous and inhaled nicotine. Journal of Pharmacology and Experimental Therapeutics, 234, 1-12.

Hickey, J. E., & Jasinski, D. R. (note 1). Protection of the rights and welfare of human subjects. Manuscript in preparation.

Himmelsbach, C. K. & Andrews, H. L. (1943). Studies on modification of the morphine abstinence syndrome by drugs. Journal of Pharmacology and Experimental Therapeutics, 77, 17-23.

Isbell, H. (1948). Methods and results of studying experimental human addiction to the newer synthetic analgesics. Annals of the New York Academy of Sciences, 51, 108-122.

Jaffe, J. H. (1980). Drug addiction and drug abuse. In A. G. Gilman, L. S. Goodman, & A. Gilman (Eds.), The pharmacological basis of therapeutics (pp. 535-584). New York: Macmillan.

Jasinski, D. R. (1977). Assessment of the abuse potentiality of morphine like drugs (methods used in man). In W. R. Martin (Ed.), Drug addiction I: Morphine, sedative/hypnotic and alcohol dependence (Handbook of Experimental Pharmacology, Vol. 45, pp. 197-258). Berlin: Springer-Verlag.

Jasinski, D. R. (1981). Opiate withdrawal syndrome: Acute and protracted aspects. Annals of the New York Academy of Sciences, 362, 183-186.

Jasinski, D. R., Griffith, J. D., & Pevnick, J. S. (1978). Human pharmacology and abuse potential of the analgesic buprenorphine. Archives of General Psychiatry, 35, 501-516.

Jasinski, D. R., Haertzen, C. R., Henningfield, J. E., Johnson, R. E., Makhzoumi, H. M., & Miyasato, K. (1982). Progress report of the Addiction Research Center. In L. S. Harris (Ed.), Problems of drug dependence, 1981 (National Institute on Drug Abuse Research Monograph 41, pp. 45-52). Washington, DC: U.S. Government Printing Office.

Jasinski, D. R., Henningfield, J. E., & Johnson, R. E. (1984). Abuse liability assessment in human subjects. Trends in Pharmacological Sciences, 5, 196-200.

Jasinski, D. R., Johnson, R. E., & Kocher, T. R. (1985). Clonidine in morphine withdrawal: Differential effects on signs and symptoms. Archives of General Psychiatry, 42, 1063-1066.

Lukas, S. E., & Griffiths, R. R. (1982). Precipitated withdrawal by a benzodiazepine receptor antagonist (RO 15-1788) after 7 days of diazepam. Science, 217, 1161-1163.

Martin, W. R. (1977). Chemotherapy of narcotic addiction. In W. R. Martin (Ed.), Drug addiction I: Morphine, sedative/hypnotic and alcohol dependence (Handbook of Experimental Pharmacology, Vol. 45, pp. 279-318). Berlin: Springer-Verlag.

Martin, W. R., & Isbell, H. (1978). Drug Addiction and the U.S. Public Health Service (DHEW Publication No. 77-434). Washington, DC: U.S. Government Printing Office.

Martin, W. R., Jasinski, D. R., Haertzen, C. A., Kay, D. C., Jones, B. E., Mansky, P. A., & Carpenter, R. W. (1973a). Methadone--a reevaluation. Archives of General Psychiatry, 28, 286-295.

Mendelson, J. H., & Mello, N. K. (1966). Experimental analysis of drinking behavior of chronic alcoholics. Annals of the New York Academy of Science, 133, 828-845.

Spealman, R. D. (1983). Maintenance of behavior by postponement of scheduled injections of nicotine in squirrel monkeys. Journal of Pharmacology and Experimental Therapeutics, 227, 154-159.

Thompson, T., & Johanson, C. E. (Eds.). (1981). Behavioral pharmacology of human drug dependence (National Institute on Drug Abuse Research Monograph 37). Washington, DC: U.S. Government Printing Office.

Thompson, T., & Schuster, C. R. (1968). Behavioral pharmacology. Englewood Cliffs, NJ: Prentice-Hall.

Wikler, A. (1952). A psychodynamic study of a patient during self-regulated readdiction to morphine. Psychiatric Quarterly, 26, 270-293.

Wise, R. A., de Wit, H., & Yokel, R. A. (1976). Both positive reinforcement and conditioned aversion from amphetamine and from apomorphine in rats. Science, 191, 1273-1275.

Woods, J. H., Herling, S., & Young, A. M. (1982). Classification of narcotics on the basis of their reinforcing, discriminative, and antagonist effects in rhesus monkeys. Federation Proceedings, 41, 221-227.

Yanagita, T. (1976). Some methodological problems in assessing dependence-producing properties of drugs in animals. Pharmacological Reviews, 27, 503-509.

Yanagita, T. (1980). Self-administration studies on psychological dependence. Trends in Pharmacological Sciences, 161-164.

CHAPTER 28

OPERATIONALIZING AND MEASURING THE ORGANIZING
INFLUENCE OF DRUGS ON BEHAVIOR

Norman M. White, Claude Messier, and Geoffrey D. Carr

Department of Psychology
McGill University
1205 Dr. Penfield Avenue
Montreal, Quebec, Canada   H3A 1B1

ABSTRACT

This paper examines the use of conditioning methods to measure the organizing influence on behavior of natural reinforcers and of the reinforcing drug amphetamine. The problems associated with the objective measurement of reward and aversion are discussed and it is suggested that the tendency to approach or to withdraw from stimuli associated with reinforcers can provide an objective index of the rewarding or aversive value of these reinforcers. However, reinforcing drugs do not provide an external reference point; consequently, researchers have used conditioning methods that promote the association of external stimuli with the internal effect of the drug. The advantages of these associative conditioning methods and the problems of interpretation associated with them are discussed. The fact that some reinforcing drugs also have the separate property of improving memory is presented as a special interpretative problem. This discussion of the measurement of the organizing influence of reinforcers on behavior is illustrated by experiments using three different associative conditioning methods: taste conditioning and two place conditioning methods (preference and runway). These methods were used to assess the organizing influence of peripheral and central d-amphetamine, sucrose, and saccharin solutions.

INTRODUCTION

Reinforcement is the process that occurs in the nervous system when contact with certain stimulus events (called reinforcers) produces a change in behavior. The administration of certain drugs (called reinforcing drugs) often produces behavioral changes that resemble those produced by naturally reinforcing events. This similarity of effect has led to the view that the influences on behavior of natural reinforcers and of reinforcing drugs can be studied using similar assumptions and techniques. Our approach involves the parallel analysis of the effect of these two types of events on behavior. This approach may help to reveal the neural basis of the influence on behavior exerted by both natural reinforcers and by reinforcing drugs.

It is generally agreed that reinforcers can have two different qualities. Although there is not agreement on terminology, these qualities have been described as positive and negative or as rewarding and punishing. The corresponding reinforcement processes initiated by these events are referred to as reward and aversion. The fact that most workers use the terms reinforcement and reward or aversion and punishment interchangeably suggests that these qualities of reinforcement form the basis of thinking about the process. A discussion of the reinforcement process can therefore begin with a consideration of these qualities.

Present notions of reward and aversion emerge from a long line of philosophical and psychological thought. The pleasure principle--the idea that individuals behave so as to maximize pleasure and minimize pain--is present in the writings of the Epicureans, the Hedonists, and the Freudians. The theory of evolution can be used to predict that behaviors promoting survival are associated with pleasure and that behaviors impeding survival are associated with pain. However, these teleological views clearly relate to the affective experience of individuals rather than to the objective measurement of the influence of events on behavior. The psychologist P.T. Young (1959, 1961, 1966) made an important contribution to thinking on this issue because he recognized both the existence of affective experience and the need to study the behavior associated with it in an objective manner.

Contributions of P. T. Young

Young developed the preference technique as a measure of the affective properties of environmental stimuli. He argued that the best measure of affect consists of brief exposures to two stimuli, followed by a test to see which of the two is preferred. He stressed that drawing conclusions about the affective value of stimuli requires that the experimenter observe the development of a preference and that this method measures only relative preference.

In one series of experiments, Young and Falk (1956) measured preference for sodium chloride solutions. They observed that preference for these solutions increased with concentration up to a certain point but decreased at higher concentrations--a conclusion confirmed electrophysiologically by Pfaffman (1960). Young and Christensen (1962) showed that preference for a sucrose solution is increased by adding a low concentration of salt and that preference for the same sucrose solution is decreased by adding a higher concentration of salt. Therefore, the affective properties of stimuli summate algebraically to determine the final level of preference. Algebraic summation of lateral hypothalamic self-stimulation (reward) and lithium chloride injections (aversion) has more recently been demonstrated by Ettenberg, Sgro, and White (1980).

One property of the affective states produced by stimuli and implied by the notion of algebraic summation is their sign: They can be rewarding or aversive. Reward and aversion exist on an affective continuum (Young, 1959), and, at any moment in time, an animal occupies one and only one position on the affective continuum with respect to a particular stimulus. The position may be rewarding, neutral, or aversive, and it may be the outcome of the summation of several different processes with different affective signs relating to the same or different stimuli. In a given environment the presence of one or more reinforcing stimuli therefore serves to organize an animal's behavior by influencing "neurobehavioral patterns" that serve to "orient the organism towards or against the stimulus object" (Young, 1961). Four issues of relevance to the problem of measuring the effects of drugs on behavior are raised by this brief summary of Young's views.

Neurobehavioral Patterns

Like other psychologists of his time (e.g., Hebb, 1949; Hull, 1951), Young understood that the behaviors he observed were mediated by events in the nervous system but was unable to discuss these events because little information about them was available. However, his approach was conducive to the eventual study and elucidation of these neural events because of his willingness to consider the existence of a (intervening) variable such as affect. With the techniques for studying the nervous system available to today's behavioral neuroscientist, the prospect of describing Young's organizing neurobehavioral patterns and substituting them for the concept of affect becomes real.

Pharmacological techniques are among those that can be of value in locating and studying the neural substrates of behavioral organization. Some reinforcing drugs may act directly on these substrates. Others may act indirectly on central or peripheral systems which influence these substrates. It is also possible for a drug to act on more than one substrate. To study these possibilities we require an objective method of measuring the affective influence of drugs on behavior.

Objective Measurement of Reward and Aversion

A preference for one of two stimuli implies either that the affect produced by the preferred stimulus is relatively rewarding or that the alternative choice produces relative aversion. Young pointed out that the actual observation in this situation is a tendency for an animal to orient towards or away from a reinforcing stimulus. It seems clear that conclusions about the affective properties of stimuli are in fact based on observation of the orientation and approach or withdrawal behaviors they produce. The tendency to orient towards, to approach, and to maintain contact with a stimulus is interpreted as evidence of a rewarding process. The tendency to orient away from a stimulus and to withdraw from it is taken as evidence of aversion. The preference method gives us an operational definition of reward and aversion in terms of approach and withdrawal, thereby allowing their objective study.

The fact that certain stimuli produce approach and others produce withdrawal must surely be among the most elementary behavioral observations that can be made. Schneirla (1959; Maier & Schneirla, 1964) has emphasized that these two behavioral tendencies are properties of the simplest living organisms (including plants and the single-celled amoeba) and that they are present in all animals including humans. Herrick (1948) describes how whole-body movements towards or away from environmental stimuli are controlled by undifferentiated nervous systems of primitive organisms and how in higher animals there is a parallel increase in the specificity of the behavioral response and the differentiation of the neural substrate controlling it.

In measuring approach and withdrawal tendencies, we study elementary properties of behavior mediated by neural substrates which, in a more or less differentiated form, are present in all living organisms and which act to organize behavior. The concepts of affect and reward or aversion that were useful to Young as substitutes for knowledge about the neural substrate of approach and withdrawal can now be put into their proper perspective as manifestations of individual experience. These manifestations are irrelevant to the objective study of affect because they are accessible only by introspection. An equally intractable question is whether or not affective states exist in the absence of behaviors such as approach and withdrawal. We can, however, answer questions about the influence of natural and pharmacological events on the neural substrates of approach and withdrawal by quantifying these behaviors.

Given that this is what we can measure, we should be careful to state what we mean by the terms reward and aversion. Reward is activity in the brain that promotes approach and maintenance of contact, and aversion is activity in the brain that promotes withdrawal. One of our major goals is, of course, to state precisely what is meant by "activity in the brain." The use of pharmacological techniques is a major tool in the effort to arrive at this definition.

It should also be noted that defining affect in terms of approach and withdrawal means that the study of these phenomena is no longer confined to the use of preference methods. Other methods of measuring the same two classes of behavior could, in principle, provide equally valid information about the effects of reinforcers on the neural substrates which organize behavior. In a later section we describe our efforts to develop a measure of approach using a runway.

The Role of Learned Associations

External stimuli play an essential role in the development and detection of approach and withdrawal. These behaviors can exist only in the presence of some external stimulus to which they can be referred by both the animal and the experimenter. In the case of experiments using food, the sight, smell, and taste of the stimulus provide the external reference point required for either of the behaviors to develop. As the animal consumes a sweet food, for example, the neural substrate mediating approach and maintenance of contact becomes activated, and the discriminable environmental stimuli become associated with this activated state. If this learned association is retained (and this memory may be facilitated by the reinforcer), the animal will exhibit the same behavior when it next encounters the same situation, leading to increased consumption of the sweet food.

Other events which do not naturally provide external stimulus reference points may also activate the neural substrates of approach or withdrawal (The question of whether or not this occurs is one that can be answered empirically.), but these behaviors cannot develop in the absence of such external stimuli. A classic instance of this problem was the discovery of the so-called "medicine effect" by Harris, Clay, Hargreaves, and Ward (1933). These workers showed that when rats deficient in vitamin B1 were offered a choice among a number of foods, they quickly learned to prefer the taste of the only one that contained B1 if the taste of that food was discriminable from the tastes of the alternate foods offered. If the vitamin was present in one of several foods with the same taste, the animals failed to exhibit a preference for it. Thus, in the absence of an external stimulus, the behavioral effects of replacement therapy were neither expressed nor measurable. In the presence of such a reference point, the animals learned a tendency to approach and maintain contact with the discriminable B1-containing food, and this tendency was observed as increased consumption of that food.

The medicine effect clearly illustrates a problem of measuring the organizing effect of reinforcing drugs on behavior. Regardless of how or where any drug may interact with the nervous system, it is clear that it cannot provide an external reference point. Therefore, neither approach nor withdrawal will be expressed or detected unless the drug is administered in an experimental situation which includes discriminable stimuli and which promotes the formation of an association between those stimuli and any effect the drug may have on the neural substrates of approach or withdrawal.

Successful techniques for measuring the rewarding or aversive properties of drugs have, in fact, used this method. The conditioned taste aversion (CTA) method (Goudie, 1979; Revusky & Bedarf, 1967) promotes the formation of an association between the organizing effects of drugs and novel tastes. Conditioned place (Kumar, 1972) and runway (White, Sklar, & Amit, 1977) methods promote the formation of associations between the effects of drugs and the visual, olfactory, and tactile stimuli that constitute a given experimental environment. Such associations are also formed in self-administration paradigms. Providing a discriminative stimulus signaling delivery of the reinforcer accelerates acquisition of bar-pressing responses for intragastric food (Holman, 1969) and for intravenous amphetamine (Thompson, Bigelow, & Pickens, 1971).

The use of associative conditioning methods to measure the organizing influence of drugs on behavior has at least one advantage. During training the influence of the drug is paired with neutral stimuli, but during testing the animal's behavior is free from any direct influence the drug may have on behavior because the drug is not administered. This is particularly important in the case of drugs thought to affect motor behavior (e.g., pimozide: Ettenberg, Cinsavitch, & White, 1979). It should be kept in mind, however, that conditioned physiological changes may occur on the test day in the absence of the drug (e.g., the temperature change produced by morphine; Eikelboom & Stewart, 1979) and that such effects could influence behavior directly.

Dual Action of Reinforcers

The fact that a learning process is required to measure the approach and withdrawal behaviors produced by reinforcing drugs necessitates a consideration of the role of reinforcers in learning. Reinforcers initiate two processes that are relevant here. The first process is the influence of the stimulus properties of reinforcers on the neural substrates of approach and withdrawal. As described in the previous section, some neutral stimulus becomes associated with this influence. The second process is the influence of reinforcers on an animal's tendency to remember this association. Young (1940) may have been the first to point out that although the stimulus properties of reinforcers serve to organize behavior, they have no influence on an animal's tendency to remember this organizing influence. However, it seems clear that some nonstimulus property of reinforcers can initiate a memory improving process.

In a series of experiments, Major and White (1978) and Coulombe and White (1980) showed that electrical self-stimulation of certain brain regions can improve memory independently of its rewarding properties. More recently, Messier and White (1984) used a conditioned taste preference (CTP) paradigm to identify solutions of sucrose and of saccharin with equivalent organizing influences on behavior (i.e., pairing a flavored solution with each of the sweet substances produced equal preferences for the paired taste). Subsequent experiments in which the animals drank these same solutions after training on a conditioned emotional response (CER) task showed that sucrose improved memory for the CER but that saccharin had no such effect. Subcutaneous injections of glucose also improved memory. These data show that although the organizing influence of the solutions depended on their stimulus properties, the memory improving action of sucrose must have been the result of some postingestional effect. It should be noted that this memory improving action of reinforcers is not essential for retention; it merely facilitates storage if it is present.

The distinction between the organizing and the memory-improving processes initiated by reinforcers is important for two reasons. First, evidence exists that some reinforcing drugs influence memory independently of their organizing influences (amphetamine: Carr & White, 1984; Doty & Doty, 1966; Krivanek & McGaugh, 1969; morphine: White, Major, & Siegal, 1978). Second, as previously discussed, techniques for measuring the organizing action of drugs rely on the formation of learned associations which must be remembered.

Problems of Interpretation with Conditioning Methods

Associative conditioning methods involving taste or place are used to obtain information about the tendency of reinforcing events, including drugs, to organize behavior by producing approach or withdrawal. Inferences about the sign and amplitude of the organizing properties of reinforcers are made from observation of animals' responses to the conditioned stimuli. However, the interpretation of responses to conditioned stimuli as measures of the organizing properties of reinforcers is constrained by certain features of the associative conditioning process itself.

As already discussed, two processes are involved when an associative conditioning procedure causes a change in behavior. First, the animal must experience the associative relationship between a neutral stimulus and the stimulus properties of the reinforcer. Second, the animal must remember this association. Both of these processes present interpretative problems.

Associative Bias

It is well-known that stimuli and responses differ in their associability (Garcia & Koelling, 1966; Glickman, 1973; Moore, 1973; Seligman, 1970; Shettleworth, 1973), a phenomenon that can be referred to as associative bias. According to this principle, variability of observed responses to conditioned stimuli in taste or in place conditioning experiments may be due to differences in the tendency of the organizing properties of a reinforcer to become associated with a given conditioned stimulus rather than to variability in the amplitudes of the organizing influences themselves. Another problem is the possibility that a drug may act at more than one site in the brain and that the behavioral influence of these different actions can be expected to summate algebraically, obscuring the fact that the observed behavior is the result of more than a single action.

Data already available for the drug amphetamine provide a good example of these problems. Peripheral administration of this drug in a taste conditioning paradigm gives evidence of aversion (Carey, 1973), but administration of similar doses in a place conditioning paradigm gives evidence of reward (Reicher & Holman, 1977). The considerations under discussion suggest the hypothesis that amphetamine may exert organizing influences with opposite signs by acting on more than one neural substrate. One of these influences is a direct or indirect activation of the substrate of withdrawal, and this activation may have an associative bias for taste stimuli. The other influence is activation of the neural substrate of approach, and this action of the drug may have an associative bias for place stimuli. In the following sections we describe our investigations of this hypothesis.

Memory of the Association

Since some drugs have a memory improving effect as well as an organizing influence on behavior, variability in observed responses to the conditioned stimuli could be due to variability in either process. It is possible to imagine two substances with equally strong organizing influences on behavior but with different memory improving properties. In such a case clear approach or withdrawal relative to the conditioned stimulus may be observed for the substance that promotes the memory of the association between its own organizing properties and the stimulus, but much weaker responses or no responses at all may be observed for the substance that does not promote retention of this memory. For example, White and Carr (1985) found that although conditioned place preferences are observed when sucrose solutions are used as the reinforcers, equally rewarding saccharin solutions have no such effect. When postpairing, memory-improving treatments (injections of glucose or amphetamine) followed the saccharin- and control-environment pairings preferences were observed, confirming the role of memory improvement in this situation.

The distinction between the organizing and the memory-improving effects of drugs must be stressed. In particular effects on memory cannot change the sign of an organizing influence. Even if a memory effect distorts the appearance of an organizing effect, such distortion cannot include changing approach into withdrawal or vice versa. Therefore, a detected behavioral tendency is a reliable index of a neural process. The problems of interpretation arise in the absence of an observed effect, or in trying to compare the organizing properties of different reinforcers, or in comparing the same reinforcer using different methods.

In our laboratory we have investigated the effects of "natural" reinforcers (cases where the nature of the organizing influence is generally accepted) and of reinforcing drugs on approach and withdrawal using taste conditioning and two types of place conditioning methods. We have tested the ability of each method to detect rewarding and aversive influences of natural reinforcers. We have also studied the effects of amphetamine on behavior in each of the paradigms. These experiments provide information on the usefulness of each of the methods for measuring the organizing properties of a reinforcing drug. They also form an initial test of the hypothesis that amphetamine has more than one organizing influence on behavior by acting at more than one site in the brain.

TASTE CONDITIONING METHOD

The use of taste conditioning methods to measure the organizing properties of reinforcing stimuli rests on the discovery of a phenomenon that has come to be known as the conditioned taste aversion (CTA: Garcia, Kimmeldorf, & Hunt, 1957; Richter, 1945, 1953). There is a large literature demonstrating that the pairing of a variety of taste stimuli with a number of different treatments causes animals to withdraw from the paired taste on future occasions (Garcia, Hawkins, & Rusiniak, 1974; Revusky & Garcia, 1970). In most cases there was already reason to believe that the treatments producing these effects were aversive, and the demonstration that these reinforcers produced CTAs served to confirm this information and to validate the method. However, the demonstration that CTAs are produced by certain self-administered drugs (e.g., morphine: Cappell, LeBlanc, & Endrenyi, 1973; Jacquet, 1973; and amphetamine: Carey, 1973) was regarded as paradoxical because the fact that they are self-administered suggests that they are rewarding, not aversive.

Natural Reinforcers

There have also been a few demonstrations that taste conditioning methods can be used to measure the rewarding effects of various reinforcers. The medicine effect (Harris et al., 1933) already described was the first example of this phenomenon. More recently, it has been shown that pairing a session of drinking a novel tasting solution with a sweetener (Holman, 1975) or with a session of electrical self-stimulation of the brain (Ettenberg & White, 1978) resulted in a subsequent preference for the solution with the novel flavor. Since we wished to validate the ability of this method to measure reward as well as aversion, we paired the drinking of flavored solutions with the sweet taste of sucrose and saccharin to determine if the approach tendencies one would expect these rewarding events to produce could be detected by this method.

Rats were presented with two flavored solutions simultaneously over a two day period: For each rat sucrose or saccharin was mixed with one of the solutions, resulting in the pairing of a novel flavor with a sweet taste. When offered a choice between the two flavors with no sweeteners, the rats drank significantly more of the solutions that had been paired with all concentrations of sucrose and saccharin (see Figure 1). Since each of the flavors was paired for half of the animals in each group, this result cannot be attributed to preferences for the flavors themselves and must therefore be attributed to the formation and retention of an association between the conditioned taste stimuli and the rewarding effect of the sweet substances.

These results show that the conditioned taste method can be used to detect the organizing properties of at least some reinforcers that tend to produce approach and maintenance of contact. The facts that both sucrose and saccharin produced approximately equal shifts in responding to the conditioned taste stimuli and that saccharin has no reliable postingestional effect (Steffens, 1969a, 1969b) suggest that the tastes of the two reinforcers were the sources of their organizing influences. This conclusion is consistent with a previous suggestion of Holman (1975).

Amphetamine

Taking this confirmation of the ability of the taste conditioning method to detect the rewarding effects of natural reinforcers together with the data on the CTA which demonstrate its ability to detect a drug's aversive effects as a validation of the method, we applied it to the study of the organizing properties of amphetamine. In our first experiment we replicated previous findings (Carey, 1973) that pairing of drinking a flavored solution with an injection of the drug produces withdrawal from the conditioned taste stimulus, suggesting aversion (see Figure 2). The conclusion that the data for the amphetamine-paired animals represent a genuine conditioned withdrawal response to the taste is supported by the fact that the animals in the unpaired group, in which plain water was paired with a drug injection, consumed more of the flavored solution on test day than did the rats in the paired group.

Our next step was to use this taste conditioning method to determine if the site of amphetamine's aversive action in the brain could be detected by injecting the drug directly into local brain sites. Wagner, Foltin, Seiden, and Schuster (1981) showed that the CTA produced by systemic injections of amphetamine is attenuated by (relatively) selective depletions of brain

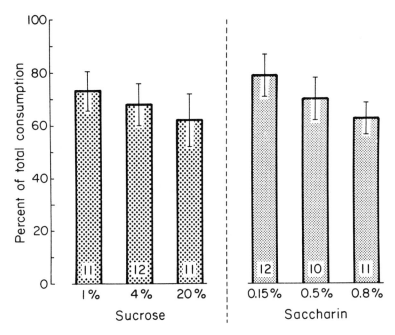

Figure 1: Effect of natural reinforcers on taste conditioning. Each bar shows consumption of paired solutions (together with standard errors and numbers of subjects) during 30-minute preference test following 48 hours of experience with almond- and chocolate-flavored solutions. During the 48-hour pairing, one of the solutions (almond for half of the subjects and chocolate for the other half) available to the rats in each group was adulterated with sucrose or saccharin. During the 30-minute test period the flavored solutions were unadulterated. Consumption of paired solution was significantly higher than consumption of unpaired solution for all groups [F (1,61) = 32.09, p < 0.01].

dopamine. Since a major pharmacological action of amphetamine in the CNS is a facilitation of endogenous dopaminergic activity (Fuxe & Ungerstedt, 1970; Sulser & Saunders-Bush, 1971), this finding suggests that dopaminergic neurotransmission may be the basis of the aversive organizing influence of amphetamine. Accordingly, we decided to inject the drug into three of the major forebrain areas known to contain dopamine: nucleus accumbens, caudate nucleus, and amygdala. There is also evidence (Berger, Wise, & Stein, 1972; McGlone, Ritter, & Kelley, 1980) that the CTAs produced by various toxins (e.g., lithium chloride, although not amphetamine) are abolished by thermal lesions of area postrema. We also selected the region around this structure as an injection site.

Pairing a session of drinking flavored solutions with direct microinjections of amphetamine into nucleus accumbens, caudate nucleus, or amygdala had no effect on the animals' subsequent behavior towards the paired tastes (see Figure 3). As discussed above, however, this result must by

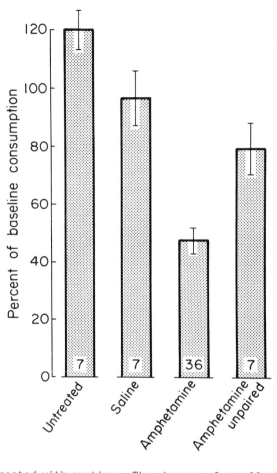

Figure 2: Effect of amphetamine on taste conditioning. Each bar shows the mean amount of solution with paired taste consumed during a 15-minute test 24 hours after pairing. On pairing day the rats in the first three groups shown all drank a solution of instant decaffeinated coffee and almond extract in water for 10 minutes. Following this the rats in the untreated group received no treatment, the rats in the saline group received subcutaneous injections of physiological saline, and the rats in the amphetamine group received subcutaneous injections of 2 mg/kg d-amphetamine sulphate in saline. The rats in the amphetamine unpaired group drank water and then received the same injection of amphetamine. Each bar shows the standard error of the mean and the number of subjects. The amount of coffee consumed by the rats in the amphetamine groups was significantly lower than the amounts consumed by the rats in the other groups [$F_{(3,53)} = 20.17$, $p < 0.001$].

treated with caution. The absence of an effect may have been caused by the lack of an organizing influence of amphetamine at these brain sites, by the inability of the animals to associate the taste stimuli with this influence, or by their inability to remember the association if it was formed. As also shown in Figure 3, pairing of a taste stimulus with microinjection of amphetamine into the region around the area postrema caused a reduction in consumption of the solution with the paired taste, suggesting that the drug acted at this site in the brain to initiate a withdrawal response.

These data suggest that the aversive action of amphetamine that is observed when taste stimuli are paired with peripheral injections may occur because of an action of the drug in the region around the area postrema. We suggest that the site of action is in the region of the area postrema but not restricted to the structure itself because lesions restricted to the structure do not block the aversive action of amphetamine observed in a taste conditioning paradigm (Berger, Wise, & Stein, 1972). This finding does not, of course, preclude the possibility that amphetamine may also have aversive or rewarding influences on behavior by acting at other brain sites.

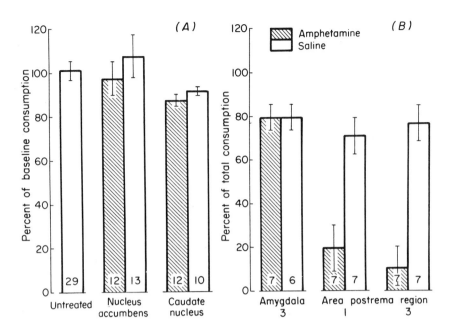

Figure 3: Effect of local microinjections of amphetamine on taste conditioning. Cannulae were aimed at the following Pellegrino, Pellegrino, and Cushman (1979) coordinates, and subsequent histological examination confirmed that the tips were clustered around these points (all referred to stereotaxic zero): Caudate 7.8 mm anterior, 4.0 mm lateral, 1.0 mm above; accumbens, 9.4, 1.5, 0.0 (cannulae angled 20 degrees to avoid ventricle); central nucleus of amygdala 6.2, 4.0, -2.0; area postrema -4.5, 0.0, -7.0. Data for rats in the untreated, accumbens, and caudate groups are shown in **A**. These animals experienced a single pairing of a coffee-almond flavored solution followed by an injection of 10 μg d-amphetamine sulphate in 0.5 μL physiological saline or saline alone. The data shown are for a 30-minute drinking period with only the flavored solution available. Data for the rats in the amygdala and area postrema groups are presented in **B**. These rats experienced one or three pairings of a maple-sucrose solution followed by 20 μg amphetamine in distilled water or an isomotic injection of saline solution. The data shown are for a 30-minute test with the flavored solution and water available. All injections were administered over 30 seconds. The numbers of subjects in each group and the standard errors of the means are shown on each bar. The only significant effects are for the area postrema injections with one pairing [t (12) = 3.48, p < 0.005] and three pairings [t (12) = 4.82, p < 0.001].

Summary

It is well known that the taste conditioning paradigm can detect the aversive consequences of various toxic substances by producing withdrawal from the conditioned taste stimuli. A smaller amount of data, including those presented here, suggest that, in some circumstances at least, the technique can also detect the rewarding effects of reinforcing events by producing approach and maintenance of contact with the conditioned taste stimuli. In our attempts to use this method to study the organizing influence on behavior of amphetamine, we replicated previous findings that the technique detects an aversive action of peripherally administered amphetamine and showed that a central microinjection of the drug into the region of area postrema produces a similar effect. No effects of microinjections into caudate nucleus, nucleus accumbens, or amygdala were detected. These data suggest that amphetamine may exert at least part of its aversive organizing influence on behavior through an action on neural tissue in the region of area postrema. Further experiments will be necessary to confirm this suggestion.

PLACE CONDITIONING: PREFERENCE METHOD

A version of the place preference method was first used to study the behavioral effects of morphine by Beach (1957). More recently, other versions of the method were used by Kumar (1972), by Rossi and Reid (1976), and by Mucha, van der Kooy, O'Shaughnessy and Bucenieks (1982). It is based on the idea that when animals experience the organizing influence of a reinforcer in the presence of the constellation of stimuli constituting a distinctive environment, they learn an association between the stimuli and the organizing influence. On future occasions these learned associations lead the animals to approach and maintain contact with or to withdraw from the conditioned stimuli. The technique has been used to detect the rewarding effect of food (Spyraki, Fibiger, & Phillips, 1982a) and the aversive effect of lithium chloride injections (Ettenberg, van der Kooy, LeMoal, Koob, & Bloom, 1983; Mucha et al., 1982). Rewarding effects of morphine (Mucha et al., 1982; Rossi & Reid, 1976) and of amphetamine (Reicher & Holman, 1977; Spyraki, Fibiger, & Phillips, 1982b) have also been detected with this method.

In our work with the place preference technique, we use the apparatus illustrated in Figure 4. On the first day of our experiments, the rats are allowed to explore the apparatus freely for 10 minutes. On each of the following 12 days, each rat is confined in one of the two large compartments and experiences a reinforcing or a control event. In each group of each experiment, half of the rats experience the reinforcer in compartment "A" on the even numbered days and the control treatment in compartment "B" on the odd numbered days. The other half of the rats experience the control event in compartment "A" and the reinforcer in compartment "B." On Day 14 each rat is placed into compartment "C" and allowed to move freely in the apparatus for 20 minutes. The amount of time each rat chooses to spend in each of the two large compartments is measured. If the rats spend significantly more time in the presence of the reinforcer-paired stimuli than with the control-paired stimuli, we conclude that the reinforcer produced a tendency to approach and to maintain contact. If the rats in a group choose to spend significantly less time in the presence of the reinforcer-paired stimuli than with the control-paired stimuli, we conclude that the reinforcer produced a tendency to withdraw. Pilot experiments have shown that rats run through this procedure with no reinforcers exhibit approximately equal preferences for the two large compartments.

Natural Reinforcers

We began our work with this method by attempting to verify its ability to detect conditioned approach and withdrawal produced by known rewarding and

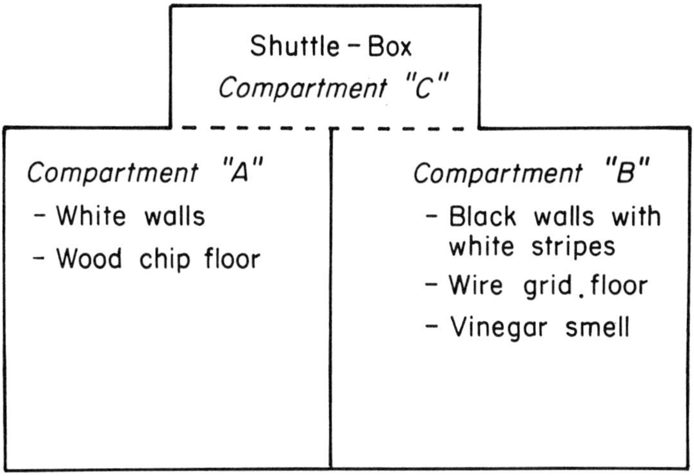

Figure 4: Plan view of the place conditioning apparatus. Compartments A and B (45 X 45 X 30 cm) have wooden walls and tops and Plexiglas fronts. The distinguishing stimulus features of the two environments are shown on the figure. Compartment C is constructed entirely of wood. The dotted line represents a removable wooden partition.

aversive events. Using the same three concentrations of sucrose we had used to test the taste conditioning method, we observed a relationship between concentration of sucrose and amount of time spent on the paired side but a clear preference for the paired side only when the 20% sucrose solution was the reinforcer (see Figure 5). By comparison, all three of these concentrations of sucrose produced significant preferences in our taste conditioning experiment, and the lowest preference was observed with the 20% solution (see Figure 1). The difference in the effect of the 20% sucrose solution can be explained by the fact that, unlike the rats in the taste experiment, the rats in the place experiment were food-deprived, a condition that is known to increase the preferred concentration of sucrose (Collier & Bolles, 1968).

It is also worth noting that the present place conditioning method detected the rewarding effect of sucrose after only six 30-minute pairings, while 48 hours of continuous pairing in our experiment and ten 60-minute pairings in Holman's (1975) experiment were required to detect reward using the taste conditioning method. Although the procedures of the various experiments do not permit precise comparisons, the suggestion that the place method may be a more sensitive measure of reward than the taste method is worth further study.

Figure 5 also shows our attempt to detect the influence of an aversive event in this apparatus, using an injection of a moderate dose of lithium chloride as the reinforcer. Our failure to detect a significant effect of this dose of lithium is in contrast to the significant aversion we observed with the same dose in using the taste conditioning method (see Figure 5, inset). Using a higher dose of lithium (60 mg/kg), however, we have observed significant aversion using our place conditioning method, confirming findings from other

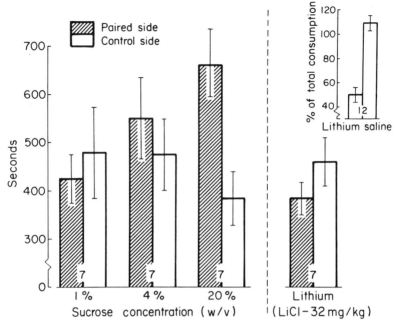

Figure 5: Effect of natural reinforcers in place conditioning. All rats in the sucrose groups were on a 22 hour food deprivation schedule. All rats were allowed to drink their reinforcing solution freely while on their paired sides of the apparatus and were given no treatment on their control sides. Each bar shows the standard error of the mean and the number of subjects in each group. The 20% sucrose reinforcer produced a significant preference [t (6) = 2.34, p < 0.05]. The rats in the lithium chloride group were given an intraperitoneal injection of 32 mg/kg (0.75 mEq/kg) lithium chloride in distilled water (15 mg/cc) before being placed into their paired sides and an injection of an equivalent volume of physiological saline before being placed into their control sides. There was no significant effect of the lithium treatment. The inset shows the significant aversion [t (11) = 6.89, p < 0.01] produced by a single pairing of a maple-flavored solution with the same dose of lithium in a taste conditioning experiment. The animals in this experiment also experienced pairings of a saccharin-flavored solution with a saline injection in random order with respect to the maple-lithium pairing. Data are for a 30-minute test with appropriate flavored solutions available.

laboratories (Ettenberg et al., 1983; Mucha et al., 1982). These findings suggest that the taste method may be a more sensitive detector of aversion than the place method.

Amphetamine

Our next step was to replicate and extend previous findings that the place preference technique can detect a rewarding effect of peripherally administered amphetamine. Using four different doses of amphetamine as reinforcers, we observed significant preferences for the paired side at the three higher doses and a significant dose-response measure of the tendency of amphetamine to produce approach and maintenance of contact (see Figure 6).

As has been noted, the finding that amphetamine produces evidence of reward in this paradigm is in contrast to the evidence of aversion the same drug gives in the taste conditioning paradigm. To continue our investigation of the hypothesis that these two effects are due to actions of the drug at different brain sites, we tested the effects of intracerebral microinjections of amphetamine, aimed at the same four sites tested with the taste method, using the place conditioning method. A significant preference for the paired

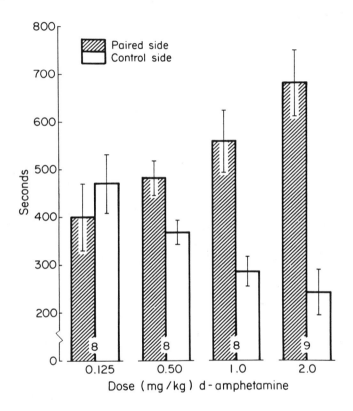

Figure 6: Effect of peripherally injected amphetamine on place conditioning. Each rat was injected subcutaneously with one of the indicated doses of amphetamine (in 1 cc/kg physiological saline) before being placed into its paired side and with an equivalent volume of saline before being placed into its control side. Each bar shows the standard error of the mean and the number of subjects. Significant preferences were observed at 0.5 [t (7) = 2.13, p < 0.05], 1.0 [t (7) = 3.74, p < 0.005], and 2.0 [t (8) = 4.07, p < 0.005] mg/kg. In addition, a significant dose-response relationship (r = 0.61, p < 0.001) was found for the four doses tested.

side was observed only for rats that experienced injections into nucleus accumbens (see Figure 7). This finding suggests that peripherally injected amphetamine may produce its rewarding effect by acting at this site, although it does not, once again, eliminate the possibility that the drug may also have a similar action at other sites. Given the fact that the primary effect of amphetamine in nucleus accumbens is release of endogenous dopamine, this finding suggests that dopaminergic function in nucleus accumbens may act to

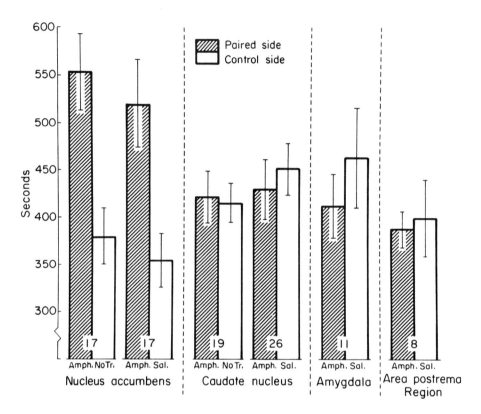

Figure 7: Effect of intracerebral microinjection of amphetamine on place conditioning. All injection parameters were the same as those used in the taste conditioning experiments (except that the dose in the amygdala groups was 10 µg). Rats tested in the amphetamine-saline condition received intracerebral injections of amphetamine before being placed into their paired sides of the place apparatus and the same volume of isotonic saline solution into the same brain areas before being placed into their control sides. Rats tested in the amphetamine-no treatment condition were injected with amphetamine before being placed into their paired sides and received no treatment before being placed into their control sides. Each bar shows the standard error of the mean and the number of subjects. Significant preferences for the paired sides were observed for both nucleus accumbens groups (saline control: t (16) = 2.01, p < 0.05; no treatment control: t (16) = 3.25, p < 0.01).

produce approach and maintenance of contact with external stimuli. This conclusion is consistent with results reported by other workers: Self-administration of amphetamine (Lyness, Friedle, & Moore, 1979) and of cocaine (Roberts, Koob, Klonoff, & Fibiger, 1980) and the conditioned place preference produced by amphetamine (Spyraki, Fibiger, & Phillips, 1982b, 1982c) are both blocked by dopamine-selective lesions of nucleus accumbens.

Injections of amphetamine into caudate nucleus, amygdala, or the region of area postrema had no influence on the animal's behavior. Once again these latter results must be interpreted with caution. These negative data may mean that the injections produced no organizing effect on behavior, or they may mean that the animals failed to acquire or to remember associations between the environmental stimuli and organizing effects of amphetamine that may have been present.

Associative Bias in the Place and Taste Methods

Our earlier failure to observe an effect of injections of amphetamine into nucleus accumbens using the taste conditioning method (see Figure 3) is in contrast to the evidence of reward detected using place conditioning. A possible cause of this difference is the fact that our place method includes six environment reinforcer pairings while only a single pairing was used in the taste experiment. Accordingly, we repeated the taste conditioning experiment, pairing eight sessions of drinking a flavored solution with nucleus accumbens injections of amphetamine. All injection parameters were the same as in the taste and place experiments already described, and the testing included a free choice with water. Nonetheless, we still failed to observe any significant shift in the animals' responses to the conditioned taste stimulus.

These data support the conclusion that injections of amphetamine into nucleus accumbens have no effect in the taste method but give evidence of reward in the place method. Conversely, injections into the region of area postrema give evidence of aversion in the taste method (one pairing) but have no effect in the place method (six pairings). It is, of course, possible that higher or lower doses of amphetamine might produce an effect where none was observed in these experiments. Nevertheless, when comparing the characteristics of different methods of measuring the effects of drugs, data for the same dose in both situations are what is required to make such comparisons.

It therefore appears that amphetamine may have at least two independent organizing influences with opposite signs at two different brain sites. The drug's rewarding action in nucleus accumbens is biased towards forming associations with place stimuli. The drug's aversive action in area postrema is biased towards forming associations with taste stimuli. None of this precludes the possibility that amphetamine may also have other actions at other brain sites.

These conclusions on associative bias with amphetamine are in line with the data for sucrose and for lithium, suggesting that the place method may be a more sensitive detector of reward and that the taste method may be a more sensitive detector of aversion. Considering the data for amphetamine and natural reinforcers together leads to the suggestion that organizing influences producing approach and maintenance of contact are more easily associable with the environmental stimuli in a place conditioning apparatus and that organizing influences producing withdrawal are more easily associable with taste stimuli.

Summary

The place preference technique appears to be an adequate measure of both the rewarding and the aversive influences on behavior of natural reinforcers. However, comparisons of the effects of the same concentrations of sucrose and of the same doses of lithium in the place and taste conditioning methods suggest that the former may be a somewhat more sensitive measure of reward than the latter. Our demonstration of a dose-response relationship for peripherally injected amphetamine suggests that the place conditioning method is a sensitive detector of the rewarding effects of this drug. Intracerebral microinjections of amphetamine at four different sites revealed a preference only with nucleus accumbens injections. Taken together with the data on intracerebral injections using the taste method, these findings suggest that amphetamine has at least two behaviorally important sites of action: a rewarding effect in nucleus accumbens and an aversive effect in area postrema. The assumption of associative bias can provide an explanation of the data on the differences in the abilities of the two methods to detect rewarding and aversive organizing influences on behavior.

PLACE CONDITIONING: RUNWAY METHOD

The two techniques for studying the organizational influences of reinforcers discussed in the previous sections measure approach and withdrawal indirectly: In one case the amount consumed of a substance flavored with the conditioned taste stimulus is measured, and in the other case the amount of time spent in the presence of the conditioned environmental stimuli is measured. An alternative type of measure commonly used in experimental psychology to measure the organizing properties of food and water makes use of a runway. In this case approach responses are directly observed and can be quantified in terms of the animals' running speeds.

Although this technique has not been widely used to measure the organizing influence of drug reinforcers on behavior, two recent studies suggest that it may be a valuable tool. White, Sklar, and Amit (1977) showed that rats' running speeds increased from day to day when they had been given one trial per day with an injection of morphine while remaining in the goal box for an hour after each trial. Increases in running speed can be interpreted as increases in the intensity of the animals' tendency to approach the goal box, suggesting that morphine has a rewarding influence on behavior. These findings are consistent with the results of place conditioning experiments using this drug. Distinctively flavored food was available in the goal box, and the animals were allowed to eat for a few minutes before receiving their drug injections. The amount of food consumed decreased from day to day while, on the same trials, the animals were showing evidence of reward. The decrease in consumption, which is consistent with the results of other taste conditioning experiments with morphine, suggests that the drug also produced aversion. Reicher and Holman (1977) reported similar results for amphetamine using a version of the place conditioning method.

These findings can be interpreted in terms of associative bias. In agreement with data presented in the previous sections, it is possible that the rewarding effect of the drugs is biased towards the formation of associations with the place stimuli in the goal box and that the aversive effect of the drugs is biased towards the formation of associations with the taste stimuli also present there. Whether or not this explanation is correct, the fact that this method appears to detect both reward and aversion simultaneously would seem to make it a useful one for studying the organizing influence of drugs on behavior.

We decided to test the value of the runway technique for measuring the organizing influence of reinforcers by using a slightly different experimental method. Water-deprived rats were trained in a runway with water in the goal box. When they had learned to run, they were given four daily home cage pairings of a flavored solution followed by a reinforcer. They were then given five runway trials per day for 2 days. On each of these two test days, there was water in the goal box on the first two trials so that the animals' running speeds on Trials 2 and 3 followed experience with this reinforcer. The speeds on these trials were used as a baseline measure. On Trial 3 and on subsequent trials, the paired solution that provided the conditioned taste stimulus was placed in the goal box. The effect of the conditioned taste stimulus on the animals' tendency to approach the goal box was measured by observing the change from baseline in running speed that its introduction caused.

Natural Reinforcers

In our first experiment we paired drinking the flavored solution with drinking a sucrose solution on the four pairing days. The effects of this pairing on running speed are shown in Figure 8. In Group A introduction of the conditioned taste stimulus on Day 1 had no effect on running speed, but its introduction on Day 2 resulted in a significant increase in running speed. The hypothesis that this increase was caused by learned properties of the conditioned taste stimulus is supported by the results for two control groups. Group B experienced pairings of the flavored solution with water on the four pairing days. Introduction of the taste stimulus into the runway had no effect on running speed. Group C experienced pairings with the sucrose solution, but the conditioned taste stimulus was never introduced into the runway. These rats showed a decrease in running speed on the trials where the rats in Group A increased. Therefore it seems likely that the increase in running speed observed in Group A was due to the conditioned properties of the taste stimulus acquired during the pairings. These findings suggest that the method is able to detect a rewarding influence on behavior.

The fact that the increase in running speed occurred only on the second day of testing in the runway might be explained by postulating a requirement for a secondary conditioning process in which the conditioned properties of the taste stimulus become associated with the environmental stimuli that constitute the goal box. If this process occurs on the first test day, then the appearance of the increase would be delayed until the second test day. To test this hypothesis, we paired the flavored solution with sucrose but did not introduce the conditioned taste stimulus into the runway on the first test day, thus preventing the occurrence of the suggested conditioning process (Group D). When the taste stimulus was introduced on the second day of testing, no change in running speed was observed, supporting the hypothesis that some process involving the conditioned taste stimulus takes place in the goal box on Day 1. As a second test the animals in Group E experienced the pairings of flavored solution and sucrose in the goal box of the runway, allowing both the primary and postulated secondary conditioning processes to occur together. The rats in this group showed a large increase in running speed when the taste was introduced into the goal box on the first test day. This suggests that the increase in running speed on Day 2 occurs when the organizing influence of the reinforcer becomes associated with the environmental stimuli of the goal box. When this process is prevented from occurring during the initial pairing (e.g., when the pairings are done in the home cage), then it occurs on the first test day and the organizing influence of the reinforcer is detected in the runway on the second test day.

These findings suggest that the rewarding influence of a sucrose reinforcer can become associated with a taste stimulus which can, in turn, become associated with place or environmental stimuli in the runway. Both of these processes are consistent with what we have observed for natural reinforcers using the taste and place conditioning methods separately, since

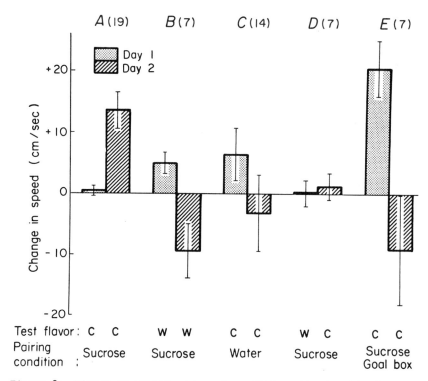

Figure 8: Effect of introduction of conditioned taste stimulus on running speed. The letters at the top of the figure are group identification labels and show the numbers of subjects in each group. In each pair of bars the first one is the mean change in running speed observed on the first test day; the second is the same data for the second test day. On pairing days the animals drank a solution of 2% instant decaffeinated coffee in distilled water for 5 minutes followed by drinking the reinforcer for 25 minutes. The experimental conditions for each group are shown on the abscissa. The line labeled "Test Flavor" shows whether coffee ("C") or water ("W") was available in the goal box on Trials 3 to 5 (Water was always used on Trials 1 and 2.). The line labeled "Pairing Condition" shows whether coffee was paired with sucrose (4% in distilled water) or water on the four pairing days. Significant changes in running speed were: Group A, Day 2: t (18) = 2.32, p < 0.05; Group E, Day 1: t (6) = 2.15, p < 0.05.

both methods are able to detect the rewarding effect of a natural reinforcer. Our next step was to test the runway method with amphetamine, and, as we had found when using the taste and place methods separately, the drug has its own properties in this situation.

Amphetamine

In this experiment the animals were pretrained in the runway and experienced four pairings of novel taste with an injection of saline or with one of two doses of amphetamine. They were then given two days of runway testing. As shown in Figure 9, a substantial aversion to the paired flavor was observed during the pairings, and large decreases in speed were observed when the conditioned taste stimulus was introduced into the runway on both test days. The interpretation of these decreases, that the reinforcer has aversive organizing properties, is consistent with previous taste conditioning data but not with previous findings using other place conditioning methods. The fact that the method detected a sizable aversive effect of 0.5 mg/kg of amphetamine suggests that it may be a very sensitive measure of aversion, and it may even be the case that the decrease in running speed observed in the saline group reflects the aversive properties of the injection procedure. Since these data are the first collected using this method, further investigation of its properties will be necessary before any of these data can be considered firm.

Summary

The present version of the place conditioning method deserves further investigation because it may provide an additional sensitive method for detecting the organizing influence on behavior of reinforcers in general and of drugs in particular. It appears to be able to detect both rewarding and aversive influences, and it has the advantage that the reinforcer need never become directly associated with the test apparatus, thus decreasing the possibility of interference with ongoing behavior by direct or conditioned peripheral actions of drug reinforcers. An apparent disadvantage of this method is that it can detect only those organizing influences which can become associated with taste stimuli; this is illustrated by the purely aversive response to amphetamine. The runway method, in which both conditioned and unconditioned stimuli are present in the goal box, has the advantage of being able to measure two organizing influences simultaneously. However, in cases where the dual method poses difficulties of interpretation, the method of pairing outside the apparatus may offer certain advantages.

CONCLUSION

Our approach to the study of the reinforcing properties of drugs is through an examination of the reinforcement process itself. Accordingly, we conduct parallel studies of the effects on behavior of both naturally occurring and drug reinforcers, using several different experimental methods. Our goal is to determine the neural basis of the change in behavior produced by reinforcers. One property of natural reinforcers is their rewarding or aversive stimulus properties, which are objectively observable as tendencies to produce approach and maintenance of contact with the reinforcer or to produce withdrawal from it. Therefore, reinforcers are viewed as organizing influences on behavior, and the tendency of animals to approach them or to withdraw from them can be observed in order to determine their stimulus properties.

Although reinforcing drugs have stimulus properties, they lack external

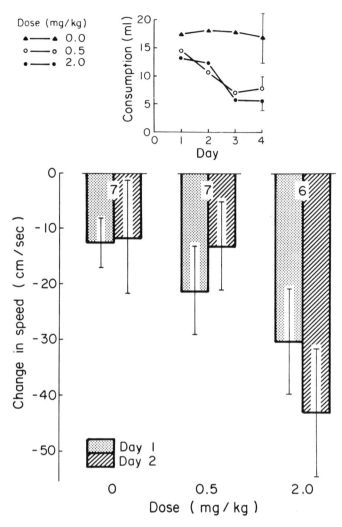

Figure 9: Effects of amphetamine on running speed. The inset shows the mean amount of coffee-flavored solution consumed by the rats in each group on the four pairing days. There is a significant difference among the means on the fourth day [F (2,17) = 3.63, p < 0.05]. The main part of the figure shows the change in running speed produced by introduction of the coffee solution (for all groups) on test Days 1 and 2, according to the format described for Figure 8. Each bar shows the standard error of the mean and the number of subjects. In the saline group there was a significant decrease on Day 1 [t (6) = 2.69, p < 0.05]. In the 0.5 mg/kg group there was a significant decrease on Day 1 [t (6) = 2.65, p < 0.05]. In the 2.0 mg/kg group there was a significant decrease on Day 1 [t (5) = 3.14, p < 0.03] and on Day 2 [t (5) = 3.79, p < 0.01].

reference points for approach or withdrawal. Therefore, the organizing influences of drugs on behavior can be detected only when they are associated with neutral stimuli in a conditioning paradigm and then inferred from responses to the conditioned stimuli. We have examined three methods for accomplishing this.

It is well known that the taste conditioning method detects the aversive properties of a variety of reinforcers, including self-administered drugs such as morphine and amphetamine. We have shown that it can also detect the rewarding properties of self-stimulation and of sucrose and saccharin solutions. However, it does not appear to detect any rewarding properties of amphetamine.

The place preference conditioning method can detect the rewarding and aversive properties of natural reinforcers, and we present data showing a linear relationship between an ascending series of sucrose concentrations and preference. Furthermore, the place preference method may be a somewhat more sensitive detector of reward than the taste conditioning method. Place conditioning is a highly sensitive detector of the rewarding effects of amphetamine; this was demonstrated by a significant dose-preference relationship for this drug.

The place conditioning runway method described here can detect the rewarding properties of a natural reinforcer, and there is some evidence that it is also a highly sensitive detector of aversion. However, the problems of interpretation posed by our data require further analysis. The runway method in which animals experience food and drug in the goal box has certain advantages over the one described here.

Some data are presented in support of the hypothesis that amphetamine's influence on behavior is mediated by actions of the drug on more than one neural substrate. Microinjections of the drug into nucleus accumbens give evidence of reward using the place preference method, and similar injections into the region of area postrema give evidence of aversion using the taste conditioning method. These data suggest that amphetamine acts at these two sites with opposite influences. More experiments will be necessary to verify this conclusion and to determine if amphetamine has additional actions at other brain sites.

We attribute the fact that the rewarding and the aversive influences of amphetamine were detected with different methods to associative bias--the notion that the brain is organized to favor the association of certain stimuli. Support for this notion comes from suggestions that reward may be better detected with the place method and aversion better detected with the taste method. However, the concept of associative bias remains an "intervening variable." It will be necessary to find independent corroborating evidence and to determine the neural basis for the proposed biases before it can be accepted as an accurate explanation of the observed phenomena.

ACKNOWLEDGMENTS

The research reported and the preparation of this manuscript were supported by grants from the Natural Sciences and Engineering Research Council of Canada and from Fonds FCAC, Province of Quebec. We thank Smith-Kline and French, Canada Ltd. for the gift of amphetamine.

REFERENCES

Beach, H. D. (1957). Morphine addiction in rats. Canadian Journal of Psychology, **11**, 104-112.

Berger, B. D., Wise, C. D., & Stein, L. (1973). Area postrema damage and bait shyness. Journal of Comparative and Physiological Psychology, **82**, 475-479.

Cappell, H., LeBlanc, A. E., & Endrenyi, L. (1973). Aversive conditioning by psychoactive drugs: Effects of morphine, alcohol and chlordiazepoxide. Psychopharmacology, **29**, 239-246.

Carey, R. J. (1973). Long-term aversion to saccharin solution induced by repeated amphetamine injections. Pharmacology Biochemistry & Behavior, **1**, 265-270.

Carr, G. D., & White, N. M. (1984). The relationship between stereotypy and memory improvement produced by amphetamine. Psychopharmacology, **82**, 203-209.

Collier, G., & Bolles, R. (1968). Hunger and thirst and their interaction as determinants of sucrose consumption. Journal of Comparative and Physiological Psychology, **66**, 633-641.

Coulombe, D., & White, N. M. (1980). The effect of post-training lateral hypothalamic self-stimulation on aversive and appetitive classical conditioning. Physiology & Behavior, **25**, 267-272.

Doty, B., & Doty L. (1966). Facilitating effects of amphetamine on avoidance conditioning in relation to age and problem difficulty. Psychopharmacology, **9**, 234-241.

Eikelboom, R., & Stewart, J. (1979). Conditioned temperature effects using morphine as the conditioned stimulus. Psychopharmacology, **61**, 31-38.

Ettenberg, A., Cinsavitch, S., & White, N. M. (1979). Performance effects with repeated measures during pimozide induced dopamine receptor blockade. Pharmacology Biochemistry & Behavior, **11**, 557-561.

Ettenberg, A., Sgro, S., & White, N. M. (1982). Algebraic summation of the affective properties of a rewarding and an aversive stimulus in the rat. Physiology & Behavior, **28**, 873-877.

Ettenberg, A., van der Kooy, D., LeMoal, M., Koob, G. F., & Bloom, F. E. (1983). Can aversive properties of (peripherally injected) vasopressin account for its putative role in memory? Behavioural Brain Research, **7**, 331-350.

Ettenberg, A., & White, N. M. (1978). Conditioned taste preference in the rat induced by self-stimulation. Physiology & Behavior, **21**, 353-368.

Fuxe, K., & Ungerstedt, U. (1970). Histochemical, biochemical and functional studies on central monoamine neurons after acute and chronic amphetamine administration. In E. Costa & S. Garattini (Eds.), Amphetamines and related compounds (pp. 257-288). New York: Plenum Press.

Garcia, J., Hawkins, W. G., & Rusiniak, K. W. (1974). Behavioral regulation of the milieu interne in man and rat. Science, **185**, 823-831.

Garcia, J., Kimmeldorf, D. J., & Hunt, E. L. (1957). Spatial avoidance in the rat as a result of exposure to ionizing radiation. British Journal of Radiation, **30**, 318-321.

Garcia, J., & Koelling, R. A. (1966). Relation of cue to consequence in avoidance learning. Psychonomic Science, **4**, 123-124.

Glickman, S. E. (1973). Responses and reinforcement. In R. A. Hinde & J. Stevenson-Hinde (Eds.), Constraints on learning, (pp. 207-242). New York: Academic Press.

Goudie, A. J. (1979). Aversive stimulus properties of drugs. Neuropharmacology, **13**, 971-979.

Harris, L. J., Clay, J., Hargreaves, F. J., & Ward, A. (1933). Appetite and diet. The ability of the vitamin B deficient rat to discriminate between diets containing and lacking the vitamin. Proceedings of the Royal Society (London), **113**, 161-190.

Hebb, D. O. (1949). The organization of behavior. New York: Wiley.

Herrick, C. J. (1948). The brain of the tiger salamander. Chicago: University of Chicago Press.

Holman, E. W. (1975). Immediate and delayed reinforcers for flavour preference in rats. Learning and Motivation, **6**, 19-100.

Holman, G. L. (1969). The intragastric reinforcement effect. Journal of Comparative and Physiological Psychology, **69**, 432-441.

Hull, C. L. (1951). Essentials of behavior. New Haven: Yale University Press.

Jacquet, Y. (1973). Conditioned aversion during morphine maintenance in mice and rats. Physiology & Behavior, **11**, 527-541.

Krivanek, J., & McGaugh, J. L. (1969). Facilitating effects of pre- and post-training amphetamine on discrimination learning in mice. Agents and Actions, **1**, 36-42.

Kumar, R. (1972). Morphine dependence in rats: Secondary reinforcement from environmental stimuli. Psychopharmacology, **25**, 971-979.

Lyness, W. H., Friedle, N. M., & Moore, K. E. (1979). Destruction of dopaminergic nerve terminals in nucleus accumbens: Effect on d-amphetamine self-administration. Pharmacology Biochemistry & Behavior, **11**, 553-556.

Maier, N. R. F., & Schneirla, T. C. (1964). Principles of animal psychology. New York: Dover.

Major, R., & White, N. M. (1978). Memory facilitation by self-stimulation reinforcement mediated by the nigro-neostriatal bundle. Physiology & Behavior, **20**, 723-733.

McGlone, J. J., Ritter, S., & Kelley, K. W. (1980). The antiaggressive effect of lithium is abolished by area postrema lesions. Physiology & Behavior, **24**, 1095-1100.

Messier, C., & White, N. M. (1984). Contingent and non-contingent actions of sucrose and saccharin reinforcers: Effects on taste preference and memory. Physiology & Behavior, **32**, 195-203.

Moore, B. R. (1973). The role of directed Pavlovian reactions in simple instrumental learning in the pigeon. In R. A. Hinde & J. Stevenson-Hinde (Eds.), Constraints on learning (pp. 159-188). New York: Academic Press.

Mucha, R. F., van der Kooy, D., O'Shaughnessy, M., & Bucenieks, P. (1982). Drug reinforcement studied by use of place conditioning in rat. Brain Research, **243**, 91-105.

Pellegrino, L. J., Pellegrino, A. S., & Cushman, A. J. (1979). A stereotaxic atlas of the rat brain (2nd ed.). New York: Plenum Press.

Pfaffman, C. (1960). The pleasures of sensation. Physiological Review, **67**, 253-268.

Reicher, M. A., & Holman, E. W. (1977). Location preference and flavor aversion reinforced by amphetamine in rats. Animal Learning and Behavior, **5**, 343-346.

Revusky, S. H., & Bedarf, E. W. (1967). Association of illness with prior ingestion of novel food. Science, **155**, 219-220.

Revusky, S. H., & Garcia, J. (1970). Learned associations over long delays. In G. H. Bower (Ed.), The psychology of learning and motivation (Vol. 4, pp. 1-84). New York: Academic Press.

Richter, C. P. (1945). The development and use of alpha-naphtyl-thiourea (ANTU) as a rat poison. Journal of the American Medical Association, **29** 927.

Richter, C. P. (1953). Experimentally produced behavior reactions to food poisoning in wild and domesticated rats. Annals of the New York Academy of Sciences, **6** 223-239.

Roberts, D. C. S., Koob, G. F., Klonoff, P., & Fibiger, H. C. (1980). Extinction and recovery of cocaine self-administration following 6-hydroxydopamine lesions of the nucleus accumbens. Pharmacology Biochemistry & Behavior, 2 781-787.

Rossi, N. A., & Reid, L. D. (1976). Affective states associated with morphine injections. Physiological Psychology, 4, 269-274.

Schneirla, T. C. (1959). An evolutionary and developmental theory of biphasic processes underlying approach and withdrawal. Nebraska Symposium on Motivation, 7, 1-42.

Seligman, M. E. P. (1970). On the generality of the laws of learning. Psychological Review, 77, 406-418.

Shettleworth, S. J. (1973). Food reinforcement and the organization of behavior in golden hamsters. In R. A. Hinde & J. Stevenson-Hinde (Eds.), Constraints on learning (pp. 243-264). New York: Academic Press.

Spyraki, C., Fibiger, H. C., & Phillips, A. G. (1982a). Attenuation by haloperidol of place preference conditioning using food reinforcement. Psychopharmacology, 77, 379-382.

Spyraki, C., Fibiger, H. C., & Phillips, A. G. (1982b). Dopaminergic substrates of amphetamine-induced place preference conditioning. Brain Research, 253, 185-193.

Spyraki, C., Fibiger, H. C., & Phillips, A. G. (1982c). Cocaine-induced place preference conditioning: Lack of effects of neuroleptics and 6-hydroxydopamine lesions. Brain Research, 253, 195-203.

Steffens, A. B. (1969a). The influence of insulin injections and infusions on eating and blood glucose level in the rat. Physiology & Behavior, 4, 823-828.

Steffens, A. B. (1969b). Rapid absorption of glucose in the intestinal tract of the rat after ingestion of a meal. Physiology & Behavior, 4, 829-832.

Sulser, F., & Sanders-Bush, E. (1971). Effects of drugs on amines in the CNS. Annual Review of Pharmacology, 11, 209-230.

Thompson, T., Bigelow, G., & Pickens, R. (1971). Environmental variables influencing drug self-administration. In T. Thompson & R. Pickens (Eds.), Stimulus properties of drugs (pp. 193-208). New York: Appleton-Century-Crofts.

Wagner, G. C., Foltin, R. W., Seiden, L. S., & Schuster, C. R. (1981). Dopamine depletion by 6-hydroxydopamine prevents conditioned taste aversion induced by methylamphetamine but not lithium chloride. Pharmacology Biochemistry & Behavior, 14, 85-88.

White, N. M., & Carr, G. D. (1985). The conditioned place preference is affected by two independent reinforcement processes. Pharmacology Biochemistry & Behavior, 23, 37-42.

White, N. M., Major, R., & Siegal, J. (1978). Effects of morphine on one-trial appetitive learning. Life Sciences, 23, 1967-1972.

White, N. M., Sklar, L., & Amit, Z. (1977). The reinforcing action of morphine and its paradoxical side effect. Psychopharmacology, 52, 63-66.

Young, P. T. (1940). Reversal of food preference of the white rat through controlled pre-feeding. Journal of General Psychology, 22, 33-66.

Young, P. T. (1959). The role of affective processes in learning and motivation. Psychological Review, 66, 104-125.

Young, P. T. (1966). Hedonic organization and regulation of behavior. Psychological Review, 73, 59-86.

Young, P. T. (1969). Motivation and emotion. New York: Wiley.

Young, P. T., & Christensen, K. R. (1962). Algebraic summation of hedonic processes. Journal of Comparative and Physiological Psychology, 55, 332-336.

Young, P. T., & Falk, J. L. (1956). The relative acceptability of sodium chloride solutions as a function of concentration and water needs. Journal of Comparative and Physiological Psychology, **49**, 569-575.

CHAPTER 29

THE MOUSE AS A SUBJECT IN THE STUDY OF NEURAL MECHANISMS OF REWARD

Hugh E. Criswell

East Tennessee State University
Johnson City, Tennessee 37614

Abstract

Mice have several properties which make them ideal subjects for studying the effect of drugs on the reward process. They are compact, inexpensive, and available in strains which vary in number of dopamine receptors, opiate receptors, or sensitivity to alcohol. Mice can be lightly restrained by taping their tails to the floor thereby allowing electrical or chemical stimulation of the brain without the use of swivel connectors or commutators. Intravenous injections can be made through a lateral tail vein while the animal is restrained and is free to emit operants. This chapter describes these techniques and suggests some pitfalls to avoid.

Introduction

Readers of this book cannot help but be aware of the pre-eminence of the laboratory rat in behavioral pharmacology. Rats are relatively inexpensive, docile, easy to maintain creatures, and there is a good file of behavioral and pharmacological literature pertaining to the rat. There is, also, a strong tradition in many behavioral testing programs to acquaint students with the laboratory rat at an early stage in their training. Having come from such a tradition, I worked with rats for some time until I found myself in a position of low funding with mice available ad libitum through an experimental breeding program in our biology department. To my surprise many of the standard procedures which have traditionally employed rats can be duplicated with mice. There are occasional problems associated with the small size of the mouse, but often the procedures are actually easier with mice than rats. In many cases the availability of strains of mice differing in the distribution of dopamine, serotonin, or opiate receptor sites makes studies possible that could not be accomplished with other species.

This chapter outlines some of the situations where mice are useful and appropriate subjects and warns of some potential problems. The emphasis will be on the positive aspect of the mouse as an experimental animal in the study of drug effects on reward.

Why Use a Mouse?

There are three basic attributes of mice which make them a valuable research tool. First, mice can be inexpensive, especially if you breed your own. Second, mice come in several strains some of which have interesting properties; for instance, CXBK mice are not analgesic at standard doses of morphine (Oliverio, Castellano, & Eleftheriou, 1975; Reith, Sershen, Vadasz, & Lajtha, 1981). And third, mice do not show stress responses when they are lightly restrained by immobilizing their tails (Moran & Straus, 1980). This makes operant work with electrical brain stimulation or microinjections much easier because there are no swivels or commutators needed. During restraint, intravenous injections can be made via the tail veins without the difficulty of surgically implanting a carotid catheter.

Electrode or Cannula Implantation

Mice can be prepared with stereotaxically implanted electrodes or guide cannulae using a slight modification of the methods used for rats. A standard Kopf small animal stereotaxic instrument or probably any small stereotaxic device can be used. On the Kopf instrument the nose clamp will have to be removed (It unscrews.) as it extends over the skull of an animal as small as a mouse. The standard ear and incisor bars work, but specially designed mouse ear and incisor bars are available. To keep the mouse's nose from rotating upward in the Kopf instrument, tape the nose down with masking tape. Stereotaxic atlases are available from either Sidman, Angevine, & Pierce (1971) or Lehmann (1974). The only differences between mouse and rat implant surgery relate to the size and metabolic rate of mice. They usually require more anesthetic (70 to 80 mg/kg of sodium pentobarbital), and screw placement is critical. The mouse skull is very thin and in order to get a good grip, the screws (0-80 by 1/8 inch) must be placed into the frontal skull over the olfactory bulbs. They can be placed immediately posterior to the lateral skull vein which is a major landmark on the mouse skull. Bilateral screws over the olfactory bulbs and one posterior screw placed laterally near the skull ridge will anchor an electrode platform securely. We rarely experience dislodged electrode platforms using this placement during the first 4 weeks of testing. Prolonged retention has not been as good. Few animals retain their electrodes longer than one year; plans to maintain animals for demonstration or screening work using this technique are not feasible. For intracranial self-stimulation (ICSS) or multiple unit recording, 36 gauge Teflon-coated, Nichrome electrodes work well. We have been able to show a fair degree of anatomical specificity in ICSS work using 36 gauge electrodes (Criswell, 1982a). Guide cannula can be implanted for microinjections using standard stereotaxic techniques or, alternatively, microinjections can be made in etherized mice by making a scalp incision, by visualizing landmarks (The junction between the inferior and superior colliculi are easily visualized through the skull.), and by inserting a 26 gauge hypodermic needle through the skull followed by a 30 gauge injection cannula with a block to regulate depth (Criswell, 1976).

The Poor Man's Skinner Box

Both ICSS and self-administration studies often use operant technology where a response at some sort of manipulandum--usually a lever press--results in delivery of a reinforcer such as ICSS, intravenous or intracerebral-ventricular administration of a drug. A peculiarity of the mouse makes it an ideal subject for operant studies of drug effects on reinforcement. A mouse can be lightly restrained by taping its tail to a surface. During restraint there is little evidence of stress (Moran & Straus, 1980). By placing a mouse inside an operant chamber with its tail protruding through a hole in one wall and by taping the tail down, you have a very useful preparation. The mouse is able to emit operant responses (We use a nosepoke, but a lever press should work also.), but it is unable to circle and its tail is always available. This means that you can do electrical stimulation or recording without a commutator. Commutators are not much of a problem for stimulation, but they are often a source of noise in recording studies. Intracranial microinjections can be performed without a swivel connector (Swivel connectors are problematic with mice.); and, best of all, you can do both at the same time or even microinject through two cannulae simultaneously while stimulating or recording through a pair of electrodes. The tail is always available, and intravenous injections through a lateral tail vein are not too difficult in a mouse. One hint here is to place the mouse under a heat lamp for a short period of time to raise its body temperature. Mice regulate body temperature in part by dilation of the tail veins, and it makes insertion of an intravenous needle much easier.

Figure 1 shows the all purpose operant chamber that we have been using for a couple of years. The dimensions of the chamber (8 cm front to back by 9 cm side to side by 10 cm high) are such that when the mouse's tail is placed through the hole in the back wall and taped down, it can reach either of the holes (manipulanda) in the front of the cage. A light and photocell are placed across the hole so that a nosepoke response breaks the light beam and darkens the photocell.

A simple and inexpensive way to interface the operant chamber to control and data acquisition facilities is via a microcomputer. Any microcomputer with

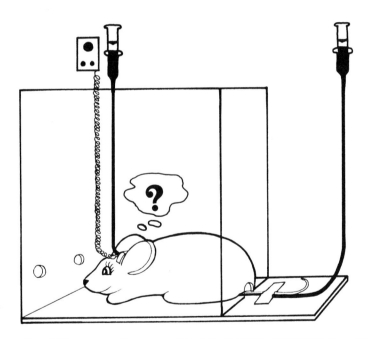

Figure 1: All-purpose two-manipulandum operant chamber with a mouse prepared for simultaneous electrical stimulation and intracerebral and intravenous injections.

a game paddle input such as the Vic-20, Commodore-64, Apple II+, or Radio Shack color computer has a built-in photocell interface. By connecting the photocell across the paddle input, you have replaced the variable resistor in the paddle with the variable resistance of the photocell. Figure 2 shows an interface for a Vic-20 microcomputer. The Vic-20 is available for under $100 in many parts of the world. This system will allow the use of two manipulanda. If you want to use a lever, just replace the photocell with the normally closed contacts of the switch. The resistors in series with the photocell are needed because the Vic-20 cannot handle a rapid decrease in resistance to near zero. It won't hurt the microcomputer to leave them out, but a fast mouse can confuse the computers analog/digital (A-D) converter resulting in an occasional missed response. The parallel input/output (I-O) port is capable of driving a transistor with each data bit, and the circuit shown allows the Vic-20 to

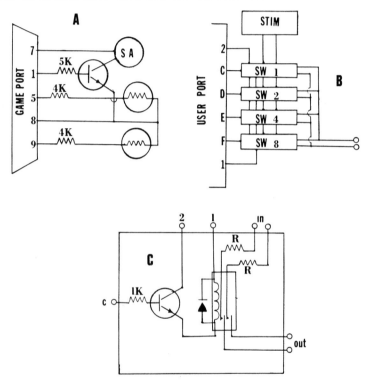

Figure 2: Interface circuitry for a Vic-20 microcomputer. **A** shows the input to the computer. Two photocells are connected to the game port. The transistor drives a Sonalert Alarm (SA) which signals a correct response. **B** is an array of switches (SW 1-4) which controls the resistance in series with a constant voltage source (STIM). Detail of the switches is shown in **C**. An NPN transistor acts as an inverting buffer for the output port and drives a S.T.D.P. relay. When the relay is on, it passes current through the resistors (R). SW1 passes the least current; SW2 passes twice as much, et cetera. The value of the resistors must be in multiples of 2. We use 8 megaohms for SW1, 4 for SW2, 2 for SW3, and 1 megaohm for SW4.

control the current of a constant voltage source by placing different resistors
in series with the voltage. As shown the output will change by 1 part in 16 as
the number poked into the output port is incremented or decremented. The
current level is controlled by the four relays. If you want more resolution,
simply add one more relay with a resistance of one half that of the lowest
shown and change the stimulation program to count to 32 instead of 16. The
program in the Appendix will run an autotitration schedule using this
apparatus. In an autotitration schedule responses at one manipulandum result
in reinforcement, but the magnitude of the reinforcer is reduced with continued
responding. A response at a second manipulandum resets the magnitude of
reinforcement to its original level. This allows determination of the
subject's preferred magnitude of reinforcement and is similar to a threshold
determination where you find the lowest reinforcement magnitude for which the
animal is willing to work. If you remove line 562, it will record response
rate at both manipulanda but reinforce responses at only one, and the current
will not be decremented every fifth response (a simple right-left
discrimination task). If you want to use this apparatus for drug self-
administration, simply connect one of the relays to an infusion pump, and you
have a right-left discrimination procedure where responses at one manipulandum
deliver the drug and responses at the other manipulandum serve as a control for
changes in activity level. Figure 3 illustrates a mouse working at an
autotitration task with this. Figure 4 shows a dose-response curve for
morphine effects on response rate at a low current (about 10% above threshold)
and high current (where response rate started to decline with increased
current). Vigorous responding was obtained at all doses using the high current
stimulation while it dropped considerably--but not to zero--at the lower
stimulation level. Using 36 gauge electrodes in the perifornical lateral
hypothalamic area, thresholds for ICSS ranged between 2 and 30 µA of 60 Hz
sinewave stimulation for 1/3 second. These levels are lower than those
obtained with rats using larger electrodes. The effectiveness may be related
to current density, and the smaller electrode tips can be an important factor

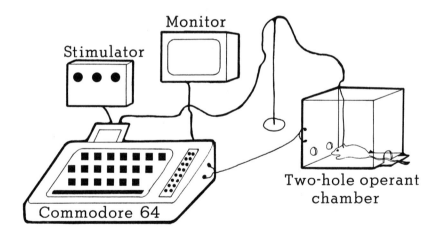

Figure 3: A typical testing station. The stimulation cable is
hanging from a ring stand. Since the mouse cannot rotate in the
cage, electrical or chemical stimulation of discrete brain sites is
a simple procedure.

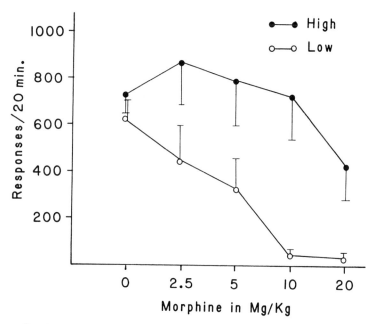

Figure 4: Dose-response curves for the effect of morphine on high and low current ICSS in ICR mice using a nosepoke response.

in regulation of current density. We usually start testing at a current of 6 μA rather than the 50 μA commonly used in rats.

Use of the nosepoke response results in a rapid acquisition of the response when ICSS is used as a reinforcer and may be superior to the more commonly used lever-press response. The nosepoke, wheel-turn (Kornetsky, Esposito, McLean, & Jacobson, 1979), and shuttling responses (Levitt, Baltzer, Evers, Stillwell, & Furby, 1978) are all natural, easily acquired responses for rats. We have found that mice rapidly acquire shuttling (Criswell & Starnes, 1980) and nosepoking (Criswell, 1983).

Shuttle-Box

Allowing animals to control ICSS duration and time between stimuli in a shuttle-box offers a convenient way to simultaneously measure appetitive and aversive aspects of ICSS. Levitt et al., (1977) have examined opiate effects on ICSS in rats using this procedure, and it has been adapted for mice by Cazala, Cazals, and Cardo (1974), Cazala and Garrigues (1980, 1983), Cazala and Guenet (1980). A workable shuttle-box for mice can be constructed by making a Plexiglas box 26 cm long, 10 cm wide, and 10 cm high with a grid floor 1 cm above the bottom of the box. A hinged top with a 1/2 cm slit running longitudinally and a similar slit joining the open side forming a "t" will allow you to place a mouse in the cage and to slide the stimulation cable into the slit in the top. If you then close the top and tape the short arm of the "t" so that the cable will not catch in it as it slides by, you will have an inexpensive and useful shuttle-box. The box can be interfaced to recording and control equipment by balancing it on a fulcrum and by resting one end on a microswitch. As the mouse shuttles, the microswitch will be on when it is on one side of the cage and off when it is on the other. The simplest interface is via a microcomputer. Our system is run by an antique SYM-1 microcomputer which is no longer in production so I cannot include a program, but it should be a simple process to program any microcomputer with a built-in clock to rack on- and off-times and to supply current at the proper times. The relay system described in Figure 2 will work for control of ICSS, and closure of a microswitch can be sensed by replacing the photocells shown in the figure with the normally closed contacts of a microswitch.

By simply counting cage crossings without stimulation, you can use the shuttle-box to measure activity level. Figure 5 shows the effects of morphine on activity level for two strains of mouse. By making electrical stimulation contingent on the mouse being in one side of the cage, you can measure the effects of drugs on the preferred duration of stimulation (on-time) and time between stimuli (off-time). In this situation it is a good idea to have your control apparatus automatically turn the stimulus on if the animal leaves it off for more than some criterion time (I use 30 seconds.) or they may just lay down on the off side and sleep or groom. As number of shuttles as a function of time is allowed to vary, on- and off-times are independent. Figure 6 shows differences in the effects of morphine on on- and off-times of two different mouse strains. You might want to compare the effects of morphine on on- and off-times to its effect on activity level for these two strains (Figure 5).

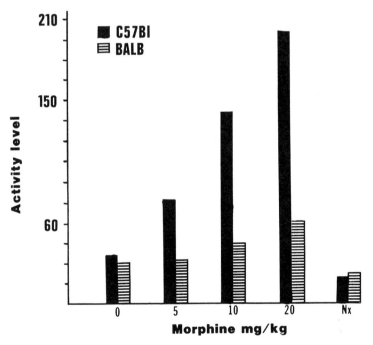

Figure 5: Dose-response curve for the effect of morphine and morphine plus naloxone on activity level of BALB/c and C57BL/6 mice.

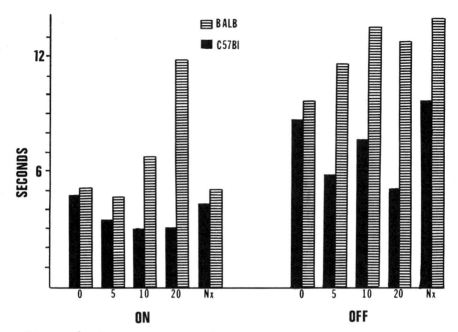

Figure 6: Dose-response curves for the effect of morphine and morphine plus naloxone on preferred stimulus duration (ON-times) and preferred time between stimuli (OFF-times) in BALB/c and C57BL/6 mice.

Note that the morphine selectively increases on-times in BALB/c mice while decreasing them in C57BL/6 mice. The BALB/c mice acted like rats (Baltzer, Levitt, & Furby, 1977), but the C57BL/6 mice acted quite differently. Off-times were not affected in either strain. We only obtain this pattern of responses reliably with electrodes within 0.5 mm of the fornix (Criswell, 1983a).

There are certainly other operant techniques which can be used with mice, and the non-operant procedures such as conditioned place preference described in previous chapters should be easily adaptable to the mouse. In cases where cost of maintaining an animal colony is important or where only small quantities of an experimental drug are available, the mouse has much to recommend it. The other prime reason for using mice as experimental subjects is the availability of several specialized strains of mouse.

The Generic Mouse

The common Swiss-Webster or ICR mouse is available through most lab animal suppliers. They breed easily and have large litters (12 to 16 pups) and are, therefore, inexpensive. Current prices from suppliers run about a dollar each. They can be bred in a standard laboratory animal facility without difficulty. They can be comfortably housed five to a cage in disposable plastic rodent cages. Mice make nests whenever possible and have sticky urine. For those reasons it is probably not wise to keep them in standard screen floored rat cages. Mice can be safely picked up by the tail but should not be carried for long distances that way. It is convenient to set the mouse on the back of a hand while transporting it between cages. These mice are albino and have rather poor vision. Other strains would be more appropriate for visual discrimination work. Also, the ICR or Swiss mouse is an outbred strain, and there is quite a bit of variability between mice. Where variability in either behavior or biochemistry is a primary concern, one of the inbred strains would be more appropriate.

The Designer Mouse

One of the most useful features of the mouse is the availability of several inbred strains which show different pharmacological and behavioral responses to abused drugs. Many of the inbred strains are difficult to breed and may be expensive or only occasionally available. They are typically designated by sometimes obscure codes. One of the more commonly used inbred strains is the BALB/c. BALB stands for Bag albino, and the letters after the slash represent a particular substrain. In spite of the origin of BALB mice from one pair, different breeding colonies produce BALBs with different characteristics. A BALB/cJ (J for Jackson Laboratories) is a different animal from a BALB/byJ. Some strains such as the CXBK are f2 backcrosses from two inbred strains and are only produced periodically and may run several dollars each when available. In general, the inbred strains are smaller (20 to 30 grams) than the Swiss or ICR mouse (30 to 40 grams). The particularly interesting areas where strain effects have been documented involve responses to opiates, dopaminergic compounds, and ethanol.

I have compiled a non-exhaustive set of references regarding the use of mice in ICSS and self-administration studies (see Table 1). I have also listed studies relating strain differences in responses to opiates, biogenic amines, and ethanol.

Table 1

Examples of Studies Using Mice as Subjects

General ICSS and Self-Administration

Cazala et al., 1974: ICSS (lever press)
Cazala & Guenet, 1980: ICSS (shuttle-box)
Cazala & Garrigues, 1980: ICSS (shuttle-box)
Cazala & Garrigues, 1983: Drug effect on ICSS
Criswell, 1982a: Self-administration
Criswell, 1982b: ICSS (shuttle-box)
Criswell & Ridings, 1983: Self-administration & ICSS
Kokkinidis & Zacharko, 1980: ICSS (nosepoke response)

Effects of Opiates

Receptor Sites

Baran, Schuster, Eleftheriou, & Bailey, 1975: 7 recombinant strains examined
Gwynn & Domino, 1984: Mu vs. kappa sites
Huidobro-Toro & Way, 1981: Rat vs. mouse
Maarten et al., 1981: Opiate receptors in mouse strains
Reggiani, Battaini, Kobayashi, Spano, & Trabucchi, 1980: DBA/2 vs. C57BL/6
Reith et al., 1981: Recombinant strains

Behavior

Carroll & Sharp, 1972: Locomotion
Castellano, 1980: Memory
Castellano, 1981: Locomotion
Cheng & Pomeranz, 1979: Analgesia
Collins & Whitney, 1978: Analgesia, locomotion
Filibeck, Castellano, & Oliverio, 1981: Analgesia, excitability
Gwynn & Domino, 1984a: Locomotion, catalepsy
Gwynn & Domino, 1984b: Analgesia
Oliverio et al., 1975: Analgesia, tolerance
Reggiani et al., 1980: Analgesia, locomotion
Siegfried, Frischknecht, & Waser, 1984: Defeat-induced analgesia

Biogenic Amines

Receptor Sites

Berger, Herve, Dolphin, Barthelemy, Gay, & Tassin, 1979: Norepinephrine
Daszuta, Faudon, & Hery, 1984: 5-HT
Daszuta, Hery, & Faudon, 1984: 5-HT
Reggiani et al., 1980: Dopamine turnover
Severson, Randall, & Finch, 1981: Dopamine

Behavior

Cazala & Garrigues, 1983: Apomorphine, clonidine, 5-meth-DMT
Kokkinidis & Zacharko, 1980: Amphetamine
Sansone, Ammassari-Teule, Renzi, & Oliverio, 1984: Apomorphine
Seale, McLanahan, Johnson, Carney, & Rennert, 1984: Apomorphine

Ethanol

Crabbe, Janowsky, Young, Kosobud, Stack, & Rigter, 1982: Hypothermia,
    locomotor, ataxia
Gilliam & Collins, 1983: Sleep hypothermia
Gentry, Rappaport, & Dole, 1983: Voluntary consumption
Kiianmaa, Hoffman, & Tabakoff, 1983: Locomotor
McSwigman, Crabbe, & Young, 1984: Withdrawal seizures
Millard & Dole, 1983: Voluntary consumption

References

Baltzer, J. H., Levitt, R. A., & Furby, J. E. (1977). Etorphine and shuttle-box self-stimulation in the rat. Pharmacology Biochemistry & Behavior, 7, 413-416.

Baran, A., Schuster, L., Eleftheriou, B. E., & Bailey, D. W. (1975). Opiate receptors in mice: Genetic differences. Life Sciences, 17, 633-640.

Berger, B., Herve, D., Dolphin, A., Barthelemy, C., Gay, M., & Tassin, J. P. (1979). Genetically determined differences in noradrenergic input to the brain cortex: A histochemical and biochemical study in two inbred strains of mice. Neuroscience, 4, 877-888.

Carroll, B. J., & Sharp, P. T. (1972). Monoamine mediation of the morphine-induced activation of mice. British Journal of Pharmacology, 46, 124-139.

Castellano, C. (1980). Dose-dependent effects of heroin on memory in two inbred strains of mice. Psychopharmacology, 67, 235-239.

Castellano, C. (1981). Strain dependent effects of the enkephalin analogue FK33-824 on locomotor activity in mice. Pharmacology Biochemistry & Behavior, 15, 729-734.

Cazala, P., Cazals, Y., & Cardo, B. (1974). Hypothalamic self-stimulation in three inbred strains of mice. Brain Research, 81, 159-167.

Cazala, P., & Garrigues, A. M. (1980). An apparent genetic relationship between appetitive and aversive effects of lateral hypothalamic stimulation in the mouse. Physiology & Behavior, 25, 357-361.

Cazala, P., & Garrigues, A. M. (1983). Effects of apomorphine, clonidine or 5-methoxy-NN-Dimethyltryptamine on approach and escape components of lateral hypothalamic and mesencephalic central gray stimulation in two inbred strains of mice. Pharmacology Biochemistry & Behavior, 18, 87-93.

Cazala, P., & Guenet, J. (1980). The recombinant inbred strains: A tool for the genetic analysis of differences observed in the self-stimulation behavior of the mouse. Physiology & Behavior, 24, 1057-1060.

Cheng, R. S., & Pomeranz, B. (1979). Correlation of genetic differences in endorphin systems with analgesic effects of D-amino acids in mice. Brain Research, 177, 583-587.

Collins, R. L., & Whitney, G. (1978). Genotype and test experience determine responsiveness to morphine. Psychopharmacology, 56, 57-60.

Crabbe, J. C., Janowsky, J. S., Young, E. R., Kosobud, A., Stack, J., & Rigter, H. (1982). Tolerance to ethanol hypothermia in inbred mice: Genotypic correlations with behavioral responses. Alcoholism: Clinical and Experimental Research, 6, 446-458.

Criswell, H. E. (1976). Analgesia and hyperactivity following morphine microinjection into mouse brain. Pharmacology Biochemistry & Behavior, 4, 23-26.

Criswell, H. E. (1982a). A simple methodology for opiate self-administration and electrical brain stimulation in the mouse. Life Sciences, 31, 2391-2394.

Criswell, H. E. (1982b). Effect of opiates on perifornical reward areas. Anatomical Record, 204, 395-396.

Criswell, H. E., & Ridings, R. (1983). Intravenous self-administration of morphine by naive mice. Pharmacology Biochemistry & Behavior, 18, 467-470.

Criswell, H. E., & Starnes, D. M. (1980). Effect of morphine on preferred duration of electrical brain stimulation in the mouse. Society for Neuroscience Abstracts, 6, 309.

Daszuta, A., Faudon, M., & Hery, F. (1984). In vitro ^{3}H-serotonin (5-HT) synthesis and release in BALBc and C57BL mice. II. Cell body areas. Brain Research Bulletin, 12, 565-570.

Daszuta, A., Hery, F., & Faudon, M. (1984). In vitro H-serotonin (5-HT) synthesis and release in BALBc and C57BL mice. I. Terminal areas. Brain Research Bulletin, 12, 559-563.

Filibeck, U., Castellano, C., & Oliverio, A. (1981). Differential effects of opiate agonists-antagonists on morphine-induced hyperexcitability and analgesia in mice. Psychopharmacology, 73, 134-136.

Frischknecht, H. R., Siegfried, B., Riggio, G., & Waser, P. G. (1983). Inhibition of morphine-induced analgesia and locomotor activity in strains of mice: A comparison of long-acting opiate antagonists. Pharmacology Biochemistry & Behavior, 19, 939-944.

Gentry, R. T., Rappaport, M. S., & Dole, V. P. (1983). Elevated concentrations of ethanol in plasma do not suppress voluntary ethanol consumption in C57BL Mice. Alcoholism: Clinical and Experimental Research, 7, 420-423.

Gilliam, D. M., & Collins, A. C. (1982). Circadian and genetic effects on ethanol elimination in LS and SS mice. Alcoholism: Clinical and Experimental Research, 6, 344-349.

Gilliam, D. M., & Collins, A. C. (1983). Concentration-dependent effects of ethanol in long-sleep and short-sleep mice. Alcoholism: Clinical and Experimental Research, 7, 337-342.

Gwynn, G. J., & Domino, E. F. (1984a). Genotype-dependent behavioral sensitivity to mu vs. kappa opiate agonists. I. Acute and chronic effects on mouse locomotor activity. Journal of Pharmacology and Experimental Therapeutics, 231, 306-311.

Gwynn, G. J., & Domino, E. F. (1984b). Genotype-dependent behavioral sensitivity to mu vs. kappa opiate agonists. II. Antinociceptive tolerance and physical dependence. Journal of Pharmacology and Experimental Therapeutics, 231, 312-316.

Huidobro-Toro, J. P., & Way, E. L. (1981). Comparative study on the effect of morphine and the opioid-like peptides in the vas deferens of rodents: Species and strain differences, evidence for multiple opiate receptors. Life Sciences, 28, 1331-1336.

Kiianmaa, K., Hoffman, P. L., & Tabakoff, B. (1983). Antagonism of the behavioral effects of ethanol by naltrexone in BALB/c, C57BL/6, and DBA/2 mice. Psychopharmacology, 79, 291-294.

Kokkinidis, L., & Zacharko, R. M. (1980). Intracranial self-stimulation in mice using a modified hole-board task: Effects of d-amphetamine. Psychopharmacology, 68, 169-171.

Kornetsky, C., Esposito, R. U., McLean, S., & Jacobson, J. O. (1979). Intracranial self-stimulation thresholds: A model for the hedonic effects of drugs of abuse. Archives of General Psychiatry, 26, 289-292.

Lehmann, A. (1974). Atlas stereotaxique du cerveau de la souris. Paris: Centre National De La Recherche Scientifique.

Levitt, R. A., Baltzer, J. H., Evers, T. M., Stillwell, D. J., & Furby, J. E. (1977). Morphine and shuttle-box self-stimulation in the rat: A model for euphoria. Psychopharmacology, 54, 307-311.

Maarten, E. A., Reith, H. S., Vadasz, C., & Lajtha, A. (1981). Differences in opiate receptors in mouse brain. European Journal of Pharmacology, 74, 377-380.

McSwigan, J. D., Crabbe, J. C., & Young, E. R. (1984). Specific ethanol withdrawal seizures in genetically selected mice. Life Sciences, 35, 2119-2126.

Millard, W. J., & Dole, V. P. (1983). Intake of water and ethanol by C57BL mice: Effect of an altered light-dark schedule. Pharmacology Biochemistry & Behavior, 18, 281-284.

Moran, R. E., & Straus, J. J. (1980). A method for establishing prolonged intravenous infusions in mice. Laboratory Animal Science, 30, 865-867.

Oliverio, A., Castellano, C., & Eleftheriou, B. E. (1975). Morphine sensitivity and tolerance: A genetic investigation in the mouse. Psychopharmacologia, **42**, 219.

Reggiani, A., Battaini, F., Kobayashi, H., Spano, P., & Trabucchi, M. (1980). Genotype-dependent sensitivity to morphine: Role of different opiate receptor populations. Brain Research, **189**, 389-294.

Reith, E. A., Sershen, H., Vadasz, C., & Lajtha, A. (1981). Strain differences in opiate receptors in mouse brain. European Journal of Pharmacology, **74**, 377-380.

Sansone, M., Ammassari-Teule, M., Renzi, P., & Oliverio, A. (1981). Different effects of apomorphine on locomotor activity in C57BL/6 and DBA/2 mice. Pharmacology Biochemistry & Behavior, **14**, 741-743.

Seale, T. W., McLanahan, K., Johnson, P., Carney, J. M., & Rennert, O. M. (1984). Systematic comparisons of apomorphine-induced behavioral changes in two mouse strains with inherited differences in brain dopamine receptors. Pharmacology Biochemistry & Behavior, **21**, 237-244.

Severson, J. A., Randall, P. K., & Finch, C. E. (1981). Genotypic influences on striatal dopaminergic regulation in mice. Brain Research, **210**, 201-215.

Sidman, R., Angevine, J. B., & Pierce, E. T. (1971). Atlas of the mouse brain and spinal cord. Cambridge, MA: Harvard University Press.

Siegfried, B., Frischknecht, H., & Waser, P. G. (1984). Defeat, learned submissiveness, and analgesia in mice: Effect of genotype. Behavioral and Neural Biology, **42**, 91-97.

Appendix

Program Listing for Brain Stimulation Reward Studies

```
  1 I = 0: OPEN 4,4
    :REM OPEN PRINTER PORT
  2 DIM C0(20), C1(20)
  5 PRINT "{SC}"
    :REM CLEAR SCREEN
  7 M = 0
    :N = 0
 10 POKE 37138,31
    :REM SET UP OUTPUT PORTS
 15 POKE 37136,31
 17 POKE 37139,132
 18 POKE 37137,4
 20 PRINT "TYPE ON TO TURN ON THE CURRENT"
 22 INPUT X$
    :REM TURN ON RELAYS TO TEST CONTINUITY
 24 IF X$ = "ON" THEN GOSUB 800
 30 POKE 37136,31
 45 PRINT "{SC}"
 50 BASE = PEEK (36872)
    :REM TEST PHOTOCELL OUTPUT < 250 = ON
 60 PRINT "ACTIVE = "; BASE
 75 B1 = PEEK (36873)
 77 PRINT "THE PASSIVE PHOTOCELL"
    :PRINT "OUTPUT = "; B1
 80 GET X$
    :IF X$ = "" THEN 45
 85 B1 = 254
 95 INPUT "STIMULUS DURATION"; LINGTH
```

```
100 TI$ = "000000"
    :REM DURATION IS IN 60THS OF A SECOND
105 PRINT "{SC}"
110 BASE = 254
200 RESP = PEEK (36872)
    :REM READ ACTIVE PHOTOCELL
210 IF RESP > BASE THEN GOSUB 500
250 R1 = PEEK (36873)
    :REM READ PASSIVE PHOTOCELL
260 IF R1 > B1 THEN GOSUB 600
300 IF TI$ > "001000" THEN GOSUB 950
    :REM PRINT DATA EVERY 10 MINUTES
310 IF I = 12 THEN PRINT #4
    :CLOSE 4
    :END
    :REM STOP AFTER 2 HOURS
390 PRINT "{HM}"; TI$
    :PRINT COUNT(I); "REINFORCED"
    :PRINT
395 PRINT C1(I); "PASSIVE"
400 GOTO 200
500 POKE 37136,N
    :REM TURN ON RELAYS
510 X = TI + LINGTH
520 COUNT(I) = COUNT(I) + 1
    :REM INCREMENT RESPONSE COUNTER
550 IF TI < X THEN 550
    :REM WAIT
560 POKE 37136,31
    :REM TURN OFF RELAYS
562 M = M + 1
565 IF (M = 5 AND N < 15) THEN M = 0
    :N = N + 1
    :IF N = 15 THEN N = 31
    :REM DECREASE CURRENT
570 IF PEEK (36872) > = BASE THEN 570
590 RETURN
600 C1(I) = C1(I) + 1
610 X = TI + LINGTH
613 IF (N > 0 OR M > 0) THEN GOSUB 900
    :REM PRINT CURRENT LEVEL
614 POKE 37137,0
    :REM TURN ON DISCRIMINATIVE STIMULUS
615 N = 0
    :M = 0
    :REM RESET CURRENT LEVEL
620 IF TI < X THEN 620
700 IF PEEK (36873) > B1 THEN 700
710 POKE 37137,4
    :REM TURN OFF DISCRIMINATIVE STIMULUS
720 RETURN
800 POKE 37136,N
810 PRINT "TO TURN THE CURRENT OFF"
    :PRINT "AND CONTINUE TYPE"
    :PRINT "RETURN"
820 GET X$
    :IF X$ = "" THEN 820
```

```
830 RETURN
900 IF N = 31 THEN N = 16
    :REM COMPUTE MEAN CURRENT LEVEL
910 PRINT #4, "N = "; N
    :A = A + N
    :NN = NN + 1
    :RETURN
950 PRINT #4, I, C0(I), C1(I)
    :I = I + 1
    :TI$ = "000000"
    :PRINT"{SC}"
960 IF NN = 0 THEN PRINT #4, "NO RESPONSES"
    :RETURN
970 PRINT #4, "THRESHOLD = "
    :(A/NN)
    :A = 0
    :NN = 0
    :RETURN
```

CHAPTER 30

AN OVERVIEW OF ASSESSING DRUG REINFORCEMENT

Michael A. Bozarth

Center for Studies in Behavioral Neurobiology
Department of Psychology
Concordia University
Montreal, Quebec, Canada H3G 1M8

ABSTRACT

The various methods used to study drug reinforcement are briefly examined, and some of the advantages and limitations of each procedure are discussed. Although some measures may seem preferable to others, each experimental technique has certain applications where it is most appropriate. The concordance of different experimental paradigms is also examined by summarizing the results of studies attempting to identify the neural substrates of psychomotor stimulant and opiate rewards. In general, there is substantial agreement among different experimental paradigms purporting to identify the brain mechanisms involved in these drug rewards. Finally, a protocol is suggested for the routine screening of new compounds for addiction liability. This protocol uses several experimental procedures, including both indirect and direct indices of drug reinforcement.

INTRODUCTION

As evidenced by the chapters in this book, there are a variety of ways to study the reinforcing properties of abused drugs. This chapter will present a brief overview of the major methods of assessing drug reinforcement, examine the concordance among several experimental techniques, and outline a protocol for screening new compounds for their addiction potential. The overviews of the different experimental methods are necessarily cursory and only a few exemplary considerations for using these methods are outlined. These topics are fully explored in the various chapters, and the reader is referred to this material for a detailed discussion of the experimental methods summarized here.

Definitions and Terms

Before proceeding to an overview of the techniques used to assess drug reinforcement and their relationships to drug addiction and drug abuse liability, it is necessary to briefly define some of the terms used in this chapter. The term drug addiction has suffered from numerous re-interpretations and a general lack of standardization in its usage. The term addict and its derivatives were used in reference to alcohol by 1612 and tobacco by 1779 (Oxford English Dictionary) and described habitual morphine use by 1909 (Oxford English Dictionary [Supplement]). Both morphine addiction (Tatum, Seevers, & Collins, 1929) and cocaine addiction (Tatum & Seevers, 1929) were described in scientific papers in 1929 without explicit definition of the term addiction. Drug addiction was defined, however, by Tatum and Seevers in 1931 as "a condition developed through the effects of repeated actions of a drug such that its use becomes necessary and cessation of its action causes mental or physical disturbances (p. 107)." The nature of these disturbances was vividly described in the literature.

The early use of the term addiction appears to have described a condition where chronic and habitual drug use develops and the individual becomes intensely preoccupied with the drug and its effects. Later definitions focused on physiological dependence, and drug addiction has come to be applied commonly to describe a condition where the organism becomes physiologically dependent on a substance. The general confusion about the use of this term has led several agencies to advocate abandoning the use of this term altogether (e.g., American Psychiatric Association; World Health Organization) and to replace it by clearly defined terms that have not yet been adopted into common usage. The obvious advantage of coining new terms is that they do not carry the connotations that have been developed over a long period of poorly defined use. However, it is difficult to totally eliminate a word from language by edict, and it is perhaps preferable to re-define the term for scientific usage if the lay usage of the term carries a similar meaning.

The general lexical definition of addiction is notably different from the special application that it has been given by many pharmacologists and clinicians. The American Heritage Dictionary defines addiction under the verb addict as follows:

> to devote or give (oneself) habitually or compulsively . . . [the term is derived from] Latin addictus 'given over,' one awarded to another as a slave. (p. 15)

Furthermore, Webster's Third New International Dictionary defines addict as follows:

> to apply or devote (as oneself or one's mind) habitually: give (oneself) up or surrender (oneself) as a constant practice . . . [also] one who habitually uses and has an uncontrollable craving for an addictive drug. (p. 24)

Addiction is defined as:

> the compulsive uncontrolled use of habit-forming drugs beyond the period of medical need or under conditions harmful to society . . . enthusiasm, devotion, strong inclination, or frequent indulgence. (p. 24)

The Oxford English Dictionary defines addict as:

> 1. To deliver over formally by sentence of a judge (to anyone). 2. To bind, attach, or devote oneself as a servant, disciple, or adherent (to any person or cause). 3. To attach (anyone) to a pursuit. 4. To devote, give up, or apply habitually to a practice . . . (A person addicts his mind, etc., or his tastes addict him.) (p. 103)

Interestingly, the term addiction is found in Roman Law describing:

A formal giving over or delivery by sentence of court. Hence, a surrender, or dedication, of any one to a master (Oxford English Dictionary, p. 104)

The confusing use of this term does not stem from the common use, from the general definition, or from the etymology of this term but rather from the scientific community's attempt to educate the lay population about the (once) presumed underlying cause of addiction. Physiological dependence appeared to be a common property of addictive drugs and was presumed to be the primary etiological factor in the development of an addiction. With more recent data showing that physiological dependence is not a necessary component or even a concomitant of addiction to some compounds, much of the scientific community has hopelessly tainted their use of this term by attempting to define it independent of its original behavioral definition.

Jaffe (1975) has provided a more precise, scientific definition of addiction:

a behavioral pattern of compulsive drug use, characterized by overwhelming involvement with the use of a drug, the securing of its supply, and a high tendency to relapse after withdrawal [abstinence]. (p. 285)

It should be noted that addiction defined in this manner is not viewed as the cause of drug-taking behavior, but rather it is a description of the behavior. The use of the term addiction as an explanation of compulsive drug-taking behavior would be circular because this term is in fact defined by the behavior that it describes. Other causes of addiction must be identified to avoid the nominal explanation of drug-taking behavior resulting from addiction.

The term drug abuse has fewer problems with its definition. The lay and scientific communities have used this term in similar fashions, although several scientific agencies have again recommended that this term be dropped from professional usage. For the purposes of this chapter, and indeed much of this book, the term drug abuse has been used as defined by Jaffe (1975):

the use, usually by self-administration, of any drug in a manner that deviates from the approved medical or social patterns within a given culture. The term conveys the notion of social disapproval, and it is not necessarily descriptive of any particular pattern of drug use or its potential adverse consequences. (p. 284)

Although the use of the term drug abuse clearly differs from the use of the term addiction and explicitly does not indicate whether there are "potential adverse consequences" of the drug's use, the use of most drugs that fall under the definition of drug abuse is usually associated with substance use that has a disruptive influence on society. The use of addictive drugs is almost invariably defined as drug abuse, even though not all instances of drug abuse involve substances that are addictive. In general, the use of a substance in a manner prohibited by the society the individual lives in attests to the strong motivational effects of that substance. These drugs are frequently drugs whose long-term use is associated with adverse psychological or medical consequences. (There are several notable exceptions to this relationship including the taboo against even moderate alcohol use in Islamic cultures.) The fact that drug use persists despite social (and usually legal) sanctions against its use aptly demonstrates the potent motivational effects of the drug and suggests a potential for addiction to that substance. Drug abuse encompasses a somewhat wider range of substances than does drug addiction, but many (and perhaps even most) drugs that are abused by a large segment of society have the potential to produce an addiction. Hence, drug addiction can usually be viewed as an extreme form of drug abuse with the added features outlined by Jaffe (1975).

Role of Drug Reinforcement in Drug Addiction

Because the term addiction is limited to a description of behavior, other factors must be identified that control the development and expression of drug addiction. One approach to studying drug addiction involves describing the relationship of the behavior to the consequences of that behavior. That is, the behavior of drug taking is governed by the direct and immediate consequence of that behavior--drug administration and the ensuing pharmacological actions of the drug. Essentially, this model of drug addiction is a simple extension of basic operant psychology. Viewed with this perspective, drug addiction is just another behavior controlled by its consequences and does not represent any special class of motivation or behavior (see Bozarth, 1986). The term reinforcement is used to describe the relationship between the behavior (i.e., drug taking) and the consequences of that behavior (i.e., drug effect). Drug self-administration is the paramount case of drug reinforcement--the operant response directly produces administration of the addictive substance. In operant terms, reinforcement is said to occur when the presentation of the reinforcing stimulus (i.e., drug) increases the probability (or frequency) of the behavior that presentation of the stimulus is contingent upon. Positive reinforcement refers to the situation where the presentation of a reinforcing stimulus increases the frequency of a behavior, and negative reinforcement refers to the cases where removal of some stimulus (usually an aversive event such as electric shock) results in an increase in the frequency of some behavior. Although the motivational properties of stimuli serving as positive and negative reinforcers would appear to be much different, the consequence of these stimuli is the same--they both increase the frequency of the behaviors they are associated with. Punishment, on the other hand, represents a much different situation where the presentation of some stimulus (again, usually aversive) suppresses the behavior that it is associated with. It is important to keep in mind the distinction between punishment and negative reinforcement. These terms are frequently used incorrectly as synonyms because they both involve aversive stimuli, but they in fact represent much different processes involved in the control of behavior.

There are two general models of drug addiction that have evolved from reinforcement theory. One model focuses on the positive reinforcing properties of a drug and is probably related to drug-induced mood elevation and euphoria. The second model focuses on the potential negative reinforcing properties of drug administration; chronic administration of many drugs can produce physiological dependence, and drug abstinence can produce an aversive motivational state that is relieved by subsequent drug intake. Although both models are derived from reinforcement theory and emphasize observable behavior and the pharmacological actions of addictive drugs, their motivational effects can be much different. Negative reinforcement models have figured prominently in some traditional theories of drug addiction, but positive reinforcement models appear to have become dominant in recent years. Indeed, most of the chapters in this book reflect the new emphasis on positive reinforcement models of drug addiction.

The use of the phrase "the role of reinforcement in drug addiction" is somewhat misleading. Any event can be studied in terms of reinforcement theory, and the use of this phrase really implies a scientific approach rather than a cause of drug-taking behavior. There is, however, an important feature that distinguishes this approach from other theoretical orientations--the emphasis of this approach is usually on the contingencies of drug self-administration and the pharmacological properties of the drug.

It may be argued that reinforcement theory offers no more than a nominal explanation of drug addiction. In fact, there does appear to be an inherent circularity in describing a behavior as "produced by" the consequences of that behavior. Reinforcement models of drug addiction have, however, transcended their strict operational definitions and generate more implicit rules governing drug-taking behavior. These models generally focus on the intrinsic reinforcing properties of the drug and place far less emphasis on special conditions that are necessary for the drug to serve as a reinforcer. In particular, the observation that most drugs that are potent reinforcers of human behavior (and hence are potentially addictive) are also potent reinforcers of animal behavior has received considerable attention and further supports the notion that some inherent property of the drug is critical for this reinforcing action. Thus, reinforcement theory does not rely strictly on nominally explaining drug-taking behavior but provides an empirical construct that has evolved from this perspective of drug addiction.

Rationale for the Study of Drug Reinforcement

Compulsive drug-taking behavior is the defining characteristic of an addiction, and drug reinforcement is a primary determinant in drug-taking behavior. Thus, the study of drug reinforcement is, in essence, the study of drug addiction. The general rationale for the study of drug reinforcement requires no explanation, but a brief outline of some of the more obvious reasons is nonetheless appropriate. The methods used to study drug reinforcement provide an instrument for:

1. the study of drug addiction qua addiction (e.g., the determination of patterns of drug-intake, motivational properties of drugs, and interactions among various addictive drugs and other reinforcers; see chapter by Mello & Mendelson);

2. the determination of brain mechanisms mediating drug addiction (see chapters by Broekkamp; Phillips & Fibiger; Roberts & Zito);

3. the screening of new compounds for potential addiction liability (see chapters by Brady, Griffiths, Hienz, Ator, Lukas, & Lamb; Reid; Weeks & Collins; Yanagita; see also chapters by de Wit & Johanson; Haertzen & Hickey; Henningfield, Johnson, & Jasinski);

4. the development of treatments for drug addiction (see chapter by Amit, Smith, & Sutherland);

5. the study of structure-activity relationships in medicinal chemistry (see chapter by Glennon & Young); and

6. an approach to studying basic motivational processes (see chapter by White, Messier, & Carr; see also Bozarth, 1982, 1986).

PRINCIPAL METHODS FOR ASSESSING DRUG REINFORCEMENT

The following section presents a brief overview of the major methods used to assess drug reinforcement in laboratory animals and in humans. Some of the main advantages and disadvantages of each technique are outlined, although no attempt is made to provide a detailed discussion of the various techniques. This section is presented only to summarize these methods, and the reader should consult the individual chapters specifically addressing the various experimental methods for details.

Intravenous Self-Administration

Intravenous self-administration involves preparing animals with intravenous catheters and allowing them to self-administer a drug (see chapters by Brady, Griffiths, Hienz, Ator, Lukas, & Lamb; Weeks & Collins; Yanagita; Yokel). Some behavioral response, usually lever pressing, is followed by intravenous drug administration, and the ability of the drug injection to directly reinforce behavior is determined. Two basic procedures are used to establish the self-administration of a drug. The cross substitution procedure involves initially training animals to self-administer a standard reinforcing drug such as cocaine and then substituting the test drug and determining if the new drug maintains self-administration. This method has the advantage of circumventing the drug's influence on learning when screening potentially reinforcing drugs, but has the disadvantage associated with possible pharmacological interactions between the training drug and the test drug. The direct acquisition method involves testing drug-naive animals for the acquisition of intravenous self-administration.

The largest advantage of the intravenous self-administration technique is that the principles of operant conditioning can be directly applied to the study of drug reinforcement. Intravenous drug self-administration can control behavior in much the same manner as traditional reinforcers such as food and water in hungry or thirsty animals (for a review, see Spealman & Goldberg, 1978; see also Katz & Goldberg, this volume; cf. Wise, this volume).

There are several specific advantages of using intravenous self-administration to study drug reinforcement. First, the patterns of drug intake can be used to distinguish reward from motoric effects of pharmacological challenges (see chapters by Yokel; Wise). Second, principles of operant conditioning can be directly applied to assess drug reinforcement. For example, progressive-ratio testing can determine the relative reinforcing strength of several compounds (see chapters by Brady, Griffiths, Hienz, Ator, Lukas, & Lamb; Weeks & Collins; Yanagita; Yokel), and persistence of drug-seeking behavior and relapse can be directly studied by examining extinction patterns of responding (see Stewart & de Wit, this volume). Third, the pattern of drug intake can be evaluated and cases of regulated drug intake and binge intake can be easily distinguished (see Yokel, this volume). Fourth, choice procedures have been developed where the animals choose one of two reinforcing drug injections; either different doses of the same compound or two different drugs can be tested with this method.

There are also several disadvantages to using intravenous self-administration, and these disadvantages are severe enough to restrict the number of laboratories currently using this technique. First, the intravenous preparation is relatively difficult to maintain; subject loss due to blocked or leaky catheters and illness can be quite high. Second, although animals learn quite quickly to self-administer some drugs (e.g., cocaine, heroin), weeks and sometimes months of testing is often required for response patterns and drug-intake levels to stabilize. Third, the dose range tested for self-administration is very important; if excessively high drug doses are tested, aversive side-effects may inhibit drug self-administration; if very low doses are tested, the drug may not be sufficiently rewarding to establish or maintain operant behavior. Fourth, possible drug interactions and learning variables can be important when the cross substitution procedure is used; abrupt decreases in the reward magnitude can produce a negative contrast effect, and animals might fail to maintain self-administration of a drug that would otherwise be reinforcing. Also, important interactions may occur between the effects of the training drug and the test drug. For example, animals initially trained to self-administer heroin would be unlikely to self-administer an agonist/antagonist like pentazocine because the latter compound would precipitate withdrawal which would presumably be aversive. In direct acquisition studies, drugs that disrupt learning may retard the acquisition of drug self-administration, even though they can serve as reinforcers.

Intravenous self-administration has a high degree of face validity. It is the most direct method of studying drug reinforcement because it directly measures the ability of a drug to reinforce behavior; it is viewed by most drug addiction specialists to be unequivocal demonstration of a drug's reinforcing action, provided certain behavioral control procedures are tested. Furthermore, there is excellent concordance between the ability of a drug to support intravenous self-administration in animals and its addiction potential in humans (see Griffiths & Balster, 1979; Weeks & Collins, this volume).

Other Self-Administration Procedures

There are several other self-administration procedures that have been used in laboratory animals. Each of these methods has been applied in special situations, although their use is generally not as widespread and they lack the consentaneous validity given the intravenous technique.

Oral self-administration has been shown for several drugs (see chapters by Amit, Smith, & Sutherland; Meisch & Carroll). This method has the advantage of being relatively easy but suffers from controversy regarding the interpretation of some data derived from this technique. Nonetheless, oral drug self-administration has three advantages that establish it as a useful technique for studying drug reinforcement. First, it is easy and does not require surgical preparation of the subjects or special apparatus. Any laboratory with animal housing facilities and drinking bottles can use this technique. Second, the experimental preparation remains viable for long periods of time. Studies that require extensive testing of the subjects can be completed where the attrition rate in intravenous self-administration would be prohibitive. Third, large numbers of subjects can be easily tested. When assessing the effects of brain lesions or pharmacological challenges, individual subject reactivity to the treatment may require that large sample sizes be used. The oral self-administration procedure, because of its low equipment and labor requirements, is especially suitable for testing such large numbers of subjects.

Intragastric self-administration has been shown for several compounds (e.g., see Yanagita, this volume), but it does not appear to have any significant advantages over intravenous self-administration for most drugs. The argument has been made that drugs abused by the oral route of administration are best studied by this technique, but that argument has not been substantiated.

Intracranial self-administration has been shown for several compounds (see Bozarth, 1983, this volume). Self-administration procedures have been modified to produce drug microinjections directly into brain tissue. This method has the distinct advantage of localizing the reinforcing action of a drug (provided certain control procedures are observed), but it is methodologically difficult and only a few laboratories have reported success with this technique. Intracranial self-administration is a valuable technique for asking certain experimental questions that cannot be addressed with other experimental methods.

The concordance of the results from these methods with the documented addiction liability of various drugs in humans has not been evaluated. Some addictive drugs are correctly categorized with each of these measures, but too few compounds have been tested to fully evaluate the overall accuracy of these methods in predicting addiction liability.

Conditioned Place Preference

Conditioned place preference is a relatively new method of assessing the rewarding effects of drugs. With this method the animal develops an association between the rewarding action of a drug and specific environmental cues. When tested in the drug-free state, the animal approaches and maintains contact with the environmental cues that have been associated with the rewarding drug. This procedure involves several conditioning trials where the animal is injected with the test compound and placed in a specific compartment of the test apparatus containing various cues (e.g., tactile, visual, and/or olfactory). The animal is later tested to determine if it increases the amount of time spent in the compartment associated with the drug injection. If so, a conditioned place preference is said to have developed, and the drug is presumed to have some rewarding action. There are numerous variations of this basic method (see chapters by Bozarth; Phillips & Fibiger; Reid; van der Kooy; White, Messier, & Carr), but all of these procedures appear to produce strikingly similar results.

The conditioned place preference method appears to be quick and easy. Only simple equipment is required, and no special surgical preparation of the animals is needed. Procedural differences do not appear to be important, although some methods of testing may be preferred over others (see van der Kooy, this volume). The motor facilitating or impairing effects of some drug treatments that adversely influence most measures of drug reward do not have a significant influence with this method, because the response requirement is very simple and because the animals are usually tested in the drug-free state when the motoric effects of these drugs are absent. Lastly, this technique offers a direct method of studying conditioning effects which are important in the control of drug-taking behavior.

The main disadvantage of this method is that little is really known about the basis of this effect. Manipulations that should have a strong influence on classical conditioning have a relatively small effect on conditioned place preference. Also, investigators using much different conditioning and testing procedures report surprisingly similar strengths of conditioning; the subjects usually show around a 200 second increase in the time spent in the conditioning environment during a 15-minute test. Finally, although not documented in the literature, the conditioned place preference technique may be prone to spurious results; that is, individual tests where rewarding drugs do not produce a preference and other tests where nonrewarding drugs produce a slight, but statistically significant, conditioned place preference may occur with an unacceptably high frequency; this makes replication of important findings derived from this technique very important.

The concordance of conditioned place preference studies with human addiction liability has not yet been established. Conditioned place preferences have been shown for a wide variety of drugs that are addictive in humans, and nonaddictive drugs generally do not produce a place preference (see Bozarth, this volume). Furthermore, the place preference produced by heroin is very reliable over numerous replications (see Bozarth, this volume). Because this technique is relatively new and because the variables controlling place preference conditioning are not well understood, caution should be exercised when interpreting the results of these studies. Specifically, the results of conditioned place preference studies should be considered in concert with the findings from more established techniques, and this method is probably most valuable as a preliminary screen for addiction liability and for answering experimental questions that cannot be suitably addressed with other methods.

Other Conditioning Procedures

There are several other conditioning procedures that have been used to study the rewarding effects of drugs. The two techniques that have received the most study are conditioned reinforcement (see Davis & Smith, this volume) and reinstatement of responding (see Stewart & de Wit, this volume).

Conditioned reinforcement studies involve developing an association between a rewarding drug injection and some stimulus (e.g., visual, auditory) that is concurrently presented with the drug infusion. The animal is later tested to determine if it will lever press to produce presentation of the drug-associated stimulus. If the drug injections were reinforcing, then lever-pressing behavior should be maintained (or established) by the presentation of the stimulus event associated with the drug reward. One of the most important applications of this technique is testing manipulations that may interfere with operant responding. Because the animal passively receives the rewarding drug injections during the conditioning trials, pharmacological treatments that interfere with response performance should not affect the establishment of the conditioned reinforcer. Testing for the putative rewarding drug effect occurs when the animal is drug-free (as in the place preference conditioning method) and thus should not be influenced by motor-impairing drug effects.

Reinstatement of operant responding involves a much different procedure with a similar conceptual basis. The animal is first trained to intravenously self-administer a drug. It is then subjected to extinction trials where the drug vehicle (usually physiological saline) is substituted for the reinforcing drug. After several extinction trials, the response rates drop to control levels. Next, a priming drug injection is given noncontingently to the animal. If the drug effect is similar to the rewarding effect of the drug that the animal was trained to self-administer, the animal will reinstate lever pressing even though it only receives the drug vehicle with each self-administered infusion. This phenomenon is probably related to the priming effect that is seen in many behavioral studies, and it may be related to the sensations of drug craving in humans. There are two important potential applications of this technique. First, this procedure may provide a model of relapse to drug self-administration (and addiction), and conditioning factors involved in drug-taking behavior can be directly studied. Second, this method appears to have a great potential as a preclinical screening tool. Animals can be trained on standard drugs such as cocaine or heroin and the abilities of new compounds to reinstatement responding determined. If the test drug produces an increase in operant responding, then it probably has properties very similar to the training drug. A major advantage of this method over other techniques that are designed to test similarities across compounds (e.g., drug discrimination) appears to be the ease of training the subjects. Another potential advantage is that pharmacologically dissimilar drugs that share similar addiction liabilities may show cross generalization. For example, animals trained on cocaine show a reinstatement of responding when given a noncontingent injection of morphine (de Wit & Stewart, 1981). This cross generalization combined with the ease of training and the fact that (unlike conditioned place preference) these animals can be repeatedly tested on various drugs makes this method of assessing drug reinforcement one of the most promising new methods for screening compounds for addiction liability.

Brain Stimulation Reward

This method of studying drug reward involves training animals to work for electrical brain stimulation and determining the effects of drugs on brain stimulation reward (see chapters by Esposito, Porrino, & Seeger; Lewis & Phelps; Reid). Addictive drugs appear to enhance or facilitate brain stimulation reward; this facilitation effect can be demonstrated as an increased rate of lever pressing for fixed intensity brain stimulation (see Reid & Bozarth, 1978) or as a lowering of current thresholds for brain stimulation (see Esposito & Kornetsky, 1978). Although many manipulations can attenuate brain stimulation reward including both reward and response-impairing manipulations, facilitation of brain stimulation reward has not been reported for pharmacological treatments that lack independently confirmed, directly reinforcing actions.

Both rate and threshold measures of brain stimulation should reveal any facilitatory effect that the test drug might produce. Rate measures are easy to obtain and require only simple equipment. The primary disadvantage seems to be that rates can vary considerably over the course of a test session. Brief pauses in responding can greatly affect the lever-pressing rate for small time samples (e.g., 1 to 5 minutes). If one attempts to determine the drug's time-course by continuously testing the subject for an hour or more and to resolve response-rate measures into short time samples (e.g., 10-minute time periods), the effects of fatigue and response pauses can adversely influence the rate measures. It is probably better to test the subject for only a few minutes of each hour (or perhaps at 30-minute time periods) to increase the likelihood that the animal will not take breaks or experience significant fatigue. Such testing has yielded stable baseline rates of responding over the course of 24 hours (e.g., Atalay & Wise, 1983). Alternatively, most threshold measures are not influenced by response pauses or fatigue, and the animal's threshold can be continuously "tracked" over the course of several hours of testing. Threshold procedures require, however, more sophisticated equipment or more laborious testing procedures although microcomputers can easily automate the procedure.

This technique is very easy and considerable experience has been gained with brain stimulation reward over the past three decades. The surgical procedure is simple and the animals are easy to maintain. The drug effect is assessed against an already established behavior so learning effects are not important. The initial drug dose tested is not critical, because the animal is working for the rewarding effects of the electrical stimulation and behavior will not be extinguished with subrewarding drug doses as in the intravenous self-administration method. Repeated drug testing does not disrupt the animal's behavior, and full time-course and dose-response data can be easily generated. The pharmacokinetics of the drug's action can provide direction to other, more direct methods of assessing drug reinforcement, and the use of this technique for determining dose and time-after-injection parameters is probably the most important application of brain stimulation reward in screening drug addiction liability.

There has been controversy regarding the use of some measures. For example, the use of response rates has been challenged (e.g., Kornetsky & Esposito, 1979), and the two-lever autotitration method appears to have some problems (see Fouriezos & Nawiesniak, this volume). The most serious limitation of this technique involves consideration of what is actually being measured--the interaction of the addictive drug with the neural substrate presumed to mediate its rewarding action. Brain stimulation reward studies provided some of the earliest evidence that addictive drugs may interact with brain reward systems, and early applications of this technique (e.g., Broekkamp, 1976; see also Broekkamp, this volume) have been very influential in subsequent work studying the neural basis of drug reward (e.g., Bozarth & Wise, 1981). Nonetheless, the effect of drugs on brain stimulation reward remains an indirect method of assessing addiction liability.

The overall concordance of the results of brain stimulation reward studies with human addiction liability data is very good (see Bozarth, 1978). In fact, brain stimulation reward studies predicted the long-term abuse liability of several compounds that were initially "missed" by intravenous self-administration studies (see Bozarth, 1978). The potential usefulness of this technique for determining the dose and time course of potentially rewarding drug-effects is probably unequaled by any other method, and this technique can potentially make a unique contribution to the preclinical screening of drugs for addiction liability.

Drug Discrimination

Drug discrimination involves training an animal to make one of two (or more) alternate responses when under the influence of a specific drug (see chapters by Colpaert; Overton). For example, the animal is injected with a training drug, and one of two possible responses (e.g., depressing the left-hand or right-hand lever; turning left or right in a T-maze) is reinforced (e.g., food reward presented to a food-deprived animal). Alternative trials are conducted under either placebo or another drug; the subject must learn to make a different response to obtain reinforcement when it has not been injected with the training drug. Once the animal has learned to discriminate the training drug effect from that of placebo and to make the correct response, new compounds can be tested for their ability to produce stimulus properties similar to the training drug. If the test drug produces similar cue properties, the subject should make the same response as when it is injected with the training drug.

Drug discrimination offers a very sensitive measure of the stimulus properties of various drugs. Animals can successfully discriminate various classes of drugs (e.g., ethanol, benzodiazepines, psychomotor stimulants, opiates), and they can even distinguish between two drugs in the same general pharmacological class (e.g., the stimulants amphetamine and apomorphine;

Hernandez, Holohean, & Appel, 1978). Dose-response effects are easily obtained, and new compounds can be fairly quickly tested once the animal has been successfully trained in the discrimination task. This general technique has been used to study structure-activity relationships for several classes of drugs (e.g., see Glennon & Young, this volume), and relatively small changes in molecular structure can produce large changes in the compound's stimulus properties. With the procedures used by most investigators, drug discrimination studies are relatively insensitive to the response-impairing effects of some drugs since a disruption of motor capacity would only decrease response rates and not influence which choice the animal makes.

Most methods of training subjects to reliably discriminate the stimulus properties of a drug involve long training periods and a substantial investment in time and effort. Retraining periods must be interspersed with test sessions to insure that the animal still makes the correct response when given the training drug. The effect of various treatments on the motivational properties of the primary reinforcer have not been evaluated, but changes in motivational level may influence response selection and this variable needs to be systematically evaluated. Most importantly, drug discrimination is based on the stimulus properties of a drug and there is no reason a priori to suppose that the most salient drug cues are necessarily related to the attributes that the investigator wishes to assess. For example, opiate drugs produce a number of effects including reward, analgesia, physiological dependence, changes in gastric motility, and changes in other autonomic nervous system functions. When a drug is reported to have stimulus properties similar to morphine, any one (or more) of the myriad of stimulus effects could be responsible for this effect. It is indeed erroneous to conclude that the test drug is an analgesic or that it will have an addiction liability similar to morphine.

The concordance of drug discrimination studies with human addiction liability appears reasonably good, but there has been no systematic evaluation conducted across a wide range of drugs. The stimulus properties of a drug in humans (as measured by instruments such as the Addiction Research Center Inventory) may be an excellent predictor of the drug's potential for abuse, but there is no reason to presuppose that similar stimulus properties in animals are responsible for the generalization in the drug discrimination method. In reporting the subjective effects of addictive drugs in humans, special attention has been directed toward identifying response items (e.g., euphoria, drug liking) that correctly classify highly addictive drugs. Thus, not all of the stimulus properties of a drug necessarily constitute its subjective-effects profile that predicts addiction liability.

Subjective-Effects Measures in Humans

Some of the earliest studies attempting to identify variables that would predict a drug's addiction liability involved assessing the subjective effects of the drug after administration in humans. Much of this work was pioneered at the Addiction Research Center in Lexington, Kentucky, and it usually involved determining the effects of various addictive drugs in ex-addict, prisoner volunteers from the local federal penitentiary.

Questionnaires have been designed to evaluate the subjective effects of drugs in humans. One of the tests, the Addiction Research Center Inventory (ARCI), has several specific scales that identify drug effects similar to prototypical addictive agents (see Haertzen & Hickey, this volume). The ARCI has been very successful in accurately classifying addictive drugs. It is an empirically keyed questionnaire based on a very large sample size, and it can be used with either single dose or chronic drug evaluation. Several other questionnaires have also been developed, some of which are based on items derived from the ARCI (see Henningfield, Johnson, & Jasinski, this volume).

The major advantage of subjective-effects questionnaires is that they have been shown to accurately classify the addiction liability of known addictive drugs. When used following a single drug injection, they also minimize the subject's exposure to the potentially addictive drug. Two important limitations of these tests are that new addictive compounds may possess properties that are not identified as "like" the prototypical addictive drugs the scoring system is based on and that repeated exposure or subject-controlled exposure may influence the addiction liability of the compound. Nonetheless, subjective-effects measures are frequently employed even where other measures of drug reinforcement are the primary interest (e.g., see de Wit & Johanson, this volume). The concordance of these measures with the observed addiction liability of most drugs is very high.

Human Drug Self-Administration

A more direct method of assessing the reinforcing properties of addictive drugs in humans involves tests for drug self-administration (see chapters by Henningfield, Johnson, & Jasinski; Mello & Mendelson). Laboratory procedures very similar to those used in animal intravenous self-administration can be adapted for use in humans. Not surprising, some of the same patterns of responding seen in animals are also seen during human drug self-administration (e.g., see Mello & Mendelson, this volume).

The major advantage of this technique is that it directly assesses the reinforcing properties of the drug. The major disadvantages are that this method is costly and that it usually involves considerable exposure to the potentially addictive substance, thus risking the development of an addiction in the experimental subjects. This technique has not been used extensively to screen new compounds (Its primary use seems to have been to study known addictive drugs.), so it is premature to judge its usefulness for predicting the addiction liability of new drugs. The face validity of this method, however, is extremely high.

Choice Testing in Humans

A relatively new procedure for assessing drug reinforcement in humans involves choice testing (see de Wit & Johanson, this volume). Subjects are given alternative trials with two or more color-coded capsules and are instructed to associate the drug effects with the different capsules. After several training trials have been completed, the subjects are tested in a choice condition where they can select one of the two (or more) color-coded capsules for ingestion. The relative preference for the capsules is used as a measure of drug reinforcement, and subjects generally show a significant preference for drugs with a known addiction liability.

The are several advantages to using this technique for assessing drug addiction liability in humans. First, relatively few drug exposures are necessary to demonstrate a preference for highly addictive drugs; this minimizes the exposure of the experimental subjects to potentially dangerous or addictive drugs. Second, choice testing can be conducted between drug and placebo or among two or more drugs. Relative measures could potentially demonstrate preferences for various addictive drugs or different dosages of the same drug. Third, subjective-effects measures can be easily taken during the training trials without disrupting the subject's performance. Thus, choice testing can be conducted concurrently with subjective-effects assessment, and the drug evaluation can be based on the outcome of both measures. Fourth, this experimental method is relatively inexpensive and does not require any special apparatus or facilities. Fifth, this technique does not require that the subjects be tested as inpatients. This greatly increases the range of subject populations that can be easily recruited for this procedure, and it can allow the subjects to experience the drug effects in their natural environment.

Most choice testing involves relatively few exposures to the test drug. Some addictive drugs may require repeated administration, higher doses, or special conditions to be reinforcing, and this technique may not accurately predict abuse liability in these situations.

Choice testing accurately classifies the addiction liability of amphetamine, but an insufficient number of other compounds has been tested with this method to determine if other classes of addictive drugs show similar effects. The technique is very promising, but considerably more work needs to be completed before its usefulness for screening new compounds can be accurately evaluated.

CROSS VALIDATION OF EXPERIMENTAL PROCEDURES

During the past decade, considerable progress has been made in identifying and characterizing the neural basis of psychomotor stimulant and opiate rewards. The ventral tegmental dopamine system appears to be involved in both classes of drug rewards (see Bozarth, 1985, 1986; Bozarth & Wise, 1983; Phillips & Fibiger, this volume; Wise & Bozarth, 1982, 1984). This system has its cell bodies in the ventral tegmental area and sends its axonal projections forward to terminate in several brain regions including the nucleus accumbens and frontal cortex. Although other brain mechanisms may also participate in reward from these compounds, the data suggesting the involvement of this brain system will be briefly examined to illustrate how various methods of assessing drug reinforcement have provided similar answers to the same general question. The concordance across markedly different methods of study provides a type of empirical test for the validity of each measure. The conclusions drawn from this research far exceed the limitations of any single method of studying drug reinforcement.

Psychomotor Stimulant Reward

No fewer than nine independent studies using four different experimental paradigms have suggested that the nucleus accumbens (NAS) terminal field of the ventral tegmental dopamine system is critically involved in the rewarding effects of psychomotor stimulants (see Table 1). Microinjections of amphetamine into the NAS facilitate brain stimulation reward (BSR). Dopamine-depleting lesions of the NAS or of the cell body region of this system (ventral tegmental area: VTA) disrupt intravenous self-administration (IVSA) of cocaine. Dopamine-depleting lesions of the NAS disrupt the acquisition and the maintenance of amphetamine self-administration. Kainic acid lesions that destroy the target cells of the NAS dopamine terminals also disrupt cocaine self-administration. Amphetamine is intracranially self-administered (ICSA) directly into the NAS. Finally, NAS microinjections of amphetamine produce a conditioned place preference (CPP), and the conditioned place preference produced by systemic amphetamine injections is attenuated by dopamine-depleting lesions of the ventral tegmental system.

Table 1

Evidence Suggesting the Involvement of Dopamine Terminal Fields
in Psychomotor Stimulant Reward

Effect	Investigator(s)
BSR/NAS amphetamine microinjections	Broekkamp et al., 1975
IVSA/NAS dopamine-depleting lesions	Lyness et al., 1979
	Roberts et al., 1977, 1980
IVSA/VTA dopamine-depleting lesions	Roberts & Koob, 1982
IVSA/NAS kainic acid lesions	Zito et al., 1985
ICSA/NAS amphetamine	Hoebel et al.; 1983
CPP/NAS amphetamine microinjections	White et al.; this volume
CPP/NAS dopamine-depleting lesions	Spyraki et al., 1982

Note: See text for abbreviations and description of studies.

Some evidence suggests that the frontal cortex projection of the ventral tegmental dopamine system may also be involved in psychomotor stimulate reward. The relative importance of the nucleus accumbens and frontal cortex terminal fields has not been established, but nine studies have suggested a role for the nucleus accumbens (see Table 1) while only three studies have suggested a role for the frontal cortex (i.e., Goeders & Smith, 1983; Glick & Marsanico, 1975; Phillips, Mora, & Rolls, 1981).

Opiate Reward

At least 14 independent studies using four different experimental paradigms have suggested that the ventral tegmental area is involved in opiate reward (see Table 2). Morphine microinjections into the ventral tegmental area (VTA) facilitate brain stimulation reward (BSR). Dopamine-depleting lesions in the VTA attenuate the facilitatory action of systemic morphine injections on BSR. The acquisition of intravenous heroin self-administration (IVSA) is disrupted by dopamine-depleting lesions of the VTA, and narcotic antagonist microinjections into the VTA disrupt heroin self-administration. Animals trained and later extinguished on intravenous morphine self-administration show a reinstatement of responding following VTA morphine microinjections. Both fentanyl and morphine are intracranially self-administered (ICSA) directly into the VTA. Morphine, an opioid peptide, and an enkephalinase inhibitor all produce a conditioned place preference when microinjected into the VTA. Finally, the conditioned place preference produced by systemic morphine injections is attenuated by dopamine-depleting lesions of the VTA system.

There is evidence that opiate reward may involve additional systems. Other brain regions that have been suggested to mediate opiate reward include the caudate nucleus (Glick, Cox, & Crane, 1975), the nucleus accumbens (Goeders, Lane, & Smith, 1984; Olds, 1982; Vaccarino, Bloom, & Koob, 1985), and the lateral hypothalamus (Olds, 1979). The periventricular gray region may also contribute to the net reinforcing impact of systemically delivered opiates (see Bozarth, 1986; Bozarth & Wise, 1983).

Table 2

Evidence Suggesting the Involvement of the Ventral Tegmental Area
in Opiate Reward

Effect	Investigator(s)
BSR/VTA morphine microinjections	Broekkamp et al., 1976, 1979
BSR/VTA dopamine-depleting lesions	Hand & Franklin, 1985
IVSA/VTA dopamine-depleting lesions	Bozarth & Wise, 1986
IVSA/VTA narcotic antagonist microinjections	Britt & Wise, 1983
IVSA/VTA morphine reinstatement of responding	Stewart, 1984, this volume
ICSA/VTA fentanyl	van Ree & De Wied, 1980
ICSA/VTA morphine	Bozarth & Wise, 1981, 1982
CPP/VTA morphine	Bozarth & Wise, 1982
	Phillips & LePiane, 1980
CPP/VTA opioid peptide	Phillips & LePiane, 1982
CPP/VTA enkephalinase inhibitor	Glimcher et al., 1984
CPP/VTA dopamine-depleting lesions	Spyraki et al., 1983

Note: See text for abbreviations and description of studies.

Conclusion

The overall concordance of these various experimental methods is excellent. Markedly different experimental paradigms and several variations of these methods of study have yielded very similar conclusions. Both psychomotor stimulants and opiates appear to derive a major part of their reinforcing effects by activation of the ventral tegmental dopamine system, although at different synaptic elements (i.e., the nucleus accumbens terminal field and the ventral tegmental area cell body region, respectively; for a review, see Bozarth, 1986). A recent study has provided a direct test of this hypothesis by demonstrating a partial cross substitution of ventral tegmental morphine microinjections for intravenous cocaine reinforcement (Bozarth & Wise, 1986). Most importantly, even though there is evidence to suggest that additional mechanisms may be involved in the reinforcing actions of both classes of drugs, the concordance among markedly different experimental techniques and among various independent laboratories provides important cross validation of these methods of assessing the reinforcing properties of abused drugs.

It is interesting to note that the neural substrates for both amphetamine and morphine reward were first identified by brain stimulation reward studies combined with microinjection methodology (see chapter by Broekkamp for a description of the experimental technique; see also Broekkamp [1976] for a description of the studies). The results of these studies seem to have been initially ignored by most drug addiction specialists because the relevance of these findings to drug reward was not generally appreciated. Ironically, later studies confirming the rewarding sites of action for these drugs (such as the work with intracranial self-administration) have helped to provide validation of the brain stimulation reward method as a technique for assessing the reinforcing properties of these abused drugs.

SCREENING DRUGS FOR ADDICTION LIABILITY

One of the most important applications of assessing drug reinforcement is screening new compounds for addiction liability. Several pharmacological classes of drugs used for specific therapeutic applications are traditionally associated with a moderate to high addiction potential. Most notable are the strong analgesics, appetite suppressants, stimulants, and hypnotic sedatives. Minor tranquilizers have also been suggested to be somewhat addictive, although their addiction liability appears far less than their abuse potential.

Medicinal chemists can generate new compounds at a rapid rate by making slight alterations in the basic drug molecule. The objective is to develop compounds that retain a high therapeutic efficacy while minimizing the undesirable side-effects such as addiction liability. Fast and effective methods are required to assess the addiction liability of these new compounds before clinical trials are begun. Probably a very high proportion of compounds never progress beyond the initial phase of drug screening because alterations in the drug molecule fail to significantly diminish the undesirable side-effects of the drug or do so by also diminishing the therapeutic efficacy.

Screening new compounds for addiction liability is divided into two phases--preclinical and clinical. Although both phases are concerned with assessing addiction liability, they differ markedly in their immediate objectives. Preclinical studies involve screening compounds using animal models and must progress at a quick pace and need not concern themselves with the long-term effects on the experimental subjects. Methods used for preclinical screening should maximize the potential for drug addiction by using a wide range of dose levels and exposures to the compound. Clinical studies must investigate the addiction liability of a compound without producing long-term adverse effects in the subjects. This poses a particularly difficult task, because clinical screening must expose the subjects to a potentially addictive compound under conditions that will maximize the probability of detecting the drug's addiction potential while minimizing the likelihood of producing an actual drug addiction. Unfortunately, the conditions that maximize the potential for detecting the addictive properties of a drug also maximize the potential for producing an addiction in the experimental subjects. This situation has led to the development of methods that detect the underlying properties of a compound that are intimately related to its addictive properties under conditions that minimize the risk of actual addiction to the compound.

Two important results ensued, in part, from this dilemma. First, methods have been developed that can directly assess addiction liability in lower animals, and these techniques provide the first line for eliminating compounds with a high addiction liability. The animal models are so good as to almost eliminate the need for screening in humans, but clinical assessment remains the final determination of whether a new compound will be advanced to clinical trials. The techniques used to assess addiction liability in humans have also greatly progressed. Instead of directly measuring the ability of the compound to produce compulsive drug use, measures have been developed that determine the subjective effects and "liking" for the compound. These variables appear to be intimately related to a drug's addiction potential and are usually, in themselves, accurate predictors of a drug's addiction potential. The limiting factors in the accuracy of clinical assessment involve conditions of drug exposure (e.g., drug dosage or days of repeated exposure) and subject variables (e.g., subjective impressions of the psychological state produced by the compound) that are not important in animal studies. Thus, preclinical screening remains an important step in the process of drug development not only for its ability to rapidly screen large numbers of compounds, but also for its ability to use higher drug doses and longer conditions of exposure that would be impractical (or unethical) in routine clinical screening. The final assessment in humans, however, may detect properties of a compound that ultimately produce an addiction that might be missed in lower animals.

Preclinical Screening

The preclinical screening of new compounds for addiction liability can be divided into three stages. The first stage determines the drug dosage and time course of the drug effects that will be studied in the subsequent tests. The second stage involves an initial demonstration that the new compound has (or is likely to have) a substantial reinforcing or rewarding effect. The third stage is the most difficult but also provides the most direct demonstration that the administration of the compound is reinforcing and, hence, is very likely to have significant addictive properties.

Stage I: Initial Determination of Drug Dosage & Time Course

The initial determination of appropriate drug dose and time course for rewarding effects should use a measure that is quick, easy, and allows repeated testing of the subject across various conditions. Brain stimulation reward is uniquely suited for this purpose. Animals with lateral hypothalamic electrodes can be maintained for long periods of time without noticeable deterioration in performance or substantial change in the rewarding effects of the electrical stimulation. A pool of trained subjects can be used to determine the relevant dose and time-course of a new compound's effect. Testing should continue for several hours after drug administration, and relatively large doses of the compound may be tested. Any delayed facilitation of brain stimulation reward should be apparent if the sessions continue 4 to 6 hours after drug injections.

Threshold-tracking measures are the best approach because they generate stable baseline values when testing the subjects for long session durations. Rate measures may also be suitable, but they would probably require that the subjects be tested periodically for short periods of time (e.g., every 30 minutes for 5-minute test durations). Otherwise, a marked deterioration in the subject's performance may result from fatigue, and the drug's effect would have to be evaluated against a changing baseline response rate. Automation of the testing procedure and data analysis is a definite asset because considerable data must be collected to fully evaluate the compound.

From this stage of testing, the dose range to be tested with the other measures can be selected. The dose most likely to be self-administered is probably the one which produces a facilitation of brain stimulation reward with the shortest latency after injections. Larger doses that produce a delayed facilitation, however, may also be self-administered.

The reinstatement of responding method may also be suitable for the initial screening of new compounds, although the feasibility of this technique for this application, particularly the effects of a delayed rewarding action, has not been evaluated. Two important disadvantages to using this technique for Stage I testing are the difficulty in maintaining intravenous subjects for repeated testing (as in the use of a subject pool for screening multiple drugs) and the possible influence that repeated extinction trials may have on this measure. Thus, until the use of the reinstatement of responding method for determining initial drug dosages and time courses of potentially addictive drugs has been evaluated, brain stimulation reward remains the preferred technique for Stage I screening of new compounds.

Stage II: Preliminary Demonstration of Directly Rewarding Drug Action

The next stage of testing a compound for addiction liability involves a preliminary assessment of the compound's directly rewarding effect. The conditioned place preference method is the preferred procedure for this stage of testing because large numbers of subjects can be quickly and easily screened. The lowest drug dose effective in facilitating brain stimulation reward should be used as the low end of the dose range, and doses one and two orders of magnitude greater than this dosage should also be tested. (There is probably no need to test intermediate doses because conditioned place preferences appear to be produced across a wide range of doses of a compound.) Unless there is evidence from the brain stimulation reward studies that the drug effect is markedly delayed following injection, the subjects can be conditioned immediately after the drug injections. Conditioning duration may be an important variable if the drug has a particularly short or long duration of action, but 30-minute conditioning sessions will probably be satisfactory for many compounds. Again, the time course determined from brain stimulation reward testing can be used to direct the duration of the conditioning trials.

An alternative procedure particularly useful for screening large numbers of compounds and obtaining dose-response data is the drug discrimination method. This method yields additional data, such as whether the test compound is similar or dissimilar to the training drug, and also shows clear dose-dependent effects. The major limitation of this technique for assessing addiction liability is that this method does not necessarily measure drug reward. It is likely that the rewarding action of a compound significantly contributes to the stimulus properties of that drug, but the relative importance of this and other interoceptive cues has not been established. Furthermore, drug discrimination studies are very laborious, and selection of an inappropriate training drug may cause the test drug's addiction liability to be missed.

The reinstatement of responding method may also be very effective for this stage of testing. A potential advantage of this method over drug discrimination testing is that the training drug and test drug can be markedly different (as in the case of opiates and psychomotor stimulants, see de Wit & Steward, 1981) and generalization may still occur. The utility of this method for screening potentially addictive drugs merits further exploration.

Stage III: Confirmation of Directly Rewarding Drug Action

The last stage of preclinical screening for addiction liability involves testing the compound for its ability to directly reinforce behavior. Intravenous self-administration is the preferred method for this, but intragastric, intraventricular, and oral self-administration may be useful in some situations. Drug substitution procedures are commonly used to determine if a new compound will maintain intravenous self-administration. This approach has the advantage that the subjects have already been trained to self-administer a drug with known reinforcing properties, so learning factors do not affect the outcome of the test. However, important pharmacological and behavioral interactions may occur that invalidate the conclusions drawn from this procedure. For example, if a compound is a partial narcotic antagonist with low intrinsic reinforcing properties, then testing this compound in an animal that has been self-administering morphine is likely to precipitate withdrawal and the animal may actively avoid lever pressing. Similarly, if a subject has been self-administering a potent reinforcer like cocaine or heroin and a compound with much lower reinforcing efficacy is substituted, then a behavioral contrast effect may be produced and the subject may fail to maintain self-administration. That is, the shift to a reinforcer of much lower incentive value is likely to produce a contrast effect where that reinforcer will be unable to maintain the behavioral response, even though the same reinforcer would normally maintain responding if the abrupt shift in reinforcement magnitude were not present. In both of these cases, the test compound is reinforcing, but its reinforcing efficacy is relatively small.

Direct acquisition of intravenous self-administration is the best approach to assessing a compound's directly reinforcing effect. This method, however, suffers from several serious limitations. First, the drug dose and pharmacokinetics must be satisfactory for the reinforcing action to be associated with the lever-pressing response. Second, the response must be learned and compounds that disrupt learning may fail to support (or severely retard the acquisition of) self-administration. Third, a drug may be reinforcing only after considerable exposure to that drug. This requires that the animals be involuntarily given drug injections prior to assessing drug self-administration. And fourth, the compound may be reinforcing only under certain circumstances or conditions. Anxiolytic compounds may not be reinforcing in normal experimental animals but may be reinforcing in stressed subjects.

It is obviously not practical to test a new compound under all of the conditions that may affect its reinforcing properties. Organismic variables or long-term drug exposure may modify a drug's reinforcing efficacy. The general pharmacological properties (e.g., analgesic, anxiolytic, or sedative effects) may provide information regarding likely conditions that will reveal a compound's reinforcing effect not seen with a simple test of direct response acquisition of intravenous self-administration.

Clinical Screening

A positive finding in any of the three stages of preclinical screening is strongly suggestive that the compound will possess a significant addiction liability. The lack of concordance across these measures does not constitute evidence that the compound is devoid of addiction potential but, rather, suggests that more extensive tests need to be conducted with the procedures that failed to reveal the drug's addiction potential. The fact that a compound has some addiction liability, however, does not preclude its further assessment as a potentially useful therapeutic agent. A surprisingly large number of medicinal compounds probably possess some addiction liability.

Stage IV: Clinical Assessment

Initial clinical screening for addiction liability should probably use psychometric assessment of the compound's subjective effects. Instruments, such as the Addiction Research Center Inventory, are very reliable and have considerable accuracy in predicting addiction liability. Single-dose administration (or limited dose-range testing) minimizes the exposure of the potentially addictive compound to human subjects.

Choice testing or drug self-administration is the final step in clinical screening before limited clinical trials are begun. Here, the subjects must be exposed to repeated administration of the compound so the risk of developing an addiction in the human subjects is significant. This approach, however, may reveal addictive properties that cannot be detected using the single dose methods of assessment. The selection of the test compound during choice testing or its voluntary self-administration remains the most direct method of demonstrating an addiction potential. As with the animal self-administration studies, the compound may be reinforcing under special conditions related to repeated exposure or specific circumstances. Even voluntary self-administration testing in humans may miss this reinforcing action.

Stage V: Clinical Trials

After the drug has progressed through the first four stages of testing and has been shown not to be reinforcing in these tests, it is ready for limited clinical trials. During this phase, it is important that dispensing and use pattern information be accurately recorded to determine if there are any indications that the compound possesses a high addiction liability. As mentioned above, conditions that cannot be duplicated in either a laboratory or outpatient settings may influence whether a drug is potentially addictive, and the fact that the earlier tests failed to reveal any addiction liability could be related to any number of variables present in "the real world" but not duplicated in the experimental conditions.

CONCLUDING COMMENT

The study of drug reinforcement is in essence the study of the motivational properties of drugs and hence the study of drug addiction. The development of better experimental methods and a full understanding of existing techniques is an important step in elucidating the mechanisms of drug addiction, the development of new, less addictive compounds, and even the identification of basic neural processes involved in motivation and reward.

Some experimental techniques have a firmer empirical basis than others, but the most compelling conclusions are drawn from studies where several different experimental methods produce similar findings. In general, methods of assessing drug reinforcement that have been adopted across several laboratories and/or have been used for some time have obvious merit documented by their widespread application. Although ease of implementing the procedure is not a substitute for a validated measure of drug reinforcement, most currently used procedures are useful in some situations and possess a certain degree of inherent validity.

This book has attempted to provide a compendium of the most important methods used to assess drug reinforcement. The individual chapters were written by authors who have extensive experience with these techniques. There is a mixture of senior investigators involved in the early development of these methods and of new scientists who are further developing and exploiting these experimental techniques. Many chapters in the book summarize considerable work with a given method, while others present original data illustrating how the techniques are actually applied. The inclusion of diverse experimental methods and of both laboratory animal and human assessment techniques appears to be unique to this volume. The topics and format were selected to provide a thorough understanding of the principles and applications of the methods of assessing the reinforcing properties of abused drugs.

ACKNOWLEDGMENT

Preparation of this chapter was facilitated by a grant from the National Institute on Drug Abuse (U.S.A.) and by a University Research Fellowship from the Natural Sciences and Engineering Research Council of Canada.

REFERENCES

American heritage dictionary. (1969). New York: American Heritage Publishing Company.

Atalay, J., & Wise, R. A. (1983). Time course of pimozide effects on brain stimulation reward. Pharmacology Biochemistry & Behavior, 18, 655-658.

Bozarth, M. A. (1978). Intracranial self-stimulation as an index of opioid addiction liability: An evaluation. Unpublished master's thesis, Rensselaer Polytechnic Institute, Troy, NY.

Bozarth, M. A. (1982). The neural substrate of opiate reward in the rat. Unpublished doctoral dissertation, Concordia University, Montreal.

Bozarth, M. A. (1983). Opiate reward mechanisms mapped by intracranial self-administration. In J. E. Smith and J. D. Lane (Eds.), The neurobiology of opiate reward processes (pp. 331-359). Amsterdam: Elsevier/North Holland Biomedical Press.

Bozarth, M. A. (1985). Biological basis of cocaine addiction. In C. J. Brink (Ed.), Cocaine: A symposium (pp. 32-36). Madison, WI: Wisconsin Institute on Drug Abuse.

Bozarth, M. A. (1986). Neural basis of psychomotor stimulant and opiate reward: Evidence suggesting the involvement of a common dopaminergic system. Behavioural Brain Research, 22, 107-116.

Bozarth, M. A., & Wise, R. A. (1981). Intracranial self-administration of morphine into the ventral tegmental area. Life Sciences, 28, 551-555.

Bozarth, M. A., & Wise, R. A. (1982). Localization of the reward-relevant opiate receptors. In L. S. Harris (Ed.), Problems of drug dependence, 1981 (National Institute on Drug Abuse Research Monograph 41, pp. 158-164). Washington, DC: U.S. Government Printing Office.

Bozarth, M. A., & Wise, R. A. (1983). Neural substrates of opiate reinforcement. Progress in Neuro-Psychopharmacology & Biological Psychiatry, 7, 569-575.

Bozarth, M. A., & Wise, R. A. (1986). Involvement of the ventral tegmental dopamine system in opioid and psychomotor stimulant reinforcement. In L. S. Harris (Ed.), Problems of drug dependence, 1985 (National Institute on Drug Abuse Research Monograph 67, pp. 190-196). Washington, DC: U.S. Government Printing Office.

Britt, M. D., & Wise, R. A. (1983). Ventral tegmental site of opiate reward: Antagonism by a hydrophilic opiate receptor blocker. Brain Research, 258, 105-108.

Broekkamp, C. L. E. (1976). The modulation of rewarding systems in the animal brain by amphetamine, morphine, and apomorphine. Druk, The Netherlands: Stichting Studentenpers Nijmgen.

Broekkamp, C. L., Phillips, A. G., & Cools, A. R. (1979). Facilitation of self-stimulation behavior following intracerebral microinjection of opioids into the ventral tegmental area. Pharmacology Biochemistry & Behavior, 11, 289-295.

Broekkamp, C. L. E., Pijnenburg, A. J. J., Cools, A. R., & van Rossum, J. M. (1975). The effect of microinjections of amphetamine into the neostriatum and the nucleus accumbens on self-stimulation behavior. Psychopharmacologia, 42, 179-183.

Broekkamp, C. L., van den Bogaard, J. H., Heynen, H. J., Rops, R. H., Cools, A. R., & van Rossum, J. M. (1976). Separation of inhibiting and stimulating effects of morphine in self-stimulation behavior by intracerebral microinjections. European Journal of Pharmacology, 36, 443-446.

de Wit, H., & Stewart, J. (1981). Reinstatement of cocaine-reinforced responding in the rat. Psychopharmacology, 75, 134-143.

Esposito, R., & Kornetsky, C. (1978). Opioids and rewarding brain stimulation. Neuroscience and Biobehavioral Reviews, 2, 115-122.

Goeders, N. E., Lane, J. D., & Smith, J. E. (1984). Self-administration of methionine enkephalin into the nucleus accumbens. Pharmacology Biochemistry & Behavior, 20, 451-455.

Goeders, N. E., & Smith, J. E. (1983). Cortical dopaminergic involvement in cocaine reinforcement. Science, 221, 773-775.

Glick, S. D., Cox, R. D., & Crane, A. M. (1975). Changes in morphine self-administration and morphine dependence after lesions of the caudate nucleus in rats. Psychopharmacology, 41, 219-224.

Glick, S. D., & Marsanico, R. G. (1975). Time-dependent changes in amphetamine self-administration following frontal cortex ablations in rats. Journal of Comparative and Physiological Psychology, 88, 355-359.

Glimcher, P. W., Giovino, A. A., Margolin, D. H., & Hoebel, B. G. (1984). Endogenous opiate reward induced by an enkephalinase inhibitor, thiorphan, injected into the ventral midbrain. Behavioral Neuroscience, 98, 262-268.

Griffiths, R. R., & Balster, R. L. (1979). Opioids: Similarity between evaluations of subjective effects and animal self-administration results. Clinical Pharmacology and Therapeutics, 25, 611-617.

Hand, T. H., & Franklin, K. B. J. (1985). 6-OHDA lesions of the ventral tegmental area block morphine-induced but not amphetamine-induced facilitation of self-stimulation. Brain Research, 328, 233-241.

Hernandez, L. L., Holohean, A. M., & Appel, J. B. (1978). Effects of opiates on the discriminative stimulus properties of dopamine agonists. Pharmacology Biochemistry & Behavior, 9, 459-463.

Hoebel, B. G., Monaco, A. P., Hernandez, L., Aulisi, E. F., Stanley, B. G., & Lenard, L. (1983). Self-injection of amphetamine directly into the brain, Psychopharmacology, 81, 158-163.

Jaffe, J. H. (1975). Drug addiction and drug abuse. In L. S. Goodman & A. Gilman (Eds.), The pharmacological basis of therapeutics (pp. 284-324). New York: MacMillan.

Kornetsky, C., & Esposito, R. U. (1979). Euphorigenic drugs: Effects on the reward pathways of the brain. Federation Proceedings, 38, 2473-2476.

Lyness, W. H., Friedle, N. M., & Moore, K. E. (1979). Destruction of dopaminergic nerve terminals in nucleus accumbens: Effect on d-amphetamine self-administration. Pharmacology Biochemistry & Behavior, 11, 553-556.

Olds, M. E. (1979). Hypothalamic substrate for the positive reinforcing properties of morphine in the rat. Brain Research, 168, 351-360.

Olds, M. E. (1982). Reinforcing effects of morphine in the nucleus accumbens. Brain Research, 237, 429-440.

Oxford English dictionary. (1933). Oxford: Oxford University Press.

Oxford English dictionary (supplement). (1933). Oxford: Oxford University Press.

Phillips, A. G., & LePiane, F. G. (1980). Reinforcing effects of morphine microinjection into the ventral tegmental area. Pharmacology Biochemistry & Behavior, 12, 965-968.

Phillips, A. G., & LePiane, F. G. (1982). Reward produced by microinjection of (D-ala ^{2}), Met ^{5}-enkephalinamide into the ventral tegmental area. Behavioural Brain Research, 5, 225-229.

Phillips, A. G., Mora, F., & Rolls, E. T. (1981). Intracerebral self-administration of amphetamine by rhesus monkeys. Neuroscience Letters, 24, 81-86.

Reid, L. D., & Bozarth, M. A. (1978). Addictive agents and pressing for intracranial stimulation (ICS): The effects of various opioids on pressing for ICS. Problems of Drug Dependence, 729-741.

Roberts, D. C. S., Corcoran, M. E., & Fibiger, H. C. (1977). On the role of the ascending catecholaminergic systems in intravenous self-administration of cocaine. Pharmacology Biochemistry & Behavior, 6, 615-620.

Roberts, D. C. S., and Koob, G. F. (1982). Disruption of cocaine self-administration following 6-hydroxydopamine lesions of the ventral tegmental area in rats, Pharmacology Biochemistry & Behavior, 17, 901-904.

Roberts, D. C. S., Koob, G. F., Klonoff, P., and Fibiger, H. C. (1980). Extinction and recovery of cocaine self-administration following 6-hydroxydopamine lesions of the nucleus accumbens. Pharmacology Biochemistry & Behavior, 12, 781-787.

Spealman, R. D., & Goldberg, S. R. (1978). Drug self-administration by laboratory animals: Control by schedules of reinforcement. Annual Reviews of Pharmacology & Toxicology, 18, 313-339.

Spyraki, C., Fibiger, H. C., & Phillips, A. G. (1982). Dopaminergic substrates of amphetamine-induced place preference conditioning. Brain Research, 253, 185-192.

Spyraki, C., Fibiger, H. C., & Phillips, A. G. (1983). Attenuation of heroin reward in rats by disruption of the mesolimbic dopamine system. Psychopharmacology, 79, 278-283.

Stewart, J. (1984). Reinstatement of heroin and cocaine self-administration behavior in the rat by intracerebral application of morphine in the ventral tegmental area. Pharmacology Biochemistry & Behavior, 20, 917-923.

Tatum, A. L., & Seevers, M. H. (1929). Experimental cocaine addiction. Journal of Pharmacology and Experimental Therapeutics, 36, 401-410.

Tatum, A. L., & Seevers, M. H. (1931). Theories of drug addiction. Physiological Reviews, 11, 107-121.

Tatum, A. L., Seevers, M. H., & Collins, K. H. (1929). Morphine addiction and its physiological interpretation based on experimental evidences. Journal of Pharmacology and Experimental Therapeutics, 36, 447-475.

Vaccarino, F. J., Bloom, F. E., & Koob, G. F. (1985). Blockade of nucleus accumbens opiate receptors attenuates intravenous heroin reward in the rat. Psychopharmacology, 86, 37-42.

van Ree, J. M., & de Wied, D. (1980). Involvement of neurohypophyseal peptides in drug-mediated adaptive responses. Pharmacology Biochemistry & Behavior, 13(Suppl. 1), 257-263.

Webster's third new international dictionary. (1981). Springfield, MA: Merrian-Webster.

Wise, R. A., & Bozarth, M. A. (1982). Action of drugs of abuse on brain reward systems: An update with specific attention to opiates. Pharmacology Biochemistry & Behavior, 17, 239-243.

Wise, R. A., & Bozarth, M. A. (1984). Brain reward circuitry: Four elements "wired" in apparent series. Brain Research Bulletin, 12, 203-208.

Zito, K. A., Vickers, G., & Roberts, D. C. S. (1985). Disruption of cocaine and heroin self-administration following kainic acid lesions of the nucleus accumbens. Pharmacology Biochemistry & Behavior, 23, 1029-1036.